# Information Technology for the Health Professions

## Fourth Edition

### Lillian Burke

### Barbara Weill

**PEARSON**

Boston  Columbus  Indianapolis  New York  San Francisco  Upper Saddle River
Amsterdam  Cape Town  Dubai  London  Madrid  Milan  Munich  Paris  Montréal  Toronto
Delhi  Mexico City  São Paulo  Sydney  Hong Kong  Seoul  Singapore  Taipei  Tokyo

**Publisher:** Julie Levin Alexander
**Executive Editor:** Joan Gill
**Development Editor:** Melissa Kerian
**Editorial Assistant:** Stephanie Kiel
**Production Manager:** Meghan DeMaio
**Design Director:** Maria Guglielmo
**Creative Director:** Jayne Conte
**Cover Designer:** Suzanne Behnke

**Cover Image:** Tiberiu Stan/Shutterstock
**Director of Marketing:** David Gesell
**Executive Marketing Manager:** Katrin Beacom
**Marketing Coordinator:** Alicia Wozniak
**Composition/Full-Service Management:** Jouve India
Private Limited/Shylaja Gattupalli
**Printer/Binder:** R. R. Donnelley & Sons
**Cover Printer:** Lehigh-Phoenix Color

**Library of Congress Cataloging-in-Publication Data**
Catalogue in Publication data available from the Library of Congress

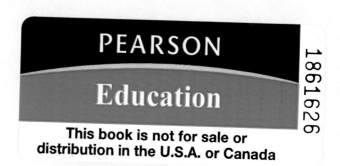

PEARSON

Education

This book is not for sale or
distribution in the U.S.A. or Canada

1861626

10 9 8 7 6 5 4 3 2 1

PEARSON

ISBN-13: 978-0-13-289764-8
ISBN-10: 0-13-289764-4

To our families, for their inspiration, understanding, patience, faith in us, and love.

*Molly and Harry, Richard, Andrea, and Daniel*
*—L.B.*

*Hazel and Rob, Mike, Buffy and Jon, Joanne and Melissa, and Sarah and Emma*
*—B.W.*

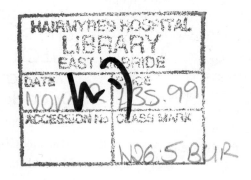

# Table of Contents

## Chapter 1

## Introduction to Information Technology— Hardware, Software, and Telecommunications   1

## Chapter 2

## Medical Informatics: The American Recovery and Reinvestment Act, HITECH, and the Health Information Technology Decade   17

# Chapter 9

# Information Technology in Dentistry   208

# Chapter 10

# Informational Resources: Computer-Assisted Instruction, Expert Systems, Health Information Online   231

# Preface

Each chapter of the fourth edition of *Information Technology for the Health Professions* has been updated with new information. Chapter 1 is a very brief introduction to computers and computer literacy with new sections on smartphones and tablet computers. Classes with any computer background should omit this chapter. Chapters 2 and 3 have been expanded with current information on the American Recovery and Reinvestment Act, HITECH, and the Patient Protection and Affordable Care Act and their impact on the expansion of the use of the electronic health record. Chapter 2 has an expanded section on the meaningful use criteria for certified electronic health records, which should become universal by 2014. Chapter 3 is expanded to include practice management software, scheduling, and accounting. Chapter 4 deals with the continuing expansion of telemedicine.

Chapter 5 has been updated to include more information on the effects of poverty and inequality on health outcomes and to include information on new problems in public health, such as the emergence of antibiotic resistance. Computers are intimately involved in public health because even to know whether an epidemic exists, counting and statistics are necessary. New disasters such as Hurricane Katrina and the unfolding tragedy in Japan are included, as well as the public health responses. We continue to deal with the problems caused by climate change and the inadequate public response.

Chapter 6 deals with radiology, stressing the expansion of interventional radiology with a new section on the dangers posed by medical radiation. Chapter 7 discusses computers in surgery with a new section on the developing field of nanotechnology. Chapter 8 on pharmacy includes new developments in biotechnology and new developments in the use of stem cells and their potential. Chapter 9 examines the use of computer technology in dentistry. Chapter 10 looks at information resources made available by networks and computers, with an added section on the many health-related applications (apps) available for smartphones and tablet computers. The very interesting expanded use of computers in psychiatry is also discussed. Chapter 11 examines computerized devices, adaptive technology, functional electrical stimulation (FES), and computers in rehabilitative therapies. Chapter 12 is on the security and privacy of information with an emphasis on medical information. New information on the enforcement of HIPAA privacy protections and the added protections of HITECH has been added, as has a section on the privacy of genetic information.

A note on point of view: Over the last several years, politics and science have clashed over many issues including climate change and whether human action is contributing to it. This is not a debate *within* the scientific community, which has achieved a consensus on the issue. We take the consensus of the scientific community as our point of view.

# Reviewers

## Reviewers of the Fourth Edition

James Bonsignore, RHIA
William Rainey Harper College
Palatine, Illinois

Mary Beth Brown, MRC, BM
Sinclair Community College
Dayton, Ohio

Michelle Buchman MA, BSN, RN
Cox College
Springfield, Missouri

Michelle Cranney
Virginia College, Online Division
Birmingham, Alabama

Tricia Elliott, MBA, CSHA
William Rainey Harper College
Palatine, Illinois

Jeri Layer, AS
Sinclair Community College
Dayton, Ohio

Deborah L. Weaver, RN, PhD
Valdosta State University
Valdosta, Georgia

## Reviewers of Previous Editions

Richard Boan, PhD
Midlands Technical College
West Columbia, South Carolina

Joseph Burke, BS, MS
Sanford-Brown College
Fenton, Missouri

Patt Elison-Bowers
Boise State University
Boise, Idaho

Pamela Greenstone, RHIA
Cincinnati State Technical
and Community College
Cincinnati, Ohio

Deedee McClain Smith, CDA, RDH, MS
York Technical College
Rock Hill, South Carolina

Heather Merkley, MEd, RHIA
Weber State University
Ogden, Utah

Nancy Powell, RHIT, BS
South Plains College
Lubbock, Texas

Diane Premeau
Chabot College
Hayward, California

Theresa Lyn Schlabach, OTR/L, BCP, MA
St. Ambrose University
Davenport, Iowa

Patricia Shaw, MEd, RHIA
Weber State University
Ogden, Utah

R. Bruce Steinbach, RRT
Pitt Community College
Greenville, North Carolina

Nick Thireos
Rochester Institute of Technology
Rochester, New York

Philip Vuchetich
Creighton University
Omaha, Nebraska

Deborah Weaver, RN, PhD
Valdosta State University
Valdosta, Georgia

James A. Yanci, MS, MT(ASCP),
CLS(NCA)
Youngstown State University
Youngstown, Ohio

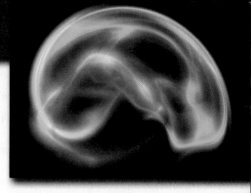

# Introduction to Information Technology— Hardware, Software, and Telecommunications

## LEARNING OBJECTIVES

Upon completion of this chapter, you will be able to:

- Define information technology, computer, and computer literacy, and understand their significance in today's society.
- Describe the classification of computers into supercomputers, mainframes, microcomputers, minicomputers, netbooks, personal digital assistants (PDAs), and embedded computers.
- Differentiate between hardware and software and discuss the different hardware components of a computer.
- Describe the difference between system and application software, know what an operating system is, and know what various application programs are used for what tasks.
- Discuss the significance of connectivity and networking.
- Discuss the recent expansion of the uses of wireless technologies including cell phones, Global Positioning System (GPS) technology, PDAs with Internet access, smartphones, and tablet computers.
- List the components necessary for telecommunications to take place.
- State the uses of telecommunications and networking.

## INFORMATION TECHNOLOGY AND COMPUTER LITERACY

The term **information technology (IT)** includes not only the use of computers but also communications networks and computer literacy—knowledge of how to use computer technology. As in other fields, the basic tasks of gathering, allocating, controlling, and retrieving information are the same. The push to use IT in all aspects of health care, from the electronic health record (EHR) to integrated hospital information technology (HIT) systems, makes it crucial for health care professionals to be familiar with basic computer concepts. In this chapter, we will focus on computer literacy, computers, and networks. Currently, computer literacy involves several aspects. A computer-literate person knows how to make use of a computer in his or her field to make tasks easier and to complete them more efficiently, has a knowledge of terminology, and understands in a broad, general fashion what a computer is and what its capabilities are. **Computer literacy** involves knowledge of the Internet and the World Wide Web and the ability to take advantage of their resources and to critically judge the information.

A **computer** is an electronic device that accepts data (raw facts) as input, processes or alters them in some way, and produces useful information as output. A computer manipulates data by following step-by-step instructions called a **program**. The program, the data, and the information are temporarily stored in memory while processing is going on and then are permanently stored on secondary storage media for future use. Computers are accurate, fast, and reliable.

## HARDWARE AND SOFTWARE

To understand the myriad uses of IT in health care, you need to familiarize yourself with computer terminology, hardware, and software applications. Every computer performs similar functions. Specific hardware is associated with each function.

**Input devices** take data that humans understand and digitize those data, that is, translate them into binary forms of ones and zeroes, ons and offs that the computer processes. A **processing unit** manipulates data. Output devices produce information that people understand. Memory and **secondary storage devices** hold information, data, and programs (Figure 1.1 ▶).

Although all computers perform similar functions, they are not the same. There are several categories based on size, speed, and processing power. Supercomputers are the largest and most

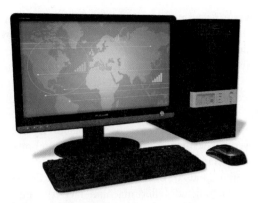

▶ **Figure 1.1**  Desktop computer.
*Source:* Oleksiy Mark/Shutterstock.com

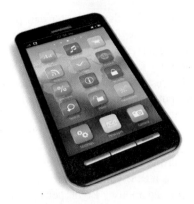

▶ **Figure 1.2**  Touchscreen smartphone.
*Source:* Oleksiy Mark/Shutterstock.com

powerful. Supercomputers are used for scientific purposes, such as weather forecasting and drug design. Supercomputers take complex mathematical data and create simulations of epidemics, pandemics, and other disasters. Mainframes are less powerful and are used in business for input/output intensive purposes, such as generating paychecks or processing medical insurance claims. Minicomputers are scaled-down mainframes; they are multiuser computers that are used by small businesses. Microcomputers (personal computers) are powerful enough for an individual's needs in word processing, spreadsheets, and database management. Netbooks are scaled-down microcomputers that are light and easy to carry; they provide a link to the Internet, and also support common application software. Small handheld computers called **personal digital assistants (PDAs)** originally could hold only a notepad, a calendar, and an address book. Today, sophisticated PDAs are used throughout the health care system. Physicians can write prescriptions on PDAs, consult online databases, and capture patient information and download it to a hospital computer. PDAs also hold reference manuals and are used in public health to gather information and help track diseases and epidemics. More recently, **smartphones** (Figure 1.2 ▶) and **tablet computers** (Figure 1.3 ▶) have been embraced by health care providers. (See later section, The Expansion of Wireless Technology.) The **embedded computer** is a single-purpose computer on a chip of silicon,

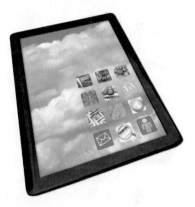

▶ **Figure 1.3**  Tablet computer.
*Source:* iQoncept/Shutterstock.com

which is embedded in anything from appliances to humans. An embedded computer may help run your car, microwave, pacemaker, or watch. A chip embedded in a human being can dispense medication, among other things.

## Hardware

The physical components of a computer are called **hardware**. Pieces of hardware may be categorized according to the functions each performs: input, process, output, and storage. As you recall, inside the computer, all data are represented by the **binary digits (bits)** 1 (one) and 0 (zero). To translate data into 1s and 0s is to **digitize**.

INPUT DEVICES Input devices function to take data that people understand and translate those data into a form that the computer can process. Input devices may be divided into two categories: **keyboards** and direct-entry devices.

**Direct-entry devices** include pointing devices, scanning devices, smart and optical cards, speech and vision input, touch screens, sensors, and human-biology input devices.

The pointing device with which you are most familiar is the **mouse**, which you can use to position the insertion point on the screen or make a choice from a menu. Other pointing devices are variations of the mouse. Light pens, digitizing tablets, and pen-based systems allow you to use a pen or stylus to enter data. The marks you make or letters you write are digitized.

Most **scanning devices** digitize data by shining a light on an image and measuring the reflection. Bar-code scanners read the universal product codes; optical mark recognition devices can recognize a mark on paper; and optical character recognition devices can recognize letters. Special scanning equipment called magnetic ink character recognition (MICR) is used by banks to read the numbers at the bottoms of checks. You are familiar with fax machines, which scan images, digitize them, and send them over telecommunication lines. Some scanning devices, called image scanners, scan and digitize whole pages of text and graphics. One scanning device of particular interest to those with impaired eyesight is the Kurzweil scanner—hardware and software—which scans printed text and reads it aloud to the user.

**Radio frequency identification (RFID) tags** (input devices) are now used to identify anything from the family dog to the sponge the surgeon left in your body, by sending out radio waves. RFIDs were approved by the U.S. Food and Drug Administration (FDA) for implanting in people. They could be used to keep track of medications and medical devices and of patients. An RFID transponder worn on a patient's wrist is being used in Florida to track patients suspected of having dementia. It tracks wandering, sudden veering, and repeated pausing.[1] People with chronic illnesses were recruited several years ago by Blue Cross/Blue Shield in New Jersey to have RFID chips implanted.

Over a 2-year period, Blue Cross/Blue Shield was going to assess whether this lowered costs by reducing duplicate tests.[2] However, dangerous side effects have been noted in animals, including cancer. There is also concern that RFIDs interfere with pacemakers and implantable cardioverter defibrillators. However, the FDA, although continuing to study the matter, sees no cause for panic.[3] By 2011, several states had prohibited employers and others from forcing implantation of RFID chips.[4] Several different kinds of cards are used as input devices: Your automated teller machine (ATM) card or charge card contains a small amount of data in the magnetic stripe. A smart card can hold more data and contains a microprocessor. Smart cards have been used as debit cards. Several states now use smart cards as driver's licenses. The card includes a biometric identifier and may include other personal information as well. Privacy advocates fear that there is so much information on the cards that they can become a target for identity thieves. An optical card holds about 2,000 pages. The optical card may be used to hold your entire medical history, including test results and x-rays. If you are hospitalized in an emergency, the card—small enough to carry in your wallet—would make this information immediately available.

Vision input systems are currently being developed and refined. A computer uses a camera to digitize images and stores them. The computer "sees" by having the camera take a picture of an object. The digitized image of this object is then compared to images in storage. This technology can be used in adaptive devices, such as in glasses that help Alzheimer's patients. The glasses include a database of names and faces; a camera sees a face, and if it "recognizes" the face, it gives the wearer the name of the subject.

Speech input systems allow you to talk to your computer, and the computer processes the words as data and commands. A speech-recognition system contains a dictionary of digital patterns of words. You say a word, and the speech-recognition system digitizes the word and compares the word to the words in its dictionary. If it recognizes the word, the command is executed. There are speech dictation packages tailored to specific professions. A system

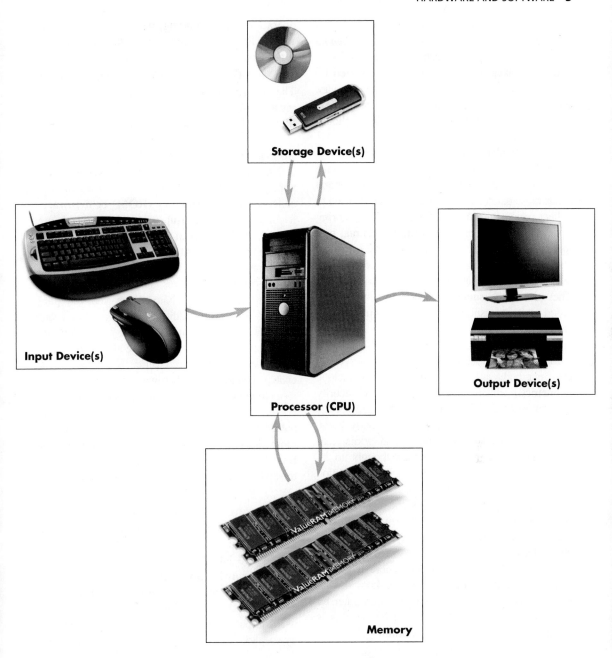

**Storage Device(s)**

**Input Device(s)**

**Processor (CPU)**

**Output Device(s)**

**Memory**

▶ **Figure 1.4** Hardware.
*Source:* Beekman, George, and Ben Beekman. *Digital Planet Tomorrow's Technology and You.* 10th ed. New York: Prentice Hall, 2011.

geared toward medicine would include an extensive vocabulary of digitized medical terms and would allow the creation of patient records and medical reports. This system can be used as an input device by physicians who, in turn, can dictate notes, even while, for example, operating. Speech recognition is also especially beneficial as an enabling technology, allowing those who do not have the use of their hands to use computers. In English, many phrases and words sound the same, for example, *hyphenate* and *-8* (hyphen eight). Speech-recognition software allows mistakes such as these to be corrected by talking. The newest speech-recognition software does not need training and gets "smarter" as you use it. It looks at context to recognize homophones (e.g., to, too, two) correctly.[5]

Of particular interest to health professionals are input devices called **sensors**. A sensor is a device that collects data directly from the environment and sends those data to a computer. Sensors are used to collect patient information for clinical monitoring systems, including physiological, arrhythmia, pulmonary, and obstetrical neonatal systems. In critical care units, monitoring systems make nurses aware of any change in a patient's condition immediately. They detect the smallest change in temperature, blood pressure, respiration, or any other physiological measurement.

The newest kinds of input devices are called human-biology input devices. They allow you to use your body as an input device. They include biometrics, which are being used in security systems to protect data from unauthorized access. **Biometrics** identify people by their body parts. Biometrics include fingerprints, hand prints, face recognition, and iris scans. Once thought to be almost 100 percent accurate, biometric identification systems are now recognized as far from perfect.

Line-of-sight input allows the user to look at a keyboard displayed on a screen and indicate the character selected by looking at it. Implanted chips have allowed locked-in stroke patients (a syndrome caused by stroke where a person cannot respond, although he or she knows what is going on) to communicate with a computer by focusing brain waves (brain wave input); this is experimental, and research is continuing.[6]

PROCESSING HARDWARE AND MEMORY Once data are digitized, they are processed. Processing hardware is the brain of the computer. Located on the **main circuit board** (or **motherboard**), the **processor** or **system unit** contains the **central processing unit (CPU)** and **memory**. The CPU has two parts: the **arithmetic-logic unit**, which performs arithmetic operations and logical operations of comparing; and the **control unit**, which directs the operation of the computer in accordance with the program's instructions.

The CPU works closely with memory. The instructions of the program being executed must be in memory for processing to take place. Memory is also located on chips on the main circuit board. The part of memory where current work is temporarily stored during processing is called **random-access memory (RAM)**. It is temporary and volatile. The other part of memory is called **read-only memory (ROM)** or **firmware**; it contains basic start-up instructions, which are burned into a chip at the factory; you cannot change the contents of ROM.

Many computers have **open architecture** that allows you to add devices. The system board contains **expansion slots**, into which you can plug expansion boards for additional hardware. The board has sockets on the outside, called **ports**. You can plug a cable from your new device into the port. The significance of open architecture is the fact that it enables you to add any hardware and software interfaces to your existing computer system. This means you can not only expand the memory of your computer but also add devices that make your computer more amenable to uses in medicine. **Expansion boards** also allow the use of virtual reality simulators, which help in teaching certain procedures.

OUTPUT DEVICES Once data are processed, **output devices** translate the language of bits into a form humans can understand. Output devices are divided into two basic categories: those that produce **hard copy**, including **printers** and **plotters**; and those that produce **soft (digital) copy**, including **monitors** (the most commonly used output device). Soft copy is also produced by speakers that produce speech, sound, or music.

SECONDARY STORAGE DEVICES The memory we have discussed so far is temporary or volatile. To save your work permanently, you need secondary storage devices. Magnetic diskettes and magnetic tape have been largely replaced by high-capacity media. Magnetic media (hard disks and high-capacity Zip disks) store data and programs as magnetic spots or electromagnetic charges. High-capacity **optical disks** (**compact disks [CDs** or **digital video disks [DVDs]**) store data as pits and lands burned into a plastic disk. **Solid-state memory devices** include flash memory cards used in notebooks, memory sticks, and very compact key chain devices; these devices have no moving parts, are very small, and have a high capacity. USB flash drives have a huge capacity for information.

## Software

**Software** refers to programs—the step-by-step instructions that tell the hardware what to do. Without software, hardware is useless. Software falls into two general categories: system software and application software.

SYSTEM SOFTWARE **System software** consists of programs that let the computer manage its resources. The most important piece of system software is the operating system. The **operating system** is a group of programs that manage and organize resources of the computer. It controls the hardware, manages basic input and output operations, keeps track of your files saved on disk and in memory, and directs communication between the CPU and other pieces of hardware. It coordinates how other programs work with the hardware and with each other. Operating systems also provide the **user interface**—that is, the way the user communicates with the computer. For example, Windows provides a **graphical user interface**, pictures or icons that you click on with a mouse. When the computer is turned on, the operating system is **booted** or loaded into the computer's RAM. No other program can work until the operating system is booted.

APPLICATION SOFTWARE **Application software** allows you to apply computer technology to a task you need done. There are application packages for many needs.

**Word-processing software** allows you to enter text for a paper, report, letter, or memo. Once the text is entered, you can format it, that is, make it look the way you want it to look. You can change the size, style, and face of the type. In addition, margins and justification can be set to any specifications. Style checkers can help you with spelling and grammar. Word-processing software also includes thesauri, headers and footers, index generators, and outlining features.

**Electronic spreadsheets** allow you to process numerical data. Organized into rows and columns intersecting to form cells, spreadsheets make doing arithmetic almost fun. You enter the values you want processed and the formula that tells the software how to process them, and the answer appears. If you made a mistake entering a value, just change it, and the answer is **automatically recalculated**. Spreadsheet software also allows you to create graphs easily—just by indicating what cells you want graphed. Electronic health records (EHRs) can use spreadsheets to graph a series of a patient's blood values over time.

**Database management software** permits you to manage large quantities of data in an organized fashion. Information in a database is organized in tables. The database management software makes it easy to enter data, edit data, sort or organize data, search for data that meet a particular criterion, and retrieve data. Once the structure of the table is defined and the data entered, that data can be used for a variety of purposes without being retyped. Eye-pleasing, businesslike reports can easily be generated by simply defining their structure.

There are also specialized software packages used in specific fields such as medicine. For example, specialized accounting programs are used in medical offices. Microsoft is considering developing a new software package for the health care industry.[7]

**Communications software** includes Web browsers, such as Internet Explorer. These programs allow you to connect your computer to other computers in a network.

## AN OVERVIEW OF NETWORKING, CONNECTIVITY, AND TELECOMMUNICATIONS

Telecommunications forms the third component of IT. The implications of telecommunications for the medical world will be more fully explored in

Chapter 4. Although you can enjoy the wonders of the Internet and surf the World Wide Web with very little technical knowledge, this section introduces you to some of the complexities behind networking, connectivity, telecommunications, and the Internet and gives you a foundation for appreciating the impact of these developments on health care.

Standing alone, your computer has access only to the data and information stored on its hard drive and on the disks you insert in its disk drives. If you can connect your personal computer to a network, however, you have access to the data and information on that network as well. The fact that computers can be connected is referred to as **connectivity**. Connectivity greatly enhances the power of your computer, bringing immense stores of information to your fingertips and making it possible for you to interact with people around the world. Connectivity is the prerequisite for developing the field of telemedicine. Computers and other hardware devices that are connected form what is called a **network**. Networks come in all sizes, from small **local area networks (LANs)**, which span one room, to **wide area networks (WANs)**, which may span a state, nation, or even the globe, like the Internet and World Wide Web. Networks can be private or connected through telephone lines, making them **telecommunications networks**. Given the right mix of hardware and software, computers are connected globally.

When computers are connected, the data and information that travel between them must follow some path. There are several communications channels—either wired or wireless. Communications can be high bandwidth (broadband or high speed) or low bandwidth (slow). Most hospitals use broadband connections such as dedicated T1–T3 lines. A slow dial-up connection, however, may be used for sending e-mail and small attachments.

Bluetooth technology is used to create small personal area networks. **Bluetooth** is a wireless technology that can connect digital devices from computers to medical devices to cell phones. For example, if someone is wearing a pacemaker and has a heart attack, his or her cell phone could automatically dial 911.

Transmission is governed by sets of technical standards or rules called **protocols**. The protocols take care of how the connection is set up between devices. Protocols also establish security procedures. You do not have to think about these factors because they are embedded in the communications software. For information on standards-setting organizations, visit ConsortiumInfo.org.

**Cloud computing** is a relatively new concept. Cloud computing allows many users to have secure access to all of their applications (for example, documents, chat, e-mail, blogs, presentations, video, calendar, pictures, address book, and training spreadsheets) from their multiple network devices (smartphones, laptops, desktops, tablets, etc.)[8] Dropbox is a service using cloud computing that allows users to share files.[9]

## USES OF TELECOMMUNICATIONS AND NETWORKING

The linking of computers and communications devices via telecommunications lines into networks of all sizes has made many things possible. A complete list is beyond the scope of this text. Networking allows such things as the electronic linking of health departments in a National Health Information Network for Public Health Officials. This linking permits the sharing of information, which can be important in containing potential epidemics. The successful sharing of information will only take place if the computers are interoperable.

## THE EXPANSION OF WIRELESS TECHNOLOGY: CELL PHONES, GLOBAL POSITIONING SYSTEMS, WI-FI, PERSONAL DIGITAL ASSISTANTS (PDAS), SMARTPHONES, AND TABLET COMPUTERS

During the last few years, the use of wireless technologies has expanded. Cell phones, Global Positioning System (GPS) technology, and PDAs with Internet access have become commonplace. In places without electricity and without landlines, wireless networks using cell phones and PDAs are both bringing health information to people and gathering information to track the spread of disease. **Wi-Fi** is a wireless technology that allows you to connect, for example, a PDA (and other devices) to a network (including the Internet) if you are close enough to a Wi-Fi access point. There are currently investigations into the possibility that wireless communication poses a radiation threat.[10]

The most common wireless device is the **cell phone**. The use of GPS technology, which can pinpoint your location to within several feet, is widely available. RFID tags are becoming more and more common. RFID tags can be incorporated into products; they receive and send a wireless signal. By identifying doorways and other objects, these tags could be used to help people with impaired vision. They can be incorporated into sponges used in surgeries, so that sponges are not left in the patient. They could also be incorporated into medication bottles, so that people could more easily locate their medications.[11]

A smartphone is a cell phone with built-in applications and Internet access. The first smartphone was introduced in 1992 by IBM. It was called Simon, and it included a calculator, note pad, and the ability to send and receive faxes and e-mail; later, games and a world clock were added. Today, smartphones provide phone service, text messaging, e-mail, Web browsing, still and video cameras, MP3 players, and video viewing. They have become smaller and more powerful—small computers. There are many health-related applications (apps) for smartphones that will be discussed in later chapters.[12]

Tablet computers, most notably the **iPad**, have become widely used by health care providers. A tablet is a "computer contained in a touch-screen."[13] Several companies produce tablets; the three major platforms are Apple, Android, and Windows. The Apple iPad has a 9.7" screen, is 0.05 inches thick, and weighs 1.5 pounds. Input is with your finger. It has no stylus. It can run programs written for the **iPhone**.[14] A variety of health-related apps for the iPad will be discussed in later chapters.

Even though the iPad is used in health care, there are some hardware drawbacks that affect its use in acute care settings. It uses non-swappable batteries—although its batteries run 10 hours on one charge. It is not drop-resistant; if dropped, it is likely that its screen would break. It can only run one program at a time, lacks a bar-code scanner, and is not easily disinfected. It is not waterproof.[15]

By 2013, some cell phone users whose phones include a specific chip and software will be able to receive emergency alerts. These alerts range from local emergencies such as tornadoes and hurricanes to national emergencies such as the terrorist attacks of 9/11. The alerts will be sent as text messages and will only be sent to the area affected.[16]

## THE INTERNET AND THE WORLD WIDE WEB

The **Internet** (short for *inter*connected *net*work) is a global network of networks, connecting innumerable smaller networks, computers, and users. It is run by a committee of volunteers; no one owns it or controls it. The Internet originated in 1969 as **ARPAnet**, a project of the Advanced Research Projects Agency of the U.S. Department of Defense. The Department of Defense was attempting to create both a national network of scientists and a communications system that could withstand nuclear attack. The network was, therefore, to be decentralized, forming a communications web with no central authority. The protocol that eventually governed ARPAnet and continues to govern the Internet today is public domain software called **transmission-control protocol/Internet protocol (TCP/IP)**. Any computer or network that subscribes to this protocol can join the Internet.

### Intranets/Extranets

Private corporate or hospital networks that use the same structure as the Internet and TCP/IP protocols are called **intranets**. Software called a **firewall** is used to protect the intranet from unauthorized users. What the user sees looks like a Web page. Companies can use the intranet to distribute information to employees in an easy, attractive format, for training videos, or to post job openings. If the intranet in one organization is linked to other intranets in other organizations, it becomes an **extranet**.

## Internet Services

Once you are connected, what services are available? You can access reliable, peer-reviewed medical information databases, such as MEDLINE using a search engine called **PubMed** (http://www.ncbi.nlm.nih.gov/PubMed/). MedlinePlus is a fairly reliable site for consumers of health care information. However reliable the site, the information should be reasonable and should be checked. For example, the FDA can provide a great deal of health information; however, much of its drug approval project budget comes from the drug

companies it regulates. Drug companies provide a large portion of the Center for Drug Evaluation's budget.[17,18] Be very careful of any information you find, whatever the source. Try to check it with another source.

You can find support groups and information on almost any disease, medication, hospital, and treatment. The information, which may or may not be accurate, can be so up to date that your physician may not even be aware of it. Internet support groups may help people cope with illness and isolation.

The **World Wide Web (WWW)** or **Web** is the part of the Internet that is most accessible and easiest to navigate. The Web is made up of information organized as documents (pages). The information on the Web is stored in files called **Web sites**. To browse the Web, you need

# IN THE NEWS

According to "Cellphone Use Tied to Changes in Brain Activity," by Tara Parker-Pope, published in *The New York Times*, on February 22, 2011, using cell phones, which emit electromagnetic waves, changes brain activity. Brain scans have recorded the changes, and the changes may or may not be harmful.

According to a study by the National Institutes of Health (NIH) that was published in *The Journal of the American Medical Association* in 2011, the radiation that cell phones emit affects the human brain. The position of the cell phone affects brain activity (the closer to the cell phone, the greater the brain activity). Nothing in the study addresses the long-term use of cell phones, and most studies agree that they are safe to use.

The research was directed by Dr. Nora D. Volkow of the National Institute on Drug Abuse.

Dr. Volkow stated, "The study is important because it documents that the human brain is sensitive to the electromagnetic radiation that is emitted by cellphones . . . . It also highlights the importance of doing studies to address the question of whether there are — or are not — long-lasting consequences of repeated stimulation, of getting exposed over five, 10 or 15 years." She continued, "Unfortunately this particular study does not enlighten us in terms of whether this is detrimental or if it could even be beneficial. It just tells us that even though these are weak signals, the human brain is activated by them."

This study, unlike others, used brain scans. They measured the effects on the brain of the cell phone's electromagnetic radiation. The study found that when a phone was on, there was a 7 percent rise in brain activity.

a connection to the Internet and software called a **Web browser**. Finding what you are looking for on the Web can be challenging. If you know the address (**uniform resource locator [URL]**), you can just type it in. However, you are just looking for information on a particular topic, you can use a program called a **search engine**.

The Internet and Web provide an enormous amount of information—some of it reliable, some not. The lack of regulation, the freewheeling quality, is also an attraction but may bring some negative consequences. *Any* information may find its way onto the Internet, and there are no safeguards for accuracy. How do you judge the reliability of medical information on the Internet? There are Web sites that rate online health information. These rating services, however, are not subject to regulation or quality control either. Recognizing the difficulty of sifting through the health information and advice on the Internet, in 1997, the Federal Department of Health and Human Services created Healthfinder (http://www.healthfinder.gov), a listing of "sites 'hand-picked'. . . by health professionals." Most of the sites it recommends are "government agencies, non-profit and professional organizations, universities, libraries," although it does list a few commercial sites. Along with a listing, **Healthfinder** provides the source of the information and a summary.

The lack of regulation applies not only to speech and information but also to commerce. Web sites promote and sell worthless remedies. These sites play on fear—for example, promoting protection from severe acute respiratory syndrome (SARS), which first appeared in February 2003.

## Chapter Summary

Chapter 1 introduces the reader to the concepts of IT and computer literacy and their significance. It also deals with computer hardware and software and how they interact to accept data as input, process the data, and produce information as output. This chapter familiarizes you with networking and connectivity, telecommunications, the Internet, and the World Wide Web and gives you the basic information you need for appreciating the significance of these developments in health care.

- IT includes not only computers, but also communications networks and computer literacy.
- Computer literacy is knowledge of computers and their functions.
- A computer is an electronic device that can accept data as input, process the data, and produce information as output following step-by-step instructions called a program.
- Inside a digital computer, all data and information are represented by combinations of binary digits (bits).
- Physical components of a computer are called hardware.

- Input devices digitize data, so that the computer can process the data.
  - Input devices include keyboards and direct-entry devices.
  - Direct-entry devices include pointing devices, scanning devices, smart cards, optical cards, sensors, and human-biology input devices.
- The system unit includes the CPU, which is comprised of the arithmetic-logic unit and the control unit, and memory, which temporarily stores the work you are currently doing. The CPU and memory work together following the instructions of a program to process data into information.
- Output devices (printers and monitors) present the processed information to the user.
- Secondary storage devices (drives) and media (diskettes, hard disks, optical disks, Zip disks, magnetic tape, and solid-state memory devices) allow you to store information permanently.
- Software (programs) is comprised of the step-by-step instructions that tell the hardware how to process data.

- Software is classified as system software, which controls the basic operation of the hardware, and application software, which completes tasks for the user.
- When computers are connected in networks, the data that are transmitted travel over a path or medium.
- Data transmission is governed by technical standards or rules called protocols.
- Wireless transmission is becoming more and more common with the widespread use of cell phones, smartphones, tablet computers, and other wireless devices.
- The connection of computers and communications devices into networks makes many things possible, including telemedicine.
- The Internet is a global network of networks, which makes vast amounts of information available.
- The World Wide Web is part of the Internet, organized as documents with links to other documents.
- Speech-recognition software is getting better and better.

# Key Terms

| | | |
|---|---|---|
| application software | extranet | output devices |
| arithmetic-logic unit | firewall | personal digital assistants (PDAs) |
| ARPAnet | firmware | |
| automatically recalculated | graphical user interface | plotters |
| binary digits (bits) | hard copy | ports |
| biometrics | hardware | printers |
| Bluetooth | Healthfinder | processing unit |
| booted | information technology (IT) | processor |
| cell phone | input devices | program |
| central processing unit (CPU) | Internet | protocols |
| Cloud computing | intranets | PubMed |
| communications software | iPad | radio-frequency identification (RFID) tags |
| compact disks (CDs) | iPhone | |
| computer | keyboards | random-access memory (RAM) |
| computer literacy | local area networks (LANs) | read-only memory (ROM) |
| connectivity | magnetic diskette | scanning devices |
| control unit | main circuit board (or | search engine |
| database management software | motherboard) | secondary storage devices |
| digital video disks (DVDs) | memory | sensors |
| digitize | monitors | smartphones |
| direct-entry devices | mouse | soft (digital) copy |
| electronic spreadsheets | network | software |
| embedded computer | open architecture | solid-state memory devices |
| expansion boards | operating system | system software |
| expansion slots | optical disks | system unit |

tablet computers

telecommunications networks

transmission-control protocol/
Internet protocol (TCP/IP)

uniform resource locator (URL)

user interface

Web browser

Web sites

wide area networks (WANs)

Wi-Fi

word-processing software

World Wide Web (WWW) or Web

# Review Exercises

## Multiple Choice

1. A computer-literate person _____ .
   a. can use a computer to perform tasks in his
      or her field
   b. is generally familiar with what a computer
      can do
   c. can program a computer
   d. A and B

2. Binary digits (ones and zeroes) are used to
   represent _____ inside the computer.
   a. words
   b. music
   c. graphics
   d. All of the above

3. A/An _____ is a computer that can solve
   complex scientific equations and may be used
   for worldwide weather forecasting.
   a. supercomputer
   b. mainframe
   c. embedded computer
   d. microcomputer

4. A/An _____ can generate a payroll for
   a large business. Several hundred users can
   access terminals at the same time.
   a. supercomputer
   b. mainframe
   c. embedded computer
   d. microcomputer

5. The type of input device that collects data
   directly from the environment and sends
   the data to the computer is called a _____ .
   It is used in clinical monitoring devices.
   a. scanner
   b. sensor
   c. mouse
   d. keyboard

6. Pointing devices include the _____ .
   a. mouse
   b. trackball
   c. light pen
   d. All of the above

7. An input device that reads printed text aloud
   is the _____ .
   a. keyboard
   b. mouse
   c. digitizing tablet
   d. Kurzweil scanner

8. The actual manipulation of data inside the
   computer is performed by the _____ .
   a. input devices
   b. output devices
   c. processing unit
   d. secondary storage devices

9. Wi-Fi _____ .
   a. is a wireless technology
   b. allows you to connect to the Internet
   c. Both A and B
   d. None of the above

10. In areas of the world that lack electricity and
    landlines, _____ bring health information
    and help track the spread of disease.
    a. cell phones
    b. smartphones
    c. PDAs
    d. All of the above

11. During the past few years, the use of _____
    technology (including smartphones, cell
    phones, and PDAs) has expanded.
    a. wired
    b. wireless
    c. Both A and B
    d. None of the above

12. Standards governing communications are called_____ .
    a. standards
    b. protocols
    c. conventions
    d. rules

13. Today, you can access medical information on a/an _____ .
    a. smartphone
    b. tablet computer
    c. A and B
    d. None of the above

14. The part of the Internet comprised of pages with hyperlinks to other pages is referred to as the _____ .
    a. public information utility
    b. bulletin board system
    c. World Wide Web
    d. None of the above

15. By 2013, some cell phone users whose phones include a specific chip and software will be able to receive _____ .
    a. e-mail
    b. emergency alerts
    c. text messages
    d. All of the above

## True/False

1. Embedded computers can be embedded in humans as well as appliances. _____
2. IT includes not only computers but also networks and computer literacy. _____
3. Information from reliable sites (such as the FDA) does not need to be checked. _____
4. A computer manipulates data by following the step-by-step instructions of a program. _____

5. Hardware refers to the physical components of the computer. _____
6. Another word for hardware is programs. _____
7. Solid-state memory devices include flash memory cards. _____
8. The main circuit board of a computer is also called the motherboard. _____
9. Application software controls the basic operations of the computer hardware including input and output. _____
10. The operating system must be booted for the computer to work. _____
11. If you are using a computer to create a budget, you would need a word-processing program. _____
12. The binary number system uses two digits: 0 and 1. _____
13. RFID tags can be incorporated into products; they send a wireless signal. _____
14. Hospitals may use broadband connections for real-time consultations. _____
15. You are sure to get reliable medical information from the Web. _____

## Critical Thinking

1. What input devices do you foresee being used in the health care field? Comment on how such devices as sensors and speech-recognition devices are especially relevant to your discipline.
2. What measures can be taken to help assure the quality of medical information one receives over the World Wide Web?
3. Critically examine the issue of implanting RFIDs into humans.
4. Critically examine the issue of conflict of interest. Discuss the FDA. Does a conflict of interest necessarily corrupt information from the organization?

## Notes

1. Joseph L. Flatley, "RFID Network Used in the Fight Against Alzheimer's," February 2, 2009, http://www.engadget.com/2009/02/02/rfid-network-used-in-the-fight-against-alzheimers/ (accessed March 19, 2011).

2. M. L. Baker, "Insurers Study Implanting RFID Chips in Patients," July 19, 2006, http://www.eweek.com/c/a/Health-Care-IT/Insurers-Study-Implanting-RFID-Chips-in-Patients/ (accessed March 19, 2011).

3. U.S. Food and Drug Administration, "Radiofrequency Identification," January 6, 2010, http://www.fda.gov/Radiation-EmittingProducts/RadiationSafety/ElectromagneticCompatibilityEMC/ucm116647.htm (accessed March 19, 2011).

4. Todd Lewan, "Chip Implants Linked to Animal Tumors," September 8, 2007, http://www.washingtonpost.com/wp-dyn/content/article/2007/09/08/AR2007090800997_pf.html (accessed March 19, 2011).

5. David Pogue, "Like Having a Secretary in Your PC," July 20, 2006, http://www.nytimes.com/2006/07/20/technology/20pogue.html?partner=rssnyt&emc=rss (accessed April 24, 2011).

6. Jeffrey Winters, "Communicating by Brain Waves," *Psychology Today,* http://psychologytoday.com/articles/PTO-20030724-000002.html (accessed April 24, 2011).

7. Steve Lohr, "Microsoft to Offer Software for Health Care Industry," July 27, 2006, http://www.nytimes.com/2006/07/27/technology/27soft.html?ex=1311652800&en=2e589acf4a87ba92&ei=5090&partner=rssuserland&emc=rss (accessed April 24, 2011).

8. "What Is Cloud Computing?" June 6, 2011, http://blog.gcflearnfree.org/2011/06/06/what-is-cloud-computing/ (accessed July 19, 2011).

9. PCMag.com, "Dropbox," March 25, 2009, http://www.pcmag.com/article2/0,2817,2343852,00.asp (accessed July 19, 2011).

10. "WiFi Could Be Health Risk at Schools," April 23, 2007, http://www.physorg.com/news96519690.html (accessed April 24, 2011).

11. John Peifer, "Mobile Wireless Technologies for Rehabilitation and Independence," *Journal of Rehabilitation Research & Development* 42, no. 2 (March–April 2005): vii–x.

12. PCMag.com, "Smartphone," http://www.pcmag.com/article2/0,2817,2331562,00.asp (accessed February 28, 2011); wiseGEEK, "What Is a Smartphone?" http://www.wisegeek.com/what-is-a-smartphone.htm (accessed February 26, 2011); R. Elizabeth and C. Kitchen, "iPhone Apps That Could Save Your Life," August 30, 2010, http://www.healthguideinfo.com/health-testing-technology/p85038/ (accessed February 16, 2011).

13. Sam Costello, "What Is the iPad?" 2010, http://ipod.about.com/od/glossary/g/ipad-defintion.htm (accessed February 26, 2011).

14. "Definition of a Tablet Computer," *PC Magazine*, April 17, 2010, http://www.pcmag.com/encyclopedia_term/0,2542,t=tablet+computer&i=52520,00.asp (accessed February 16, 2011); Ryan Faas, "How the iPad Is Changing Mobile Health Care," October 5, 2010, http://www.enterprisemobiletoday.com/features/management/article.php/3906771/How-the-iPad-is-Changing-Mobile-Health-Care.htm (accessed February 15, 2011); Sam Costello, "What Is the iPad?" 2010, http://ipod.about.com/od/glossary/g/ipad-defintion.htm (accessed February 26, 2011).

15. Brian Dolan, "9 Reasons the iPad Falls Short for Acute Care," January 28, 2010, http://mobihealthnews.com/6299/9-reasons-the-ipad-falls-short-for-acute-care/ (accessed February 16, 2011).

16. Edward Wyatt, "Emergency Alert System Expected for Cellphones," May 9, 2011, http://www.nytimes.com/2011/05/10/us/10safety.html (accessed May 14, 2011).

17. Manette Loudon, "The FDA Exposed: An Interview with Dr. David Graham, the Vioxx Whistleblower," Newstarget.com, August 30, 2005, http://www.newstarget.com/011401.html (accessed April 24, 2011).

18. Sidney Wolfe, "How Independent Is the FDA?" *Frontline,* November 13, 2003, http://www.pbs.org/wgbh/pages/frontline/shows/prescription/hazard/independent.html (accessed April 24, 2011).

# Additional Resources

Anderson, Sandra. *Computer Literacy for Health Care Professionals.* Albany, NY: Delmar, 1992.

Austen, Ian. "A Scanner Skips the ID Card and Zeroes In on the Eyes." May 15, 2003. http://topics.nytimes.com/2003/05/15/technology/circuits/15howw.html (accessed April 25, 2011).

Baase, Sara. *A Gift of Fire: Social, Legal, and Ethical Issues in Computing.* Upper Saddle River, NJ: Prentice Hall, 1996.

Baker, M. L. "Insurers Study Implanting RFID Chips in Patients." July 19, 2006. http://www.eweek.com/c/a/Health-Care-IT/Insurers-Study-Implanting-RFID-Chips-in-Patients/ (accessed March 19, 2011).

Beekman, George. *Computer Confluence: Exploring Tomorrow's Technology.* 5th ed. Upper Saddle River, NJ: Prentice Hall, 2002.

Bureau of Labor Statistics. *Occupational Outlook Handbook (OOH), 2006–07 Edition.* http://www.bls.gov/oco/ (accessed April 25, 2011).

Costello, Sam. "What Is the iPad?" 2010. http://ipod.about.com/od/glossary/g/ipad-defintion.htm (accessed February 26, 2011).

"Definition of a Tablet Computer." *PC Magazine.* April 17, 2010. http://www.pcmag.com/encyclopedia_term/0,2542,t=tablet+computer&i=52520,00.asp (accessed February 16, 2011).

Divis, Dee Ann. "Bill Would Push Driver's License with Chip." May 1, 2002. http://www.upi.com/Science_News/2002/05/01/Bill-would-push-drivers-license-with-chip/UPI-66261020227215/ (accessed April 25, 2011)

Dolan, Brian. "9 Reasons the iPad Falls Short for Acute Care." January 28, 2010. http://mobihealthnews.com/6299/9-reasons-the-ipad-falls-short-for-acute-care/ (accessed February 16, 2011).

Eisenberg, Anne. "When the Athlete's Heart Falters, a Monitor Dials for Help." January 9, 2003. http://query.nytimes.com/gst/

fullpage.html?res=9B03E0DE113EF93AA35752C0A9659 C8B63 (accessed April 25, 2011).

Elizabeth, R., and C. Kitchen, "iPhone Apps That Could Save Your Life." August 30, 2010. http://www.healthguideinfo.com/health-testing-technology/p85038/ (accessed February 16, 2011).

Evans, Alan, Kendall Martin, and Mary Anne Poatsy. *Technology in Action.* Upper Saddle River, NJ: Prentice Hall, 2006.

Faas, Ryan. "How the iPad Is Changing Mobile Health Care." October 5, 2010. http://www.enterprisemobiletoday.com/features/management/article.php/3906771/How-the-iPad-is-Changing-Mobile-Health-Care.htm (accessed February 15, 2011).

Feder, Barnaby. "Face-Recognition Technology Improves." March 14, 2003. http://query.nytimes.com/gst/fullpage. html?res=9805E0D9103EF937A25750C0A9659C8B63 (accessed April 25, 2011 ).

Fein, Esther B. "For Many Physicians, E-Mail Is the High-Tech House Call." *The New York Times,* November 20, 1997, A1, B8.

Flatley, Joseph L. "RFID Network Used in the Fight Against Alzheimer's." February 2, 2009. http://www.engadget.com/2009/02/02/rfid-network-used-in-the-fight-against-alzheimers/ (accessed March 19, 2011).

Harmon, Amy. "U.S., in Shift, Drops Its Effort to Manage Internet Addresses." *The New York Times,* June 6, 1998, A1, D2.

Lewan, Todd. "Chip Implants Linked to Animal Tumors." September 8, 2007. http://www.washingtonpost.com/wp-dyn/content/article/2007/09/08/AR2007090800997_pf.html (accessed March 19, 2011).

Markoff, John. "High-Speed Wireless Internet Network Is Planned." December 6, 2002. http://query.nytimes.com/gst/fullpage.html?res=9807EEDB133BF935A35751 C1A9649C8B63 (accessed April 25, 2011 ).

Oakman, Robert L. *The Computer Triangle.* 2nd ed. New York: Wiley, 1997.

PCMag.com. "Smartphone." http://www.pcmag.com/article2/0,2817,2331562,00.asp (accessed February 28, 2011).

Petersen, Melody. "A Respiratory Illness: Cashing In; The Internet Is Awash in Ads for Products Promising Cures or Protection." April 14, 2003. http://query. nytimes.com/gst/fullpage.html?res=950DE5DA133BF937A25757C0A9659 C8B63 (accessed April 25, 2011).

Race, Tim. "What Do They Mean by Digital, Anyhow?" *The New York Times,* March 19, 1998, G11.

Senn, James A. *Information Technology in Business: Principles, Practices, and Opportunities.* 2nd ed. Upper Saddle River, NJ: Prentice Hall, 1998.

U.S. Food and Drug Administration. "Radiofrequency Identification." January 6, 2010. http://www.fda.gov/Radiation-EmittingProducts/RadiationSafety/ElectromagneticCompatibilityEMC/ucm116647.htm (accessed March 19, 2011).

"What Is Bluetooth?" Palowireless. http://www.palowireless.com/infotooth/whatis.asp (accessed April 25, 2011).

wiseGEEK. "What Is a Smartphone?" http://www.wisegeek.com/what-is-a-smartphone.htm (accessed February 26, 2011).

# Related Web Sites

The following Web sites provide research information on medical matters. We cannot, however, vouch for the accuracy of the information.

Healthfinder.gov (http://www.healthfinder.gov), for a government listing of nonprofit and government organizations that provide you with health-related information.

Medicine OnLine (http://www.meds.com), for information on pharmaceutical and medical device companies.

OncoLink (http://www.oncolink.org), for information on cancer.

PubMed (http://www.ncbi.nlm.nih.gov/PubMed), for access to reliable medical information databases.

U.S. National Library of Medicine (http://www.nlm.nih.gov/). Services include Health Information, MEDLINE/PubMed, MedlinePlus, NLM Gateway, Library Services, Catalog, Databases, Historical Materials, MeSH, Publications. Description: The world's largest medical library.

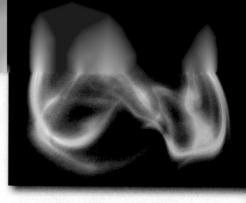

## CHAPTER 2

# Medical Informatics: The American Recovery and Reinvestment Act, HITECH, and the Health Information Technology Decade

## CHAPTER OUTLINE

- Review Exercises
- Notes
- Additional Resources

## LEARNING OBJECTIVES

Upon completion of this chapter, the reader will be able to:

- Define medical informatics.
- Discuss The American Recovery and Reinvestment Act (ARRA) and Health Information Technology for Economic and Clinical Health Act (HITECH) and their effects on health information technology (HIT).
- Define the decade of HIT.
- Define the electronic medical record (EMR) and electronic health record (EHR) and discuss the differences between the two.
- Define interoperability.
- Define the Nationwide Health Information Network (NHIN).
- Describe computer information systems used in health care settings.
  - Hospital information systems (HIS)
  - Financial information systems (FIS)
  - Clinical information systems (CIS)
  - Pharmacy information systems (PIS)
  - Nursing information systems (NIS)
  - Laboratory information systems (LIS)
  - Radiology information systems (RIS)
  - Picture archiving and communication systems (PACS)
- Discuss the issues raised by several studies of the computerization of health records.
- Discuss the introduction of and resistance to computer systems in health care environments.

## MEDICAL INFORMATICS

Medical informatics is a rapidly expanding discipline. It has a long history in which it has sought to improve the way medical information is managed and organized. Medical informatics is located at the "intersection of information technology and medicine and health care."[1]

Medical informatics has many definitions. The common emphasis in all definitions is on the use of technology to organize information in health care. That information includes patient records, diagnostics, expert or decision support systems, and therapies. The stress is not on the actual application of computers in health care, but the theoretical basis. **Medical informatics** is an interdisciplinary science "underlying the acquisition, maintenance, retrieval, and application of biomedical knowledge and information to improve patient care, medical information, and health science research."[2] The tool used to perform these tasks is the computer. Medical informatics focuses on improving all aspects of health care. Some of the aspects it focuses on include improving the clarity of diagnostic images, improving image-guided and minimally invasive surgery, developing simulations that allow health care workers to improve treatments without practicing on human subjects, developing low-cost diagnostic tests, treating physical handicaps, providing consumers with information, coordinating international medical reporting, developing and improving information systems used in health care settings, and developing decision-support systems.

There are several subspecialties of medical informatics. A few are bioinformatics, which uses computers to solve biological problems; dental informatics, which combines computer technology with dentistry to create a basis for research, education, and the solution of real-world problems in dentistry; and nursing informatics, which uses computers to support nurses.[3] Public health informatics uses computer technology to support public health practice, research, and learning.[4]

Currently one important focus of medical informatics is the integration of **hospital information systems (HIS)**, so that radiological images, for example, are available in real time in the operating room. Once the system in one institution is integrated, another important focus of medical informatics is creating regional and then national (and even international) **interoperability** (the connection of people and diverse computer systems). The application of computer technology continues to contribute to the achievement of these goals.

This entire book is about medical informatics; in this chapter, we will focus on the health information technology (HIT) decade, electronic medical record (EMR), electronic health record (EHR), and various **computer information systems** used in hospitals. In the next chapter, we will focus on accounting in a health care environment. In the rest of the book, specific clinical applications will be emphasized. All of these applications are the focus of medical informatics.

# THE AMERICAN RECOVERY AND REINVESTMENT ACT (ARRA), THE HEALTH INFORMATION TECHNOLOGY FOR ECONOMIC AND CLINICAL HEALTH ACT (HITECH), AND THE HEALTH INFORMATION TECHNOLOGY DECADE

On July 21, 2004, the Bush Administration declared 2004–2014 the decade of health information technology (HIT). By 2014, the EHR and electronic prescribing (e-prescribing) would be universal. The administration established an Office of the National Coordinator of Health Information Technology (ONCHIT) whose mission is to "provide leadership for the development and nationwide implementation of an interoperable health information technology infrastructure to improve the quality and efficiency of health care and the ability of consumers to manage their care and safety."[5] ONCHIT was later funded by the **Health Information Technology for Economic and Clinical Health Act (HITECH)**, part of the **American Recovery and Reinvestment Act (ARRA)**, signed into law on February 17, 2009, by President Barack Obama.[6]

The ONCHIT asserts that every health care provider and institution needs to computerize. It predicts that HIT will save money, reduce errors, allow the easy tracking of public health data, and protect privacy.[7] ONCHIT has the task of overseeing the adoption and meaningful use of EHRs, setting standards, and judging the impact. The goal is the universal use of EHRs by 2014 along with the establishment of a national HIT infrastructure.[8]

The Bush Administration (2001–2009) requested $169 million for HIT for 2007, including $116 million for ONCHIT. The specific tasks proposed for 2007 included the following: promote interoperability; find ways to improve collecting public health surveillance data; find ways for patients to keep their own medical records; "define key elements of basic EHRs"; increase e-prescribing; and attempt to solve privacy and security issues.[9] With computerized physician order entry (CPOE), a doctor enters a prescription electronically and it is checked against a hospital database of patients' allergies and drug interactions. Using bar-code medication administration, each patient is given a bar code, which is scanned to identify the patient. Each medication is also bar coded. E-prescribing is seen as a way to reduce medication errors. It is discussed in Chapter 8 on pharmacy. A short definition of **e-prescribing** is the use of computers and software to enter prescriptions and send them to pharmacies electronically.

## Medicare and Medicaid Timeline

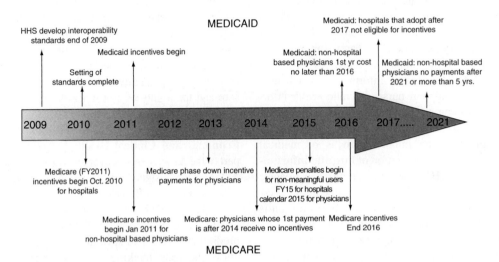

▶ **Figure 2.1**   Timeline for adoption of electronic health record (EHR).
*Source:* © The Northwest Regional Telehealth Resource Center, http://www.nrtrc.org/.

When the American Recovery and Reinvestment Act (ARRA) was signed into law on February 17, 2009, by President Obama, it included billions of dollars for the expansion of HIT. Through Medicare and Medicaid, monetary incentives would be offered to doctors and hospitals to adopt EHRs (Figure 2.1 ▶). (There are also incentives for adopting e-prescribing; however, there are conflicts between these two programs. The Centers for Medicare and Medicaid Services [CMS] is attempting to integrate the two programs.[10])

In March 2011, according to ONCHIT, 25 percent of doctors' offices and 15 percent of hospitals are using EHRs.[11] HITECH, which is a part of the ARRA, encourages the "meaningful use of electronic medical records," with $19 billion in incentives through Medicare and Medicaid for doctors and hospitals to adopt them. Medicare EHR payments can be up to $44,000 for a single doctor between 2011 and 2015. Doctors who treat many Medicaid patients can receive $65,000.[12] After 2014, monetary penalties can be assessed against doctors who fail to adopt certified EHRs.[13] After 2014, doctors who do not adopt EHRs will lose 1 percent of Medicare reimbursements in 2015–2016; in 2017, they will lose

3 percent.[14] HITECH "seeks to improve American health care delivery and patient care through an unprecedented investment in health information technology. The provisions of the HITECH Act are specifically designed to work together to provide the necessary assistance and technical support to providers, enable coordination and alignment within and among states, establish connectivity to the public health community in case of emergencies, and assure the workforce is properly trained and equipped to be meaningful users of EHRs."[15] Billions of dollars of ARRA money have already been spent on health information technology (Figure 2.2 ▶).

A study done by the American Hospital Association and the National Center for Health Statistics (part of the Centers for Disease Control and Prevention), commissioned by ONCHIT, was released in January 2011. It showed that 80 percent of U.S. hospitals and 41 percent of physicians "intend to take advantage of federal incentive payments for adoption and meaningful use of certified electronic health records (EHR) technology." According to the study, there is a significant increase in primary care physicians adopting EHRs (increasing from 19.8 percent in 2008 to 29.6 percent in 2010). However, many

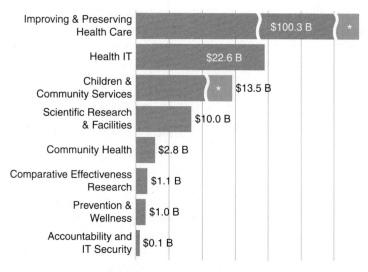

**▶ Figure 2.2**  Funding levels for health information technology (HIT).
*Source:* Courtesy of U.S. Department of Health and Human Services, www.hhs.gov.

of these do not meet the criteria for meaningful use of EHRs.[16]

The Veterans Administration (VA), as part of a federal initiative, is to play a key role in developing electronic records. Between 1997 and 2007, the VA invested $4 billion in HIT, but saved $7 billion. The savings resulted from fewer medical errors and duplicate tests. It is requesting $3.2 billion for 2012 for HIT.[17]

## THE HEALTH INSURANCE PORTABILITY AND ACCOUNTABILITY ACT (HIPAA) OF 1996: A BRIEF INTRODUCTION

The Health Insurance Portability and Accountability Act of 1996 (HIPAA) was passed by the U.S. Congress and signed into law by President Bill Clinton in 1996. Its goal was to make health insurance portable from one job to another and to secure the privacy of medical records. Its privacy provisions went into effect gradually in 2003, and the Enforcement Rule went into effect in 2006. Its primary purpose is to protect the privacy of individually identifiable health information. Basically, patients must be aware of the privacy policy of the health care provider and be notified

when their information is shared (with major exceptions detailed in the Patriot and Homeland Security Acts). Patients are guaranteed the right to see and request changes and corrections in their medical records. The information may be used for research, but software exists to remove all personal identifiers. Staff must be trained to respect the privacy of patients; they should not discuss patients in a public area. Measures must be taken to ensure that only authorized people in the office see the record. These measures may include **biometrics** (using body parts to identify the user), **encryption**, and password protection. When data are sent over the Internet, they are encrypted using software; that is, they are scrambled; the data can only be seen by someone with a decryption key.[18] HITECH increases the penalties for violating the HIPAA Privacy Rule.[19] (For a more detailed discussion of HIPAA and HITECH's privacy and security provisions, see Chapter 12.)

## THE PATIENT INFORMATION FORM

At or before a patient's first visit, he or she fills out a patient information or registration form. It includes personal data like name, address, home, cell and work phones, date of birth, Social Security number, and student status. The patient is also asked to fill in information about his or her spouse or partner.

Medical information is required: allergies, medical history, and current medications. The patient is also asked for the reason for the visit, such as accident or illness, and the name of a referring physician.

In addition, the patient is asked to provide insurance information for him or herself and a spouse or partner. This information includes the names of the primary, secondary, and tertiary insurance carriers; name and birth date of the policyholder; the co-payment; and policy and group numbers.

## THE PAPER MEDICAL RECORD

The information on the patient information forms will then be entered onto the patient's record. The traditional patient record was on paper, stored in one doctor's office. One of the problems with paper records is that they may be illegible, which can lead to serious errors in diagnosis, treatment, and billing. There is only one copy of a paper record, leading to difficulty in sharing patient information and the possibility of misplacing the record. There can be a time delay between the examination and the completion of the doctor's notes on the record. A transcribed record or a record typed using a word processor may include human errors also. A paper record is hard to search for specific information. The use of electronic records may help solve some of these problems.

## THE ELECTRONIC MEDICAL RECORD

In a computerized office, the information that was gathered and entered onto a patient information form will then be entered into a computer into EMRs. This will form the patient's medical record. Encouraged by HIPAA and the federal government, the EMR is very gradually replacing the paper record. The federal government has set a goal of 2014 for universal adoption of electronic records and e-prescribing. The EMR may be stored in a hospital's private network, but it may also be kept on the Internet.[20]

Software has been developed that makes it possible to store medical information on cell phones, smartphones, and tablet computers. The records include prescribed medications, insurance, and names of doctors, among other relevant data. It also contains digital photo identification.[21]

## THE PERSONAL HEALTH RECORD

Patients may establish their own records through the iHealth Record. The **iHealth Record** is a personal medical record that the patient can create and maintain at no cost. An electronic **personal health record (PHR)** is a person's health information in electronic form. It belongs to the individual and is available to him or her on any Web-enabled device. It may include any relevant health information, including: the primary care doctor's name and phone number; allergies, including drug allergies; medications, including dosages; any chronic health problems, such as high blood pressure; major surgeries, with dates; and the living will or advance directives. The PHR can be used in emergencies to alert emergency personnel to necessary information, as well as during routine doctor visits. The patient is in control of his or her PHR and can share it with whomever he or she chooses. The patient can also add information that he or she gathers between doctor visits on blood pressure, exercise habits, and smoking. It can help the patient keep track of appointments, necessary vaccinations and screening tests, and preventive services.[22] As of August 2, 2010, veterans are able to download their PHRs from their MyHealthVet accounts, allowing them to both control the information and share it with health care providers.[23]

## THE ELECTRONIC HEALTH RECORD

The information on a patient's EMR will form the basis of the EHR (Figure 2.3 ▶). Although the terms EMR and EHR are used interchangeably, their meanings are not the same. According to the Healthcare Information Management Systems Society, an organization that promotes the expansion of the use of information technology in health care, "[t]he Electronic Health Record (EHR) is a

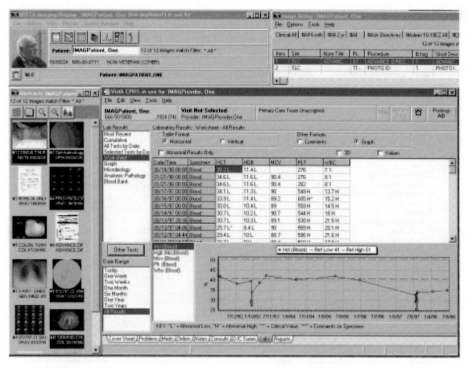

▶ **Figure 2.3** Electronic health record.
*Source:* Courtesy of U.S. Department of Veterans Affairs, www.va.gov.

longitudinal electronic record of patient health information generated by one or more encounters in any care delivery setting. Included in this information are patient demographics, progress notes, problems, medications, vital signs, past medical history, immunizations, laboratory data, and radiology reports. The EHR automates and streamlines the clinician's workflow. The EHR has the ability to generate a complete record of a clinical patient encounter, as well as supporting other care-related activities directly or indirectly...."[24]

There are specific differences between the EMR and EHR. The EMR belongs to one health care institution—a doctor's office or hospital; it must be interoperable (be able to communicate and share information with the other computers and information systems) within that institution only. Ideally, the EHR is not the property of any one institution or practitioner. Eventually, it must be interoperable nationally and internationally.[25] It

is the property of the patient who can access the record and add information. It must include information from all the health care providers and institutions that give care to the patient. It thus eases communication among many practitioners and institutions. It is a source for research in clinical areas, health services, patient outcomes, and public health. It is also an educational source.[26] A fully developed EHR automatically sends an alert to a doctor, for example, to warn of any adverse drug interactions. It will also send reminders to a patient who needs a particular test. EHRs also provide decision support in the form of medical references.[27]

**Meaningful use** of EHRs is defined by ONCHIT. It refers to meeting a required 15 criteria and meeting an additional 5 out of 10 other criteria (Figure 2.4, A–F ▶).[28] These certification criteria were developed by the Secretary of Health and Human Services. The meaningful use criteria may be adopted over a 5-year period. The record

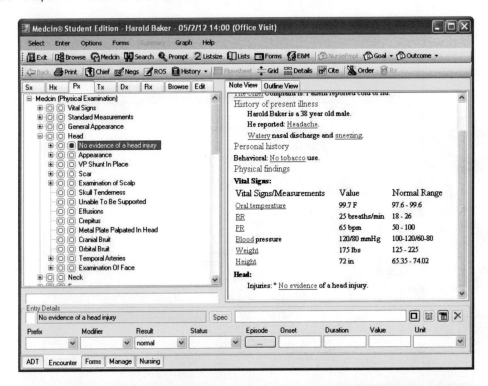

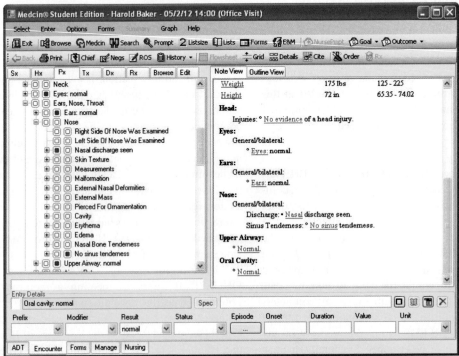

▶ **Figure 2.4** (A) (B) An office visit: MEDCIN electronic health record (EHR) meeting the criteria for meaningful use.

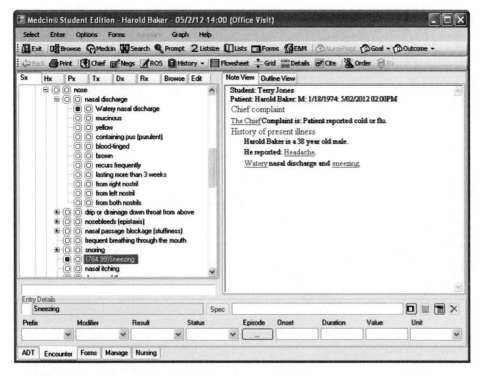

▶ **Figure 2.4** (C) Office visit, symptom list.

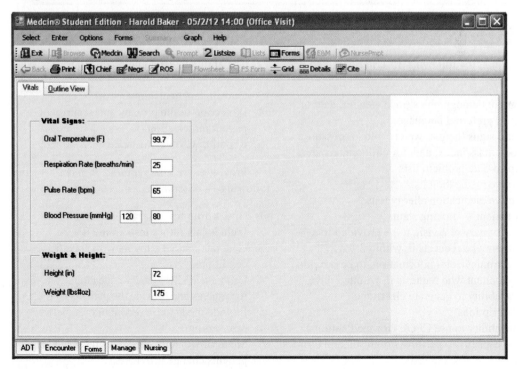

▶ **Figure 2.4** (D) Form for recording vital signs.

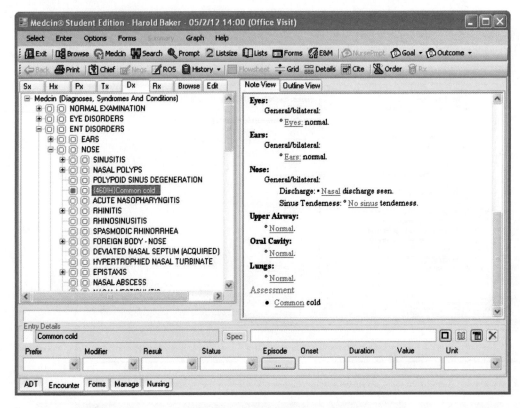

▶ **Figure 2.4** (E) Diagnosis list.

must include the following 15 criteria, which are mandatory:

1. Patient demographics (race, gender, date of birth, preferred language)
2. Vital signs (height, weight, blood pressure, body mass index, and, for children, growth)
3. Up-to-date problem lists
4. Active medication lists
5. Active medication allergy lists
6. A patient's smoking status
7. A summary of a visit, to be provided to a patient who requests it, within 3 days
8. Electronic health information, to be provided to a patient who requests it, within 3 days
9. The ability to generate electronic prescriptions
10. The ability to use CPOE (for medications)
11. The capacity to perform drug/drug and drug/allergy interaction tests
12. The ability to send and receive information electronically
13. One clinical decision-support rule
14. Protection of the privacy and security of patient information
15. Report to CMS or the state

Providers are also required to meet 5 of the following 10 criteria:

1. Check drug formulary.
2. Include laboratory tests in the EMR.
3. Generate lists of patients with specific conditions.
4. Using the EMR, identify education resources for patients and provide the patients with them.
5. Provide medication reconciliation between care settings.
6. Share EMRs with other providers when patients change providers.

```
Harold Baker                                                   Page 1 of 1

Student: your name or ID here
Patient: Harold Baker: M: 1/18/1974: 5/02/2012 02:00PM
Chief complaint
The Chief Complaint is: Patient reported cold or flu.
History of present illness
      Harold Baker is a 38 year old male.
He reported: Headache.
Watery nasal discharge and sneezing.
Personal history
Behavioral: No tobacco use.
Physical findings
Vital signs:
Vital Signs/Measurements               Value              Normal Range
Oral temperature                       99.7 F             97.6 - 99.6
RR                                     25 breaths/min     18 - 26
PR                                     65 bpm             50 - 100
Blood pressure                         120/80 mmHg        100-120/60-80
Weight                                 175 lbs            125 - 225
Height                                 72 in              65.35 - 74.02
Head:
Injuries:  No evidence of a head injury.
Eyes:
General/bilateral:
      Eyes: normal.
Ears:
General/bilateral:
      Ears: normal.
Nose:
General/bilateral:
Discharge: • Nasal discharge seen.
Sinus Tenderness:  No sinus tenderness.
Upper Airway:
             Normal.
Oral Cavity:
             Normal.
Lungs:
      Normal.
Assessment
    • Common cold
Therapy
    • Fluids.
    • Bed rest.
```

▶ **Figure 2.4** (F) Printed encounter note.
*Source:* Courtesy of MEDCIN (Figures 2.4 (A–F)).

7. Give local registries electronic immunization information.

8. Give public health agencies electronic syndromic surveillance.

9. Send patients reminders.

10. Allow patients to have access to their records.

(This list is taken from www.practice fusion.com, (2010; accessed November 11, 2010.)

HITECH established the Health Information Technology Extension Program, which funds **regional extension centers (RECs)**. It also funds the National Health Information Technology Research Center (HITRC) to help physicians adopt EHRs. The more than 60 RECs will give technical help and information.[29] In February 2011, ONCHIT announced an additional $12 million to help the 1,777 critical access and rural hospitals in the United States adopt EHRs.[30]

There are many benefits predicted from the EHR: As records become interoperable, the patient's record will be available anywhere there is a computer on the network; this helps guarantee continuity of care. Each of the patient's health care providers will know the patient's full medical history and can therefore provide better care. If the patient is in an accident in New Jersey, for example, but lives in California, the patient's record is a mouse click away. The EHR is legible and complete. However, despite its benefits, the EHR raises serious privacy issues. Any network can be broken into, and the medical information can be stolen and misused; a great deal of medical information is private. No one wants their psychiatric diagnosis, human immunodeficiency virus (HIV) status, or children's head lice infestation broadcast to the neighborhood. HIPAA provides the first federal protection for medical records. (See Chapter 12 for a full discussion of HIPAA and HITECH and the privacy of medical information.) Despite the problems of privacy and security, a survey of 1,004 Americans found that 78 percent of patients whose doctors used an EHR thought it led to improved care and that 38 percent of patients whose doctors did not use EHRs wanted them to.[31]

According to the U.S. Department of Health and Human Services (HHS), the EHR has been shown to improve health care and should be universally adopted.[32] There are some studies indicating that this is true. A study was done in 2010 of 40 Northwestern Medicine primary care physicians using smart EHRs that alerted doctors during exams when something was wrong with the patient's care: "[A] . . . yellow light on the side of the . . . computer alerts him or her that something is awry . . . . When the doctor clicks on the light, she may learn that Mr. Jones, who has congestive heart failure, hasn't gotten his recommended pneumonia shot. Or, perhaps he was taken off his beta-blockers during a recent hospitalization and needs to start them again." The study found that

doctors' performance was significantly improved. According to the study, simply using EHRs does not automatically improve care. For example, simple reminders on prescribing produce small improvements. Later studies (see below), although mixed, were more positive in their results.[33]

## THE NATIONWIDE HEALTH INFORMATION NETWORK (NHIN)

To be effective in improving care, EHRs have to be fully interoperable (have to be able to communicate with each other) nationally. A first step toward national interoperability would be regional interoperability. Regional cooperation is being fostered through the establishment of **regional health information organizations (RHIOs)** in which data could be shared within a region. The **Nationwide Health Information Network (NHIN)** is the infrastructure that would allow communication between RHIOs. Finally, a nationally interoperable system would be established, where any patient record would be available anywhere on the national network.

Eventually, the NHIN will permit the exchange of all medical information in the United States. However, until NHIN is complete, the ONCHIT is proposing a scaled-down network called NHIN Direct, which will allow the simple exchange of medical information on the Internet using stripped-down Connect software. The NHIN is not a hard-wired network, but a set "of resources . . . the standards, policies, and services that are necessary to enable the secure exchange of health information using the Internet." Local RHIOs or health information exchanges would be connected so that their providers could exchange health information electronically. Eventually, these regional networks would be linked in a national network using Connect software. This NHIN is years away from completion. Until then, NHIN Direct is "a starting point that will evolve with time," according to Micky Tripathi, co-chair of Office of the National Coordinator's Health Information Exchange Workgroup.[34] Currently, ONCHIT is testing information exchanges using NHIN Direct.[35]

In March 2011, ONCHIT announced a 5-year strategy to integrate the information from EHRs with information from other federal agencies including the Food and Drug Administration's (FDA) Sentinel Initiative, "which will track and monitor all FDA-regulated products; the Center for Disease Control's health surveillance network; and an HHS database that will use insurance claims as a basis for medical research." Under this plan, if patients request it, they must be given written summaries of office visits and electronic copies of hospital discharge instructions. ONC plans to create "a learning health system" in which information on individual patient care, potential pandemics, and fruitful avenues of research will be easily available throughout the nation's health care system.[36]

## COMPUTER INFORMATION SYSTEMS IN HEALTH CARE

Computerized information systems are used in some hospitals and other health care facilities to help manage and organize relevant patient, financial, pharmacy, laboratory, and radiological information. To receive the full benefits of computer technology, each of these separate information systems needs to be linked under the hospital information system (HIS). Very few hospitals have reached this point of computerization. Issues such as the high cost of introducing and maintaining computerized systems, the resistance of staff to systems for which they are not adequately trained, and the imposition of systems designed without worker participation and knowledge of the work process have to be dealt with.[37]

The first information systems introduced into hospitals (in the 1960s) were used for administrative purposes (managing finances and inventory). Today, the HIS attempts to integrate the administrative and clinical functions in a hospital. Ideally, the HIS includes clinical information systems, financial information systems, laboratory information systems, nursing and pharmacy information systems, picture archiving and communication systems, and radiology information systems. Systems may be technically perfect. However, if the people in the hospital do not use them, they are a failure.[38]

A **financial information system (FIS)** is concerned with the financial details of running a hospital. These include payroll, patient accounting (all charges that a person generates as an inpatient or outpatient), accounts payable, accounts receivable, general ledger and asset, claims, and contract management.[39] FIS are among the oldest and most widely used computerized information systems in health care. Although FIS are not the most important use of computers in health care, Chapter 3 examines accounting systems in detail.

A **clinical information system (CIS)** uses computers to manage clinical information. This information includes medical history and other relevant information that helps health care personnel make decisions.

The information in a computerized information system is legible and accessible. The U.S. government states that these systems will lead to improved patient outcomes by improving decision making using computerized decision-support systems and reducing adverse drug events by eliminating handwritten prescriptions. Actual studies are divided on these questions. However, these systems are expensive to adopt, raise privacy questions, and may be resisted by doctors who believe that their workload will increase.[40]

**Pharmacy information systems (PIS)** monitor drug allergies and interactions and fill and track prescriptions. They also track inventory and create patient drug profiles. Because the PIS receive prescriptions, they need to be able to interact with the CIS. For billing purposes, they need to be able to interact with the FIS.[41]

**Nursing information systems (NIS)** are supposed to improve nursing care by using computers to manage charting, staff scheduling, and the integration of clinical information. NIS are not common and may meet with resistance from nurses. The resistance may stem from a lack of adequate training, the imposition of a system by the management, or the perception (which may be accurate) that the new system will add to their workload.[42]

**Laboratory information systems (LIS)** use computers to manage both laboratory tests and their results.[43] Ideally, the LIS can interact with the EHR. However, this is often not the case; laboratory results may be mailed or faxed to the doctor's office to be entered into the EHR manually. In 2005, the California HealthCare

Foundation EHR-Lab Interoperability and Connectivity (ELINCS) project "developed the EHR-Lab Interoperability and Connectivity Specification (ELINCS) as a national standard for the exchange of lab results data."[44]

Clinical laboratory personnel (including histologists, cytotechnologists, and phlebotomists) do such work as analyzing body fluids and cells, matching blood samples, and testing for drug levels in blood. Besides microscopes and cell counters, they use computerized instruments, which can do many tests at the same time. Some laboratory personnel specialize: "Cytotechnologists prepare slides of . . . cells and examine [them] . . . microscopically for abnormalities. . . . Molecular biology technologists perform complex protein and nucleic acid testing. . . . Phlebotomists collect blood samples, . . . and histotechnicians cut and stain tissue specimens for microscopic examination by pathologists."[45] Tissue is analyzed by computerized equipment. Cytologists may scan microscopic images into computers and view them on a screen instead of a slide. These images can be viewed on site or telemedically. Although phlebotomists still draw blood, computers currently perform most blood tests.[46]

**Radiology information systems (RIS)** manage patients in the radiology department including scheduling appointments, tracking film, and reporting results. To add images to a patient's electronic record, the RIS must be able to interact with the EMR.[47]

**Picture archiving and communication systems (PACS)** manage digital images (Figure 2.5 ▶). Digital images are immediately available on the monitor and can be shared over a network. PACS can enhance images and eliminate film.[48] The standard communication protocol of imaging devices is called digital imaging and communications in medicine (DICOM).

## DOES COMPUTERIZATION IMPROVE PATIENT OUTCOMES?

Although the HHS mandates the EHR and e-prescribing by 2014 and states that this will improve patient care, it does not cite particular studies. Some studies support the position of the HHS, whereas others question it. A study published in *Health Affairs* did find that the EHR and e-prescribing improved health care by

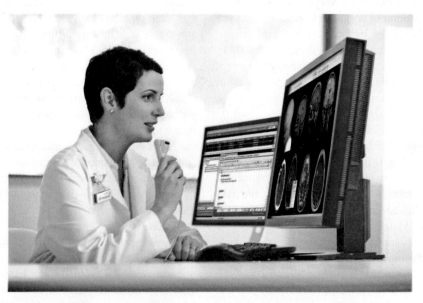

▶ **Figure 2.5** Picture archiving and communication system (PACS).
*Source:* Courtesy of Carestream.

decreasing errors caused by illegible handwriting and improving preventive medicine by generating reminders.[49] Another study, completed in 2006, found that alerts led to a "22% relative decrease in prescribing of non-preferred medications."[50] However, the authors point to the fact that not enough providers are using the EHR to see the full benefit of computerization, and an editorial in *Health Affairs* asserted that more testing is needed before "embarking on a widespread program."[51] A later study, conducted by Kaiser Permanente, concluded that when EHRs send targeted alerts, this can help decrease unnecessary tests.[52]

With all the positive reports on the effects of information technology in health care, there are many dissenting voices. In 2005, research published in *The Journal of the American Medical Association* (*JAMA*) and reported in *The New York Times* warns of some unintended and negative consequences; although decreasing some medication errors, computerized order entry systems can introduce other kinds of errors. One of the causes of errors was that "information on patients' medications was scattered in different places in the computer system. To find a single patient's medications, the researchers found, a doctor might have to browse through up to 20 screens of information." (See Chapter 8.) Computer crashes can also cause errors. Another study published in *JAMA* examined 100 decision-support systems. It found that "most of the glowing assessments of those clinical decision support systems came from technologists who often had a hand in designing the systems."[53]

In 2011, the Institute of Medicine (IOM) announced that it would be conducting a 1-year study to "ensur[e] that health information technology (HIT) will achieve its full potential for improving patient safety." It will focus on preventing errors caused by HIT and reporting of "HIT-related patient safety issues."[54] A recent review of studies of HIT done by ONCHIT in 2011 looked at 154 articles published between July 2007 and February 2010. It found positive results in 96 articles (62 percent), mixed results in 46 articles (30 percent), and negative or partly negative results in 10 articles. Among the issues

examined by the articles were EHRs, CPOE, and clinical decision-support systems. Some of the findings were that ". . . patient mortality and nurse staffing levels decreased by as much as 48 percent and 25 percent . . ." in the 3 years after New York City started using EHRs in three dialysis centers. A clinical decision support system decreased unnecessary transfusions but did not affect either length of stay or mortality. In a study of 41 Texas hospitals using HIT it was "found that hospitals with more advanced HIT had fewer complications, lower mortality, and lower costs than hospitals with less advanced HIT." Some of the negative outcomes included the finding that at one hospital e-prescribing took longer and another found that interaction between health care providers and patients was inhibited by using electronic records. Many of the negative findings had to do with the implantation of HIT.[55] However, a study of private practices, published in January 2011, in the *Archives of Internal Medicine*, found that the adoption of EHRs had little effect on outcomes. Only diet counseling did significantly better when EHRs were used. They also found no difference in outcomes between practices using "advanced function" EHRs and those using simpler systems. Physicians using clinical decision systems (CDS) did significantly better on avoiding unnecessary electrocardiographs, but on no other measure. This study has been criticized for the quality of the survey data it used.[56]

## THE INTRODUCTION OF COMPUTER SYSTEMS

Computer systems may have the potential of improving the management of health care information, but only if they are accepted by the people who need to use them. There is no one comprehensive study of the introduction of computer information systems into health care environments. However, the studies that do exist suggest that the most successful systems are created with the participation of those who will use them. Systems imposed from above are not as readily accepted. Any system that is perceived to add work or change workflow is resisted. One

# IN THE NEWS

According to "Carrots, Sticks and Digital Health Records," by Steve Lohr (published February 26, 2011 in *The New York Times*), the 2009 stimulus included $27 billion to encourage medical institutions to adopt EMRs.

To improve our health care system and lower costs, the government is attempting to encourage doctors to use electronic medical records. Several large medical institutions have successfully adopted the EMR. These include the Mayo Clinic and Kaiser. Less than 30 percent of doctors, however, have adopted the EMR. Part of the problem is the high cost and the lack of technical expertise.

Monetary incentives from the federal government are trying to remedy this. In 2010, the Obama Administration issued a plan for the adoption of the EMR and included incentives of up to $44,000 for doctors and institutions that adopt approved EMRs.

Canadian study of three hospitals (published in *Canadian Medical Association Journal*) found that the response to physician resistance to the introduction of computer systems was a crucial variable.[57] If the response addressed the real issues that physicians were concerned with, resistance dropped. However, a lack of response or antagonistic response increased resistance to the point of having to discontinue the use of the new information systems (in two of the three hospitals studied). A commentary on this article points out that in all three cases the introduction of the new computerized system "meant that clinicians would need to take more time to care for a patient during a particular encounter."[58] The commentary further points out that those systems that reduce or are perceived to reduce workload (for example, PACS) are readily accepted.[59]

## Chapter Summary

- The Bush Administration (2001–2009) declared 2004–2014 the decade of health information technology (HIT) and established an Office of the National Coordinator of Health Information Technology (ONCHIT) to promote the universal use of the EHR and e-prescribing.
- ONCHIT is funded by the HITECH Act (part of ARRA signed by President Obama) and will provide monetary incentives and technological help for doctors and hospitals to adopt meaningful use of EHRs.
- Meaningful use is defined as meeting 20 criteria.
- The EMR is a computerized record of a patient's health information within one health care facility.

- The EHR is a patient's record of all of his or her health care and will eventually be interoperable nationally.
- The first step for national interoperability is to enable regional interoperability through the establishment of RHIOs.
- Eventually a fully interoperable NHIN will be constructed.
- Computerized information systems (hospital information systems that should include FIS, CIS, PIS, LIS, and RIS) are used in some hospitals and other health care facilities to help manage and organize relevant information.
- There is not yet a consensus based on studies on the effects of computerization on patient outcomes.

- The introduction of computer systems may be resisted by those who are supposed to use them.

- Under HITECH there are financial incentives for adopting EHRs.

# Key Terms

American Recovery and Reinvestment Act (ARRA) of 2009

biometrics

clinical information system (CIS)

computer information systems

encryption

e-prescribing

financial information system (FIS)

Health Information Technology for Economic and Clinical

Health Act (HITECH) of 2009

hospital information systems (HIS)

iHealth Record

interoperability

laboratory information systems (LIS)

meaningful use

medical informatics

Nationwide Health Information Network (NHIN)

nursing information systems (NIS)

personal health record (PHR)

pharmacy information systems (PIS)

picture archiving and communication systems (PACS)

radiology information systems (RIS)

regional extension centers (RECs)

regional health information organizations (RHIOs)

# Review Exercises

## Multiple Choice

1. _____ information systems use computers to manage both laboratory tests and their results.
   a. Custom
   b. Financial
   c. Laboratory
   d. All of the above

2. _____ informatics focuses on the use of technology to organize information in health care in order to improve health care; it includes the administrative, clinical, and special purpose uses of computers.
   a. Financial
   b. Chemo-
   c. Medical
   d. None of the above

3. _____ informatics uses computer technology to support public health practice, research, and learning.

   a. Public health
   b. Research
   c. Pediatric
   d. Laboratory

4. One important focus of medical informatics is the _____ of HIS, so that the results of one system are immediately available to the others. For example, radiological images would be available in real time in the operating room.
   a. separation
   b. integration
   c. All of the above
   d. None of the above

5. _____ has the tasks of overseeing the adoption and meaningful use of EHR, setting standards, and judging the impact.
   a. The Public Health Institute
   b. ONCHIT
   c. The House Committee on Health
   d. None of the above

6. The _____ is a longitudinal electronic record of patient health information generated by one or more encounters in any care delivery setting.
   a. EMR
   b. EHR
   c. EPR
   d. Both A and B

7. The _____ belongs to one health care institution—a doctor's office or hospital.
   a. electronic medical record (EMR)
   b. electronic health record (EHR)
   c. electronic personal record (EPR)
   d. Both A and B

8. ONCHIT was funded by the Health Information Technology for Economic and Clinical Health Act (HITECH), part of the _____ signed into law on February 17, 2009, by President Barack Obama.
   a. Health Insurance Portability and Accountability Act (HIPAA)
   b. American Recovery and Reinvestment Act (ARRA)
   c. The Americans with Disabilities Act (ADA)
   d. None of the above

9. Some of the obstacles in the way of introducing the EHR are _____ .
   a. the absence of convincing proof that EHR improves health care
   b. resistance from medical personnel
   c. the initial cost
   d. All of the above

10. Regional cooperation is being fostered through the establishment of _____ in the United States.
    a. national health organizations (NHOs)
    b. international health organizations (IHOs)
    c. regional health information organizations (RHIOs)
    d. None of the above

11. A _____ information system is concerned with the financial details of running a hospital.
    a. clinical
    b. radiology
    c. patient
    d. financial

12. _____ information systems are supposed to improve nursing care by using computers to manage charting, staff scheduling, and the integration of clinical information.
    a. Clinical
    b. Radiology
    c. Nursing
    d. Financial

13. _____ will permit the exchange of all medical information in the United States.
    a. ARRA
    b. ONCHIT
    c. RHIOs
    d. None of the above

14. _____ information systems manage patients in the radiology department including scheduling appointments, tracking film, and reporting results.
    a. Clinical
    b. Radiology
    c. Patient
    d. Financial

15. PACS is a system associated with _____ information systems.
    a. Clinical
    b. Radiology
    c. Patient
    d. Financial

## True/False

1. The EHR is the property of any one institution or practitioner. _____

2. The EMR belongs to one health care institution—a doctor's office or hospital. _____

3. There are no specific differences between the EMR and EHR. _____

4. Regional cooperation is being fostered through the establishment of RHIOs. _____

5. In March 2011, ONCHIT announced a 15-year strategy to integrate the information from EHRs with information from other federal agencies. _____

6. One of the problems with paper records is that they may be illegible. _____

7. HIPAA's goal was to make health insurance portable from one job to another and to secure the privacy of medical records. _____

8. The Nationwide Health Information Network (NHIN), which will permit the exchange of all medical information in the United States, was completed in 2009. _____

9. The common emphasis in all definitions of medical informatics is on the use of technology to organize information in health care. _____

10. When medical data are sent over the Internet, they are encrypted using software; that is, they are scrambled; the data can only be viewed by someone with a decryption key. _____

## Critical Thinking

1. Describe and discuss the meaningful use criteria of the certified EHR.

a. What criteria would you add? Why?
b. What criteria would you delete? Why?

2. Define the following:
   - Hospital information systems (HIS)
   - Laboratory information systems (LIS)
   - Nationwide Health Information Network (NHIN)
   - Nursing information systems (NIS)
   - Picture archiving and communication systems (PACS)
   - Pharmacy information systems (PIS)
   - Radiology information systems (RIS)

3. What does interoperability mean? Why is it crucial for the EHR to be nationally interoperable?

4. What are the differences between the EMR and the EHR? How are they interdependent?

# Notes

1. Daniel C. Davis and William G. Chismar, "Tutorial Medical Informatics," http://www.hicss.hawaii.edu/hicss_32/tutdesc.htm (accessed April 24, 2011).

2. John Gennari, "Biomedical Informatics Is the Science Underlying the Acquisition, Maintenance, Retrieval, and Application of Biomedical Knowledge and Information to Improve Patient Care, Medical Education, and Health Sciences Research," July 22, 2002, http://faculty.washington.edu/gennari/MedicalInformaticsDef.html (accessed April 24, 2011).

3. "Become a Nursing Informatics Specialist," 2011, http://www.allnursingschools.com/nursing-careers/career/nursing-informatics (accessed April 24, 2011).

4. "$3.68 Million Grant to Boost Public Health 'Informatics,'" June 5, 2005, http://www.nlm.nih.gov/news/press_releases/pubhlth_inform_grants05.html (accessed April 24, 2011).

5. "ONC – Office of the National Coordinator for Health Information Technology," February 24, 2010, http://searchhealthit.techtarget.com/definition/ONC (accessed April 25, 2011); "Health Industry Insights Survey Reveals Consumers Are Unaware of Government's Health Records Initiative," February 15, 2006, http://www.crm2day.com/news/crm/117351.php (accessed April 25, 2011).

6. "HITECHEMR Stimulus Information for Physicians," 2010, http://www.practicefusion.com/pages/HITECH.html (accessed November 10, 2010).

7. "Office of the National Coordinator for Health Information Technology (ONC) Executive Summary," October 8, 2006, http://www.himss.org/handouts/executive Summary.pdf (accessed April 25, 2011).

8. "HHS Imposes a $4.3 Million Civil Money Penalty for Violations of the HIPAA Privacy Rule," February 22, 2011, http://www.hhs.gov/news/press/2011pres/02/20110222a.html (accessed February 22, 2011).

9. Scott Weier, "Subcommittee Recommends $98M for ONCHIT in 2007," iHealthbeat, June 15, 2006, http://www.ihealthbeat.org/articles/2006/6/15/Subcommittee-Recommends-98M-for-ONCHIT-in-2007.aspx (accessed April 25, 2011).

10. David Perera, "Two Health IT Programs Crosswise, Says GAO," February 23, 2011, http://www.fiercegovernmentit.com/story/two-health-it-programs-crosswise-says-gao/2011-02-23 (accessed March 28, 2011).

11. David Perera, "Big Data Will Transform Healthcare," March 27, 2011, http://www.fiercegovernmentit.com/story/big-data-will-transform-healthcare-says-onc/2011-03-27 (accessed March 28, 2011).

12. "HITECH EMR Stimulus Information for Physicians," 2010, http://www.practicefusion.com/pages/HITECH.html (accessed November 10, 2010).

13. Mary Mosquera, "Electronic Health Record, GAO: CMS Should Reconcile E-Prescribing, EHR Incentive Reporting," http://govhealthit.com/newsitem.aspx?tid=10&nid=76363 (accessed March 5, 2011).

14. "The EHR Stimulus: A Complete Primer–Physicians Practice," July 15, 2009, http://www.physicianspractice.com/ehr/content/article/1462168/1589230 (accessed March 5, 2011).

15. "HITECH Programs," January 27, 2011, http://healthit.hhs.gov/portal/server.pt?open=512&objID=1487&mode=2 (accessed March 4, 2011).

16. "Surveys Show Significant Proportions of Hospitals and Doctors Already Plan to Adopt Electronic Health Records

and Qualify for Federal Incentive Payments," January 31, 2011, http://www.hhs.gov/news/press/2011pres/01/20110113a.html (accessed March 5, 2011).

17. Department of Veterans Affairs, "VA Announces Budget Request for 2012," February 14, 2011, http://www.va.gov/opa/pressrel/pressrelease.cfm?id=2054 (accessed March 31, 2011).

18. Laurinda Harman, "HIPAA: A Few Years Later," *Online Journal of Issues in Nursing*, July 21, 2005, http://www.medscape.com/viewarticle/506841 (accessed April 25, 2011); "Health Information Privacy: Enforcement Rule–Final Rule," FR Doc 06-1376, *Federal Register*, February 16, 2006 (Volume 71, Number 32), http://www.hhs.gov/ocr/privacy/hipaa/administrative/enforcementrule/enforcement-finalrule.html (accessed April 25, 2011).

19. "HHS Imposes a $4.3 Million Civil Money Penalty for Violations of the HIPAA Privacy Rule," February 22, 2011, http://www.hhs.gov/news/press/ 2011pres/02/20110222a.html (accessed February 22, 2011).

20. "Medem to Launch No-Cost, Electronic Personal Health Records System," May 10, 2005, http://www.medicalnewstoday.com/articles/24123.php (accessed April 25, 2011).

21. Roy Whittington, "New Electronic Medical Records Device Can Save Lives in an Emergency," April 24, 2007, http://www.prwebdirect.com/releases/2007/4/prweb520655.htm (accessed April 25, 2011).

22. "Personal Health Record: A Tool for Managing Your Health—An Electronic Personal Health Record Makes It Easy to Gather and Manage Your Medical Information in One Accessible and Secure Location," June 16, 2011, http://www.mayoclinic.com/health/personal-health-record/MY00665 (accessed July 6, 2011).

23. "Download Your MyHealtheVet Personal Health Record," May 5, 2011, http://www. va.gov/ (accessed May 6, 2011).

24. Healthcare Information Management Systems Society (HIMSS), "EHR: Electronic Health Record," 2011, http://himss.org/asp/topics_ehr.asp (accessed April 25, 2011).

25. A. Virginia Sharpe, "Perspective: Privacy and Security for Electronic Health Records," December 19, 2005, http://www.medscape.com/viewarticle/517403 (accessed April 25, 2011).

26. Peter C. Waegmann, "Status Report 2002: Electronic Health Records," http://www.medrecinst.com/uploaded-Files/MRILibrary/StatusReport.pdf (accessed April 25, 2011); Dave Garets and Mike Davis, "Electronic Medical Records vs. Electronic Health Records: Yes, There Is a Difference," A HIMSS Analytics White Paper, January 26, 2006, http://www.himssanalytics.org/docs/WP_EMR_EHR.pdf (accessed April 25, 2011).

27. Richard W. Gartee, *Electronic Health Records: Understanding and Using Computerized Medical Records* (Upper Saddle River, NJ: Prentice Hall, 2007), 6–8.

28. "EHR Meaningful Use Criteria," http://www.practicefusion.com/pages/ehr-meaningful-use-criteria.html?utm_source=ehrbloggers&utm_medium=internal&utm_campaign=PFLS (accessed November 11, 2010).

29. "HITECH Programs," January 27, 2011, http://healthit.hhs.gov/portal/server.pt?open=512&objID=1487&mode=2 (accessed March 4, 2011).

30. "ONC to Provide Additional Funding to Accelerate Critical Access and Rural Hospitals' Switch to Electronic Health Records," February 8, 2011, http://www.hhs.gov/news/press/ 2011pres/02/2011 0208b.html (accessed March 10, 2011).

31. Molly Merrill, "Survey: 78 Percent of Patients Believe EHRs Boost Care," March 8, 2011, http://healthcareitnews.com/news/survey-78-percent-patients-believe-ehrs-boost-care (accessed March 30, 2011).

32. "Get the Facts About Using Electronic Health Records to Improve Health Care in Your Practice and Community," ONCHIT, http://search.yahoo.com/r/_ylt=A0oG7kbjFjVP7AoADopXNyoA;_ylu=X3oDMTE1amNkODF2BHNlYwNzcgRwb3MDMQRjb2xvA2FjMgR2dGlkA1ZJUDA3N18yNTI-/SIG=15vvocvfd/EXP=1328908131/**http%3a//healthit.hhs.gov/portal/server.pt/gateway/PTARGS_0_12811_953725_0_0_18/Get_the_Facts_about_%2520Using_EHRs_to_Improve_Health_Care_in_Your_Practice_and_Community.pdf (accessed April 25, 2011).

33. Marla Paul, "Research: Smarter Systems Help Busy Doctors Remember: Yellow Light During Exam Alerts Doctors to Problems in a Patient's Care," December 21, 2010, http://www.northwestern.edu/newscenter/stories/2010/12/smarter-systems-help-doctors-remember.html (accessed March 19, 2011).

34. Chris Dimick, "NHIN Direct: ONC Keeps It Simple in Effort to Jumpstart Data Exchange," June 2010, *Journal of AHIMA* 81, http://library.ahima.org/xpedio/groups/public/documents/ahima/bok1_047551.hcsp?dDocName=bok1_047551 (accessed November 11, 2010).

35. "ONC Gearing Up for Testing NHIN Direct Health Data Exchange," October 29, 2010, http://www.ihealthbeat.org/articles/2010/10/29/onc-gearing-up-for-testing-of-nhin-direct-health-data- exchange.aspx (accessed November 12, 2010).

36. David Perera, "Big Data Will Transform Healthcare," March 27, 2011, http://www.fiercegovernmentit.com/story/big-data-will-transform-healthcare-says-onc/2011-03-27 (accessed March 28, 2011).

37. Garets and Davis, "Electronic Medical Records vs. Electronic Health Records."

38. "Hospital Information Systems," 2006, http://www.biohealthmatics.com/ technologies/intsys.aspx (accessed April 25, 2011).

39. "Financial Information System," 2006, http://www.biohealthmatics.com/ technologies/his/fis.aspx (accessed April 25, 2011).

40. "Clinical Information Systems," 2006, http://www.biohealthmatics.com/ technologies/his/cis.aspx (accessed April 25, 2011).

41. "Pharmacy Information Systems," 2006, http://www.biohealthmatics.com/ technologies/his/pis.aspx (accessed April 25, 2011).

42. "Nursing Information Systems," 2006, http://www.biohealthmatics.com/technologies/his/nis.aspx (accessed April 25, 2011).

43. "Laboratory Information Systems," 2006, http://www.biohealthmatics.com/technologies/his/lis.aspx (accessed April 25, 2011).

44. "ELINCS: The National Lab Data Standard for Electronic Health Records," March 2011, http://www.chcf.org/projects/2009/elincs-the-national-lab-data-standard-for-electronic-health-records (accessed April 25, 2011).

45. Bureau of Labor Statistics, U.S. Department of Labor, "*Occupational Outlook Handbook*, 2010–11 Edition, Clinical Laboratory Technologists and Technicians," http://www.bls.gov/oco/ocos096.htm (accessed July 7, 2011).

46. "Histologist Career Info," 2011, http://diplomaguide.com/articles/Histologist_Career_Info.html (accessed July 7, 2011); Mark Orwell, "How Cytologists Use Computers," January 16, 2011, http://www.ehow.com/info_7792529_cytologists-use-computers.html (accessed July 7, 2011); "Phlebotomy and You!" 2011, http://www.squidoo.com (accessed July 7, 2011).

47. "Radiology Information System," 2006, http://www.biohealthmatics.com/technologies/his/ris.aspx (accessed April 25, 2011).

48. "PACS (Picture Archiving and Communication System)," 2006, http://www. biohealthmatics.com/technologies/his/pacs.aspx (accessed April 25, 2011).

49. Kim Krisberg, "Improved Medical Technology Could Affect Health, Lower Cost," November 1, 2005, *Nations Health* 35, no. 9 (2005), © 2005 American Public Health Association (accessed March 10, 2011).

50. Kate Ackerman, "EHR Alerts Reduce Prescription Oversights," June 2, 2006, http://www.ihealthbeat.org/articles/2006/6/2/EHR-Alerts-Reduce-Prescription-Oversights.aspx?a=1 (accessed April 25, 2011).

51. Krisberg, "Improved Medical Technology Could Affect Health, Lower Cost."

52. "Study: Targeted EHR Alerts Can Help Decrease Unneeded Tests," November 8, 2010, http://www.ihealthbeat.org/articles/2010/11/8/study-targeted-ehr-alerts-can-help-reduce-unneeded-tests.aspx (accessed November 12, 2010).

53. Steve Lohr, "Doctors' Journal Says Computing Is No Panacea," *The New York Times,* March 9, 2005.

54. "Institute of Medicine Will Study Best Policies and Practices for Improving Health Care Safety with Health Information Technology," January 3, 2011, http://www.hhs.gov/news/press/2010pres/09/20100929b.html (accessed February 19, 2011).

55. Melinda Beeuwkes Buntin, Matthew F. Burke, Michael C. Hoagland, and David Blumenthal, "The Benefits of Health Information Technology: A Review of the Recent Literature Shows Predominantly Positive Results," 2011, http://content.healthaffairs.org/content/30/3/464.abstract (accessed March 8, 2011); "News Release: A Review of the Recent Studies Shows Predominantly Positive Results for Health Information Technology," March 8, 2011, http://www.hhs.gov/news/press/2011pres /03/20110308a.html (accessed March 8, 2011); David Blumenthal, "Important New Evidence on the Journey to HIT-Assisted Health Care," March 8, 2011, http://www.healthit.gov/buzz-blog/electronic-health-and-medical-records/important-new-evidence-on-the-journey-to-hit-assisted-health-care/ (accessed March 8, 2011).

56. David Perera, "Study Says EHRs Don't Improve Outpatient Care," February 3, 2011, http://www.fiercegovernmentit.com/story/study-says-ehrs-dont-improve-outpatient-care/2011-02-03 (accessed March 28, 2011).

57. Liette Lapointe and Suzanne Rivard, "Getting Physicians to Accept New Information Technology: Insights from Case Studies," May 23, 2006, http://www.cmaj.ca/cgi/content/full/174/11/1573 (accessed April 25, 2011).

58. David Zitner, "Physicians Will Happily Adopt Information Technology," May 23, 2006, http://www.cmaj.ca/cgi/content/full/ 174/11/1583 (accessed April 25, 2011).

59. Erica Danielson, "A Qualitative Assessment of Changes in Nurses' Workflow in Response to the Implementation of an Electronic Charting Information System," A thesis presented to the Division of Medical Informatics and Outcomes Research and the Oregon Health & Science University School of Medicine in partial fulfillment of the requirements of the degree of Master of Science, June 2002; John F. Hurdle, "Can the Electronic Medical Record Improve Geriatric Care?" *Geriatric Times,* March/April 2004, http://www.cmellc.com/geriatrictimes/g040425.html (accessed April 25, 2011); Seth Schiesel, "In the E.R., Learning to Love the PC," *The New York Times,* October 21, 2004; "Latest News in Minimally Invasive Medicine," no date, http://sirweb.org/news/newsPDF/Media_Alert_Round-up.pdf (accessed April 25, 2011); "MTCC to Host 5000 Interventional Radiologists in Professional Society's International Meeting," 2006, http://www.google.com/search?q=cache:v6FA0L1ZszEJ:www.mtccc.com/admin/contentEngine/dspDocumentDownload.cfm%3FPCVID%3D41885715-1422-0efc-51ff-674cc3e1d3ec+MTCC+to+Host+5000+Interventional+Radiologists&hl=en&ct=clnk &cd=3&gl=us (accessed April 25, 2011).

# Additional Resources

"$3.68 Million Grant to Boost Public Health 'Informatics.'" June 5, 2005. http://www.nlm.nih.gov/news/press_releases/pubhlth_inform_grants05.html (accessed April 24, 2011).

Ackerman, Kate. "EHR Alerts Reduce Prescription Oversights." June 2, 2006. http://www.ihealthbeat.org/articles/ 2006/6/2/EHR-Alerts-Reduce-Prescription-Oversights.aspx?a=1 (accessed April 25, 2011).

"Become a Nursing Informatics Specialist." 2011. http://www.allnursingschools.com/nursing-careers/career/nursing-informatics (accessed April 24, 2011).

Blumenthal, David. "Important New Evidence on the Journey to HIT-Assisted Health Care." March 8, 2011. http://www.healthit.gov/buzz-blog/electronic-health-and-medical-records/

important-new-evidence-on-the-journey-to-hit-assisted-health-care/ (accessed March 8, 2011).

Buntin, Melinda Beeuwkes, Matthew F. Burke, Michael C. Hoagland, and David Blumenthal. "The Benefits of Health Information Technology: A Review of the Recent Literature Shows Predominantly Positive Results." 2011. http://content.healthaffairs.org/content/30/3/464.abstract (accessed March 8, 2011).

"Clinical Information Systems." 2006. http://www.biohealthmatics.com/technologies/his/cis.aspx (accessed April 21, 2006).

Danielson, Erica. "A Qualitative Assessment of Changes in Nurses' Workflow in Response to the Implementation of an Electronic Charting Information System." A thesis presented to the Division of Medical Informatics and Outcomes Research and the Oregon Health & Science University School of Medicine in partial fulfillment of the requirements of the degree of Master of Science. June 2002.

Davis, Daniel C., and William G. Chismar. "Tutorial Medical Informatics." http://www.hicss.hawaii.edu/hicss_32/tutdesc.htm (accessed April 25, 2011).

Department of Veterans Affairs. "VA Announces Budget Request for 2012." February 14, 2011. http://www.va.gov/opa/ pressrel/pressrelease.cfm?id=2054 (accessed March 30, 2011).

Dimick, Chris. "NHIN Direct: ONC Keeps It Simple in Effort to Jumpstart Data Exchange." June 2010. *Journal of AHIMA* 81. http://library.ahima.org/xpedio/groups/public/documents/ahima/bok1_047551.hcsp?dDocName=bok1_047551 (accessed November 11, 2010)

"ELINCS: The National Lab Data Standard for Electronic Health Records." March 2011. http://www.chcf.org/projects/2009/elincs-the-national-lab-data-standard-for-electronic-health-records (accessed April 25, 2011).

"Financial Information System." 2006. http://www.biohealthmatics.com/technologies/his/fis.aspx (accessed April 25, 2011).

Garets, Dave, and Mike Davis. "Electronic Medical Records vs. Electronic Health Records: Yes, There Is a Difference." A HIMSS Analytics White Paper, January 26, 2006. http://www.himssanalytics.org/docs/WP_EMR_EHR.pdf (accessed April 25, 2011).

Gartee, Richard W. *Electronic Health Records: Understanding and Using Computerized Medical Records* (Upper Saddle River, NJ: Prentice Hall, 2007), 6–8.

Gennari, John. "Biomedical Informatics Is the Science Underlying the Acquisition, Maintenance, Retrieval, and Application of Biomedical Knowledge and Information to Improve Patient Care, Medical Education, and Health Sciences Research." July 22, 2002. http://faculty.washington.edu/gennari/MedicalInformaticsDef.html (accessed April 24, 2011).

"Get the Facts about Using Electronic Health Records to Improve Health Care in Your Practice and Community."

ONCHIT. no date. http://search.yahoo.com/r/_ylt=A0oG7 kbjFjVP7AoADopXNyoA;_ylu=X3oDMTE1amN kODF2BHNlYwNzcgRwb3MDMQRjb2xvA2FjM gR2dGlkA1ZJUDA3N18yNTI-/SIG=15vvocvfd/ EXP=1328908131/**http%3a//healthit.hhs.gov/portal/ server.pt/gateway/PTARGS_0_12811_953725_0_0_18/ Get_the_Facts_about_%2520Using_EHRs_to_Improve_ Health_Care_in_Your_Practice_and_Community.pdf (accessed April 25, 2011).

Harman, Laurinda. "HIPAA: A Few Years Later." July 21, 2005. *Online Journal of Issues in Nursing.* http://www.medscape.com/viewarticle/506841 (accessed accessed April 25, 2011).

"Health Industry Insights Survey Reveals Consumers Are Unaware of Government's Health Records Initiative." February 15, 2006. http://www.crm2day.com/news/crm/117351.php (accessed April 25, 2011).

"Health Information Privacy: Enforcement Rule–Final Rule." FR Doc 06-1376 [*Federal Register* February 16, 2006 (Volume 71, Number 32)]. http://www.hhs.gov/ocr/privacy/hipaa/administrative/enforcementrule/enforcementfinalrule.html (accessed April 25, 2011).

Healthcare Information Management Systems Society (HIMSS). "EHR: Electronic Health Record." http://himss.org/asp/topics_ehr.asp (accessed April 25, 2011).

"HHS Imposes a $4.3 Million Civil Money Penalty for Violations of the HIPAA Privacy Rule." February 22, 2011. http://www.hhs.gov/news/press/2011pres/02/20110222a.html (accessed February 22, 2011),

"HITECH EMR Stimulus Information for Physicians." 2010. http://www.practicefusion.com/pages/HITECH.html (accessed November 10, 2010).

"HITECH Programs." January 27, 2011. http://healthit.hhs.gov/portal/server.pt?open=512&objID=1487&mode=2 (accessed March 4, 2011).

"Hospital Information Systems." 2006. http://www.biohealthmatics.com/technologies/intsys.aspx (accessed April 25, 2011).

Hurdle, John F. "Can the Electronic Medical Record Improve Geriatric Care?" *Geriatric Times,* March/April 2004. http://www.cmellc.com/geriatrictimes/g040425.html (accessed April 25, 2011).

"Institute of Medicine Will Study Best Policies and Practices for Improving Health Care Safety with Health Information Technology." January 3, 2011. http://www.hhs.gov/news/press/2010pres/09/20100929b.html (accessed February 19, 2011).

Krisberg, Kim. "Improved Medical Technology Could Affect Health, Lower Cost." November 1, 2005. *Nations Health* 35, no. 9 (2005). © 2005 American Public Health Association (accessed March 10, 2011).

"Laboratory Information Systems." 2006. http://www.biohealthmatics.com/technologies/his/lis.aspx (accessed April 25, 2011).

Lapointe, Liette, and Suzanne Rivard. "Getting Physicians to Accept New Information Technology: Insights from Case Studies." May 23, 2006. http://www.cmaj.ca/cgi/content/full/174/11/1573 (accessed April 25, 2011).

"Latest News in Minimally Invasive Medicine." 2006. http://sirweb.org/news/newsPDF/Media_Alert_Round-up.pdf (accessed April 25, 2011).

Lohr, Steve. "Doctors' Journal Says Computing Is No Panacea." *The New York Times.* March 9, 2005.

"Medem to Launch No-Cost, Electronic Personal Health Records System." May 10, 2005. http://www.medicalnewstoday.com/articles/24123.php (accessed April 25, 2011).

Merrill, Molly. "Survey: 78 Percent of Patients Believe EHRs Boost Care." March 8, 2011. http://healthcareitnews.com/news/survey-78-percent-patients-believe-ehrs-boost-care (accessed March 30, 2011).

Mosquera, Mary. "Electronic Health Record, GAO: CMS Should Reconcile E-Prescribing, EHR Incentive Reporting." http://govhealthit.com/newsitem.aspx?tid=10&nid=76363 (accessed March 5, 2011).

"MTCC to Host 5000 Interventional Radiologists in Professional Society's International Meeting." 2006. http://www.google.com/search?q=cache:v6FA0L1ZszEJ:www.mtccc.com/admin/contentEngine/dspDocumentDownload.cfm%3FPCVID%3D41885715-1422-0efc-51ff-674cc3e1d3ec+MTCC+to+Host+5000+Interventional+Radiologists&hl=en&ct=clnk&cd=3&gl=us (accessed April 25, 2011).

"News Release: A Review of the Recent Studies Shows Predominantly Positive Results for Health Information Technology.'" March 8, 2011. http://www.hhs.gov/news/press/2011pres/03/20110308a.html (accessed March 8, 2011),

"Nursing Information Systems." 2006. http://www.biohealthmatics.com/technologies/his/nis.aspx (accessed April 25, 2011).

"Office of the National Coordinator for Health Information Technology (ONC) Executive Summary." October 8, 2006. http://www.himss.org/handouts/executiveSummary.pdf (accessed April 25, 2011).

"ONC Gearing Up for Testing NHIN Direct Health Data Exchange." October 29, 2010. http://www.ihealthbeat.org/articles/2010/10/29/onc-gearing-up-for-testing-of-nhin-direct-health-data-exchange.aspx (accessed November 12, 2010).

"ONC – Office of the National Coordinator for Health Information Technology." February 24, 2010. http://searchhealthit.techtarget.com/definition/ONC (accessed April 25, 2011).

"ONC to Provide Additional Funding to Accelerate Critical Access and Rural Hospitals' Switch to Electronic Health Records." February 8, 2011. http://www.hhs.gov/news/press/ 2011pres/02/20110208b.html (accessed March 10, 2011).

"PACS (Picture Archiving and Communication System)." 2006. http://www.biohealthmatics.com/technologies/his/pacs.aspx (accessed April 21, 2006).

Paul, Marla. "Research: Smarter Systems Help Busy Doctors Remember: Yellow Light During Exam Alerts Doctors to Problems in a Patient's Care." December 21, 2010. http://www.northwestern.edu/newscenter/stories/2010/12/smarter-systems-help-doctors-remember.html (accessed March 19, 2011).

Perera, David. "Big Data Will Transform Healthcare." March 27, 2011. http://www.fiercegovernmentit.com/story/big-data-will-transform-healthcare-says-onc/2011-03-27 (accessed March 28, 2011).

Perera, David. "Study Says EHRs Don't Improve Outpatient Care." February 3, 2011. http://www.fiercegovernmentit.com/story/study-says-ehrs-dont-improve-outpatient-care/2011-02-03 (accessed March 28, 2011).

Perera, David. "Two Health IT Programs Crosswise, Says GAO." February 23, 2011. http://www.fiercegovernmentit.com/story/two-health-it-programs-crosswise-says-gao/2011-02-23 (accessed March 28, 2011).

"Pharmacy Information Systems." 2006. http://www.biohealthmatics.com/technologies/his/pis.aspx (accessed April 25, 2011).

"Radiology Information System." 2006. http://www.biohealthmatics.com/technologies/his/ris.aspx (accessed April 25, 2011).

Schiesel, Seth. "In the E.R., Learning to Love the PC." *The New York Times,* October 21, 2004.

Sharpe, A. Virginia. "Perspective: Privacy and Security for Electronic Health Records." December 19, 2005. http://www.medscape.com/viewarticle/517403 (accessed April 25, 2011).

"Study: Targeted EHR Alerts Can Help Decrease Unneeded Tests." November 8, 2010. http://www.ihealthbeat.org/articles/2010/11/8/study-targeted-ehr-alerts-can-help-reduce-unneeded-tests.aspx (accessed November 12, 2010).

"Surveys Show Significant Proportions of Hospitals and Doctors Already Plan to Adopt Electronic Health Records and Qualify for Federal Incentive Payments." January 31, 2011. http://www.hhs.gov/news/press/2011pres/01/20110113a.html (accessed March 5, 2011).

"The EHR Stimulus: A Complete Primer–Physicians Practice." July 15, 2009. http://www.physicianspractice.com/ehr/content/article/1462168/1589230 (accessed March 5, 2011).

Waegmann, Peter C. "Status Report 2002: Electronic Health Records." http://www.medrecinst.com/uploadedFiles/MRI Library/ StatusReport.pdf (accessed April 25, 2011).

Weier, Scott. "Subcommittee Recommends $98M for ONCHIT in 2007." June 15, 2006. http://www.ihealthbeat.org/articles/2006/6/15/Subcommittee-Recommends-98M-for-ONCHIT-in-2007.aspx (accessed April 25, 2011).

Whittington, Roy. "New Electronic Medical Records Device Can Save Lives in an Emergency." April 24, 2007. http://www.prwebdirect.com/releases/2007/4/prweb520655.htm (accessed April 25, 2011).

Zitner, David. "Physicians Will Happily Adopt Information Technology." May 23, 2006. http://www.cmaj.ca/cgi/content/full/174/11/1583 (accessed April 25, 2011).

CHAPTER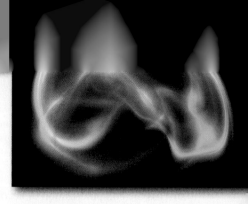

# 3

# An Introduction to the Administrative Applications of Computers: Practice Management, Scheduling, and Accounting

## CHAPTER OUTLINE

## LEARNING OBJECTIVES

Upon completion of this chapter, the reader will be able to:

- Define clinical, special-purpose, and administrative applications of computer technology in health care and its delivery.
- Define telemedicine.
- Discuss electronic scheduling
- Discuss the computerization of accounting tasks in the medical office.
  - Define bucket billing.
  - Discuss coding systems, insurance, and the various accounting reports used in the medical office.
- Discuss the Patient Protection and Affordable Care Act (2010).

## INTRODUCTION

As you recall, **medical informatics** refers to the use of computers to organize health-related information to improve patient care. It addresses all aspects of health care. The first (and most widely) used application is financial; many health care facilities have computerized accounting functions.

Traditionally, the application of computer technology in health care is divided into three categories. The **clinical** use of computers includes anything that has to do with direct patient care, such as diagnosis, monitoring, and treatment. **Special-purpose applications** include the use of computers in education, research, and some aspects of pharmacy. **Administrative applications** include office management, scheduling, and accounting tasks. Many programs are specifically designed for medical office **practice management**. **Telemedicine**—the delivery of health care over telecommunications lines—includes clinical, special-purpose, and administrative applications.

## ADMINISTRATIVE APPLICATIONS OF COMPUTER TECHNOLOGY IN THE MEDICAL OFFICE

Beginning with the computerization of hospital administrative tasks in the 1960s, the role of digital technology in medical care and its delivery has expanded at an ever-increasing pace. Today, computers play a part in every aspect of health care.

As you recall, administrative applications include office management tasks, scheduling, and accounting functions. These are tasks that need to be performed in any office. However, some of these activities are slightly different in a health care environment, so programs are needed that take into account the special needs of a medical office.

Many programs are specifically designed to computerize basic administrative functions in a health care environment—the coding systems, insurance information, and payment information. Such programs allow the user to organize information by patient, by case, and by provider. These programs enable the user to schedule patient appointments with a computer; take electronic progress notes; create lists of codes for diagnosis, treatment, and insurance; submit claims to primary, secondary, and tertiary insurers; and receive payment electronically. These programs must allow the bucket (balance) billing that medical offices must use to accommodate two or three insurers, who must be billed in a timely fashion before the patient is billed. Moreover, because these programs establish **relational databases** (organized collections of related data), information input in one part of the program can be linked to information in another part of the program. Billing information and financial status are easily available. Tables can be searched for any information, and this information can be presented in finished form in one of the many report designs provided, including various kinds of billing reports. If no report design meets the user's need, a customized report can easily be designed and generated by the user. Medical accounting software can be used by medical administrators and office workers, doctors and other health care workers, and students. It can ease the tasks of administering a practice using a computer. The amount of data and information a modern practice has to collect and organize is overwhelming. These programs allow the user to computerize tasks performed every day in any medical environment. All the disparate tasks and pieces of data and information need to be well organized, accessible, and easily linked. The user may quickly and easily organize, access, and link information from one part of the program to information in any other part of the program.

A **database** is an organized collection of information. **Database management software (DBMS)** allows the user to enter, organize, and store huge amounts of data and information. The information is then linked, updated, sorted, resorted, and retrieved. To use DBMS efficiently, the user should be familiar with certain concepts and definitions. A database **file** holds all related information on an entity, for example, a medical practice. For instance, the "Doctors' Practice of Anywhere" would store all of its data and information in a database file stored on a computer. Within the file, there can be several tables. Each **table** holds related information; for example, one table might hold information on the doctors working for the "Doctors' Practice of Anywhere"; another holds information on its patients; and another holds information on its insurance carriers. All of the tables are stored in the practice's file. A table is made up of related **records**; each record holds all the information on one item in the table. Each patient has a record in the practice's patient table. All the information on one patient makes up that patient's record. Each record is made up of related **fields**. One field holds one piece of information, such as a patient's last name, Social Security number (SSN), or chart number. One field—the **key field**—uniquely identifies each record in a table. The information in that field cannot be duplicated. SSN is a common key field because no two people have the same SSN. Chart number uniquely identifies each patient's chart. In a relational database, related tables are linked by sharing a common field. If a practice is completely computerized, a patient's electronic record may contain several pages for personal information, medical history, insurance information, notes, appointments, radiological images, alerts and reminders, and allergies. The structure of a database makes it possible to enter information in one table (say, the appointments table), and that appointment is automatically entered into the patient's electronic record.

# MEDICAL OFFICE ADMINISTRATIVE SOFTWARE: AN OVERVIEW

Medical office administration software allows the user to create one database file for each practice. Within each database, information is organized into tables. The tables are linked by sharing a common field.

## Coding and Grouping

Each category of information (personal, medical, and insurance) provided by a patient is entered into a form and becomes part of a record in a table in a database. Some of it is translated into codes before it is entered. Codes provide standardization, which allows the easy sharing of information. Because codes of diagnoses and procedures are precise and universally used, one physician recognizes another's diagnoses and procedures immediately.

Standard coding systems include the **DRG (diagnosis-related group)**. Today, hospital reimbursement by private and government insurers is determined by diagnosis. Each patient is given a DRG classification, and a formula based on this classification determines reimbursement. If hospital care and cost exceed the prospective cost determination, the hospital absorbs the financial loss.

Services including tests, laboratory work, exams, and treatments are coded using CPT (*Current Procedural Terminology,* Fourth Edition) codes. ICD-10-CM (or ICD-9-CM) provides three-, four-, or five-digit codes for more than 1,000 diseases. The **ICD** is the *International Classification of Diseases*. These coding systems make electronic claim forms easier to file because each condition or disease and each service, procedure, or diagnostic test are identified by a widely agreed-on several-digit number. These codes are standardized, but no practice uses all of them. When a new practice is set up, only codes that relate to its specialty are entered in one of the tables of codes; these tables can always be amended. The **CPT** is used on the **superbill** or **encounter form** (list of diagnoses and procedures common to the specialty) to identify all procedures performed by that practice. The codes are also used in the **electronic health record** (discussed in Chapter 2) and in data collection on public health issues (see Chapter 5).

Other coding systems have also been developed. **MEDCIN** provides 250,000 codes for such things as symptoms, history, physical exams, tests, diagnoses, and treatments. MEDCIN codes can be integrated with other coding systems. **SNOMED** (Systematized Nomenclature of Medicine) makes a common, consistent language available for health information. **LOINC** (Logical Observation Identifiers, Names,

and Codes) standardizes laboratory and clinical codes. The national drug codes (NDCs), which were developed by the Food and Drug Administration (FDA), identify drugs.[1]

## SCHEDULING

Making appointments in today's medical office involves using an electronic appointment book resembling the one in Figure 3.1▶.

MediSoft is one example of practice management software. Office Hours is its scheduling software. We will be using it as an example of scheduling software. Office Hours displays one month's calendar with today's date highlighted in the left pane. The right pane displays several columns for appointments. Each column is for one practitioner. The calendar can be moved backward or forward by using the arrow keys on the left pane. On the right pane, blocks of time can be set aside and color-coded for activities that occur every day, for instance, lunch, and for appointments with patients and other events. A provider

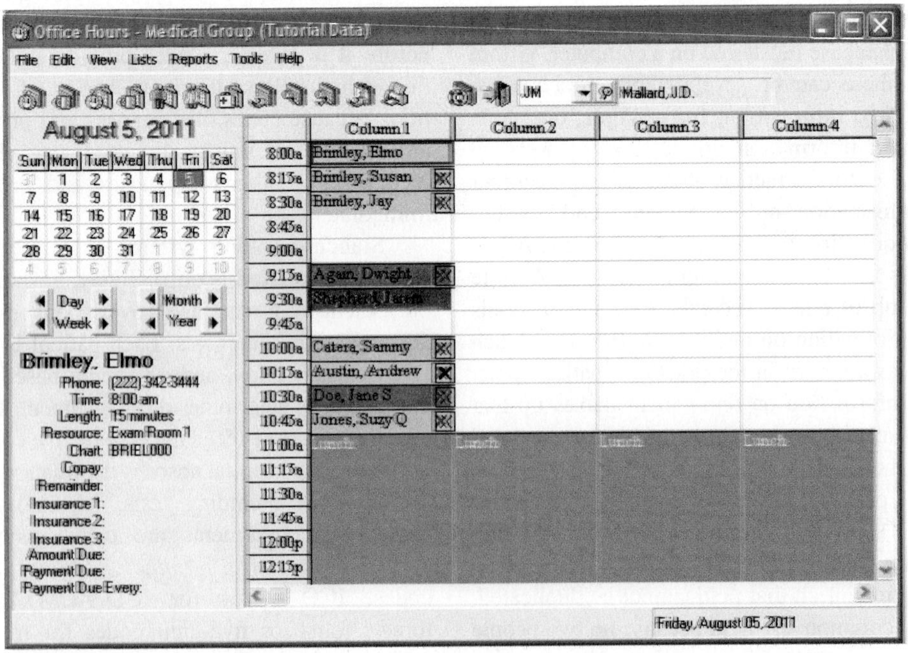

▶ **Figure 3.1**  MediSoft electronic appointment book.
*Source:* Courtesy of MediSoft.

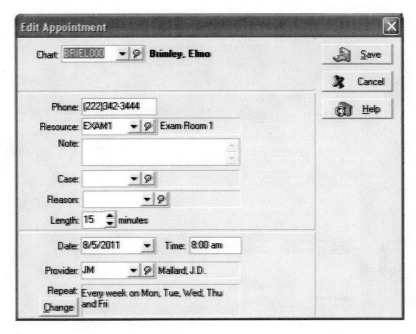

**► Figure 3.2**  MediSoft new appointment entry screen.
*Source:* Courtesy of MediSoft.

(in a multiprovider practice) can be selected from the drop-down list in the right pane. A time can also be selected, and a dialog box will open for a new appointment entry (Figure 3.2 ►).

As soon as the dialog box is filled in and saved, the appointment will appear on the schedule. Electronic scheduling also makes it easy to schedule repeating appointments and to find the next available date for an appointment.[2]

## ACCOUNTING

Many of the computerized tasks in a health care environment have to do with accounting. Therefore, several definitions are required. **Charges**, **payments**, and **adjustments** are called **transactions** (Figure 3.3 ►). A charge is simply the amount a patient is billed for the provider's service. A payment is made by a patient or an insurance carrier to the practice. An adjustment is a positive or negative change to a patient account. Transactions are organized around cases. A **case** is the condition for which the patient visits the doctor. This information is entered by the medical

office staff and stored in the practice's database tables. There can be several visits associated with one case. The case can be closed when the condition is resolved. And there can be several cases (one for each diagnosis) for one patient.

## INSURANCE

Today, many people are covered by medical insurance. A **guarantor** is the person responsible for payment; it may be the patient or a third party. There are a variety of options for those with insurance. Some carriers have a **schedule of benefits**—a list of services that the carrier will cover. This is called an **indemnity plan**. Indemnity plans are becoming less and less common, because they are **fee-for-service plans** and therefore very expensive. The patient is never restricted to a network of providers and needs no referrals for specialists. After fulfilling a **deductible** (a certain amount the patient is required to pay each year before the insurance begins paying), every visit to a doctor is paid for by the insurance company. The doctor, not the

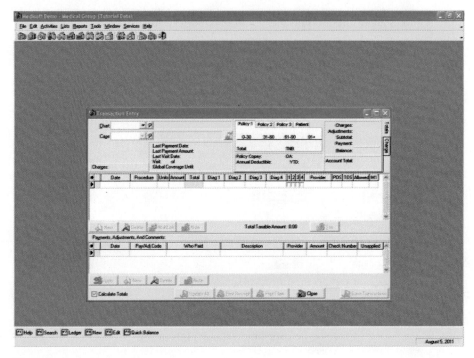

▶ **Figure 3.3**    Patient transaction entry (MediSoft 14).
*Source:* Courtesy of MediSoft.

insurance company, determines necessary care and treatment, so there is no financial reason for a health care worker to deny necessary care. **Managed care** also has a schedule of benefits for out-of-network providers. Managed care plans and **preferred provider organizations (PPOs)** may require that the provider get **authorization** before a procedure is performed. This is simply permission by the insurance carrier for the provider to perform a medical procedure.

In 2010, some private insurance companies began trying to pay doctors for performance—"evaluating physicians and paying them according to their 'quality ranking.'" However, a study published in *The Journal of the American Medical Association* found that results are influenced as much by "whom the doctors care for" as by what doctors do.[3]

A patient with PPO insurance can seek care within an approved network of health care providers who have agreed with the insurance company to lower their charges and accept **assignment** (the amount the insurance company pays). The patient may pay a **co-payment**, the part of the charge for which the patient is responsible. The patient may choose, however, to go out-of-network and pay the provider's customary charges. The insurance company may then reimburse the patient a small amount. There are several government insurance plans. They are administered by the federal **Centers for Medicare and Medicaid Services (CMS)**, formerly the Health Care Financing Administration (HCFA). **Worker's compensation** is a government program that covers job-related illness or injury. Millions of Americans receive their health care through government insurers—some through fee-for-service plans and some through managed care. According to CMS, **Medicaid** is "jointly funded, federal-state health insurance for certain low-income and needy people." As of 2010, Medicaid covers 29 million children and 15 million adults, 14 million old people and people with disabilities, and 19 million people on Medicare. Medicaid gives long-term care assistance to 1.4 million people in nursing homes and 2.8 million "community-based residents."[4] *Community-based* refers to people living in their own homes.

Medicaid resembles managed care, in that the patient is restricted to a network of providers, must get a preauthorization for procedures, and needs referrals to see any specialists. **Medicare** serves people age 65 years and over and disabled people with chronic renal disorders. Medicare allows patients to choose their physicians; referrals are not needed. Some Medicare patients choose to belong to **health maintenance organizations (HMOs)**. Many people supplement Medicare with private fee-for-service plans in which they are not restricted to a network of providers; they do not need referrals to specialists. The patient is required to pay a cost-sharing amount, and the provider bills the insurance for the remainder. Starting in 2006, people insured by Medicare received some minimal coverage for medication (Medicare Prescription Drug Coverage), which was expanded by the Patient Protection and Affordable Care Act in 2010. **TRICARE** is the health program for U.S. armed service members and their families. **CHAMPUS** covers medical necessities for those eligible: retired military, dependents of active duty retired or dead military. Run by the Department of Veterans Affairs, **CHAMPVA** covers the immediate families of veterans who are totally disabled; the surviving spouse and children of a veteran who died from a service-connected disability; the surviving spouse or children of a veteran who was permanently disabled; and the surviving spouse and children of a member of the military who died in the line of duty.[5]

With managed care, it is the insurance carrier that determines what treatment is necessary and pays for it. There are several forms of managed care. In managed care, patients pay a fixed yearly fee, and the insurance company pays the participating provider.

A patient who uses an HMO pays a fixed yearly fee and must choose among an approved network of health care providers and hospitals. The patient needs a referral from his or her primary care provider to see any specialist. If a patient goes out of network without the HMO's approval, the patient must pay out of pocket. However, this may change in light of a Supreme Court decision of April 2, 2003. Under the ruling, states may require HMOs to open their networks, allowing patients more choice.

In a **capitated plan**, a physician is paid a fixed fee (the capitation), and the physician is paid regardless of the amount of treatment he or she provides. Some patients may seek no treatment; some may visit several times.

Under the Patient Protection and Affordable Care Act, states may develop **health insurance exchanges (HIEs)**, which are marketplaces "that allow individuals and small-business owners to pool their purchasing power to negotiate lower rates."[6] In February 2011, seven states received "early innovator" grants to design the information technology infrastructure necessary for the HIEs. The states include Kansas, Maryland, New York, Oklahoma, Wisconsin, Oregon, and a multistate consortium in New England.

## Claims

To receive payment for services from an uninsured patient, the practice simply bills the patient. To receive payment for services rendered to an insured patient, the practice must submit a claim to the insurance carrier. A **claim** is a request to an insurance company for payment for services. If an insurance carrier requires a treatment plan, the accounting software you use enables you to create one. There are many claim forms, but the most widely accepted forms are the **CMS-1500** (Figure 3.4 ▶) and **UB-04** (Figure 3.5 ▶) for hospital-based claims. The CMS-1500 is the standard claim form for institutional providers. Institutional providers include hospitals, skilled nursing facilities, and home health agencies. The UB-04 (CMS-1450) is the only hardcopy claim form that CMS accepts from institutional providers.

An **electronic media claim (EMC)** is an electronically processed and transmitted claim. To create a claim to submit to an insurance company, the practice needs to gather certain information: the patient's condition, the physician's diagnosis, and the procedures performed in the office or hospital.

PLEASE DO NOT STAPLE IN THIS AREA

CARRIER

PICA **HEALTH INSURANCE CLAIM FORM** PICA

1. MEDICARE (Medicare #) MEDICAID (Medicaid #) CHAMPUS (Sponsor s SSN) CHAMPVA (VA File #) GROUP HEALTH PLAN (SSN or ID) FECA BLK LUNG (SSN) OTHER (ID)
1a. INSURED S I.D. NUMBER (FOR PROGRAM IN ITEM 1)
2. PATIENT S NAME (Last Name, First Name, Middle Initial)
3. PATIENT S BIRTH DATE MM DD YYYY SEX M F
4. INSURED S NAME (Last Name, First Name, Middle Initial)
5. PATIENT S ADDRESS (No., Street)
6. PATIENT RELATIONSHIP TO INSURED Self Spouse Child Other
7. INSURED S ADDRESS (No., Street)
CITY STATE
8. PATIENT STATUS Single Married Other; Employed Full-Time Student Part-Time Student
CITY STATE
ZIP CODE TELEPHONE (Include Area Code) ( )
ZIP CODE TELEPHONE (INCLUDE AREA CODE) ( )
9. OTHER INSURED S NAME (Last Name, First Name, Middle Initial)
10. IS PATIENT S CONDITION RELATED TO:
11. INSURED S POLICY GROUP OR FECA NUMBER
a. OTHER INSURED S POLICY OR GROUP NUMBER
a. EMPLOYMENT? (CURRENT OR PREVIOUS) YES NO
a. INSURED S DATE OF BIRTH MM DD YYYY SEX M F
b. OTHER INSURED S DATE OF BIRTH MM DD YYYY SEX M F
b. AUTO ACCIDENT? YES NO PLACE (State)
b. EMPLOYER S NAME OR SCHOOL NAME
c. EMPLOYER S NAME OR SCHOOL NAME
c. OTHER ACCIDENT? YES NO
c. INSURANCE PLAN NAME OR PROGRAM NAME
d. INSURANCE PLAN NAME OR PROGRAM NAME
10d. RESERVED FOR LOCAL USE
d. IS THERE ANOTHER HEALTH BENEFIT PLAN? YES NO *If yes*, return to and complete item 9 a-d.

**READ BACK OF FORM BEFORE COMPLETING & SIGNING THIS FORM.**

12. PATIENT S OR AUTHORIZED PERSON S SIGNATURE I authorize the release of any medical or other information necessary to process this claim. I also request payment of government benefits either to myself or to the party who accepts assignment below.
SIGNED DATE
13. INSURED S OR AUTHORIZED PERSON S SIGNATURE I authorize payment of medical benefits to the undersigned physician or supplier for services described below.
SIGNED

PATIENT AND INSURED INFORMATION

14. DATE OF CURRENT: MM DD YYYY ILLNESS (First symptom) OR INJURY (Accident) OR PREGNANCY(LMP)
15. IF PATIENT HAS HAD SAME OR SIMILAR ILLNESS. GIVE FIRST DATE MM DD YYYY
16. DATES PATIENT UNABLE TO WORK IN CURRENT OCCUPATION FROM MM DD YYYY TO MM DD YYYY
17. NAME OF REFERRING PHYSICIAN OR OTHER SOURCE
17a. I.D. NUMBER OF REFERRING PHYSICIAN
18. HOSPITALIZATION DATES RELATED TO CURRENT SERVICES FROM MM DD YYYY TO MM DD YYYY
19. RESERVED FOR LOCAL USE
20. OUTSIDE LAB? YES NO $ CHARGES
21. DIAGNOSIS OR NATURE OF ILLNESS OR INJURY. (RELATE ITEMS 1,2,3 OR 4 TO ITEM 24E BY LINE)
1. ___ . ___ 3. ___ . ___
2. ___ . ___ 4. ___ . ___
22. MEDICAID RESUBMISSION CODE ORIGINAL REF. NO.
23. PRIOR AUTHORIZATION NUMBER

| 24. A DATE(S) OF SERVICE From MM DD YYYY To MM DD YYYY | B Place of Service | C Type of Service | D PROCEDURES, SERVICES, OR SUPPLIES (Explain Unusual Circumstances) CPT/HCPCS MODIFIER | E DIAGNOSIS CODE | F $ CHARGES | G DAYS OR UNITS | H EPSDT Family Plan | I EMG | J COB | K RESERVED FOR LOCAL USE |
|---|---|---|---|---|---|---|---|---|---|---|
| 1 | | | | | | | | | | |
| 2 | | | | | | | | | | |
| 3 | | | | | | | | | | |
| 4 | | | | | | | | | | |
| 5 | | | | | | | | | | |
| 6 | | | | | | | | | | |

25. FEDERAL TAX I.D. NUMBER SSN EIN
26. PATIENT S ACCOUNT NO.
27. ACCEPT ASSIGNMENT? (For govt. claims, see back) YES NO
28. TOTAL CHARGE $
29. AMOUNT PAID $
30. BALANCE DUE $
31. SIGNATURE OF PHYSICIAN OR SUPPLIER INCLUDING DEGREES OR CREDENTIALS (I certify that the statements on the reverse apply to this bill and are made a part thereof.)
SIGNED DATE
32. NAME AND ADDRESS OF FACILITY WHERE SERVICES WERE RENDERED (If other than home or office)
33. PHYSICIAN S, SUPPLIER S BILLING NAME, ADDRESS, ZIP CODE & PHONE #
PIN# GRP#

PHYSICIAN OR SUPPLIER INFORMATION

(APPROVED BY AMA COUNCIL ON MEDICAL SERVICE 8/88) ***PLEASE PRINT OR TYPE*** APPROVED OMB-0938-0008 FORM CMS-1500 (12/90), FORM RRB-1500, APPROVED OMB-1215-0055 FORM OWCP-1500, APPROVED OMB-0720-0001 (CHAMPUS)

▶ **Figure 3.4** CMS-1500 Form.

# UB-04 claim form and instructions

The Office of Management and Budget and the National Uniform Billing Committee have approved the UB-04 claim form, also known as the CMS-1450 form. The UB-04 claim form accommodates the National Provider Identifier (NPI) and has incorporated other important changes. Sample UB-04 forms for inpatient and outpatient claims can be found on pages 3 and 4.

*The UB-04 claim form and NPI*

The UB-04 claim form includes several fields that accommodate the use of your NPI. Although the form accommodates the NPI, you may continue to report your current provider identification numbers in the appropriate areas of the form until otherwise notified. If you have obtained your NPIs and submitted them to us, you must report them on the UB-04 claim form.

If you have any questions regarding the UB-04 claim form, the NPI application process, or reporting your NPI to us, please call your Network Coordinator or contact Customer Service at 1-800-ASK-BLUE.

*UB-04 data field requirements*

| Field location UB-04 | Description | Inpatient | Outpatient |
|---|---|---|---|
| 1 | Provider Name and Address | Required | Required |
| 2 | Pay-To Name and Address | Situational | Situational |
| 3a | Patient Control Number | Required | Required |
| 3b | Medical Record Number | Situational | Situational |
| 4 | Type of Bill | Required | Required |
| 5 | Federal Tax Number | Required | Required |
| 6 | Statement Covers Period | Required | Required |
| 7 | Future Use | N/A | N/A |
| 8a | Patient ID | Situational | Situational |
| 8b | Patient Name | Required | Required |
| 9 | Patient Address | Required | Required |
| 10 | Patient Birthdate | Required | Required |
| 11 | Patient Sex | Required | Required |
| 12 | Admission Date | Required | Required, if applicable |
| 13 | Admission Hour | Required | Required, if applicable |
| 14 | Type of Admission/Visit | Required | Required |
| 15 | Source of Admission | Required | Required |
| 16 | Discharge Hour | Required | N/A |
| 17 | Patient Discharge Status | Required | Required |
| 18-28 | Condition Codes | Required, if applicable | Required, if applicable |
| 29 | Accident State | Situational | Situational |
| 30 | Future Use | N/A | N/A |
| 31-34 | Occurrence Codes and Dates | Required, if applicable | Required, if applicable |
| 35-36 | Occurrence Span Codes and Dates | Required, if applicable | Required, if applicable |
| 37 | Future Use | N/A | N/A |
| 38 | Responsible Party Name and Address | Required, if applicable | Required, if applicable |
| 39-41 | Value Codes and Amounts | Required, if applicable | Required, if applicable |
| 42 | Revenue Code | Required | Required |
| 43 | Revenue Code Description | Required | Required |
|  | NDC Code | Required, if applicable | Required, if applicable |

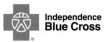

▶ **Figure 3.5** UB-04 Form. (*Continued*)

| Field location UB-04 | Description | Inpatient | Outpatient |
|---|---|---|---|
| 44 | HCPCS/Rates | Required, if applicable | Required, if applicable |
| 45 | Service Date | N/A | Required |
| 46 | Units of Service | Required | Required |
| 47 | Total Charges (By Rev. Code) | Required | Required |
| 48 | Non-Covered Charges | Required, if applicable | Required, if applicable |
| 49 | Future Use | N/A | N/A |
| 50 | Payer Identification (Name) | Required | Required |
| 51 | Health Plan Identification Number | Situational | Situational |
| 52 | Release of Info Certification | Required | Required |
| 53 | Assignment of Benefit Certification | Required | Required |
| 54 | Prior Payments | Required, if applicable | Required, if applicable |
| 55 | Estimated Amount Due | Required | Required |
| 56 | NPI | Required | Required |
| 57 | Other Provider IDs | Optional | Optional |
| 58 | Insured's Name | Required | Required |
| 59 | Patient's Relation to the Insured | Required | Required |
| 60 | Insured's Unique ID | Required | Required |
| 61 | Insured Group Name | Situational | Situational |
| 62 | Insured Group Number | Situational | Situational |
| 63 | Treatment Authorization Codes | Required, if applicable | Required, if applicable |
| 64 | Document Control Number | Situational | Situational |
| 65 | Employer Name | Situational | Situational |
| 66 | Diagnosis/Procedure Code Qualifier | Required, if applicable | Required, if applicable |
| 67 | Principal Diagnosis Code/Other Diagnosis Codes | Required | Required |
| 68 | Future Use | N/A | N/A |
| 69 | Admitting Diagnosis Code | Required | Required, if applicable |
| 70 | Patient's Reason for Visit Code | Situational | Situational |
| 71 | PPS Code | Situational | Situational |
| 72 | External Cause of Injury Code | Situational | Situational |
| 73 | Future Use | N/A | N/A |
| 74 | Principal Procedure Code/Date | Required, if applicable | Required, if applicable |
| 75 | Future Use | N/A | N/A |
| 76 | Attending Name/ID-Qualifier 1G | Required | Required |
| 77 | Operating ID | Situational | Situational |
| 78-79 | Other ID | Situational | Situational |
| 80 | Remarks | Situational | Situational |
| 81 | Code-Code Field/Qualifiers | | |
| | *0-A0 | N/A | N/A |
| | *A1-A4 | Situational | Situational |
| | *A5-AB | N/A | N/A |
| | AC - Attachment Control number | Situational | Situational |
| | AD-B0 | N/A | N/A |
| | *B1-B2 | Situational | Situational |
| | *B3 | Required | Required |

2 12.09

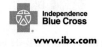

**www.ibx.com**

▶ **Figure 3.5** UB-04 Form. (*Continued*)

# INPATIENT

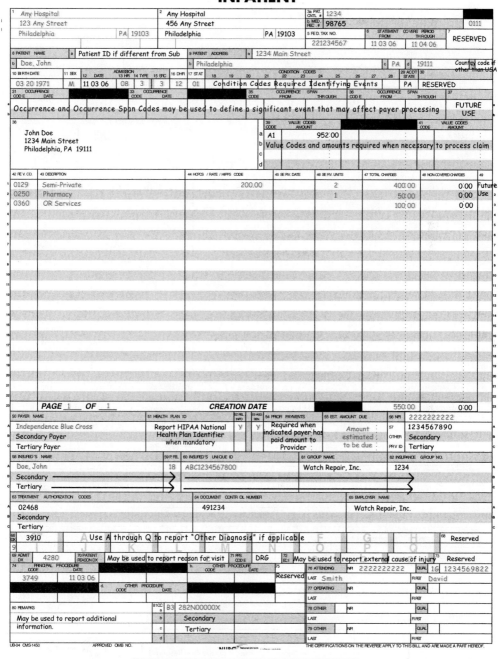

| 1 Any Hospital | 2 Any Hospital | | 3a PAT. CNTL # 1234 | | | |
|---|---|---|---|---|---|---|
| 123 Any Street | 456 Any Street | | b. MED REC # 98765 | | | 0111 |
| Philadelphia PA 19103 | Philadelphia PA 19103 | 5 FED. TAX NO. 221234567 | 6 STATEMENT COVERS PERIOD FROM 11 03 06 THROUGH 11 04 06 | | 7 RESERVED | |

| 8 PATIENT NAME a | Patient ID if different from Sub | 9 PATIENT ADDRESS a | 1234 Main Street | | | |
|---|---|---|---|---|---|---|
| b Doe, John | | b Philadelphia | | c PA | 19111 | Country code if other than USA |

| 10 BIRTHDATE | 11 SEX | 12 DATE ADMISSION 13 HR 14 TYPE 15 SRC | 16 DHR | 17 STAT | 18 19 20 21 CONDITION CODES 22 23 24 25 26 27 28 | 29 ACDT STATE | 30 |
|---|---|---|---|---|---|---|---|
| 03 20 1971 | M | 11 03 06 08 3 3 | 12 | 01 | Condition Codes Required Identifying Events | PA | RESERVED |

| 31 OCCURRENCE CODE DATE | 32 OCCURRENCE CODE DATE | 33 OCCURRENCE CODE DATE | 34 OCCURRENCE CODE DATE | 35 OCCURRENCE SPAN CODE FROM THROUGH | 36 OCCURRENCE SPAN CODE FROM THROUGH | 37 FUTURE USE |
|---|---|---|---|---|---|---|
| Occurrence and Occurrence Span Codes may be used to define a significant event that may affect payer processing | | | | | | |

| 38 | 39 CODE | VALUE CODES AMOUNT | | 41 CODE | VALUE CODES AMOUNT |
|---|---|---|---|---|---|
| John Doe 1234 Main Street Philadelphia, PA 19111 | a A1 | 952 00 | | | |
| | b Value Codes and amounts required when necessary to process claim | | | | |
| | c | | | | |
| | d | | | | |

| 42 REV. CD. | 43 DESCRIPTION | 44 HCPCS / RATE / HIPPS CODE | 45 SERV. DATE | 46 SERV. UNITS | 47 TOTAL CHARGES | 48 NON-COVERED CHARGES | 49 |
|---|---|---|---|---|---|---|---|
| 1 0129 | Semi-Private | 200.00 | | 2 | 400 00 | 0 00 | Future 1 |
| 2 0250 | Pharmacy | | | 1 | 50 00 | 0 00 | Use 2 |
| 3 0360 | OR Services | | | | 100 00 | 0 00 | 3 |
| 4 | | | | | | | 4 |
| 5 | | | | | | | 5 |
| 6 | | | | | | | 6 |
| 7 | | | | | | | 7 |
| 8 | | | | | | | 8 |
| 9 | | | | | | | 9 |
| 10 | | | | | | | 10 |
| 11 | | | | | | | 11 |
| 12 | | | | | | | 12 |
| 13 | | | | | | | 13 |
| 14 | | | | | | | 14 |
| 15 | | | | | | | 15 |
| 16 | | | | | | | 16 |
| 17 | | | | | | | 17 |
| 18 | | | | | | | 18 |
| 19 | | | | | | | 19 |
| 20 | | | | | | | 20 |
| 21 | | | | | | | 21 |
| 22 | | | | | | | 22 |
| 23 PAGE 1 OF 1 | | CREATION DATE | | | 550 00 | 0 00 | 23 |

| 50 PAYER NAME | 51 HEALTH PLAN ID | 52 REL INFO | 53 ASG BEN | 54 PRIOR PAYMENTS | 55 EST. AMOUNT DUE | 56 NPI 2222222222 | |
|---|---|---|---|---|---|---|---|
| A Independence Blue Cross | Report HIPAA National | Y | Y | Required when indicated payer has paid amount to Provider | Amount estimated to be due | 57 1234567890 | A |
| B Secondary Payer | Health Plan Identifier when mandatory | | | | | OTHER Secondary | B |
| C Tertiary Payer | | | | | | PRV ID Tertiary | C |

| 58 INSURED'S NAME | 59 P. REL | 60 INSURED'S UNIQUE ID | 61 GROUP NAME | 62 INSURANCE GROUP NO. | |
|---|---|---|---|---|---|
| A Doe, John | 18 | ABC1234567800 | Watch Repair, Inc. | 1234 | A |
| B Secondary | | | | | B |
| C Tertiary | | | | | C |

| 63 TREATMENT AUTHORIZATION CODES | 64 DOCUMENT CONTROL NUMBER | 65 EMPLOYER NAME | |
|---|---|---|---|
| A 02468 | 491234 | Watch Repair, Inc. | A |
| B Secondary | | | B |
| C Tertiary | | | C |

| 66 DX 3910 | Use A through Q to report "Other Diagnosis" if applicable | | 68 Reserved |
|---|---|---|---|

| 69 ADMIT DX 4280 | 70 PATIENT REASON DX May be used to report reason for visit | 71 PPS CODE DRG | 72 ECI May be used to report external cause of injury | 73 Reserved |
|---|---|---|---|---|

| 74 PRINCIPAL PROCEDURE CODE DATE | b. OTHER PROCEDURE CODE DATE | 75 | 76 ATTENDING NPI 2222222222 QUAL 1G 1234569822 |
|---|---|---|---|
| 3749 11 03 06 | | Reserved | LAST Smith FIRST David |
| d. OTHER PROCEDURE CODE DATE | | | 77 OPERATING NPI QUAL |
| | | | LAST FIRST |

| 80 REMARKS | 81CC a B3 282N00000X | 78 OTHER NPI QUAL |
|---|---|---|
| May be used to report additional information. | b Secondary | LAST FIRST |
| | c Tertiary | 79 OTHER NPI QUAL |
| | d | LAST FIRST |

UB-04 CMS-1450   APPROVED OMB NO.   NUBC National UB form   THE CERTIFICATIONS ON THE REVERSE APPLY TO THIS BILL AND ARE MADE A PART HEREOF.

**3**  12.09

Red = Required
Black = Situational/Required, if applicable/Reserved

Independence **Blue Cross**
www.ibx.com

▶ **Figure 3.5**   UB-04 Form. (*Continued*)

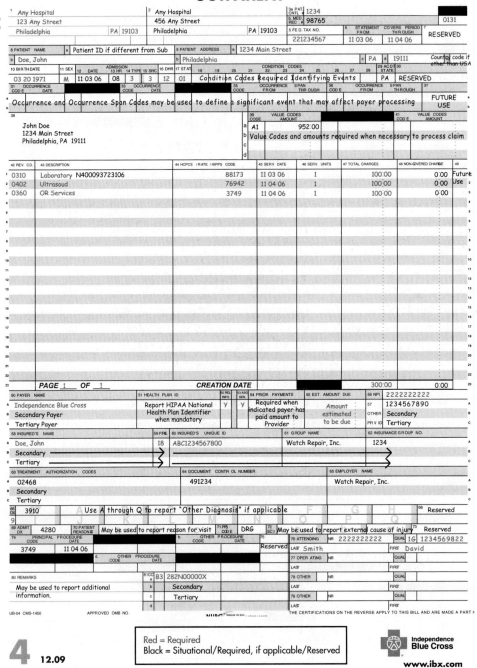

► **Figure 3.5** UB-04 Form.
*Source:* Independence Blue Cross/Blue Shield.

**TEXAS CARDIOLOGY     877 555-1212**

| Patient Number | Ticket Number | Service Date | Prior Balance |
| --- | --- | --- | --- |
| | | | Pat |
| Patient Name | | Gender | Ins |
| Address | | Phone | Other |
| SSN | Referring Dr. | | Total |
| Primary Insurance Co. | Policy/Group ID | | Paymt |
| Secondary Insurance Co. | Policy/Group ID | | Bal Due |

**Location** (checkboxes)
**Cardiologist** (checkboxes)

| X | Code | Service |
| --- | --- | --- |
| | | **New Patient** |
| | 99203 | Limited/Simple (30m) |
| | 99204 | Comprehensive (45m) |
| | 99205 | Complex (60m) |
| | | **New Patient Consult** |
| | | (Need Referring MD) |
| | 99243 | Brief (40m) |
| | 99244 | Full Consult (60m) |
| | 99245 | Very Complex (80m) |
| | | **Established Patient** |
| | 99211 | Nurse Visit |
| | 99212 | Very Brief FU (10m) |
| | 99213 | Limited/Simple FU (15m) |
| | 99214 | Comprehensive FU (25m) |
| | 99215 | Complex FU (40m) |
| | | **New Cons. 2nd Opin.** |
| | 99274 | Moderate 2nd Opinion |
| | 99275 | Complex 2nd Opinion |
| | | **Home Health** |
| | 99375 | Home Health 30 days |
| | | **Drugs:** |
| | J3420 | B-12 Injection |
| | J1940 | Lasix |
| | 90724 | Flu (Dx V-04.8) |
| | G0008 | MC Flu Admin Fee |
| | | Misc Rx |
| | 90782 | IM Injections |
| | 90784 | IV Injections |
| | A4615 | O2 Cannula |

| X | Code | Service |
| --- | --- | --- |
| | | **Office Procedures** |
| | 93000 | EKG w/ Interp |
| | 93015 | Stress Tread w/ Interp |
| | 93040 | Rhythm strip w/ Interp |
| | 93307 | 2D Echo Compl. |
| | 93320 | Doppler Compl. |
| | 93325 | Color Flow Compl. |
| | 93308 | 2D Echo F/U |
| | 93321 | Doppler F/U |
| | ES | Stress Echo |
| | BUB | Echo/Bubble/Doppler |
| | | **Event Monitor** |
| | 93268 | Loop- Non MC |
| | G0005 | Loop - Hookup - MC |
| | G0007 | Loop - Interp - MC |
| | 93012 | Chest Plate Tech - Non MC |
| | 93014 | Chest Pl - Interp Non MC |
| | G0016 | Chest Pl - Interp MC |
| | | **Holter Monitor** |
| | 93224 | Holter w/ Interp Global |
| | | **Other** |
| | 92960 | Cardioversion |
| | 93734 | Pacer Eval - Single |
| | 93735 | Pacer Eval - Sngl w/ Prg |
| | 93731 | Pacer Eval - Dual |
| | 93732 | Pacer Eval - Dual w/ Prg |
| | 99499 | Review outside records |
| | 99080 | Special Reports |

| X | Code | Service |
| --- | --- | --- |
| | | **Diagnostic w/o Interp** |
| | | **(Technical only)** |
| | 93005 | EKG |
| | 93017 | Stress Tread |
| | 93225 | Holter Hookup |
| | 93226 | Holter Scan |
| | 93307-TC | 2D Echo |
| | 93320-TC | Doppler Compl. |
| | 93325-TC | Color Flow |
| | 93308-TC | 2D Echo F/U |
| | 93321-TC | Doppler F/U |
| | 93880-TC | Carotid Doppler |
| | **Phys** | **Interpretation-Supervision,** |
| | | Interpretation & Report Only |
| | 93010 | EKG Interp & Reortt only |
| | TR | Regular Stress Test–S, I & R |
| | NU | Nuclear Stress Test–S, I & R |
| | ES-26 | Stress Echocardiogram–S, I & R |
| | 307 | Echocardiogram 2-D |
| | 320-26 | Doppler Echocardiogram |
| | 325-26 | Color Flow |
| | 308 | Echocardiogram 2-D F/U |
| | 321-26 | Doppler F/U |
| | 227 | Holter Monitor - I & R only |
| | 71250-26 | UltraFast CT |
| | XXXXX | **LAB ORDERED** |
| | | (see attached sheet) |
| | 36415 | VeniPuncture (non MC) |
| | 99000 | Specimen Collection (Lab) |

**Next Appointment:**
Return in: _____ (Wks) (Mo) (Yr)

**Before next appointment:**
☐ Ekg ☐ Echo ☐ Doppler ☐ CXR ☐ Event Monitor
☐ TM ☐ Stress Echo ☐ CFD ☐ Holter ☐ Lab

BI:

**Hospital Admission:**
☐ Admit Cath
☐ Admit to _____ unit at:
☐ BAP ☐ WMC ☐ CMC ☐ SHMC
☐ Other: _____

Notes:

**Cardiac Diagnoses**

▶ **Figure 3.6**   The Superbill or Encounter Form lists procedures and tests common to the practice.

The patient record can provide them with personal data, medical history, and insurance information. The provider table can supply information about the physician. Claims are submitted on paper or electronically. Practices that submit electronic claims use a **clearinghouse**—a business that collects insurance claims from providers and sends them to the correct insurance carrier. An insurance company can reject the claim or send a check for partial or full payment. The response to a paper claim includes an **explanation of benefits (EOB)**, which explains why certain services were covered and others not; an **electronic remittance advice (ERA)** accompanies the response to an EMC.

The practice records the claim and applies it to the charge. It then bills the secondary insurer; the EOB from the first insurer is sent to the secondary insurer with the bill. The secondary insurer responds with a check and EOB or ERA. After the response is received from the secondary insurer, the tertiary insurance company is billed. It is only after the response is received from all of a patient's carriers that the patient is billed. This is called **bucket billing** or **balance billing**.

From the time a patient is charged for a procedure to the time when all payments have been received and credited to the patient's account, there is a sequence of accounting events that occur. **Accounts receivable (A/R)** include any invoice or any payment from the patient or insurance carriers to the medical practice. The diagnoses and procedures relevant to a patient's visit are recorded on a superbill (also called an encounter form). A superbill (Figure 3.6 ▶) is a list of diagnoses and procedures common to the practice. Superbills for each patient on a day's schedule are printed that morning or the night before. Information taken from the superbill is utilized in several medical accounting reports.

## THE PATIENT PROTECTION AND AFFORDABLE CARE ACT (2010)

Although, as of 2011, the **Patient Protection and Affordable Care Act (2010)** is in the courts and could possibly be declared wholly or in part unconstitutional, the act was debated in Congress and the nation for months, was passed by both houses of Congress and signed by President Obama, and can thus be seen to represent some kind of American consensus on health care. Therefore, it is important to discuss and to see what is currently in the bill.

On March 23, 2010, the Patient Protection and Affordable Care Act was signed into law by President Obama. Basically the new law expands health insurance coverage to 32 million more people by requiring them to buy health insurance. It also expands Medicaid coverage and reforms current insurance practices. U.S. citizens and legal residents would be required to buy "minimal essential coverage." If their employer does not offer insurance, the insurance would be bought through state HIEs, which would be established by 2014. An HIE is a marketplace where you can buy insurance. The exchanges are supposed to lower the price of insurance by allowing people to band together to get lower prices than an individual would have to pay. The exchanges will be state-based, but established with federal start-up funds. The exchanges have the power to require that the plans sold are "in the interest" of purchasers. Although the exchange cannot set premiums, they can require insurers to justify rate hikes, and if the exchange is not satisfied with the reason, it can refuse to sell that plan. The exchanges are not open to all customers. You can buy from an exchange if you work for a company with fewer than 100 employees, if you are unemployed, or if you are retired and not eligible for Medicare. The exchanges are not monopolies. An individual can buy insurance on the open market, but the insurer would have to charge the same price within and outside of the exchange. If a person failed to buy insurance, he or she would have to pay a tax penalty of $695 per uninsured person (maximum of $2,085 per family) or 2.5 percent of the family's income. Certain categories of people would be exempt, including those with religious objections, Native Americans, illegal immigrants, and prisoners.[7]

Under the Patient Protection and Affordable Care Act, although most people are required to buy insurance, millions would qualify for subsidies. Of the estimated 25 million people who would shop in the HIEs, about 19 million could be eligible for subsidies. Anyone with an income below four times the federal poverty level (federal poverty level: $22,000 for a family of four, $10,800 for an individual; four times the federal poverty level: $88,000 for a family of four, $44,000 for an individual) would be eligible for some sort of subsidy. If you earn three to four times the poverty level, you would not have to pay more than 10 percent of your income for health insurance. People who earn less would be required to pay a smaller percentage of their income; for example, individuals who make $14,000 and four-person families who make $29,000 would pay no more than 3 to 4 percent of their incomes. The federal subsidies would be paid to the insurance companies. Medicaid will be extended to those who earn less than 133 percent of the poverty level.[8]

If your employer offers insurance, the federal government would still offer a subsidy so that your insurance premiums are less than 9.8 percent of your income, and you would have to buy your insurance on an exchange.[9]

For businesses that do not offer health insurance as a benefit and employ more than 50 people, if one employee buys insurance and qualifies for a subsidy, the business would be taxed $2,000 for each full-time employee (less the first 30 workers).[10]

The bill closes the donut hole in drug coverage for those over age 65, with a $250 rebate in 2010. In 2011, people in the "hole" can purchase brand name drugs at a 50 percent discount. By 2014, states must expand Medicaid to cover childless adults. Through 2016, the federal government will pay all costs for those newly eligible for Medicaid.[11]

The bill reforms some of the practices of private insurance. Children cannot be denied coverage because of pre-existing conditions; this went into effect 6 months after the bill's signing. No one can be denied coverage for pre-existing conditions starting in 2014. Children can stay on their parents' insurance plans until age 26. With certain exceptions, there can be no annual or lifetime dollar limits on coverage.[12]

The Patient Protection and Affordable Care Act also created the **Pre-Existing Conditions Insurance Plan**. It provides insurance for people with pre-existing conditions at the same rates as healthy people would pay. You have to be without insurance for 6 months to qualify. The Department of Health and Human Services is attempting to increase popular awareness of the plan. It is a temporary plan designed to bridge the gap until 2014, when private insurance companies are no longer allowed to deny insurance to people with pre-existing conditions. As of February 2011, 12,000 people are enrolled.[13]

## ACCOUNTING REPORTS

Medical accounting software allows the user to create various kinds of reports that are generated on a daily, monthly, or yearly basis. Daily reports include a patient day sheet, a procedure day sheet, and a payment day sheet. A **patient day sheet** lists the day's patients, chart numbers, and transactions. It is used for daily reconciliation. A **procedure day sheet** is a grouped report organized by procedure. Patients who underwent a particular procedure, such as a blood sugar laboratory test, are listed under that procedure. This report is used to see what procedures a health care worker is performing. It also can be used to find the most profitable procedures. A **payment day sheet** is a grouped report organized by providers. Each patient is listed under his or her provider. It shows the amounts received from each patient to each provider.

A **practice analysis report** is generated on a monthly basis and is a summary total of all procedures, charges, and transactions. A **patient aging report** is used to show a patient's outstanding payments. Current and past due balances are listed on this report based on the number of days late. For example, an account can be past due 30–60 days, 60–90 days, and over 90 days.

The administrative and accounting tasks of a health care environment can be computerized using medical accounting software. It allows the user to enter all necessary information into tables, link the information, and present it in one of the many reports it provides. Computerizing the accounting transactions allows the office to avoid being buried in paper and keeps all accounts in an accurate, up-to-date, and well-organized structure.

# IN THE NEWS

According to "Paying Doctors for Patient Performance," by Pauline W. Chen, published September 30, 2010, in *The New York Times*, some insurance companies are ranking doctors and paying them according to patient outcomes. However, there are questions as to the effects of "paying for performance." Some of the early goals physicians had to meet were screening for breast cancer and colon cancer.

Now, however, many are questioning the validity of pay-for-performance programs. An article was published by *The Journal of the American Medical Association* of a study concluded in September 2010 whose goal was as follows: "To determine if pay for performance was associated with either improved processes of care and outcomes or unintended consequences for acute myocardial infarction at hospitals participating in the CMS pilot project." The study concluded that, "Among hospitals participating in a voluntary quality-improvement initiative, the pay-for-performance program was not associated with a significant incremental improvement in quality of care or outcomes for acute myocardial infarction. Conversely, we did not find evidence that pay for performance had an adverse association with improvement in processes of care that were not subject to financial incentives. Additional studies of pay for performance are needed to determine its optimal role in quality-improvement initiatives."[14]

It seems that the types of patients and conditions treated by a doctor have more to do with outcomes than the physician's skill. Doctors who treat low-income patients, for example, rank lower.

## Chapter Summary

- Medical informatics refers to the use of computers in the management and organization of medical information. Its goal is the improvement of patient care, administration, and research through the use of computers.

- The earliest use of computers was the use of administrative applications, including the use of computers in the medical office for scheduling and accounting.

- Electronic appointment books make scheduling appointments easier.

- Medical accounting programs allow the user to computerize medical office management functions.

  - Bucket billing (or balance billing) is specific to health care office environments, where each insurer must be billed and payment received before the patient is billed.

- In today's medical office, coding systems are used to identify conditions, tests, and procedures.

- Various types of insurance need to be understood.

- The Patient Protection and Affordable Care Act (2010) expanded the number of people covered by insurance.

- Different kinds of accounting reports are used in the medical office.

- Accounting programs allow the user to computerize medical office management functions.

# Key Terms

accounts receivable (A/R)

adjustments

administrative applications

assignment

authorization

balance billing

bucket billing

capitated plan

case

Centers for Medicare and
Medicaid Services (CMS)

CHAMPUS

CHAMPVA

charges

claim

clearinghouse

clinical

CMS-1500

co-payment

CPT

database

database management software
(DBMS)

deductible

DRG (diagnosis-related group)

electronic health record

electronic media claim (EMC)

electronic remittance advice
(ERA)

encounter form

explanation of benefits (EOB)

fee-for-service plans

fields

file

guarantor

health insurance exchanges
(HIEs)

health maintenance
organizations (HMOs)

ICD

indemnity plan

key field

LOINC

managed care

MEDCIN

Medicaid

medical informatics

Medicare

patient aging report

patient day sheet

Patient Protection and
Affordable Care Act (2010)

payment day sheet

payments

practice analysis report

practice management

Pre-Existing Conditions
Insurance Plan

preferred provider organizations
(PPOs)

procedure day sheet

records

relational databases

schedule of benefits

SNOMED

special-purpose applications

superbill

table

telemedicine

transactions

TRICARE

UB-04

worker's compensation

# Review Exercises

## Define the Following Terms

administrative applications

bucket billing

Centers for Medicare and Medicaid Services

Patient Protection and Affordable Care Act
(2010)

## Multiple Choice

1. The _____ is a code used by private and
government insurers to determine insurance
reimbursement.

a. CPT
b. DRG
c. ICD
d. None of the above

2. Managed care plans and _____ may require
that the provider get authorization before a
procedure is performed.

a. fee-for-service plans
b. MediSoft
c. preferred provider organizations (PPOs)
d. DentiSoft

3. Centers for Medicare and Medicaid Services (CMS) administers _____ .
   a. MediSoft
   b. Medicare
   c. Medicaid
   d. Both B and C

4. _____ provides 250,000 codes for such things as symptoms, history, physical exams, tests, diagnoses, and treatment.
   a. Medline
   b. MediSoft
   c. Medicode
   d. MEDCIN

5. _____ applications include the use of computers in office management, accounting, scheduling, and planning.
   a. Clinical
   b. Administrative
   c. Special-purpose
   d. None of the above

6. Medicare serves _____ .
   a. people age 65 years and over
   b. people under age 65 years with broken legs
   c. people with chronic renal disorders
   d. Both A and C

7. A _____ is used to show a patient's outstanding payments.
   a. patient aging report
   b. practice analysis report
   c. patient day sheet
   d. procedure day sheet

8. A _____ is generated on a monthly basis and is a summary total of all procedures, charges, and transactions.
   a. patient aging report
   b. practice analysis report
   c. patient day sheet
   d. procedure day sheet

9. A _____ lists the day's patients, chart numbers, and transactions. It is used for daily reconciliation.
   a. patient aging report
   b. practice analysis report
   c. patient day sheet
   d. procedure day sheet

10. A _____ is a grouped report organized by procedure.
    a. patient aging report
    b. practice analysis report
    c. payment day sheet
    d. procedure day sheet

11. A _____ is a grouped report organized by providers.
    a. patient aging report
    b. practice analysis report
    c. payment day sheet
    d. procedure day sheet

12. Practices that submit electronic claims use a/an _____ , a business that collects insurance claims from providers and sends them to the correct insurance carrier.
    a. insurance collector
    b. collection agency
    c. clearinghouse
    d. None of the above

13. The insurance company's response to a paper claim includes a/an _____ , which explains why certain services were covered and others were not.
    a. explanation of benefits (EOB)
    b. electronic remittance advice (ERA)
    c. lawyer's letter
    d. All of the above

14. _____ are marketplaces "that allow individuals and small-business owners to pool their purchasing power to negotiate lower rates."
    a. Health insurance exchanges (HIEs)
    b. Centers for Medical Exchanges
    c. Centers for Insurance Services
    d. None of the above

15. The insurance company's response to an electronic claim includes a/an _____ , which explains why certain services were covered and others were not.
    a. explanation of benefits (EOB)
    b. electronic remittance advice (ERA)
    c. lawyer's letter
    d. All of the above

## True/False

1. A superbill or encounter form is a list of diagnoses and procedures common to the practice. _____

2. A patient is not responsible for the co-payment. _____

3. Charges, payments, and adjustments are called transactions. _____

4. Under fee-for-service insurance plans, the patient is required to pay a deductible before the insurance company will cover medical costs. _____

5. A patient who uses a health maintenance organization (HMO) pays a fixed yearly fee and can choose among any health care provider or hospital. _____

6. ICD-9-CM and ICD-10-CM provide codes for more than 1,000 diseases. _____

7. Today, hospital reimbursement by private and government insurers is determined by diagnosis (DRG). _____

8. Bucket billing is used by medical offices to accommodate two or three insurers, who must be billed in a timely fashion before the patient is billed. _____

9. Doctors who accept assignment require payment by the patient, not the insurance company. _____

10. Medicaid finances health care for millions of low-income people, with money provided by the federal government and the states. _____

## Critical Thinking

1. The computerization of medical records has advantages and disadvantages. Comment on this statement. Do the advantages outweigh the disadvantages? Support your answer.

2. Some insurance companies want to pay doctors by their performance. Discuss.

3. Comment on how the computerization of administrative tasks may affect a medical office. Bear in mind both efficiency and the fact that an office can print out reports that show the most profitable procedures and practitioners.

# Notes

1. "MedcomSoft Record 2006 Is Released," 2006, http://home.nestor.minsk.by/computers/news/2006/02/2217.html (accessed April 25, 2011).

2. Lillian Burke and Barbara Weill, *MediSoft Made Easy* (Upper Saddle River, NJ: Prentice Hall, 2004), 35–44.

3. Pauline W. Chen, "Paying Doctors for Patient Performance," September 30, 2010, http://www.nytimes.com/2010/10/01/health/01chen.html (accessed October 1, 2010).

4. Kaiser Commission on Medicaid and the Uninsured, "Medicaid Today," January 25, 2011, http://facts.kff.org/chart.aspx? ch=463 (accessed April 22, 2011).

5. Sidath Viranga Panangala and Susan Janeczko, "Health Care for Dependents and Survivors of Veterans," http://congressionalresearch.com/RS22483/document.php?study=Health+Care+for+Dependents+and+Survivors+of+Veterans (accessed April 25, 2011). "Understanding TRICARE," 2011, http://www.military.com/benefits/tricare (accessed April 25, 2011).

6. "States Leading the Way on Implementation: HHS Awards 'Early Innovator' Grants to Seven States," February 16, 2011, http://www.hhs.gov/news/press/ 2011pres/02/20110216a.html (accessed March 10, 2011).

7. Jill Jackson and John Nolan, "Health Care Reform Bill Summary: A Look at What's in the Bill," March 23, 2010, http://www.cbsnews.com/8301-503544_162-20000846- 503544.html (accessed November 11, 2010); Peter Grier, "Health Care Reform Bill 101: Who Must Buy Insurance?" March 19, 2010, http://www.csmonitor.com/USA/Politics/2010/0319/Health-care-reform-bill-101-Who-must-buy-insurance (accessed November 11, 2010); Peter Grier, "Health Care Reform Bill 101: Who Gets Subsidized Insurance?" March 20, 2010, http://www.csmonitor.com/USA/Politics/2010/0320/Health-care-reform-bill-101-Who-gets-subsidized-insurance (accessed November 11, 2010); Peter Grier, "Health Care Reform Bill 101: What's a Health 'Exchange'?" March 20, 2010, http://www.csmonitor.com/USA/Politics/2010/0320/Health-care-reform-bill-101-What-s-a-health-exchange (accessed November 11, 2010); "HealthReform.gov," June 2010, http://healthreform.gov/ (accessed November 11, 2010); "Health Reform Talk," March 29, 2010, http://healthcare-legislation.blogspot.com/(accessed November 11, 2010).

8. Jackson and Nolan, "Health Care Reform Bill Summary: A Look at What's in the Bill"; Grier, "Health Care Reform Bill 101: Who Must Buy Insurance?"; Grier, "Health Care Reform Bill 101: Who Gets Subsidized Insurance?"; Grier, "Health Care Reform Bill 101: What's a Health 'Exchange'?"; "HealthReform.gov"; "Health Reform Talk."

9. Jackson and Nolan, "Health Care Reform Bill Summary: A Look at What's in the Bill"; Grier, "Health Care Reform Bill 101: Who Must Buy Insurance?"; Grier, "Health Care Reform Bill 101: Who Gets Subsidized Insurance?"; Grier, "Health Care Reform Bill 101: What's a Health 'Exchange'?"; "HealthReform.gov"; "Health Reform Talk."

10. Jackson and Nolan, "Health Care Reform Bill Summary: A Look at What's in the Bill"; Grier, "Health Care Reform Bill 101: Who Must Buy Insurance?"; Grier, "Health Care Reform Bill 101: Who Gets Subsidized Insurance?"; Grier, "Health Care Reform Bill 101: What's a Health 'Exchange'?"; "HealthReform.gov"; "Health Reform Talk."

11. Jackson and Nolan, "Health Care Reform Bill Summary: A Look at What's in the Bill"; Grier, "Health Care Reform Bill 101: Who Must Buy Insurance?"; Grier, "Health Care Reform Bill 101: Who Gets Subsidized Insurance?"; Grier, "Health Care Reform Bill 101: What's a Health

'Exchange'?"; "HealthReform.gov"; "Health Reform Talk."

12. Jackson and Nolan, "Health Care Reform Bill Summary: A Look at What's in the Bill"; Grier, "Health Care Reform Bill 101: Who Must Buy Insurance?"; Grier, "Health Care Reform Bill 101: Who Gets Subsidized Insurance?"; Grier, "Health Care Reform Bill 101: What's a Health 'Exchange'?"; "HealthReform.gov"; "Health Reform Talk."

13. "Uninsured Americans with Pre-existing Conditions Continue to Gain Coverage through Affordable Health Care Act," February 10, 2011, http://www.hhs.gov/news/press/2011pres/02/20110210a.html (accessed February 22, 2011).

14. Meredith B. Rosenthal, Richard G. Frank, Zhonghe Li, and Arnold M. Epstein, "Early Experience with Pay-for-Performance: From Concept to Practice," *The Journal of the American Medical Association* 294, no. 14 (2005): 1788–1793.

## Additional Resources

Anderson, Sandra. *Computer Literacy for Health Care Professionals*. New York: Delmar Publishers Inc., 1992.

Baase, Sara. *A Gift of Fire: Social, Legal, and Ethical Issues in Computing*. Upper Saddle River, NJ: Prentice Hall, 1996.

Ball, Marion J., and Kathryn J. Hannah. *Using Computers in Nursing*. Norwalk, CT: Appelton-Century-Crofts, 1984.

Burke, Lillian, and Barbara Weill. *MediSoft Made Easy: A Step-by-Step Approach*. Upper Saddle River, NJ: Prentice Hall, 2004.

Chen, Pauline W. "Paying Doctors for Patient Performance." September 30, 2010. http://www.nytimes.com/2010/10/01/health/01chen.html (accessed October 1, 2010).

Davis, Daniel C., and William G. Chismar. "Tutorial Medical Informatics." http://www.hicss.hawaii.edu/hicss_32/tutdesc.htm (accessed August 18, 2006).

Felton, Bruce. "Technologies That Enable the Disabled." *The New York Times,* September 14, 1997.

Grier, Peter. "Health Care Reform Bill 101: Who Must Buy Insurance?" March 19, 2010. http://www.csmonitor.com/USA/Politics/2010/0319/Health-care-reform-bill-101-Who-must-buy-insurance (accessed November 11, 2010).

Grier, Peter. "Health Care Reform Bill 101: What's a Health 'Exchange'?" March 20, 2010. http://www.csmonitor.com/USA/Politics/2010/0320/Health-care-reform-bill-101-What-s-a-health-exchange (accessed November 11, 2010).

Grier, Peter. "Health Care Reform Bill 101: Who Gets Subsidized Insurance?" March 20, 2010. http://www.csmonitor.com/

USA/Politics/2010/0320/Health-care-reform-bill-101-Who-gets-subsidized-insurance (accessed November 11, 2010).

"HealthReform.gov." June 2010. http://healthreform.gov/ (accessed November 11, 2010).

"Health Reform Talk." March 29, 2010. http://healthcare-legislation.blogspot.com/ (accessed November 11, 2010).

Holland, Gina. "Court Backs Regulation of HMOs." *The Star-Ledger,* April 3, 2003, 43.

Jackson, Jill, and John Nolan. "Health Care Reform Bill Summary: A Look at What's in the Bill." March 23, 2010. http://www.cbsnews.com/8301-503544_162-20000846-503544.html (accessed November 11, 2010).

Kaiser Commission on Medicaid and the Uninsured. "Medicaid Today." January 25, 2011. http://facts.kff.org/chart.aspx?ch=463 (accessed April 22, 2011).

"MedcomSoft Record 2006 Is Released." 2006. http://home.nestor.minsk.by/computers/news/2006/02/2217.html (accessed April 25, 2011).

*MediSoft Training Manual*. Mesa, AZ: NDC Health.

Newby, Cynthia. *Computers in the Medical Office Using MediSoft*. New York: Glencoe, McGraw-Hill, 1995.

Panangala, Sidath Viranga, and Susan Janeczko. "Health Care for Dependents and Survivors of Veterans." http://congressionalresearch.com/RS22483/document.php?study=Health+Care+for+Dependents+and+Survivors+of+Veterans (accessed April 25, 2011).

"States Leading the Way on Implementation: HHS Awards 'Early Innovator' Grants to Seven States." February 16, 2011.

http://www.hhs.gov/news/press/2011pres/02/20110216a. html (accessed March 10, 2011).

"Understanding TRICARE." 2011. http://www.military.com/ benefits/tricare (accessed April 25, 2011).

"Uninsured Americans with Pre-existing Conditions Continue to Gain Coverage through Affordable Health Care Act." February 10, 2011. http://www.hhs.gov/news/press/2011pres/ 02/20110210a.html (accessed February 22, 2011).

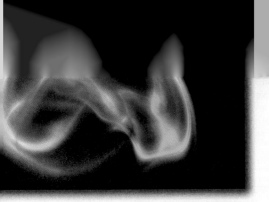

# Telemedicine

## CHAPTER OUTLINE

## LEARNING OBJECTIVES

Upon completion of this chapter, the reader will be able to:

- Define telemedicine.
- Discuss store-and-forward technology and interactive videoconferencing.
- Define the various subspecialties of teleradiology, telepathology, teledermatology, telecardiology, teleneurology, telestroke, telepsychiatry, telewound care, telehome care, and the use of smartphones and tablet computers as mobile computing devices.
- Discuss the use of telemedicine in prisons.
- Discuss the changing role of the telenurse.
- Discuss the legal, licensing, insurance, and privacy issues involved in telemedicine.

## OVERVIEW

**Telemedicine** uses computers and telecommunications equipment to deliver medical care at a distance. It should be noted at the outset, however, that because the telecommunications equipment (hardware and software), the knowledge and training, and the financial resources are not evenly distributed within the nation or throughout the world, telemedicine is not universally available.

Some doctors do not use computers. Various computer systems that are in use are not compatible or interoperable (cannot communicate with each other). Where telemedicine is in place, it is used in various medical specialties.

Several technologies are used in telemedicine: from plain old telephone service, to high-speed dedicated lines, to the Internet. The medical information transmitted can be in any form, including voice, data, still images, and video. Telemedicine delivers the whole range of medical care from diagnosis to patient monitoring to treatment. It gives patients remote access to experts who in turn have access to patient information. Today, some doctors have stopped using transcriptionists to type their notes; instead, they send their dictation over the Internet. Some dictation is sent overseas. The transcription is returned by e-mail or downloaded from a Website as word-processed documents. The linking of computers and other devices into networks forms the foundation for telemedicine.

The field of telemedicine is growing but has not yet been adopted as widely as it could,

according to a report by the California HealthCare Foundation published in February of 2011. In 2003, the American Telemedicine Association (ATA) estimated that about 200 networks connecting 2,000 health care facilities were linked via telecommunications lines.[1] The production of telehome care products grew more quickly in the 1990s than that of any other medical device. There is no comprehensive current study of the extent of telemedicine in the United States. However, a study of its use in California concluded that 37 percent of health clinics and one-third of hospitals were using videoconferencing. By 2006, the U.S. Department of Veterans Affairs (VA) had spent $20 million to install some 15,000 home health monitors; it expected to have 50,000 in place by 2009. By 2010, there were about 200 telehealth networks in place in the United States. They linked more than 2,500 institutions. The Veterans Health Administration has 50 health management programs in 18 integrated networks (2011). It has found that remote monitoring reduces the number of bed days by 25 percent and the number of admissions by 20 percent.[2] The VA has found the systems cut patient care costs by about one-third.[3] The positive outcomes found by the VA have not been found in several other studies of telemedicine. (See later section, Is Telemedicine Effective?)

Telemedicine encompasses many subspecialties of medicine including radiology, pathology, oncology, ophthalmology, cardiology, neurology (including stroke), dermatology, and psychiatry. It may involve the sending of still images or real-time conferences, the use of **remote monitoring devices**, and the remote operation of medical equipment such as microscopes. Varieties of telemedicine are now being used to treat everything from psychiatric disorders (telepsychiatry) to skin rashes (teledermatology) to cancer (teleoncology). Remote surgery is in an early phase and will be discussed in Chapter 7. The field of telemedicine is changing and developing. One of the reasons that telemedicine continues to expand is the growth of the prison population; telemedicine is increasingly used in prisons. Telemedicine has the potential of making high-quality medical care available to anyone in an urban or rural area regardless of distance from major medical centers, specialists, physicians, and visiting nurses. It can dramatically decrease the time a patient must wait and the miles the patient must travel to consult a specialist. Telemedicine transfers medical expertise instead of medical experts and patients. Many studies have found that patient satisfaction with telemedicine is high. Because there is less travel involved, telemedicine has the potential of making health care more environmentally friendly.[4]

Medical consultations and exams at a distance have been attempted from the time that people were able to talk to each other from a distance. Early endeavors were made to send heart and lung sounds to experts over the newly invented telephone. However, this failed because of poor transmission. Later, doctors tried to transmit electrocardiograms (ECGs) through the telephone. After World War II, pictures could be transmitted. However, it was only with the development of computers and telecommunications networks capable of transmitting high-resolution digital images and accurate sound that telemedicine could become a practical medical reality.

The field is expanding so quickly that it is only possible to touch on major uses of telemedicine here. This chapter introduces the student to basic definitions in the field and presents examples of some of the more interesting uses of distance medicine. It also discusses some of the technical, legal, privacy, and insurance issues that need to be addressed in order for telemedicine to fulfill its promise.

## STORE-AND-FORWARD TECHNOLOGY AND INTERACTIVE VIDEOCONFERENCING

Telemedicine projects may be based on store-and-forward technology or interactive videoconferencing. Some projects use both. **Store-and-forward technology** involves sharing information in a time- and place-independent way over the Internet. The information is stored, digitized, and then sent. If a medical specialty is image based, store-and-forward technology may be appropriate. The information may include digital images and clinical information. It may be as simple and inexpensive as attaching an image to an e-mail and sending it over telephone lines. Store-and-forward technology does not require the sophisticated telecommunications links required by videoconferencing, so it tends to be cheaper. The earliest use of store-and-forward technology was in teleradiology.

Store-and-forward technology is appropriate to specialties where diagnosis is based on images, such as dermatology and pathology. Images can be created by digital camera and sent over the Internet. This technique is used, for example, in some teleophthalmology programs; others use videoconferencing. Because store-and-forward technology is cheaper and does not require sophisticated equipment or broadband lines, it is being used simply to introduce telemedicine at low cost to developing countries in specialties that had traditionally used videoconferencing. For example, a small teleneurology program using store-and-forward technology was created between the United Kingdom and Bangladesh. The program was used with 12 patients to deliver expert advice; it was found to be effective.

**Interactive videoconferencing** or **teleconferencing** allows doctors to consult with each other and with patients in real time, at a distance. (Figure 4.1, A and B▶) A patient may be in his or her primary

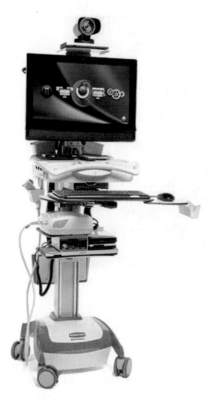

▶ **Figure 4.1** (A) MEDI PORT

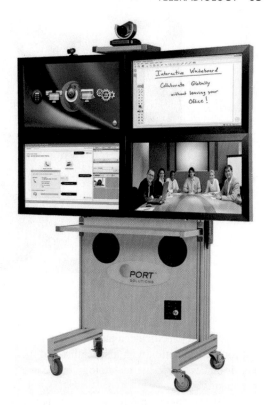

▶ **Figure 4.1** (B) QUADPORT are "mobile computing platforms enabled with high definition video conferencing capability . . . . The device allows remote medical specialists to interact with patients and provide expert counsel, which is especially important for rural clinics and field hospitals with limited medical staff. Live surgeries can be shared remotely for purposes of mentoring and better clinical outcomes are enabled via bedside access to patient data and web-based resources."
*Source:* Courtesy of C-PORT Solutions.

physician's office with a camera and a telecommunications link to a specialist's office. All can see and hear each other in real time (Figure 4.2 ▶). Teleconferencing might require only a videophone and a connection to the Internet. However, the most sophisticated systems involve microphones, scanners, cameras, medical instruments, and dedicated telephone lines. One form of video teleconferencing is the remote house call, involving only one medical practitioner and a patient in another location.

## TELERADIOLOGY

The oldest form of telemedicine using computers and telecommunications equipment is teleradiology. Today, **teleradiology** involves the sending of radiological images in digital form over telecommunications lines. Teleradiology uses store-and-forward technology; the data to be sent are digitized, stored, and transmitted over a telecommunications network. If the image is

compressed for storage and transmission, and if, as a result, any data are lost, the consultant is responsible for determining whether the image is useful. The images can be sent any distance—from across the street to across the world. Store-and-forward teleradiology can be combined with interactive videoconferencing for immediate consultation when a problem is detected in pregnancy. The specialist sees the patient and ultrasound on a split screen and controls the exam from miles

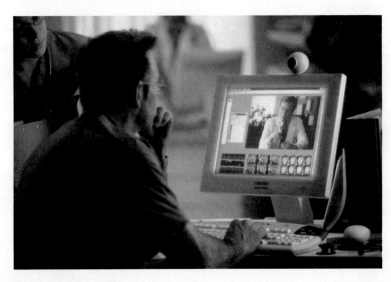

▶ **Figure 4.2** A telemedical consultation.
*Source:* Corbis Bridge/Alamy.

away. Before telemedicine, a patient might have to wait for a consultation with a specialist and travel long distances. Now, the technology can come to the patient.

In 2010, patients in remote rural areas where optimal colonoscopy is of limited availability could be screened for colon cancer via virtual colonoscopy or **computed tomography colonography (CTC)** and teleradiology. Three hundred twenty-one virtual colonoscopies were sent to the University of Arizona Hospital. The reports were returned via teleradiology. Ninety-two percent were diagnostic quality images.[5]

Today, many radiological images are telecommunicated to India for interpretation, especially at night. The turnaround time can be as little as 30 minutes. However, there are limits because of licensure issues. "Only those doctors who have relocated from [the] U.S. can do offshoring to America." In other words, a doctor has to be licensed in both the United States and India.[6]

## TELEPATHOLOGY

**Telepathology** is the transmission of microscopic images over telecommunications lines. The pathologist sees images on a monitor instead of under a microscope. Telepathology

requires a microscope, camera, and monitor, as well as a connection to a telemedicine system. Telepathology can use real-time videoconferencing for consultation during an operation. But in daily practice, store-and-forward technology is common. Pathology is based on the study of images; diagnosis is based on the study of images on slides from a microscope looking for diagnostic features. If a second opinion is needed from a distant expert, telepathology may be used. The images are taken from the slides by camera. Still images usually are at a higher resolution than those sent in real time. The images and other clinical data are used for a complete case description and then sent, in many cases, over the Internet. One of the problems of store-and-forward telepathology is the choice of images sent. They may not show a complete picture, and this may lead to misdiagnosis. In Europe, researchers are attempting to organize and consolidate information in order to create an international Web search engine for a telepathology network by November 2011.[7]

## TELEDERMATOLOGY

**Teledermatology** (the practice of dermatology using telecommunications networks) is also based partly on the study of images. It uses both videoconferencing and store-and-forward technology. Both methods appear effective. The advantage of videoconferencing is that it closely resembles the traditional visit to the doctor; however, it is more expensive. Studies have shown that diagnoses made via videoconferencing agree with diagnoses made at face-to-face dermatology visits in 59 to 88 percent of cases. A small study comparing store-and-forward teledermatology with face-to-face dermatology found 61 to 91 percent agreement. Certain skin conditions were found to be more difficult to diagnose via teledermatology. Diagnostic confidence was lower, and the rate of biopsies was higher. The advantages of store-and-forward technology are the high quality of the images and the low cost. To date, there have been no definitive outcomes studies. Some small studies have found that although there are limitations with store-and-forward technology (image quality and lack of patient interaction), teledermatology reduced unnecessary visits to dermatologists by more than 50 percent. In 2005, the "consensus on the diagnostic accuracy and clinical effectiveness of Store and Forward teledermatology appears to be growing, [however] outcome studies are needed to measure cost effectiveness and patient outcomes."[8] In a letter urging Medicare to cover teledermatology services, in March 2011, the American Academy of Dermatology and the American Telemedicine Association (ATA) stated that, "With comprehensive patient information and clear images, the dermatologist can often make a diagnosis and advise the local doctor how to care for the patient . . . ." The letter also states that teledermatology cuts costs and gives patients better access to care. It refers to the "proven quality of store-and-forward technology."[9]

## TELECARDIOLOGY

Prior to the 1800s, a doctor would listen to the heart by placing his ear on the patient's chest. Listening to the heart at a distance has a long history. Since the time of Hippocrates, physicians listened directly to patients' chests as they tried to assess cardiac health. The inventor of the stethoscope, Rene Theophile-Hyacinthe Laennec, relied on this method, too.

> One day, [in 1816] when he needed to examine an obese young woman, Laennec hesitated to put his head to her chest. Remembering that you can hear a pin scraping one end of a plank by putting your ear to the other end, he came up with the idea for a stethoscope prototype. He rolled a stack of paper into a cylinder, pressed one end to the patient's chest, and held his ear to the other end.[10]

Since the invention of the telephone, doctors have attempted to send heart and lung sounds over long distances. But the quality of the sound was not good enough. During the 1960s, it became possible to transmit heart sounds more accurately, and faxes could be used to send ECGs. By the 1990s, echocardiograms could be telecommunicated. Second opinions via telecardiology are one of the most common requests in telemedicine. Telecardiology lets a remote specialist interpret electrocardiograms (ECGs) via a telephone connection.[11] People come into rural emergency rooms (ERs) with chest pains, and many ER doctors want an expert consultation. Telemedicine is becoming more and more widely used in cardiology. One study evaluated five programs in North America: two used store-and-forward technology, and three used real-time videoconferencing. The study concluded that both real-time and store-and-forward tele-echocardiography were effective; both transmit diagnostic quality information.

Other telecommunications technology contributes to cardiac care. The Department of Veterans Affairs (VA) will be able to use an Internet-based service that connects patients wearing pacemakers with their doctors. Patients can use a monitoring device to collect information from the pacemaker by holding an antenna over it. The data are sent by telephone to the CareLink Network. Doctors then have access to it. This system will work anywhere in the United States. Another technology that can be used to connect digital devices is **Bluetooth**. Bluetooth technology can link devices such as a pacemaker and a cell phone.

In 2006, in Japan, a group of scientists began using a mobile phone–based heart monitor. "When a heart discomfort is felt, the patient pushes the data transmission switch."[12] The ECG is sent to a server at the hospital, which sends it to a doctor. This system can be used to monitor hospitalized patients and patients at home.

In 2009, a study in Italy found that telemedicine could correctly diagnose heart attacks in elderly people at home. Patients called an emergency number and were evaluated via ECGs in their homes. Phones transmitted the data to telecardiologists. The use of telecardiology both improved diagnosis and delivered treatment more quickly.[13]

In 2010, a major area of growth for telecardiology was in the diagnosis of infant congenital heart disease. Thirty percent of infant mortality in the United States is caused by congenital heart disease. Although time is essential in its diagnosis and treatment, most hospitals lack specialists. Children's Memorial Hospital in Chicago has operated a pediatric cardiology system since 1993. It now treats 1,200 to 1,500 cases per year telemedically. Children's Memorial Hospital uses a video conferencing system to consult with the hospital calling in and can see and hear the technologist and the sonogram. The specialist can direct the exam.[14]

## TELENEUROLOGY

Neurology was slower to use telemedicine when compared to other specialties. Now, however, e-mail and videoconferencing are replacing the letter and telephone call. One of the first subspecialties to use telemedicine in neurology is stroke diagnosis.[15]

### Telestroke

One of the recognized benefits of telemedicine is saving time. Time is essential in treating strokes. So is expertise. There are almost three-quarters of a million new strokes per year in the United States. According to the American Stroke Association, in 2009, "only two to three percent [of stroke patients are] treated by a specialist."[16] In 2009, in the United States, there was one neurologist per 18,000 people.[17] Telemedicine can provide stroke specialists remotely. If the stroke is caused by a clot (determined by a computed tomography [CT] scan), the victim may be helped by the administration of a clot-busting drug called tissue plasminogen activator (tPA) if it is given within a few hours. However, if the stroke is caused by excessive bleeding, tPA can kill the patient. Immediate and accurate diagnosis is crucial. However, many small hospitals do not have experts. One study showed that 70 percent of stroke patients did not receive tPA either because they arrived at the hospital too late or because the hospitals could not provide the correct therapy.

Massachusetts General Hospital began a **telestroke** program. Many people die of strokes just because they are taken to small hospitals without the capability of evaluating the stroke quickly. The telestroke program connects small local hospitals with Massachusetts General's stroke experts. When a stroke victim appeared at the local hospital in Martha's Vineyard, the doctors would do CT scans and forward them to stroke specialists at Massachusetts General. Both the local doctors and the specialists would evaluate the tests and interview the patient via a teleconferencing system to determine whether tPA was needed. Other hospitals are currently using this technology.

By 2005, Massachusetts passed a law requiring "emergency medical technicians to bring patients exhibiting signs of a stroke to a hospital *that has a neurologist on staff 24 hours a day, bypassing nearby hospitals that might not meet the requirement*" (emphasis added). Telemedicine programs that allow neurologists to consult with the patient and doctor at the remote site via dedicated lines may be used to meet this requirement.[18] By 2006, telestroke in Massachusetts had further expanded. Hospitals in New Jersey, California, Georgia, and Utah also have telestroke programs, and Vermont and New Hampshire are considering instituting such programs.[19] In 2007, in Georgia, using Remote Evaluation of Acute Ischemic Stroke (REACH), tPA was used for about 20 percent of stroke cases.[20] The federal Stop Stroke Act, which was introduced in Congress in 2001 and again in 2005, has not yet become law. It would provide funding to build telestroke systems. Telestroke has been found effective in reducing the time to administer tPA and in improving outcomes.[21]

A 2010 survey of hospitals and healthcare providers in the Northwest United States found that 88 percent thought they had a shortage of stroke neurologists. Sixty-four percent are currently in the process of developing or considering the development of telestroke programs. They exhibited a great deal of interest in regional cooperation.[22] In January 2011, Central Maine Health Care and Massachusetts General Hospital announced a partnership that will begin in spring 2011 for a telestroke program. Patients in central Maine will be able to have their strokes diagnosed by a Massachusetts General neurologist without leaving the Lewiston, Maine ER. This will allow quicker diagnosis, so that tPA may be administered when needed. The two hospitals are cooperating on a second program to diagnose and treat other neurological disorders like seizures.[23] In 2011, the U.S. Department of Agriculture (USDA) awarded a telehealth grant to a hospital in Oklahoma to institute a telestroke program.[24]

NeuroCall, Inc., provides emergency neurological telemedical services worldwide. In Texas, by February 8, 2011, it had performed 400 telemedical consults in 11 months. Twenty percent of its cases are strokes; of 107 strokes treated, tPA was administered in 27 percent of the cases. There is a shortage of neurologists in Texas, and teleneurologists sometimes diagnose patients from a distance of 2,000 miles. The service is available 24 hours a day at local hospitals via video monitor. It has lowered the transfer rate for stroke patients and enabled them to be treated in a timely manner, which is crucial.[25]

Telemedicine was also found to be effective in a stroke rehabilitation program. It improved both balance and functioning. Using an e-mail triage system for new referrals halved the number of people attending clinics.[26]

## Epilepsy

**Teleneurology** uses e-mail and videoconferencing for real-time meetings. The patient is with a nurse at one location; the neurologist is at a distant location. Using videoconferencing, the neurologist can take a history and direct and see the physical examination of the patient. The neurologist can also diagnose the patient and create a treatment plan.[27]

A recent study found no difference in the frequency of seizures, hospitalizations, or ER visits between patients getting traditional face-to-face care and patients visited via video. A comparison of new patients seen via video "had similar investigation and review rates to patients seen face-to-face."[28] In 2005, a study found that outcomes were the same for patients treated by telemedicine accompanied by a nurse as for those treated in person by a physician. In 2008, the authors of the study planned to use telemedicine to treat 800 people with epilepsy at eight telemedicine sites.[29]

Teleneurology helps to cope with some common problems of people with epilepsy. Many patients with epilepsy live in areas with no or little access to neurologists. Restrictions on driving for people with epilepsy can limit care. Thus, teleneurology, which brings the care to the patient, is crucial. A study[30] was completed of a system where a distant neurologist managed epileptic patients at a local rural hospital. Each patient was accompanied by a nurse case manager who managed medication and compliance and reinforced the neurologist's advice. When this group was compared to a traditionally managed group, it was found that "telemedicine provided an acceptable alternative."

A 2010 survey of Canadian doctors found that "although 61.5% of the physicians acknowledged need for tele-epilepsy services, the majority (64.1%) had not used telemedicine." The study found that telemedicine was available to almost 80 percent of the doctors and that more than 60 percent recognized a need for telemedicine in treating epilepsy, but that most of them did not use it.[31]

## Parkinson's Disease

Recent studies and pilot programs (2009–2011) have shown that telemedicine can be useful in the evaluation, monitoring, and treatment of patients with **Parkinson's disease**. Parkinson's disease involves damage to brain cells that hampers brain communication having to do with balance, movement, walking, and speech. Telemedicine evaluations of patients' motor skills were equivalent to in-person evaluations according to a small but randomized study. Some of the patients lived in a nursing home in Rochester, New York, and some lived in the community. They were randomly divided into two groups. One group received traditional care, and the other received telemedicine visits. The patients were also asked about "their PD [Parkinson's disease] medications, function, and complications of therapy." According to the designers of the study, "Patients in the study with Parkinson's disease (PD) who received telemedicine care over the course of 6 months showed improvements in quality of life, mood, satisfaction with care, cognition, and motor function, compared with those who received standard care." Patients at the nursing home who were treated telemedically were more highly satisfied with their care. They liked the convenience. However, some community-based patients "had mixed feelings about completing . . . visits at home without medical and technical support staff."[32]

The telemedicine visits in the nursing home were conducted in a room with a flat-screen television on which the patients could see their doctors. A nurse accompanied the patient. The neurologist was at a remote site at the University of Rochester Medical Center. The researchers plan to use telemedicine at other sites and evaluate the programs in clinical trials. The number of nursing homes using telemedicine for Parkinson's disease continues to expand in 2011.[33]

### E-mail and Digital Cameras in Teleneurology

Low-cost teleneurology programs can make use of e-mail for referral. In one study, two groups were compared, one referred by e-mail and one referred in the traditional way. The study concluded that "teleneurology by e-mail is sustainable . . . and . . . that it is safe, effective and efficient."[34]

Digital cameras that can produce high-quality video clips were successfully used to study gait. The video clips were sent to neurologists via e-mail. It was concluded that "[a]dequate-quality video clips

of movement disorders can be produced with low-cost cameras and transmitted by e-mail for teleneurology purposes."[35]

## TELEPSYCHIATRY

**Telepsychiatry** involves the delivery of therapy using teleconferencing. It usually makes use of some sort of hardware that can transmit and receive both voice and picture. However, to cut costs, psychiatrists are trying to find out if a poor image—or no image at all—makes therapy less effective. Experts warn that therapy at a distance is not a substitute for the human contact involved in face-to-face counseling. However, sometimes it is the only choice, for example, in rural areas where there are very few therapists and patients would have to travel long distances to see them.

During the 1960s, the first telepsychiatry sessions were conducted at the Nebraska Psychiatric Institute. Researchers found that the fact that the therapist was not physically present had little effect on group therapy. Studies of psychiatric consults between primary care providers and psychiatrists in New Hampshire came to the same conclusion—that videoconferencing and face-to-face consults were similar. A study of telemedicine for diagnosing patients with obsessive-compulsive disorder found it as successful as face-to-face therapy. A small study compared videoconferencing and face-to-face cognitive behavioral therapy in treating childhood depression and found them equally effective.[36]

Some studies have found that patients are more comfortable talking to a distant psychiatrist. Others have found that using a telenurse and a traditional psychiatrist improved depression more than using only a psychiatrist, although there was no improvement in the numbers of clients taking their medication properly. Telepsychiatry was also found to be successful in delivering therapy to the family of a girl suffering from anorexia. It contributed to her recovery. The family was satisfied with the teletherapy.[37] In Australia, telepsychiatry is being used to treat panic disorders with cognitive behavioral therapy. So far, the project is "as effective as . . . therapy."[38]

However, there are some negative aspects to telepsychiatry: The technology limits the therapist's perception of nonverbal clues, and the equipment can be distracting; the therapist has to be sensitive to distortions in eye contact and the fact that a patient can appear to have stopped speaking when in fact he or she has not. That is, eye contact must be maintained with the camera, not the monitor, and the patient's mouth may stop moving before the patient has stopped speaking.

One 18-month study of telepsychiatry in a prison setting found that patients were comfortable with the technology, but that many of the therapist's recommendations were not followed by prison personnel. This was a unique situation: The psychiatrist did not have some of the clients' medical records, and so some recommendations (that a woman in a wheelchair ride a bike) could not be carried out. Other recommendations were not carried out either because the doctor had little knowledge of prison rules and routines or because the doctor had no relationship with prison personnel. The psychiatrist had never been to the prison, and the medical records (which were paper records) had to stay at the prison. This points out some of the limitations of telepsychiatry—the clues that would be easily available in person are not obvious via telecommunications lines.[39]

The University of Vermont and its rural health centers are instituting a pilot family-based approach using telemedicine to treat children with psychiatric problems. According to the health centers, the program has been "extremely helpful . . . and without this pilot children and families would have had a very difficult time getting services." A second Vermont project is using Web cameras in psychiatric consults.[40]

A pilot program at Weill Cornell Medical College and Rhode Island Hospital used telemedicine to treat elderly depressed homebound patients. The patients liked it and felt it improved their care. Before the program, 19 patients suffered from major depression; in a follow-up after the study, the mean depression score was mild.[41]

Telepsychiatry is the fastest growing specialty in psychiatry. In states and areas where there are shortages of mental health workers, such as Texas

and rural Illinois, telepsychiatry is filling the gap. In Texas, telepsychiatry is used in prisons and serves school districts and women's shelters. It is also used to conduct emergency evaluations. In rural Illinois, a local hospital provides video visits from psychiatrists, including pediatric psychiatrists. Patients like the care, and fewer are seeking mental health care from their primary providers. In 1 year, 45 adults and 40 children and adolescents received telepsychiatric visits. Ninety-five percent were partially covered by Medicaid.[42]

There are questions of whether telepsychiatry is appropriate for some forms of serious mental illness. For example, can it make schizophrenia worse by reinforcing the delusion that the television is talking to the patient?

## REMOTE MONITORING DEVICES

Spending on chronic diseases, such as chronic heart failure, chronic obstructive pulmonary disease (COPD), and diabetes, adds up to about $1.7 trillion annually in the United States. This comprises 75 percent of our annual health care costs. Remote monitoring can help patients manage these chronic conditions.[43] Remote monitoring devices deal with prevention, chronic disease management, acute care and rehabilitation, and aging at home. Prevention is concerned with weight, tobacco use, and exercise. Many of these conditions are monitored by applications on smartphones (see later section, Smartphones and Tablet Computers). Chronic disease management is concerned with diabetes, hypertension, COPD, and medication compliance. Telemedicine devices allow patients to monitor themselves and "adjust lifestyle behaviors." Some studies show that home care can be as effective as hospital care for illness; good telemedical home care will, it is hoped, reduce hospital readmissions, which is one goal of the Patient Protection and Affordable Care Act. In rehabilitation, "treadmills . . . with Wi-Fi enabled sensors can transmit exercise and physiological signals" allowing physical therapists to monitor a patient's progress telemedically.[44]

Remote monitoring devices used in the home include scales, devices that measure blood sugar, implantable cardioverter defibrillators, blood pressure monitors, devices that measure blood oxygen levels, devices that measure clotting time, thermometers, electrocardiographs, stethoscopes, spirometers for patients with asthma, and pedometers. These devices gather data and communicate them to a remote computer. Some of the data can be directly downloaded into electronic health records (Figure 4.3►). Some devices give the patient a reminder. Certain home monitoring devices that used to be big and expensive can now be replaced by smartphones.[45]

Remote monitoring devices are also used in ambulances. The condition of the patient can be directly transmitted to the ER so that care can begin immediately on arrival. In September 1998, a "smart stretcher" was introduced. Weighing 135 pounds, but only 5 inches high, the stretcher includes a respirator, heart machine, intravenous drugs, and monitors that transmit all the data they gather immediately to the hospital. Using the smart stretcher means that no time needs to be wasted transporting the patient. Monitoring and treatment can begin immediately. The Defense Advanced Research Projects Agency of the U.S. Department of Defense has created a smart t-shirt, which

can monitor vital signs at a distance. Distance monitoring of blood glucose levels has improved outcomes in diabetes patients. In 2002, the U.S. Food and Drug Administration (FDA) approved an implantable cardiac device that enables a doctor to evaluate a patient over the Internet. Not all distance monitoring is successful, however. Distance monitoring of high-risk pregnancies has been a failure.[46]

Several devices are in development to monitor the blood glucose levels of people with diabetes without finger pricks. At the University of Florida, researchers developed a sensor that amplifies glucose signals in breath moisture to measure glucose levels. Other researchers use nanotechnology for the same purpose. The same technology could possibly predict asthma attacks and detect some forms of breast cancer. At the Massachusetts Institute of Technology, researchers are in the very early stages of developing a "tattoo" to detect blood glucose levels. The tattoo is created by "saline-based ink particles [injected under the skin] that release different wavelengths of light in response to different concentrations of blood glucose." A watch-like device that patients would wear over the tattoo would interpret the data. Although there are skin-based devices for monitoring blood

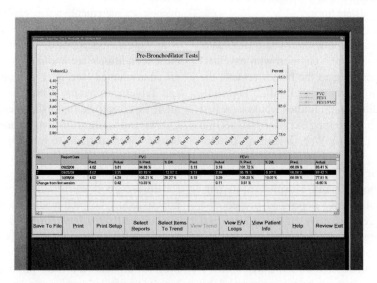

► **Figure 4.3**    Data from a digital spirometer can be directly transferred to the electronic health record.
*Source:* Courtesy of Midmark Diagnostics Group.

glucose, these last only 7 days, whereas the new tattoo would last 6 months. An implantable nano-sensor that "changes color in response to glucose levels" is under development; its nanoparticles draw blood glucose. A small handheld device is used to shine a light on the particle and interpret the results.[47]

Many of the newest, still experimental, monitoring devices use sensors embedded in fabric. The Wearable Health Care System (WEALTHY) has completed several years of research. These wearable systems are comfortable. Sensors, electrodes, and advanced signal-processing techniques are embedded in the yarn. One wearable system monitors blood oxygen during sleep. One detects sleep apnea. Another measures ECG. Other wearable systems can measure respiration and temperature.[48]

It is difficult to get the information that helps doctors adjust heart medication as needed. A remote monitoring device was in the testing stage in 2010. It is "an implantable, permanent monitor with communications technologies that measures and transmits daily pulmonary artery levels, a key indicator of heart health." In one trial on patients with Class III heart failure, it reduced the rate of hospitalization 30 percent after 6 months and 38 percent per year.[49]

It is not easy to judge the effectiveness of remote monitoring. Although many studies have been done, the results have been mixed. Proponents state that telemedicine could save money by reducing readmissions to hospitals, avoiding doctor visits, and improving both medication compliance and communications between doctors and patients. They even predict $200 billion cost savings over 25 years. However, other studies find no support in the data for either the savings or the health improvements predicted. The greatest cost savings, proponents say, will be in the reduction of the 18 percent of patients who are readmitted to hospitals within 30 days of discharge. They believe that 75 percent of these readmissions are preventable with follow-up care. According to the Centers for Medicare and Medicaid Services (CMS), half of these patients had no follow-up care. One group of studies states that Medicare could save $12 billion with telemedical follow-up care. Other studies disagree. As of 2011, there is no

"definitive evidence for the usefulness of remote monitoring."[50] (See later section, Is Telemedicine Effective?, for an extensive discussion of studies.)

## TELEWOUND CARE

**Telewound care** is relatively new; only a few programs are currently in existence in 2011. Telemedicine has been successful in treating other chronic conditions. Telewound care can benefit from the use of both store-and-forward and videoconferencing technology. Teleconferencing is appropriate for home care. Store-and-forward technology would be helpful in treating postoperative patients and in follow-up care. The care provided would be less expensive and should improve outcomes.[51] Assessment of the wound may not have to wait for a hospital appointment; access to specialists via telemedicine may be quicker. According to Wound Care Solutions Telemedicine (a company providing telemedical wound care) in the United Kingdom, it "has been demonstrated that telemedicine can have a positive outcome when used in a home care setting . . . . [T]elemedicine has demonstrated that healing rates have increased and the number of home visits and hospitalization due to wound complications has decreased."[52]

Elderly, frail patients and patients in poor health are more likely than others to suffer from problematic wounds. Telewound care can increase access to specialists not only in rural areas, but also in cities. It has the potential of reducing travel time and making an assessment of the wound more quickly. In treating problematic wounds "prompt access to specialists when needed [is] crucial to improve outcomes."[53]

Chronic wound care requires constant assessment and, therefore, frequent visits to the doctor. In rural areas, the distance can be a burden on the patient. Together with the lack of availability of wound care specialists, this can make telemedicine appropriate. Medicare reimburses live videoconferencing at certain sites. Doctors in federally designated Physician Shortage Areas who use telemedicine earn a 5 percent bonus. However, the undated 2011 CMS fee schedule "requires that debridement services be billed by area surface, and not the number of wounds."[54] Founded in 2000, the Wound Care Network treats chronic wounds. Nurses visit the patient and telecommunicate with wound care experts at a telehealth center.[55]

## TELEHOME CARE

A recent survey showed that 83 percent of Americans agree with the statement, "What I'd really like to do is stay in my current residence for as long as possible." The most widely used telehome care product is the personal emergency response system like the one that responds to "I've fallen and I can't get up."[56] However, there are many other devices. **Telehome care** involves the monitoring of vital signs from a distance via telecommunications equipment and the replacement of home nursing visits with videoconferences. It is usually used to manage chronic conditions such as congestive heart failure and diabetes, but it should be noted that it is beginning to be used for remote monitoring by intensive care unit (ICU) doctors at home. The cost of medical care for chronic conditions represents about 75 percent of medical costs in the United States, and some believe that home monitoring can lower these costs. Some large hospitals have received grants from the Centers for Medicare and Medicaid Services (CMS) to expand telehome care. Some of this money will be used for demonstration projects and randomized trials. The increasing aging population and the shortage of doctors increase the need for telehome care. (Sixty million people in the United States had no access to a primary care provider in 2010.) Forty-five percent of the population suffers from chronic conditions, and telemedicine has been effective in treating them, notably COPD and diabetes. According to a study published in *The Wall Street Journal* in 2008, the annual cost saving of using telemedicine to treat congestive heart failure was $10.1 billion; treating diabetes saves $6.1 billion; and treating COPD saves $4.9 billion.[57]

The American Telemedicine Association (ATA) conducted a survey that showed "that commercial reimbursement of 'telemed' services other than teleradiology is more widespread than even many industry participants had thought."[58] Many payers cover telemedicine, but payments for e-visits remain in their infancy.

Telehome care involves a link between the patient's home and a hospital or central office that collects the data. Equipment in the patient's home links the home or nursing home via telecommunications lines with a central office. The units differ from one another, but generally allow the patient and nurse to see and hear each other and allow the patient to push a button on the monitor, enabling the nurse to hear heart, lung, and bowel sounds; another button allows the nurse to monitor blood pressure. The machines also assess blood oxygen level and pulse rate. Many units give voice reminders to take medication and ask the patient questions. An early example is HANC (home-assisted nursing care), which yells more and more loudly until the patient responds. The most sophisticated units show a doctor on the screen to check the patient's vital signs. The patient is able to aim a camera at an injury so that the doctor can advise how to dress and care for it. Some of the programs include extensive education about home management of chronic illness and even provide a tele–social worker for end-of-life planning. HANC and other big bulky machines are being replaced by small, smart devices such as the smartphone.

In 2010, approximately 31,000 people used VA telehome care. The VA's proposed 2012 budget would let 50,000 people per day use telehome care.[59] There have not been any large-scale randomized studies of telehome care. Pilot studies have indicated that telehome care does increase access to health care in rural areas and that it may decrease unnecessary hospital and ER visits. It allows a nurse to make many more visits in a day—15 to 20 instead of five to six. A small study from the United States and United Kingdom concluded that 45 percent of U.S. home visits could be remote.

Many small studies have found that both nurses and patients like the video visits, and one study found that telehospice care was quite cost effective. A study in Italy found that home telemonitoring for patients with severe respiratory illness decreased hospital admissions; patients were satisfied. The study concluded that telemonitoring can provide high-quality home care.[60] Another small study found telemedicine effective in reducing hospital admissions for patients with congestive heart failure; patients had their vital signs and general appearance telemonitored, while maintaining regular video contact with health care professionals who offered advice on drug use and diet. In California, a study compared the use of face-to-face therapy with videoconferencing in control and intervention groups. No differences in medication compliance, knowledge of disease, and ability for self-care were found. Patients were satisfied with the videoconferencing. Further, it costs less to treat patients via teleconferencing than face-to-face therapy.[61] A study of congestive heart failure patients in Knoxville, Tennessee, found that "in comparison to a national 30-day readmission rate of 23 percent for CHF complications, only 14 percent of CHF program participants were hospitalized during the program's first six months. Further, their length of hospital stay was reduced from the national benchmark 6.2 days to four days, and their hospitalization rate for CHF was reduced from 1.7 to 0.6 per patient per year."[62] A pilot study of another home monitoring system (E-Care) used to manage patients with chronic illness by keeping track of activity, temperature, pulse, blood pressure, and glucose using sensors was done in 2003–2004. The system also includes medication reminders and checks current data against the patient's record. "Users praised its practicability, reliability, effectiveness and patient acceptance."[63] Several factors retard the adoption of telehome care, including the attitudes of home health agencies, the initial cost of the equipment, reimbursement rates, and the fact that there are few studies demonstrating that it is cost effective.

In 2006, the Visiting Nurse Service of Western New York found that using home monitoring devices reduced rehospitalizations. The national rate of rehospitalization for patients with chronic illnesses is 26 percent; in western New York, it dropped by 50 percent to 13 percent.[64] In 2010, a year-long study was begun by Intel, GE, and the Mayo Clinic to see whether remote monitoring of patients in their homes could keep them out of ERs. Although they estimate that telemedical technology could save as much as $700 billion over 10 to 15 years, they also point to obstacles such as doctors' reluctance to use the technology, Medicare reimbursement (or lack thereof), and a broadband network that is not good enough.[65]

NowClinic by OptimumHealth, a part of United Health Group, connects patients and doctors via video chat. The service will be introduced state by state. Today, in Texas, anyone can visit a doctor for $45 for 10 minutes using NowClinic. This is facing legal problems in states that require an actual physical visit to a doctor before a doctor–patient relationship is established. Other private companies are also introducing telemedical services. GoogleHealth and MDLiveCare are going to provide access to doctors and therapists via video phone and e-mail 24 hours a day, 7 days a week, 365 days a year.[66]

In Warren County, New York, small (alarm clock–sized) home monitors greet 31 patients with "Good morning. It is now time to record your vital signs." The device monitors the patients and transmits its findings via the telephone line. Among these 31 patients, hospital visits have dropped by over 70 percent.[67] Other pilot programs found that telehome care reduces travel time, improves patient outcomes, and decreases hospitalizations and ER visits. An experimental program is being used to help veterans with spinal cord injuries.[68]

Automated robots, some with your doctor's face on the monitor, are starting to make house calls. A 5-foot tall robot named RP-7 can perform remote checkups. "From more than 100 miles away, [the doctor] can carry on a face-to-face video conversation with his [or her] patient and control a high-definition camera. He [or she] can also drive the robot around the facility." The robots can help with checkups and help care for elderly patients in their homes. One manufacturer even suggests that they could be used to visit the homebound elderly sometime in the future. This could remove that onerous burden from middle-aged children.[69] On the other hand, the patient could use the robot to visit friends and family and even museums and libraries.[70]

For those who want a closer relationship with their elderly parents, homes can be equipped with sensors that allow adult children to monitor their parents' movements. When the parent opens a door, a medicine cabinet, or a refrigerator, this is transmitted to the child. If the parent records blood pressure, this is also sent.[71] Research is also being done into using webcams to measure pulse and respiration from the patient's home. CardioCam uses "slight variation in skin tone" to measure the pulse.[72]

## TELEMEDICINE IN PRISON

Telemedicine is now widely used in state prisons in at least 27 states including Arizona, Iowa, Maryland, Texas, Massachusetts, Virginia, Pennsylvania, Wisconsin, Utah, Missouri, Kansas, and New York, and in the federal prison system. In 2006, South Carolina introduced the use of tele-psychiatry.[73] The stated reasons for introducing telemedicine are cost containment, security, and enhanced medical care for inmates. A recent study of teleophthalmology in prisons found it to be cost effective and to reduce blindness caused by diabetic retinopathy.[74]

Telemedicine is used to provide specialist care, not primary care, which is delivered onsite. Although no comprehensive study exists, there are some comparisons of traditional to telemedical care in specific areas. The Arizona Department of Corrections did a cost–benefit analysis in fiscal year 2000 and found a $200.89 savings per case, which came to a total savings of $156,694.20. A review of the literature on Texas indicates that both patients and providers are satisfied with the care and that the vast majority of systems experienced reductions in travel and security costs. One preliminary study found that 95 percent of the telemedical consults had saved a trip to a clinic. A teleconsult clinic for human immunodeficiency

virus (HIV)-positive inmates was established in Texas in 1999; it was found to cut costs but had no effect on outcomes. Massachusetts also introduced a telemedicine program for HIV-positive prisoners and found no significant differences in health outcomes. However, HIV patients became increasingly concerned about privacy. Further study of this project is planned.

There seems to be a consensus that telemedicine in prisons saves money and increases security by decreasing off-site visits. Survey data also indicate that both prisoners and prison administrators are satisfied with telemedicine. It may be that more prisoners seek treatment because they do not have to travel; in states like Texas, a visit to a clinic can mean 4 days of travel shackled in a truck. However, there are no comprehensive studies on the effect on the health of prisoners.

California has used telemedicine in its prisons for more than 10 years, beginning with telepsychiatry. As of 2010, California used telemedicine for cardiology, dermatology, endocrinology, gastroenterology, infectious diseases, neurology, and transgender medicine, as well as psychiatry. According to the director of California Prison Health Care Services, the use of telemedicine services has saved $13 million, or about $800 per televisit. If telemedicine were not used, the money would be spent transporting and guarding prisoners. At the telemedical consult, a nurse is at the prison, but the doctor may be miles away.[75]

## OTHER TELEMEDICINE APPLICATIONS

In 1996, the federal government funded 19 pilot projects in telemedicine. Many are now taken-for-granted aspects of telemedicine, such as attempts to bring health care to rural areas and attempts to link small hospitals with medical centers for sharing of information. Others sent medication reminders to the elderly, and one tested an adverse drug event monitor. These programs are now in common use and will be discussed in Chapter 8.

One of the more interesting and highly successful programs is **Baby CareLink**. Baby CareLink was originated in Massachusetts. Its purpose was to compare high-risk, premature infants receiving traditional care with an experimental group that, in addition to traditional care, received a telemedicine link to the hospital while the babies were hospitalized and for 6 months after. The families could see and hear their babies in the nursery, although they were at home. They could log on to a secure Web page with up-to-date information about their babies. Once home, the families had access to the nursery and experts and could ask any question they pleased. The doctor or nurse could see the baby and reassure the parent. One purpose of Baby CareLink was to see whether parents felt more comfortable and knowledgeable about their babies' care, so that the hospital stay would be shorter. The experimental group did have shorter hospital stays. In a later case study of Baby CareLink in Chicago, it was found that the average length of stay for the experimental group was 2.73 days shorter, only 18 percent were readmitted (less than the expected 40 percent), medical staff were happy with the program, and parents were more comfortable with their infants. Baby CareLink is now covered by several state Medicaid programs and at least one private insurer. Baby CareLink is currently established in many hospitals throughout the country.[76]

In 2006, Dr. Darius Moshfeghi began using RetCam II Digital Imaging System to diagnose retinopathy of prematurity (ROP), a condition that can leave premature babies blind if not treated early. Almost 20 percent of very premature babies develop signs of ROP; it is one of the leading causes of blindness among babies. Very few doctors can screen for ROP. Using a telemedicine network called SUNDROP (Stanford University Network for Diagnosis of Retinopathy of Prematurity), the doctor can examine his or her patients from afar.[77]

Telemedical devices are also being developed to help people with Alzheimer's disease. Some of the devices include "visual prompts by the telephone that showed . . . the caller's name, picture, relationship, and reminders of their last interaction." Special "Presence" lamps would light up in an adult child's home when the parent sat in his or her favorite chair. The senior and his or her family would be able to see a representation of his or her social network.[78]

In Texas and Kansas, day care centers have brought teledoctors to day care. An onsite nurse uses a video camera and stethoscope and other equipment. A doctor diagnoses the child. In the vast majority of cases, the child is allowed to stay at day care and a prescription is called in. The parent does not have to leave work. In Rochester, New York, a federal grant is helping to set up a telemedicine system serving day care centers. By 2005, the program was considered successful. Studies report that "there has been a 63 percent drop in sickness-related absences at the pilot centers [and] that 92 percent of parents said the program enabled them to go to work when they otherwise would have needed to take their children to a family physician or emergency department."[79]

Telemedicine is currently being used in almost every aspect of health care. One of the more interesting uses of telemedicine is found in Vermont and Arizona in teletrauma projects that link trauma surgeons' homes with hospital emergency departments, providing immediate expert service at any time.[80]

It is especially common for rural areas to lack high-speed communications, although this varies and there is a lack of hard data on the issue. Presently, several rural states, including Alaska, Maine, Nebraska, and Tennessee, are using telemedicine applications. In Arkansas, "41 percent of patients who use telemedicine services would not have been able to see a doctor because of a doctor shortage and travel costs."[81] In 2011, several telehealth grants from the federal government to rural areas are attempting to address these issues.[82]

Telemedicine is being used in weight management, pain management, spinal cord injury, and podiatry. **Teleoncology** systems are helping cancer patients avoid lengthy trips to the doctor and feel more secure because they have a 24-hour link to health care. Telemedicine programs are using motion detectors to monitor elderly people in a nursing home; with the motion detectors, "atypical days" when activity was less than normal could be detected.[83]

In hospitals and even operating rooms, health care personnel (including 17 percent of doctors) are making use of personal digital assistants (PDAs) for writing prescriptions, quickly accessing patient information, and finding facts in online databases of medical articles and journals.

Information is crucial in fighting disease—access to the latest journal articles and newest treatment is necessary. However, in developing countries, access to the best information is limited at best. In 1989, **SATELLIFE** was founded. Its purpose was to deliver journals and other information to health care workers in developing areas. It "meets the . . . needs of health workers where the diseases of poverty are decimating entire communities . . . ." In 1994, SATELLIFE began using e-mail and discussion groups. Approximately 100,000 health care workers in 159 countries use SATELLIFE each day.[84] Today (2011), SATELLIFE uses smartphones and PDAs for collecting data and disseminating information. They "can now package local and international health and medical information and put it in the hands of health workers in environments where electricity, telephone lines and books are not readily available, and the Internet may still be years away."[85] In the United States, 10 percent of hospital patients are in ICUs; they account for 30 percent of hospital costs. There is a lack of doctors specializing in intensive care (intensivists), and only 10 percent to 15 percent of hospitals employ a doctor full time. Telenurses and doctors are using the eICU Smart Alerts or other eICU systems to monitor 9 percent of intensive care patients from afar. In an ICU, onsite personnel are busy and can be distracted. Remote intensive care specialists and nurses can act as adjuncts, spotting patients in trouble immediately and sending alerts to the ICU. One of the largest teleICU systems is at St. John's Mercy Health Care System in Missouri where two doctors and nine nurses watch 400 patients in different hospitals from a central location. They can see vital signs and lab results on a bank of monitors, operate cameras watching patients' doors, and zoom in on the patients themselves. They can talk to bedside nurses and patients. Using money from a recent federal grant, Mercy will install telehome devices that will record blood sugar, weight, and activity for 900 patients. The devices will transmit these to a doctor.[86] According to Terry Davis, an operations director of an eICU, "Because the eICU physician and nurse are always watching trends for the patient, the remote monitoring decreases the number of complications and . . . the length of stay in the ICU." However, his conclusion is not backed up by hard data.[87]

Veterans of modern wars have been returning home with myriad injuries. This is because of the nature of the weaponry on one hand and the medical care they receive on or near the battlefield on the other. Blast injuries lead to multiple problems or polytrauma: visual and hearing impairments, head trauma, amputations, spinal cord injuries, and posttraumatic stress disorder. These people need so many forms of rehabilitation that only telemedicine can keep track of them.[88]

In July 2006, the FDA approved a wireless electronic capsule to help diagnose stomach disorders. The capsule, which is small enough to be easily swallowed, is used to diagnose gastroparesis—a condition that causes the stomach to empty slowly. The capsule transmits to a receiver that the patient wears while it travels through the intestinal tract. "When [it] is passed, the patient brings the cell-phone-sized receiver back to the physician, who downloads the data to a computer."[89]

Other telemedical devices are in the development or experimental stages. In Switzerland, a robot is helping perform virtual autopsies. Virtobot scans the body and takes high-definition images, which are then combined with images from the CT scanner "to create a 3D image of the cadaver." It can be viewed at all angles, and repeated autopsies can be performed. Virtobot is being used in the United States at one air force base on troops who were killed in Afghanistan.[90]

Silken brain implants to monitor and control epileptic seizures have been developed at the University of Illinois, Tufts, and the Pennsylvania School of Medicine. The silk molds to the brain and could detect the beginning of a seizure and possibly stop it. It is remotely powered and could be designed to dissolve.[91] For people with sleep apnea, the iBrain uses a "single brainwave-seeking electrode [on an elastic harness] . . . [to] collect . . . brain activity overnight" and delivers it to a sleep specialist's computer via cell phone. In the future, the iBrain may be used to diagnose such disorders as Alzheimer's disease, schizophrenia, and autism and to gauge the effect of drugs and the recovery of brain trauma patients. iBrain is in clinical trials. The Q Sensor measures stress levels by contact with the skin. It can be worn like a watch. At the end of the day, data can be downloaded onto a computer and reviewed. It is being used with autistic children.[92] Researchers are working on ways to use a person's face as an indicator of health or illness. "An ongoing video camera . . . is monitoring changes in a person's vitals by tracking the way light reflects off their face as blood flows under the skin." This could be used with a webcam or cell phone camera. It can already take a pulse; eventually, its developer hopes it can take blood pressure and measure respiration and blood oxygen levels. Other researchers, using nanotechnology, are working on a contact lens that displays health-related readings on a cell phone.[93]

## THE TELENURSE

Telemedicine is changing the role of the nurse. **Telenursing** involves teletriage and the telecommunication of health-related data, the remote house call, and the monitoring of chronic disease. Teletriage starts with a call from a worried patient or parent with a question to the nurse. Software helps the nurse ask a series of questions to aid in diagnosis and make a recommendation to the patient. Telenursing increases access to medical advice by making it available in the home. Nurses may be in more autonomous positions in telemedicine programs. In England, there is a 24-hour telephone line staffed by nurses. The nurses use diagnostic software and are linked to databases, hospitals, primary care providers, and ambulances. The nurses staffing these lines need to know how to use the software and how to get the correct information; the nurses also need knowledge of local health care services. In the United States, the VA telephone care program is staffed by registered

nurses (RNs) only. The nurses have access to the patient records and to the primary care provider through e-mail. Patients appreciate the immediate attention from an expert. One study of patients whose doctors allowed secure e-mail found 90 percent of patients who used it rated their doctors as good, very good, or excellent, compared to 80 percent of a group that did not use e-mail. Those using e-mail found it to be convenient and felt free to talk about more personal issues.[94]

In teleconferencing, the nurse takes the patient's vital signs from a distance and assesses the patient via a monitor. Although the televisit is similar to the actual visit, it is not identical. Nurses lead many telemedicine programs. In some programs, nurses perform diagnostic services. Nurses need to be familiar with computerized equipment and comfortable using it. When telemedicine is used in schools, the school nurse becomes responsible for the referral and follows up on home care. Nurses involved in a study of the role of **telehealth** in psychiatry needed knowledge of management of depression, medication, counseling, and the ability to provide emotional support. In a telemedicine project examining diabetes, the nurse case manager performed weekly consultations and the doctor monthly consultations. The nurse would recommend changes in diet and exercise and participate in the doctor's monthly consult.

Telephone triage and advice services staffed by nurses are rapidly expanding, and they change the way nurses work: First, they work in call centers, not clinical settings, and second, they do not examine the patient. In a review of 16 studies of 700 telenurses in Canada, the United Kingdom, the United States, and Sweden, it was found that telenurses share some common concerns: They are concerned with their own skill level, their autonomy, the work environment (which is not a clinical setting), assessment of the patients' needs, and stress. They attempt to "build a picture" of the patient and his or her health concerns. "Telenurses who took part in half of the studies expressed a conflict between what they thought was best for the caller and what healthcare services could provide." In the end, their advice is "influenced by balancing the conflicting demands of being both carer and gatekeeper to limited healthcare services."[95]

## SMARTPHONES AND TABLET COMPUTERS

Smartphones and tablet computers, such as the iPhone and iPad (Figures 4.4 and 4.5 ▶), are among the newest additions to mobile health care. The use of these small, mobile devices can put into a patient's hands what used to be centralized in hospitals—imaging devices. The fact that healthcare providers can use phones with video means that computers are not necessary for online consultations or prescriptions.[96] Small and portable, smartphones and tablet computers have many healthcare applications. Any application (app) for the iPhone can be used on the iPad. By late 2009, two-thirds of doctors and 42 percent of consumers were using smartphones. By February 2010, 6,000 health-related apps were in use, 73 percent for the consumer and 27 percent for healthcare providers. Apps for providers include alerts, medical references, diagnostic tools, educational materials, and patient record programs. Airstrip OB for obstetricians sends information about the patient's vital signs to the doctor's smartphone. In India, a pilot program that will allow the telemedicine diagnosis of retinopathy of prematurity (ROP) is being used. Retinal images from remote locations will be shown on doctors' iPhones. Doctors will be able to send diagnoses from the iPhone. According to a recent Pew study, 64 percent of doctors and 99 percent of residents carry smartphones.[97] A new smartphone ultrasound imaging system can "provide a live image of various organs." The smartphone can be used almost anywhere and can transmit to a specialist wirelessly.[98] NETRA (Near-Eye Tool for Refractive Assessment) is using smartphones to give eye tests.[99]

At Massachusetts General Hospital, a device that hooks up to a smartphone can analyze tissue "to determine in one hour whether a patient's . . . [tumor] is malignant." The device is portable and inexpensive ($200.00). Its findings are displayed on a phone's monitor. In an early clinical test, the device correctly predicted whether 48 out of 50 patients who had had stomach tissue biopsied had cancer. It may be able to test for other kinds of cancers in the future.[100]

The consumer can use medication compliance programs, mobile and home monitoring programs, and many fitness and weight control programs. A Wi-Fi body scale can wirelessly

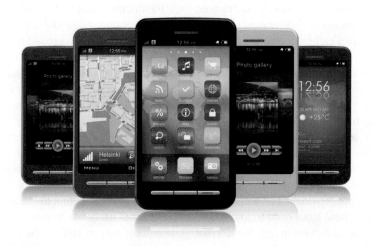

▶ **Figure 4.4** Set of touch-screen smartphones.
*Source:* Oleksiy Mark/Shutterstock.com

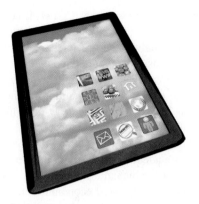

▶ **Figure 4.5** A modern tablet computer with application icons ready for mobile connectivity.
*Source:* iQoncept/Shutterstock.com

synch with a smartphone's personal health record app. An iPhone blood pressure app also synchs with a smartphone, recording your weight and body mass index into a personal health record app. Other apps for consumers help manage diabetes, high blood pressure, and stress, and give first aid information and hearing and vision assistance. Two of the stress reduction apps are iBreath and Rage Eraser. iBreath was designed by the Defense Department's National Center for Telehealth and Technology to teach troops to use deep breathing. Rage Reducer lets you record your "rant" and then listen to it. It also lets you track trigger situations and identify distorted thoughts. There are voices to talk you down and techniques for using your anger more productively. A recent Pew study found that 17 percent of cell phone users look up health information on the phone. Another survey found that about one-third of Americans would use their phones to track personal health information and 40 percent would pay for a remote monitoring device that would send health information to their doctors.[101] One of the newest and perhaps smartest phones started being sold in 2010. It can check your pulse and includes a mini-ECG, which can be transferred to a telenurse or other medical facility. If necessary, the phone calls you and says, "[A]n ambulance is on the way."[102]

In California, researchers from the University of California Los Angeles and Caltech are creating "ultrasmall, ultralow-cost microscopes for use in telemedicine applications." The images can be sent to a smartphone or other device and become part of a telemedical network. The microscope can image blood among other things. The microscope weighs 46 grams and costs only $3.00 to produce. Other tiny microscopes are also under development.[103]

Tablet computers, specifically iPads, have been a great success with health care professionals. They are used as "telehealth mobile computing device[s]." According to the chief information officer at Harvard Medical School, "the combination of lower hardware acquisition costs and relative lack of a learning curve . . . could foster widespread adoption of the iPad in health-care settings and pave the way for electronic health records to become the norm." It can be used for taking notes, accessing medical records and medical references, and viewing some medical images. There are clinical reference apps that include drug databases, interactive medication checkers, and a medical calculator. There is a program to help students track their inpatients. It is easy to use and provides access to online information from anywhere. It is light and small enough to carry, but the screen is large enough to see electronic health records and prescribing systems. It integrates with many health care systems and can switch between them in a doctor's office or hospital. Because it is the size of a piece of paper, it does not intrude between doctor and patient the way a laptop might. It allows the immediate viewing of radiographic images and can be used to show patients both these images and photos from reference books. It can hold interactive textbooks. It is Health Insurance Portability and Accountability Act (HIPAA) compliant because it does not store anything on the device and uses secure remote connections.[104]

One of the issues in the adoption of telemedicine concerns the attitudes of patients and physicians toward remote health care. Regarding the use of smartphones, attitudes seem to be positive. A PricewaterhouseCoopers survey of 2,000 consumers and 1,000 physicians in 2010 showed the following results:

- Thirty-one percent of consumers would use a smartphone app that tracked their personal health information.
- Forty percent of consumers would buy a device and pay a subscription for an app that would send them reminders to take medication and refill prescriptions and that would track their health and give them access to their health information.
- Forty percent of consumers would buy a device and pay for a service that sent data (heart rate, blood pressure, blood sugar, weight) to their doctors.
- Fifty-six percent like remote health care.
- Forty-one percent would like more of their health care delivered remotely.
- Eighty-eight percent of doctors would like their patients to monitor their health at home.
- Fifty-seven percent of doctors would like to monitor their patients via remote devices outside the hospital, but they do not want all the information, just exceptional information.[105]

## IS TELEMEDICINE EFFECTIVE?

This chapter has mentioned a few studies of the effectiveness of telemedicine. There are now many studies but few solid conclusions. One weakness in the studies is the lack of a standard definition of telemedicine, covering everything from "a phone and a bathroom scale" to a fully computerized system that connects patients in their homes with remote facilities using electronic health records. The evidence on telecardiology is most compelling. It is both effective and cuts costs. Most studies are not "randomized, clinical, controlled trials;" most have small samples, and studies do not agree on how to measure the possible benefits. Published clinical trials do not agree with each other. A 2008 study (funded by AT&T) states that remote patient monitoring "could save $200 billion . . . in the United States over the next 25 years." Yet a RAND study (funded by Royal Phillips Electronics) stated that the evidence was limited and that good outcomes and disappointing results both occurred. In September 2010, an article in the *Journal of Evaluation in Clinical Practice* analyzed 40 studies of telemonitoring of COPD. It concluded that "evaluations of home telemonitoring to date are of low quality and are undertaken by those who are enthusiastic about the potential of remote patient assessment." Much more work needs to be done to evaluate home monitoring, the article added. In 2007, a European study recognized the utility of home monitoring for people suffering from chronic disease, but pointed to the dearth of studies with adequate numbers of people and adequate time to evaluate the procedures. It also mentioned that the supposed economic benefits have not been proven. Some studies have concluded that better patient outcomes are due to nurses' interventions, not the telemedical monitoring itself. In Germany, the United Kingdom, and the Scandinavian countries, remote monitoring of chronic heart failure is standard.[106]

Between 2000 and 2002, a randomized study of 426 heart failure patients was conducted. The patients received either standard care from primary care providers; nurse phone support; or home telemonitoring, which involved the patient weighing him or herself and taking blood pressure and heart rate and rhythm twice daily using devices linked to a cardiology center. When the three groups were compared, it was found that the group that used remote monitoring spent 26 percent fewer days in the hospital compared to the group that received nurse support. There was also a 10 percent cost savings.[107] A similar study in 2010 also found that heart failure patients benefited from telemonitoring services.[108]

The Veterans Health Administration (VHA) in the United States is the leading user of remote health services in the world, that is, the biggest and the most advanced. Its Care Coordination Home Telehealth program is supposed to "improve accessibility and to provide timely and appropriate care for veterans with chronic diseases." Each day, the patients send updates, and a care coordinator might respond with a phone call, a referral, help with medication or schedule, or a reminder of the patients' appointments. If the patients have any problems with the technology, the nurse will help solve them. The VHA, with 50 programs in 18 networks, is in a position to conduct large studies of the effectiveness of telemonitoring. One study found "a 25% reduction in bed days and a 20% reduction in hospital admissions." Another study focusing on VHA telemonitoring of diabetes found reduced admissions and lower rates of other diabetes-related conditions.[109]

A review of 25 studies of 9,500 patients with chronic heart failure found that telemonitoring reduced the number of patients hospitalized to 225 per 1,000 from 285 per 1,000. A 2008 study by the New England Healthcare Institute of remote physiological monitoring for patients with heart failure found that telemonitoring reduced hospital readmissions by 60 percent compared with standard care where patients are given information regarding diet, medication, and exercise. With standard care, the patient also receives doctor visits and phone calls from a nurse. Telemonitoring reduced readmissions by 50 percent compared to patients in a traditional disease management program.[110]

A study in 2010 in central New Jersey also found that using remote monitoring resulted in a reduction in readmissions for heart failure patients. Patients would receive an automated call every day and answer questions about their health. If a patient was identified as needing help, a human nurse would call. In England, a study of 30 COPD patients using remote monitoring resulted in a 59 percent decrease in hospital admissions and an 85 percent decrease in home health visits.

In November 2010, *The New England Journal of Medicine* published a study of 1,653 patients with heart failure after they had been released from the hospital. The patients were divided into two groups: One group received traditional care, and "the other half participated in a remote monitoring program that required them to make daily phone calls to a computerized system" and report their symptoms. The study found "*no significant difference* between the two groups in any outcomes" (emphasis added). The study found that telemonitoring was no better than traditional care.[111]

Telemonitoring is used for only 9 percent of ICU beds. A small study was done that found that those who worked in eICUs were "enthusiastic about the technology's impact on ICU performance, particularly on quality and safety." They like the immediate response and earlier detection of complications by software due to continuous monitoring. However, the eICU software could not communicate with most hospitals' information technology systems. This created some problems. The study found no evidence that eICU had any effect on complications or hospital stay.[112]

With the disagreement among these studies and their conclusions, it is impossible to make a definitive statement regarding the effectiveness of telemedical care, with the exception of tele-cardiology. Also, there are no large-scale studies of telestroke or other aspects of telemedicine, including such expanding fields as telepsychiatry. The only obvious conclusion is that more large-scale, long-term, randomized clinical trials are necessary.

## ISSUES IN TELEMEDICINE

For telemedicine to fulfill its promise, certain technical, legal, insurance, human, and privacy issues need to be addressed. On the technical side, an appropriate telecommunications infrastructure must be in place. The Telecommunications Act of 1996 proposed that access be increased, but did not specify how. Certain aspects of telemedicine require high-speed, broadband media, because the files transmitted may be so huge. This applies particularly to the utilization of real-time interactive video teleconferencing, which transmits voice, sound, images, text, and motion video.

In addition, legal issues such as licensing, medical liability, and privacy concerns need to be addressed. Furthermore, there are problems of insurance. The issues of concern to telemedicine have not changed much since the inception of telemedicine as evidenced by a Washington, DC, symposium, "Balancing Access, Safety, and Quality in a New Era of Telemedicine," held on March 10, 2011.[113] Currently, there is some insurance coverage for telemedicine. As of January 1,

1999, the Balanced Budget Act of 1997 required that Medicare pay for telemedical services in medically underserved areas. However, after 2 years of this expanded reimbursement, Medicare had only reimbursed $20,000 for 301 teleconsultation claims. In an attempt to expand coverage further, Congress passed the Medicare, Medicaid, and State Children's Health Insurance Program (SCHIP) Benefits Improvement and Protection Act. It went into effect in October of 2001.

In 2011, reimbursement for telemedicine was still restricted and complex. Medicare reimbursement is limited to doctors, physician assistants, nurse practitioners, clinical nurse specialists, nurse-midwives, clinical psychologists, clinical social workers, and registered dieticians. The patient must be seen in a practitioner's office, critical access hospital, rural health clinic, federally qualified health center, hospital, certain renal dialysis centers, skilled nursing facility, or community health center. There is no reimbursement for patients seen at home. However, the Patient Protection and Affordable Care Act did create the Center for Medicare and Medicaid Innovation to test aspects of telemedicine. The office opened January 1, 2011. As of 2010, there were two bills in Congress that would expand reimbursement. The states of Virginia, California, Colorado, Georgia, Hawaii, Kentucky, Louisiana, Maine, New Hampshire, Oklahoma, Oregon, and Texas mandate insurance coverage for telemedicine. The 2011 Medicare Physician Fee Schedule expands coverage of telemedicine. The Patient Protection and Affordable Care Act of 2010 will start reducing payments to hospitals for "excessive readmission rates" for certain conditions. Some of these conditions, including chronic heart failure and COPD, have been successfully treated telemedically. If studies show that telemedical care is effective, that might push government and private insurers to cover more telemedicine. Medicaid, because it is a state-federal program, reimburses in some states and not others.[114] In January 2011, Medicaid coverage was expanded to cover telemedical "disease management training for patients with diabetes or kidney disease."[115] In 2011, the U.S. Department of Agriculture awarded 45 telehealth grants as "part of the more than $34.7 million in USDA grants that will go toward 106 health care and education projects in 38 states and one territory."[116] More than 100 private insurers provide some coverage for some aspect of telemedicine.[117] Whatever the obstacles, telemedicine continues to expand.

One of the most serious legal obstacles to the development of telemedicine is state licensing. Medical personnel are required to be licensed by the state in which they practice. Acquiring a license is a costly and time-consuming process. Practicing without a license is a crime. Licensing laws are different in each state. Some states allow consultations across state lines. However, the American Medical Association supports requiring physicians to be licensed in any state in which they practice telemedicine. Some states have reciprocity agreements with other states. Some states require telemedicine providers to be separately licensed in each jurisdiction. Not all the states have agreements that make it easier for nurses to practice across state lines. There are now licensing services that advertise (for example, in April 2011) "Get Your State Medical License as Soon as *May 9th, 2011*" (emphasis original). For a fee, the service will help doctors get licensed in any state. It is "like having a nationwide medical license."[118]

Telemedicine raises many privacy issues; medical information routinely crosses state lines, some of it via e-mail, which is not private. There are typically nonmedical personnel involved including technicians and camera operators. According to the final Health Insurance Portability and Accountability Act (HIPAA) Privacy Rules, several privacy issues are relevant: Under HIPAA, "Federal laws preempt state laws that are in conflict with regulatory requirements or those that provide less stringent privacy protections. But those states that have *more* stringent privacy laws would preempt Federal law." This leads to a "patchwork" of different standards. In a telemedical consultation, many people (both medical and nonmedical) may be present—but not apparent to the patient. Telemedicine requires greater concern with patient privacy and more complicated consent from patients. To be HIPAA-compliant,

# IN THE NEWS

In the article, "Are Doctors Ready for Virtual Visits?" by Pauline W. Chen published on January 7, 2010, in *The New York Times*, the author indicates that one obstacle to the widespread adoption of telemedicine is doctors' resistance.

Research was completed in Texas to evaluate telemedicine in an ICU. The ICU patients had both traditional care and the opportunity to be monitored by a critical care specialist. The patients' doctors could decide whether the remote doctor (a critical care specialist) could participate in direct care. For example, a doctor could choose to have the remote specialist only intervene in emergencies, or the doctor could choose to have the remote specialist give direct patient care, for instance, issue orders. Most doctors opted for the least possible involvement of the remote specialists. Most nurses also disliked having what they saw as someone looking over their shoulders.

Although the research was originally meant to measure the effect of telemedicine on the mortality of ICU patients, the attitudes of physicians made this impossible. The researchers did, however, find that that telemedicine improved the survival rate of patients who were sickest.

e-mail should be encrypted, facial recognition systems should allow the doctor to identify the patient on a network, digital identity cards should be used, and the computers and networks should be protected.[119]

The laws concerning telemedicine today are ambiguous; legal liability is not clear. It is not even clear what pieces of equipment used in a telemedical consult or exam are considered medical devices and are therefore subject to regulation by the FDA. Some of the legal ramifications are made clear by the following:

- If a doctor in one state sends an x-ray to a specialist in another state and the specialist misreads it, leading to the death of the patient, who is liable?
- If a reporter gains access to a database, finds records of a telepsychiatric consult, and publicizes them, who is liable?

The answers to these questions are not yet clear.

Another obstacle to telemedicine adoption is the human factor. Will doctors and patients accept telemedicine? One recent study reported in *The New York Times* found that the resistance of doctors was the greatest obstacle to the introduction of telemedicine. In the study, patients in the ICU had both traditional care and distance monitoring. The onsite doctors were allowed to choose whether the remote specialists could deliver such care as issuing orders. Most of the doctors "chose to have as little remote involvement as possible." Because of the resistance of doctors and nurses, the overall effect of remote monitoring could not be judged. However, among the sickest patients, telemedicine "significantly improve[d] survival."[120]

A 2010 survey of 1,202 consumers found a "slow adoption" of telemedicine technology. Of the 1,202 respondents, only 4.6 percent had used videoconferencing in health care. Among the 4.6 percent who had, 6.3 percent were 35 years old or younger as compared to 0.8 percent who were 65 or older. The report also found that people who used smartphones are three times more likely to use them for medical scheduling than people who use other kinds of mobile phones. The survey also found that "9.7 percent . . . were more likely to use their smartphones for reminders to schedule a medical appointment" compared to 3 percent of users of other mobile phones.[121]

## Chapter Summary

- Chapter 4 introduces the reader to the field of telemedicine and some of its subspecialties. In addition, its effectiveness and some of the issues that must be addressed for telemedicine to fully develop are discussed.
- Telemedicine uses computers and telecommunications technology to deliver health care including diagnosis, patient monitoring, and treatment at a distance. As such, it has the potential of making high-quality health care available to anyone regardless of distance from major medical centers. It may use store-and-forward technology for transmission of still images or interactive videoconferencing for real-time consultations.
- It encompasses subspecialties such as teleradiology, telepathology, telecardiology, teleneurology, telestroke, telewound care, telehome care, and telepsychiatry, as well as the use of remote monitoring devices and remote operation of medical equipment.
- Remote monitoring devices allow patients to be monitored at home or in an ambulance; the information is transmitted to a remote location.
- Telemedicine is changing the role of the nurse.
- Smartphones and tablet computers have many health-related applications.
- Telemedicine is currently being evaluated, and the assessments tend to be mixed. It is used in prison settings where its efficacy is being judged. Several studies have been completed and more are under way. The federal government has funded several projects to be evaluated.
- For the promise of telemedicine to be fulfilled, certain problems have to be solved. These include the establishment of adequate high-bandwidth communications lines, barriers posed by state licensing, the lack of insurance coverage in many instances, human resistance, and the insecurity of the electronic medical record. HIPAA addresses some of the privacy problems posed by telemedicine.

## Key Terms

Baby CareLink
Bluetooth
computed tomography colonography (CTC)
interactive videoconferencing
Parkinson's disease
remote monitoring devices
SATELLIFE

store-and-forward technology
teleconferencing
teledermatology
telehealth
telehome care
telemedicine
teleneurology

telenursing
teleoncology
telepathology
telepsychiatry
teleradiology
telestroke
telewound care

## Review Exercises

### Multiple Choice

1. Telemedicine involves _____ .
   a. the linking of doctors and patients at a distance
   b. the transmission of radiologic images via telecommunications lines
   c. the transmission of patient data in any form
   d. All of the above

2. The technology used in teleradiology is called
   _____ .
   a. send-and-receive
   b. receive-and-send
   c. store-and-forward
   d. None of the above

3. Before telemedicine can deliver high-quality
   medical services at a distance, _____ .
   a. a reliable broadband telecommunications
      network has to be in place
   b. state licensing barriers have to be overcome
   c. every patient needs to own a printer
   d. A and B only

4. The transmission of microscopic images over
   telecommunications lines is called _____ .
   a. teleradiology
   b. telepsychiatry
   c. telepathology
   d. remote monitoring

5. Telemedicine projects in prisons have been
   found to _____ .
   a. improve health care
   b. cut costs
   c. improve security
   d. All of the above

6. _____ allows doctors and patients to consult
   in real time, at a distance.
   a. Telepathology
   b. Teleradiology
   c. Teleoncology
   d. Interactive videoconferencing

7. Elderly, frail patients and patients in poor
   health are more likely than others to suffer
   from problematic injuries. _____ can increase
   access to specialists.
   a. Telepsychiatry
   b. Teleneurology
   c. Telewound care
   d. None of the above

8. Telemedicine is used in some way in the
   treatment of _____ .
   a. psychiatric disorders
   b. cancer
   c. skin rashes
   d. All of the above

9. Remote medical consultations and exams
   were first tried _____ .
   a. after World War II
   b. in 1997
   c. as soon as the telephone was invented
   d. in 1977

10. A remote house call by a visiting nurse is an
    example of _____ .
    a. telepathology
    b. teleradiology
    c. video teleconferencing
    d. None of the above

11. _____ technology is used to link electronic
    devices (e.g., a pacemaker with a cell phone).
    a. Telephone
    b. Bluetooth
    c. Video teleconferencing
    d. Store-and-forward

12. The _____ program at Massachusetts General
    allows quick diagnosis and can determine if
    tPA should be used in treatment.
    a. telestroke
    b. telecardiology
    c. telenurse
    d. teledoctor

13. One of the most successful telemedicine pro-
    grams links hospitalized premature infants
    with their parents at home. It is called _____ .
    a. telebaby
    b. computer parenting
    c. telepreemie
    d. Baby CareLink

14. Many telemedicine programs have been found
    to be effective; however, _____ is not.
    a. distance monitoring of problem pregnancies
    b. telehome care
    c. telemedicine in prisons
    d. a teletriage program run by telenurses

15. In Vermont and Arizona, _____ projects link
    trauma surgeons' homes with hospital emer-
    gency departments.
    a. telestroke
    b. teletrauma
    c. telecardiology
    d. teleoncology

## True/False

1. Medical insurance has limited and restricted telemedicine. _____

2. The broadband links are in place to deliver telemedicine all over the world. _____

3. State licensing of doctors is an obstacle to the development of telemedicine. _____

4. The electronic patient record is absolutely secure. _____

5. The oldest form of telemedicine is teleradiology. _____

6. Telemedicine has the potential of giving immediate access to specialists regardless of distance. _____

7. Establishing a telemedicine site is so inexpensive that any clinic can afford it. _____

8. Telepsychiatry is the recommended therapy for anyone regardless of mental disorder. _____

9. In 2006, in Japan, a group of scientists began using a mobile phone–based heart monitor. _____

10. Remote monitoring devices make it possible for patients to be monitored at home. _____

## Critical Thinking

1. Cite some examples of the current usage of aspects of telemedicine technologies in the diagnosis and treatment of patients. Can you suggest future uses of telemedicine that would improve health care?

2. How can patient confidentiality be safeguarded, given the establishment of a vast national database of medical records?

3. Discuss who should be held accountable for mistakes in diagnosis and treatment when there are several parties involved including (but not limited to) the onsite physician, remote specialist and other medical personnel, and the telecommunications equipment manufacturer.

4. Should medical personnel involved in telemedicine be licensed in every state or licensed nationally? Discuss the advantages and disadvantages of each.

5. Today, medical personnel need to be retrained in certain telemedicine technology areas. How would you convince them to retrain?

# Notes

1. "Telemedicine Defined," 2010, http://www.americantelemed. org/i4a/pages/index.cfm?pageID=3333 (accessed April 25, 2011).

2. Jane Sarasohn-Kahn, "The Connected Patient: Charting the Vital Signs of Remote Health Monitoring," February 2011, http://www.chcf.org/publications/2011/02/the-connected-patient (accessed April 9, 2011).

3. Stephen Heuser, "'Telehealth' Systems Slowly Gaining: Devices Help Curb Visits to Hospital," July 26, 2006, http://www.boston.com/yourlife/health/aging/articles/2006/07/26/telehealth_systems_slowly_gaining/ (accessed April 25, 2011).

4. Heinrich J. Audebert, Thomas Meyer, and Fabian Klostermann, "Potentials of Telemedicine for Green Health Care," 2010, http://www.frontiersin.org/teleneurology/10.3389/fneur.2010.00010/abstract (accessed March 2, 2011); Sarasohn-Kahn, "The Connected Patient: Charting the Vital Signs of Remote Health Monitoring."

5. "Virtual Colonoscopy and Teleradiology Bring Colorectal Cancer Screening to Patients in Rural Areas," October 21, 2010. http://esciencenews.com/articles/2010/ 10/21/ virtual.colonoscopy.and.teleradiology.bring.colorectal. cancer.screening.patients.rural.areas (accessed March 2, 2011).

6. "X-Rays Outsourced to India," 2011, http://health.india-times.com/articleshow/1435209.cms (accessed April 25, 2011); "Outsourcing Radiology Services to India," 2011, http://www.outsource 2india.com/services/radiology.asp (accessed April 9, 2011).

7. "Anatomic Telepathology Network," August 28, 2008, http://www.cost.eu/domains_actions/ict/Actions/IC0604 (accessed April 9, 2011).

8. Gunter Burg, "Store-and-Forward Teledermatology," August 25, 2005, http://www.emedicine.com/derm/topic560.htm (accessed April 25, 2011).

9. "Groups Urge CMS to Cover Tele_dermatology Under Medicare Part B," March 1, 2011, http://www.ihealthbeat.org/articles/2011/3/1/groups-urge-cms-to-cover teledermatology-under-medicare-part-b.aspx (accessed April 9, 2011).

10. "History of Stethoscopes and Sphygmomanometers," October 7, 2003, http://www.hhmi.org/biointeractive/museum/exhibit98/content/b6_17info.html (accessed April 26, 2011).

11. W. Backman, D. Bendel, and R. Rakhit, "The Telecardiology Revolution: Improving the Management of Cardiac Disease in Primary Care," November 2010, *Journal of the Royal Society of Medicine*, http://www.ncbi.nlm.nih.gov/pubmed/20959351 (accessed March 2, 2011).

12. J. Iwamoto, Y. Yonezawa, H. Maki, H. Ogawa, I. Ninomiya, K. Sada, S. Hamada, A. W. Hahn, and W. M. Caldwell, "A Mobile Phone-Based ECG Monitoring System," [Abstract] 2006, http://www.ncbi.nlm.nih.gov/pubmed/16817611?ordi nalpos=2&itool=EntrezSystem2.PEntrez.Pubmed.Pubmed_ResultsPanel.Pubmed_RVDocSum (accessed April 26, 2011).

13. Natale Daniele Brunetti, Luisa De Gennaro, Gianfranco Amodio, Giulia Dellegrottaglie, Pier Luigi Pellegrino, Matteo Di Biase, and Gianfranco Antonelli, "Telecardiology Improves Quality of Diagnosis and Reduces Delay to Treatment in Elderly Patients with Acute Myocardial Infarction and Atypical Presentation," [Abstract] August 9, 2009, http://www.ncbi.nlm.nih.gov/pubmed/ 20729737 (accessed April 9, 2011).

14. Dave Fornell, "Telecardiology Growth Mainly in Infant Congenital Heart Disease," March–April, 2009, http://www.dicardiology.com/article/telecardiology-growth-mainly-infant-congenital-heart-disease (accessed March 2, 2011).

15. Victor Patterson and Richard Wooten, "How Can Teleneurology Improve Patient Care?" July 17, 2006, http://www.medscape.com/viewarticle/540191 (accessed April 26, 2011).

16. "GlobalMedia Partners with NeuroCall to Offer Remote Neurology Services Anywhere in the World," May 6, 2009, http://www.neurocall.com/press.html (accessed April 9, 2011).

17. "GlobalMedia, NeuroCall, Reach Call Partner to Provide Fully Integrated Telemedicine Solution," September 21, 2009, http://www.neurocall.com/press.html (accessed April 9, 2011).

18. Jason Meserve, "Telemedicine Helps Victims of Stroke," May 23, 2005, http://www.networkworld.com/news/2005/052305-stroke.html (accessed April 25, 2011).

19. Liz Kowalczyk, "Going the Distance in Stroke Treatment," *Boston Globe*, April 3, 2006, http://www.boston.com/yourlife/health/diseases/articles/2006/04/03/going_the_distance_in_stroke_treatment/ (accessed April 26, 2011).

20. Susan Jeffrey, "Telemedicine System May Increase tPA Use in Stroke," July 17, 2007, http://www.medscape.com/viewarticle/559914 (accessed April 26, 2011).

21. "Detailed Technology Analysis, Tele-Stroke," June 2009, http://www.nehi.net/ publications/43/detailed_technolgy_analysis_telestroke (accessed March 2, 2011).

22. Molly Merrill, "Interest in Telestroke Care Runs High," September 13, 2010, http://www.healthcareitnews.com/news/interest-telestroke-care-runs-high (accessed March 2, 2011).

23. John Farrell, "Telemedicine Progress Advances," January 26, 2011, http://www.mhimss.org/blog/telemedicine-progress-advances (accessed March 3, 2011).

24. "USDA to Award Grants for Telehealth Programs in Rural US Locations," January 25, 2011, http://www.ihealthbeat.org/articles/2011/1/25/usda-to-award-grants-for-telehealth-programs-in-rural-us-locations.aspx (accessed April 9, 2011).

25. "NeuroCall Conducts 400th Teleconsultation in El Paso, TX," February 8, 2011, http://www.neurocall.com/press.html (accessed April 9, 2011).

26. Patterson and Wooten, "How Can Teleneurology Improve Patient Care?"

27. Victor Patterson and Ena Bingham, "Telemedicine for Epilepsy: A Useful Combination," *Epilepsia* 44, no. 5 (2005): 614–5.

28. Patterson and Wooten, "How Can Teleneurology Improve Patient Care?"

29. "Remote Telemedicine for Epilepsy," 2011, https://www.epilepsy.com/epilepsy/telemedicine (accessed April 9, 2011).

30. **Telemedicine for Epilepsy: A Useful Contribution, Victor Patterson, Ena Bingham. Epilepsia, Volume 46, Issue 5, pages 614–615, May 2005.**

31. S. N. Ahmed, S. Weibe, C. Mann, and A. Ohinmaa, "Telemedicine and Epilepsy Care," [Abstract] November 2010, http://www.ncbi.nlm.nih.gov/pubmed/21059544 (accessed April 9, 2011).

32. "Telemedicine Expands Reach of Care for Parkinson's Patients," June 17, 2009, https://www.urmc.rochester.edu/news/story/index.cfm?id=2521 (accessed April 26, 2011); Renee Matthews, "Pilot Study Shows Feasibility of Telemedicine for Parkinson's," July 2009, http://www.entrepreneur.com/tradejournals/article/205586270.html (accessed April 26, 2011); "Telemedicine Helps Monitor Parkinson's Symptoms in Patients," June 23, 2009, http://medgadget.com/2009/06/telemedicine_helps_monitor_parkinsons_symptoms_in_patients.html (accessed April 26, 2011); Brian Downs, "Parkinson's Disease Care Through Telemedicine," April 22, 2011, http://www.lvhn.org/news/updates/parkinson%E2%80%99s-disease-care-through-telemedicine/123101 (accessed April 26, 2011).

33. "Telemedicine Expands Reach of Care for Parkinson's Patients"; Matthews, "Pilot Study Shows Feasibility of Telemedicine for Parkinson's"; "Telemedicine Helps Monitor Parkinson's Symptoms in Patients"; Downs, "Parkinson's Disease Care Through Telemedicine."

34. V. Patterson, J. Humphreys, and R. Chua, "Teleneurology by Email," *Journal of Telemedicine and Telecare* 9, no. 2 (2003): S42–3, http://www.ncbi.nlm.nih.gov/sites/entrez?cmd=Retrieve&db=PubMed&list_uids=14728758&dopt=AbstractPlus (accessed April 26, 2011).

35. Kerrie L. Schoffer, Victor Patterson, Stephen J. Read, et al., "Guidelines for Filming Digital Camera Video Clips for the Assessment of Gait and Movement Disorders by Teleneurology," *Journal of Telemedicine and Telecare* 11, no. 7 (October 2005): 368–71, http://www.ncbi.nlm.nih.gov/pubmed/16238839 (accessed April 26, 2011).

36. E. L. Nelson, M. Barnard, and S. Cain, "Treating Childhood Depression over Videoconferencing," *Telemedicine Journal and e-Health Spring* 9, no. 1 (2003): 49–55, http://ebookbrowse.com/treating-childhood-depression-over-videoconferencing-pdf-d41415583 (accessed April 26, 2011).

37. G. S. Goldfield and A. Boachie, "Delivery of Family Therapy in the Treatment of Anorexia Nervosa Using Telehealth: A Case Report," November 1, 2003, http://www.hawaii.edu/hivandaids/Case_Report__Delivery_of_Family_Therapy_in_the_Tx_of_Anorexia_Using_Telehealth.pdf (accessed April 26, 2011).

38. Kenneth Lane, "Telemedicine News," *Telemedicine and e-Health* 12, no. 2 (2006): 81–4.

39. Jeanine Turner, "Telepsychiatry as a Case Study of Presence: Do You Know What You Are Missing?" *Journal of Computer-Mediated Communication* 6, no. 4 (2001), http://jcmc.indiana.edu/vol6/issue4/turner.html (accessed April 26, 2011).

40. "Enhancing Vermont's Healthcare Delivery System: Telemedicine Child Psychiatry," Winter 2010, http://www.bistatepca.org/VT-Government-Relations/Telemedicine-Child-Psychiatry-Winter-Spring-2008.pdf (accessed February 16, 2011).

41. "Telemedicine Can Help Address Mental Health Needs of Elderly Homebound Individuals: Findings of a Pilot Study to Be Presented at National Meeting," October 2010, http://www.news-medical.net/news/20101004/Telemedicine-can-help-address-mental-health-needs-of-elderly-homebound-individuals.aspx (accessed February18, 2011).

42. "Telepsychiatry Helps Address Mental Health Worker Shortage," September 10, 2008. http://www.ihealthbeat.org/articles/2008/9/10/Telepsychiatry-Helps-Address-Mental-Health-Worker-Shortage.aspx?topicID=60 (accessed May 16, 2011); "Telemedicine Can Help Address Mental Health Needs of Elderly Homebound Individuals: Findings of a Pilot Study to Be Presented at National Meeting."

43. Sarasohn-Kahn, "The Connected Patient: Charting the Vital Signs of Remote Health Monitoring."

44. Ibid.

45. Ibid.

46. Carol Lewis, "Emerging Trends in Medical Device Technology: Home Is Where the Heart Monitor Is," *FDA Consumer*, May–June 2001, http://findarticles.com/p/articles/mi_m1370/is_3_35/ai_75608871/ (accessed April 26, 2011).

47. Alan Naditz, "Medical Connectivity: New Frontiers: Telehealth Innovations of 2010," *Telemedicine and e-Health* 16, no. 10 (December 2010): 986–8.

48. "'Smart' Fabrics to Keep Patients Healthy," March 16, 2005, http://www.medicalnewstoday.com/articles/21338.php (accessed April 26, 2011); Sarah Wright, "Media Lab Hosts Workshop on Body Sensors," April 12, 2006, http://web.mit.edu/newsoffice/2006/media-sensors.html (accessed April 26, 2011); S. Milior, "A Wearable Health Care System Based on Knitted Sensors," [Abstract] September 2005, http://ieeexplore.ieee.org/xpl/freeabs_all.jsp?arnumber=1504803 (accessed April 26, 2011).

49. "Top 10 Medical Innovations for 2011: #6 Telehealth Monitoring for Individuals with Heart Failure/Implanted Wireless Cardiac Device for Monitoring Heart Failure," 2010, http://www.clevelandclinic.org/innovations/summit2010/topten11/six.html (accessed February 28, 2011).

50. Sarasohn-Kahn, "The Connected Patient: Charting the Vital Signs of Remote Health Monitoring."

51. C. A. Ong, "Telemedicine and Wound Care," [Abstract] 2008, http://www.ncbi.nlm.nih.gov/pubmed/18305332 (accessed March 3, 2011).

52. "Wound Care Solutions Telemedicine," 2011, http://woundcaresolutions-telemedicine.co.uk (accessed March 3, 2011).

53. Marek Dobke, Alicja Renkielska, Joan De Neve, James Chao, and Dhaval Bhavsar, "Telemedicine for Problematic Wound Management: Enhancing Communication Between Long-Term Care, Skilled Nursing, and Home Caregiver," September 4, 2001, http://www.woundsresearch.com/article/ (accessed March 3, 2011).

54. Ibid.

55. Trisha Carlson, "Highlighting Tele medicine," May/June 2009, *Todays Wound Clinic*, http://www.today-swoundclinic.com/highlighting-telemedicine-0 (accessed November 12, 2010); Steve Lohr, "AT&T's Bet on Health Technology," November 4, 2010, http://bits.blogs.nytimes.com/2010/11/04/atts-bet-on-health-technology/ (accessed February 16, 2011).

56. Sarasohn-Kahn, "The Connected Patient: Charting the Vital Signs of Remote Health Monitoring."

57. "Telemedicine Trends and Technologies," February 8, 2010, http://www.impact-advisors.com/UserFiles/file/IA%20Telemedicine%20Overview%2020100208.pdf (accessed February 18, 2011).

58. Physician Compensation Report. FindArticles.com. 18 Feb, 2012. © 2003 Atlantic Information Services, Inc.

59. "VA Announces Budget Request for 2012," February 14, 2011, http://www.va.gov/opa/pressrel/pressrelease.cfm?id=2054 (accessed March 26, 2011).

60. C. Maiolo, E. I. Mohamed, C. M. Fiorani, and A. De Lorenzo, "Home Telemonitoring for Patients with Severe Respiratory Illness: The Italian Experience," [Abstract] *Journal of Telemedicine and Telecare* 9, no. 2 (2003): 67–71, http://www.ncbi.nlm.nih.gov/pubmed/12699574 (accessed April 26, 2011).

61. B. Johnson, L. Wheeler, J. Deuser, and K. H. Sousa, "Outcomes of the Kaiser Permanente Tele-Home Health Research Project," January 2000, http://archfami.ama-assn.org/cgi/content/full/9/1/40 (accessed April 26, 2011).

62. Max E. Stachura and Elena V. Khasanshina, "Telemedicine and Tele-Health: An Outcomes Overview," no date (but after 2007), http://www.viterion.com/web_docs/Telehomecarereport%20Diabetes%20and%20CHR%20Meta%20Analyses.pdf (accessed April 26, 2011).

63. "Remote Healthcare Monitoring Not So Distant," March 21, 2005, http://www.prweb.com/releases/2005/03/prweb220375.htm (accessed April 26, 2011).

64. "Monitoring Devices Help Reduce Rehospitalizations," June 26, 2006, http://www.ihealthbeat.org/articles/2006/6/26/Monitoring-Devices-Help-Reduce-Rehospitalizations.aspx?topicID=53 (accessed April 26, 2011).

65. Claire Cain Miller, "The Virtual Visit May Expand Access to Doctors," December 21, 2009, http://www.nytimes.com/2009/12/21/technology/start-ups/21doctors.html (accessed February 16, 2011); Stacey Higginbotham, "Will US TeleMedicine Be DOA?" February 23, 2010, http://gigaom.com/2010/02/23/will-u-s-telemedicine-be-doa/ (accessed February 16, 2011).

66. "Telemedicine Trends and Technologies."

67. Lane, "Telemedicine News."

68. Marinella Galea, Janine Tumminia, and Lisa Garback, "Telerehabilitation in Spinal Cord Injury Persons: A Novel Approach," *Telemedicine and e-Health* 12, no. 2 (2006): 160–2; Stanley M. Finkelstein, Stuart M. Speedie, and Sandra Potthof, "Home Telehealth Improves Clinical Outcomes at Lower Cost for Home Healthcare," *Telemedicine and e-Health* 12, no. 2 (2006): 128–36; Thomas S. Nesbitt, Stacy L. Cole, Lorraine Pellegrin, and Patricia Keast, "Rural Outreach in Home Telehealth: Assessing Challenges and Reviewing Successes," *Telemedicine and e-Health* 12, no. 2 (2006): 107–13.

69. John Markoff, "The Boss Is Robotic, and Rolling Up Behind You," September 4, 2010, http://www.nytimes.com/2010/09/05/science/05robots.html (accessed November 11, 2010); "Mobile Robots Offer New Ways to Assess Patients from Remote Locations," September 8, 2010, http://www.ihealthbeat.org/articles/2010/9/8/mobile-robots-offer-new-ways-to-assess-patients-from-remote-locations.aspx (accessed November 11. 2011); Justin Corr, "Robot Helps Patients with Checkups," February 2, 2011, http://www.ktvb.com/news/health/Patients-in-Idaho-and-Oregon-get-checkups-through-robot-115138214.html (accessed February 15, 2011).

70. Markoff, "The Boss Is Robotic, and Rolling Up Behind You."

71. Hilary Stout, "Technologies Help Adult Children Monitor Aging Parents," July 28, 2010, http://www.nytimes.com/2010/07/29/garden/29parents.html (accessed February 16, 2011).

72. Raphael Cariou, "Recent Trends in Tele-health," November 15, 2010, http://www.realityfrontier.com/tele-health-trends-2010/ (accessed April 2, 2011).

73. "Upstate Prison to Use Telemedicine for Mentally Ill Inmates," August 8, 2006, http://www.wistv.com/Global/story.asp?S=5256538 (accessed April 26, 2011).

74. Noriaki Aoki, Kim Dunn, Tsuguya Fukui, J. Robert Beck, William J. Schull, and Helen K. Li, "Cost-Effectiveness Analysis of Telemedicine to Evaluate Diabetic Retinopathy in a Prison Population," *Diabetes Care* 27, no. 5 (2004): 1095–101, http://care.diabetesjournals.org/content/27/5/1095.full (accessed April 26, 2011); John Gramlich, "Telemedicine: Lessons from State Prison," May 12, 2009, http://ts-si.org/medical-horizons/4755-telemedicine-lessons-from-state-prison.html (accessed April 9, 2011).

75. Cheryl Clark, "A Captive Audience—and Providers—Benefit from Telemedicine," February 3, 2010, http://www.healthleadersmedia.com/content/COM-245964/A-Captive-Audiencemdashand-ProvidersmdashBenefit-from-Telemedicine (accessed April 9, 2011).

76. James E. Gray, Charles Safran, Roger B. Davis, Grace Pompilio-Weitzner, Jane E. Stewart, Linda Zaccagnini, and DeWayne Pursley, "Baby CareLink: Using the Internet and Telemedicine to Improve Care for High-Risk Infants," July 3, 2000, http://pediatrics.aappublications.org/cgi/content/abstract/106/6/1318 (accessed April 26, 2011); "Baby CareLink Installed in Special Care Nurseries," December 3, 2002, http://www.news-releases.uiowa.edu/2002/december/1203baby-carelink.html (accessed April 26, 2011).

77. "Using Telemedicine to Save Babies' Vision," April 11, 2006, http://www.genengnews.com/news/bnitem.aspx?name=356247 (accessed April 26, 2011); "Clarity Medical Systems Announces Major Move into Adult Eye Care Market: Company to Introduce New Technology Aimed at Revamping How Eye Exams Are Performed," June 23, 2006, http://www.claritymsi.com/news/060623.html (accessed April 26, 2011).

78. "High Technology Improves Alzheimer's Care and Diagnosis," July 17, 2006, http://www.hoise.com/vmw/06/articles/vmw/LV-VM-08-06-17.html (accessed April 16, 2011).

79. "Rochester Expands Use of Telemedicine in Day Care Centers," May 5, 2005, http://www.ihealthbeat.org/index.cfm?Action=dspItem&itemID=110905 (accessed April 26, 2011).

80. Jennifer Nachbur, "Improving Major Trauma Survival in Vermont," November 8, 2001, http://www.uvm.edu/~uvmpr/?Page=News&storyID=3146 (accessed April 26, 2011); "Saving Lives with Teletrauma Video Communications: Trauma Surgeons Provide Consultative Services to Rural Communities Using State-of-the-Art Videoconferencing Technology," September 2005, http://findarticles.com/p/articles/mi_m0DUD/is_9_26/ai_n15377639/ (accessed April 26, 2011); "Southern Arizona Telemedicine and Telepresence (SATT) Program," 2007, http://umcaz.org/body.cfm?id=953 (accessed April 26, 2011).

81. Nancy Ferris, "The Missing Last Mile," April 17, 2006, http://www.govhealthit.com/news/missing-last-mile (accessed April 26, 2011).

82. "USDA to Award Grants for Telehealth Programs in Rural US Locations."

83. Ryoji Suzuki, Sakuto Otake, Takeshi Izutsu, Masaki Yoshida, and Tsutomu Iwaya, "Monitoring Daily Living Activities of Elderly People in a Nursing Home Using an Infrared Motion-Detection System," [Abstract] *Telemedicine and e-Health* 12, no. 2 (2006), http://www.ncbi. nlm.nih.gov/pubmed/16620169 (accessed April 26, 2011).

84. "Harnessing the Power of ICT for Health," May 2005, http://www.i4don-line.net/may05/healthNet.pdf (accessed April 26, 2011).

85. "Moving Information into the Hands of Those Who Heal: ICT for Health: Empowering Health Workers to Save Lives," May 21, 2009, http://www.health-net.org/ict (accessed April 11, 2011).

86. Jim Doyle, "Care Command Centers: Missouri Hospital System Leads the Way in Telemedicine," *The Sunday Star-Ledger*, April 3, 2011, section 3, 3.

87. Mark Cantrell, "Nurses Keep Watch for Miles Away or at the Bedside," January 10, 2005, *Nursing Spectrum*, http://community.nursingspectrum.com/MagazineArticles/article.cfm?AID=13378/ (accessed April 26, 2011); Robert A. Berenson, Joy M. Grossman, and Elizabeth A. November, "Do Does Telemonitoring of Patients—The eICU—Improve Intensive Care?" August 2009, *Health Affairs*, http://content. healthaffairs.org/content/28/5/w937.short (accessed April 10, 2011).

88. "ATA Emergency Prep and Response," 2007, http://media. americantelemed.org/ICOT/sigemergency.htm (accessed April 26, 2011); Andre Pennardt, "Blast Injuries," May 28, 2010, http://emedicine.medscape.com/article/822587-overview (accessed April 26, 2011); Erik Eckholm, "The New Kind of Care in a New Era of Casualties," January 31, 2006, http://www.nytimes.com/2006/01/31/national/31wounded. html (accessed April 26, 2011).

89. "E-Messaging Enhances Patient Satisfaction, Research Shows," August 15, 2005, http://www.health-itworld.com/newsletters/index_08172005.html (accessed April 26, 2011).

90. Naditz, "Medical Connectivity: New Frontiers: Telehealth Innovations of 2010," December 2010, *Telemedicine and e-Health* 16, no. 10 (December 2010): 990.

91. Ibid.

92. Ibid., 990–91.

93. Ibid., 989.

94. "FDA Approves Electronic Capsule for Stomach Disorder," July 21, 2006, http://www.ihealthbeat.org/articles/2006/7/21/FDA-Approves-Electronic-Capsule-for-Stomach-Disorder.aspx?topicID=53 (accessed April 26, 2011).

95. Rebecca J. Purc-Stephenson and Christine Thrasher, "Telenurses Struggle with Patient Care and Available Services: Nurses' Experiences with Telephone Triage and Advice: A Meta-Ethnography," *Journal of Advanced Nursing* 66, no. 3 (2010): 482–94, http://ts-si.org/healthcare/23129-telenurses-struggle-with-patient-care-and-available-services.html (accessed March 9, 2011).

96. James J. Egidio, "Online Doctor Visits? A Look at Telemedicine Trends of 2009," 2009, http://ezinearticles .com/?Online-Doctor-Visits?-A-Look-at-Telemedicine-Trends-of-2009&id=2669593 (accessed March 8, 2011).

97. Pauline W. Chen, "Are Doctors Ready for Virtual Visits?" January 7, 2010, http://www.nytimes.com/2010/01/07/health/07chen.html (accessed February 16, 2011); R. Iltifat Husein, "Withings WiFi Body Scale Can Now Wirelessly Sync with Your Smartphone's Personal Health Record App," February 15, 2011, http://www.imedicalapps.com/2011/02/withings-wifi-body-scale-wireless-personal-health-record/ (accessed February 16, 2011); Jane Sarasohn-Kahn, "How Smartphones Are Changing Healthcare for Consumers and Providers," April 2010, http://www.chcf.org/publications/2010/04/how-smartphones-are-changing-health-care-for-consumers-and-providers (accessed February 16, 2011); "Smartphone Apps for Health," December 6, 2010, http://thistimethisspace.com/2010/12/06/smartphone-apps-for-health/ (accessed February 16, 2011); R. Elizabeth and C. Kitchen, "iPhone Apps That Could Save Your Life," August 30, 2010, http://www.healthguideinfo.com/health-testing-technology/p85038/ (accessed February 16, 2011); "iPhone Takes Up a New and at the Same Time an Important Role in Application in India," September 8, 2010, http://technology.globalthoughtz.com (accessed March 3, 2011).

98. Cariou, "Recent Trends in Tele-health."

99. Ibid.

100. Carolyn Y. Johnson, " Device Linked to Smartphone Helps Diagnose Cancer: Early Trials Show Promising Results, Researchers Say," *The Boston Globe*, February 24, 2011, http://articles.boston.com/2011-02-24/business/29343388_1_ovarian-cancer-cancer-care-smartphone (accessed February 25, 2011).

101. Chen, "Are Doctors Ready for Virtual Visits?"; Husein, "Withings WiFi Body Scale Can Now Wirelessly Sync with Your Smartphone's Personal Health Record App"; Sarasohn-Kahn, "How Smartphones Are Changing Healthcare for Consumers and Providers"; "Smartphone Apps for Health"; Elizabeth and Kitchen, "iPhone Apps That Could Save Your Life"; "iPhone Takes Up a New and at the Same Time an Important Role in Application in India."

102. "New Mobile Can Check Pulse, Send Ambulance," February 17, 2011, http://www.physorg.com/print217169 458.html (accessed March 2, 2011).

103. Naditz, "Medical Connectivity: New Frontiers: Telehealth Innovations of 2010."

104. Ryan Faas, "How the iPad Is Changing Mobile Health Care," October 5, 2010, http://www.enterprisemobiletoday.com/features/management/article.php/3906771/How-the-iPad-is-Changing-Mobile-Health-Care.htm (accessed February 16, 2011); Martha C. White, "With the iPad, Apple May Just Revolutionize Health Care," April 11, 2010, http://www.washingtonpost.com/wp-dyn/content/article/2010/04/09/AR2010040906341.html (accessed February 16, 2011); Iltifat Husein, "The First Interactive

Medical Textbook for the iPad: Ganong's Review of Medical Physiology," February 15, 2011, http://www.imedicalapps.com/2011/02/medical-textbook-ipad-ganong-medical-physiology-app-review-learning/ (accessed February 16, 2011); Felasfa Wpodajo, "Scutsheet Aims to Help Students Replace Their Note Cards with iPads to Better Track Their Inpatients," February 9, 2011, http://www.imedicalapps.com/2011/02/scutsheet-aims-to-help-students-and-residents-replace-their-note-cards-with-ipads-to-better-track-their-inpatients/ (accessed February 16, 2011); Amit Patel, "Lexi-Complete Clinical Reference Medical App Reviewed for the iPhone and iPad: Worth the Cost?" February 8, 2011. http://www.imedicalapps.com/2011/02/lexi-comp-app-review-iphone-medical/ (accessed February 16, 2011); Pamela Lewis, "Health Care Embraces the iPad: Doctors Jump on New Technology," 2011, http://www.ama-assn.org/amednews/m/2011/02/07/bsa0207.htm (accessed February 16, 2011).

105. Molly Merrill, "PwC Survey: Three in 10 Americans Would Track PHI with Their Phones," September 7, 2010, http://www.healthcareitnews.com/news/pwc-survey-three-10-americans-would-track-phi-their-phones (accessed November 11, 2010).

106. Sarasohn-Kahn, "The Connected Patient: Charting the Vital Signs of Remote Health Monitoring."

107. J Healthc Manag. 2010 Sep-Oct;55(5):312-22; discussion 322-3. A randomized trial of telemonitoring heart failure patients. Tompkins C, Orwat J.

108. Ibid.

109. Ibid.

110. Ibid.

111. Ibid.

112. Berenson, Grossman, and November, "Do Does Telemonitoring of Patients—The eICU—Improve Intensive Care?"

113. Carolyn Bloch, "Telemedicine Issues Discussed." March 30, 2011. http://telemedicinenews.blogspot.com/2011/03/telemedicine-issues-discussed.html (accessed April 9, 2011).

114. "Telemedicine and Telehealth," August 23, 2010, http://www.cms.gov/Telehealth/ (accessed November 12, 2010); "Telemedicine Services Expanded under Medicare, Mandated in 12 States," 2010, http://www.aapa.org (accessed November 12, 2010); K. Romanow and J. A. Brannon, "Telepractice Reimbursement Is Still Limited," November 2, 2010, *The ASHA Leader*, http://www.asha.org/Publications/leader/2010/101102/BottomLine-101102/ (accessed Apri 26, 2011); Sarasohn-Kahn, "The Connected Patient: Charting the Vital Signs of Remote Health Monitoring."

115. "Medicare Making Changes to Acknowledge Telemedicine's Growing Use," November 22, 2010, http://www.kaiserhealthnews.org/Daily-Report.aspx?reportdate=11-22-2010#Health Information Technology-0 (accessed March 3, 2011).

116. Farrell, "Telemedicine Progress Advances."

117. Sarasohn-Kahn, "The Connected Patient: Charting the Vital Signs of Remote Health Monitoring."

118. "Healthcare Licensing Services," 2011, Healthcare Licensing.com (accessed March 9, 2011).

119. Jason Gaya, " Telemedicine—Enhancing Network Security to Achieve HIPAA Compliance," March 18, 2010, http://ezinearticles.com/?Telemedicine--Enhancing-Network-Security-to-Achieve-HIPAA-Compliance&id=3950233 (accessed April 9, 2011).

120. Chen, "Are Doctors Ready for Virtual Visits?"

121. Nicole Lewis, "Telemedicine Searches for Strategy, Adoption," April 28, 2010, http://www.informationweek.com/news/ 224700094 (accessed March 7, 2011).

# Additional Resources

Ahmed S. N., S. Weibe, C. S, Mann, C., and A. Ohinmaa. "Telemedicine and Epilepsy Care." [Abstract] November 2010. http://www.ncbi.nlm.nih.gov/pubmed/21059544 ncbi.nlm.nih.gov (accessed April 9, 2011).

Aitken, Robyn L., Robyn Faulkner, Tracey Bucknall, and Judith Parker. "Literature Review on Aspects of Nursing Education: The Types of Skills and Knowledge Required to Meet the Changing Needs of the Labour Force Involved in Nursing." December 14, 2001. http://www.dest.gov.au/archive/highered/nursing/pubs/aspects_nursing/1.htm (accessed April 26, 2011).

"Anatomic Telepathology Network." August 28, 2008. http://www.cost.eu/domains_actions/ict/Actions/IC0604 (accessed April 9, 2011).

Audebert, Heinrich J., Thomas Meyer, and Fabian Klostermann. "Potentials of Telemedicine for Green Health Care." http://www.frontiersin.org/teleneurology/10.3389/fneur.2010.00010/abstract (accessed March 2, 2011).

Austen, Ian. "For the Doctor's Touch, Help in the Hand." August 22, 2002. http://query.nytimes.com/gst/fullpage.html?res=9A0CE2DD163CF931A1575BC0A9649C8B63 (accessed April 26, 2011).

Baby CareLink in the News. "Iowa Hospitals to Use CST's Baby CareLink to Improve Care of Premature Infants." December 3, 2002. http://www.babycarelink.com/news (accessed April 26, 2011).

Backman, W, D. Bendel, and R. Rakhit. "The Telecardiology Revolution: Improving the Management of Cardiac Disease in

Primary Care." November 2010. *Journal of the Royal Society of Medicine.* http://www.ncbi.nlm.nih.gov/pubmed/20959351 (accessed March 2, 2011).

Berenson, Robert A., Joy M. Grossman, and Elizabeth A. November. "Does Telemonitoring of Patients—The eICU—Improve Intensive Care?" August 2009. *Health Affairs.* http://content.healthaffairs.org/content/28/5/w937.short (accessed April 10, 2011).

Bloch, Carolyn. "Telemedicine Issues Discussed." March 30, 2011. http://telemedicinenews.blogspot.com/2011/03/telemedicine-issues-discussed.html (accessed April 9, 2011).

Brunetti, Natale Daniele, Luisa De Gennaro, Gianfranco Amodio, Giulia Dellegrottaglie, Pier Luigi Pellegrino, Matteo Di Biase, and Gianfranco Antonelli. "Telecardiology Improves Quality of Diagnosis and Reduces Delay to Treatment in Elderly Patients with Acute Myocardial Infarction and Atypical Presentation." [Abstract] August 9, 2009. http://www.ncbi.nlm.nih.gov/pubmed/20729737 (accessed April 9, 2011).

Burg, Gunter. "Store-and-Forward Teledermatology." August 25, 2005. http://www.emedicine.com/derm/topic560.htm (accessed April 25, 2011).

Cariou, Raphael. "Recent Trends in Tele-Health." November 15, 2010. http://www.realityfrontier.com/tele-health-trends-2010/ (accessed April 2, 2011).

Carlson, Trisha. "Highlighting Telemedicine." May/June 2009. *Todays Wound Clinic.* http://www.todayswoundclinic.com/highlighting-telemedicine-0 (accessed November 12, 2010).

Chen, Pauline W. "Are Doctors Ready for Virtual Visits?" January 7, 2010. http://www.nytimes.com/2010/01/07/health/07chen.html (accessed February 16, 2011).

Clark, Cheryl. "A Captive Audience—and Providers—Benefit from Telemedicine." February 3, 2010. http://www.healthleadersmedia.com/content/COM-245964/A-Captive-Audiencemdashand-ProvidersmdashBenefit-from-Telemedicine (accessed April 9, 2011).

Corr, Justin. "Robot Helps Patients with Checkups." February 2, 2011. http://www.ktvb.com/news/health/Patients-in-Idaho-and-Oregon-get-checkups-through-robot-115138214.html (accessed February 15, 2011).

"Department of Corrections Brief History." http://www.vadoc.state.va.us/about/history.shtm (accessed April 26, 2011).

"Detailed Technology Analysis, Tele-Stroke New England Health Care Institute." June 2009. http://search.yahoo.com/r/_ylt=A0oG7lbJNTpP6wUAH4VXNyoA;_ylu=X3oDMTE1amNkODF2BHNlYwNzcgRwb3MDMQRjb2xvA2FjMgR2dGlkA1ZJUDA3N18yNTI-/SIG=1389qc4k3/EXP=1329243721/**http%3a//www.nehi.net/uploads/full_report/detailed_technology_analysis__telestroke.pdf (accessed March 2, 2011).

Dobke, Marek, Alicja Renkielska, Joan De Neve, James Chao, and Dhaval Bhavsar. "Telemedicine for Problematic Wound Management: Enhancing Communication Between Long-Term Care, Skilled Nursing, and Home Caregiver." September 4, 2001. http://www.woundsresearch.com/article/ (accessed March 3, 2011).

Doolittle, G. C., A. Allen, C. Wittman, E. Carlson, and P. Whitten. "Oncology Care for Rural Kansans via Telemedicine: The Establishment of a Teleoncology Practice (Meeting Abstract)." 1996. http://www.asco.org/portal/site/ASCO/template.ERROR/;jsessionid=H1NrHhql9VtMhGpGZZF7qCs2GZP7rT2VfZyfhQY7QWz9Bc0xTpyq!-1886814676 (accessed April 26, 2011).

Doolittle, G. C., A. R. Williams, and D. J. Cook. "An Estimation of Costs of a Pediatric Telemedicine Practice in Public Schools." *Medical Care* 41, no. 1 (2003): 100–9. http://www.ncbi.nlm.nih.gov/sites/entrez?db=pubmed&uid=12544547&cmd=showdetailview (accessed April 25, 2011).

Doyle, Jim. "Care Command Centers: Missouri Hospital System Leads the Way in Telemedicine." *The Sunday Star-Ledger.* April 3, 2011, section 3, 3.

Elizabeth, R., and C. Kitchen. "iPhone Apps That Could Save Your Life." August 30, 2010. http://www.healthguideinfo.com/health-testing-technology/p85038/ (accessed February 16, 2011),

"Enhancing Vermont's Healthcare Delivery System: Telemedicine Child Psychiatry." Winter 2010. http://www.bistatepca.org/VT-Government-Relations/Telemedicine-Child-Psychiatry-Winter-Spring-2008.pdf (accessed February 16, 2011).

Faas, Ryan. "How the iPad Is Changing Mobile Health Care." October 5, 2010. http://www.enterprisemobiletoday.com/features/management/article.php/3906771/How-the-iPad-is-Changing-Mobile-Health-Care.htm (accessed February 16, 2011).

Farrell, John. "Telemedicine Progress Advances." January 26, 2011. http://www.mhimss.org/blog/telemedicine-progress-advances (accessed March 3, 2011).

"Federal Legislative Issues Update—July 2005." The Stop Stroke Act. July 27, 2005. http://www.arota.org/pdfs/July2005legupdate.pdf (accessed April 26, 2011).

"Federal Telemedicine Legislation 105th Congress." Arent Fox. http://www.thecre.com/fedlaw/legal17/105.htm (accessed April 26, 2011).

Fornell, Dave. "Telecardiology Growth Mainly in Infant Congenital Heart Disease." March–April, 2009. http://www.dicardiology.com/article/telecardiology-growth-mainly-infant-congenital-heart-disease (accessed March 2, 2011).

Gaya, Jason. "Telemedicine—Enhancing Network Security to Achieve HIPAA Compliance." March 18, 2010. http://ezinearticles.com/?Telemedicine---Enhancing-Network-Security-to-Achieve-HIPAA-Compliance&id=3950233 (accessed April 9, 2011).

"Globalmedia, NeuroCall, Reach Call Partner to Provide Fully Integrated Telemedicine Solution." September 21, 2009. http://www.neurocall.com/press.html (accessed April 9, 2011).

Goldberg, Howard S., and Alfredo Morales. "Improving Information Prescription to Parents of Premature Infants through An OWLBased Knowledge Mediator." 2004. citeseerx.ist.psu.edu/viewdoc/download?doi=10.1.1.112.8988 (accessed April 26, 2011).

Goldfield, G. S., and A. Boachie. "Delivery of Family Therapy in the Treatment of Anorexia Nervosa Using Telehealth: A Case Report." November 1, 2003. http://www.hawaii.edu/hivandaids/Case_Report_Delivery_of_Family_Therapy_in_the_Tx_of_Anorexia_Using_Telehealth.pdf (accessed April 26, 2011).

Gramlich, John. "Telemedicine: Lessons from State Prison." May 12, 2009. http://ts-si.org/medical-horizons/4755-tele-medicine-lessons-from-state-prison.html (accessed April 9, 2011).

Gray, James E., Charles Safran, Roger B. Davis, Grace Pompilio-Weitzner, Jane E. Stewart, Linda Zaccagnini, and DeWayne Pursley. "Baby CareLink: Using the Internet and Telemedicine to Improve Care for High-Risk Infants." July 3, 2000. http://pediatrics.aappublications.org/cgi/content/abstract/106/6/1318 (accessed April 26, 2011).

"Groups Urge CMS to Cover Teledermatology Under Medicare Part B." March 1, 2011. http://www.ihealthbeat.org/articles/2011/3/1/groups-urge-cms-to-cover-teledermatology-under-medicare-part-b.aspx (accessed April 9, 2011).

Hafner, Katie. "'Dear Doctor' Meets 'Return to Sender.'" June 6, 2002. http://query.nytimes.com/gst/fullpage.html?res=9C0CE1DC1F3AF935A35755C0A9649C8B63 (accessed April 26, 2011).

"Healthcare Licensing Services." 2011. HealthcareLicensing.com (accessed March 9, 2011).

Heuser, Stephen. "'Telehealth' Systems Slowly Gaining: Devices Help Curb Visits to Hospital." July 26, 2006. http://www.boston.com/yourlife/health/aging/articles/2006/07/26/tele-health_systems_slowly_gaining/ (accessed April 25, 2011).

Higginbotham, Stacey. "Will U.S. TeleMedicine Be DOA?" February 23, 2010. http://gigaom.com/2010/02/23/will-u-s-telemedicine-be-doa/ (accessed February 16, 2011).

"History of Stethoscopes and Sphygmomanometers." October 7, 2003. http://www.hhmi.org/biointeractive/museumexhibit98/content/b6_17info.html (accessed April 26, 2011).

Hoffmann, Allan. "Is There a Doctor in the Net." *Star-Ledger*, April 6, 1998, 21, 25.

Husein, Iltifat. "The First Interactive Medical Textbook for the iPad: Ganong's Review of Medical Physiology." February 15, 2011. http://www.imedicalapps.com/2011/02/medical-textbook-ipad-ganong-medical-physiology-app-review-learning/ (accessed February 16, 2011).

Husein, R. Iltifat. "Withings WiFi Body Scale Can Now Wirelessly Sync with Your Smartphone's Personal Health Record App." February 15, 2011. http://www.imedicalapps.com/2011/02/withings-wifi-body-scale-wireless-personal-health-record/ (accessed February 16, 2011).

"iPhone Takes Up a New and at the Same Time an Important Role in Application in India." September 8, 2010. http://technology.globalthoughtz.com (accessed March 3, 2011).

Jeffrey, Susan. "Telemedicine System May Increase tPA Use in Stroke." July 17, 2007. http://www.medscape.com/view-article/559914 (accessed April 26, 2011).

Johnson, Carolyn Y. "Device Linked to Smartphone Helps Diagnose Cancer: Early Trials Show Promising Results, Researchers Say." *The Boston Globe.* February 24, 2011. http://articles.boston.com/2011-02-24/business/29343388_1_ovarian-cancer-cancer-care-smartphone (accessed February 25, 2011).

Joseph, Amelia M. "Care Coordination and Telehealth Technology in Promoting Self-Management Among Chronically Ill Patients." *Telemedicine and e-Health* 12, no. 2 (2006): 156–9.

Kim, Hyungjin, Julie C. Lowery, Jennifer B. Hamill, and Edwin G. Wilkins. "Patient Attitudes Toward a Web-Based System for Monitoring Wounds." [Abstract] *Telemedicine Journal and e-Health* 10, no. 2 (2004): S-26–34. http://deepblue.lib.umich.edu/handle/2027.42/63370 (accessed April 26, 2011).

Kowalczyk, Liz. "Going the Distance in Stroke Treatment." *Boston Globe*. April 3, 2006. http://www.boston.com/yourlife/health/diseases/articles/2006/04/03/going_the_distance_in_stroke_treatment/ (accessed April 26, 2011).

"Latest News in Minimally Invasive Medicine." Society of Interventional Radiology. March 23, 2006. http://www.news-wise.com/articles/view/518995/ (accessed December 28, 2007).

Lesher, Jack L., Jr., L. S. Davis, F. W. Gourdin, D. English, and W. O. Thompson. "Telemedicine Evaluation of Cutaneous Diseases: A Blinded Comparative Study." [Abstract] *The Journal of the American Academy of Dermatology* 38, no. 1 (1998). http://www.ncbi.nlm.nih.gov/sites/entrez?db=pubmed&uid=9448201&cmd=showdetailview (accessed April 26, 2011).

Lewis, Carol. "Emerging Trends in Medical Device Technology: Home Is Where the Heart Monitor Is." *FDA Consumer*. May–June 2001. http://findarticles.com/p/articles/mi_m1370/is_3_35/ai_75608871/ http://www.fda.gov/Fdac/features/2001/301_home.html (accessed April 26, 2011).

Lewis, Nicole. "Telemedicine Searches for Strategy, Adoption." April 28, 2010. http://www.informationweek.com/news/224700094 (accessed March 7, 2011).

Lewis, Pamela. "Health Care Embraces the iPad: Doctors Jump on New Technology." 2011. http://www.ama-assn.org/amednews/m/2011/02/07/bsa0207.htm (accessed February 16, 2011).

Lohr, Steve. "AT&T's Bet on Health Technology." November 4, 2010. http://bits.blogs.nytimes.com/2010/11/04/atts-bet-on-health-technology/ (accessed February 16, 2011).

Maddox, Peggy Jo. "Ethics and the Brave New World of E-Health." November 21, 2002. http://www.nursingworld.org/Main MenuCategories/ANAMarketplace/ANAPeriodicals/OJIN/Columns/Ethics/Ethicsandehealth.aspx (accessed April 26, 2011).

Markoff, John. "The Boss Is Robotic, and Rolling Up Behind You." September 4, 2010. http://www.nytimes.com/2010/09/05/science/05robots.html (accessed March 11, 2010).

"Medicare Making Changes to Acknowledge Telemedicine's Growing Use." November 22, 2010. http://www.kaiserhealthnews.org/Daily-Report.aspx?reportdate=11-22-2010#Health Information Technology-0 (accessed March 3, 2011).

Merrill, Molly. "Interest in Telestroke Care Runs High." September 13, 2010. http://www.healthcareitnews.com/news/interest-telestroke-care-runs-high (accessed March 2, 2011).

Merrill, Molly. "PwC Survey: Three in 10 Americans Would Track PHI with Their Phones." September 7, 2010. http://www.healthcareitnews.com/news/pwc-survey-three-10-americans-would-track-phi-their-phones (accessed November 11, 2010).

Meserve, Jason. "Telemedicine Helps Victims of Stroke." May 23, 2005. http://www.networkworld.com/news/2005/052305-stroke.html (accessed April 25, 2011).

Miller, Claire Cain. "The Virtual Visit May Expand Access to Doctors." December 21, 2009. http://www.nytimes.com/2009/12/21/technology/start-ups/21doctors.html (accessed February 16, 2011).

"Mobile Robots Offer New Ways to Assess Patients from Remote Locations." September 8, 2010. http://www.ihealthbeat.org/articles/2010/9/8/mobile-robots-offer-new-ways-to-assess-patients-from-remote-locations.aspx (accessed November 11. 2011).

Montana Office of Rural Health. "Rural Community-Based Home Health Care and Support Services—A White Paper." [Abstract] August 2001. http://jobfunctions.bnet.com/abstract.aspx?docid=103613 (accessed April 26, 2011).

"Moving Information into the Hands of Those Who Heal: ICT for Health: Empowering Health Workers to Save Lives." May 21, 2009. http://www.healthnet.org/ict (accessed April 11, 2011).

Murphy, Kate. "Telemedicine Getting a Test in Efforts to Cut Costs of Treating Prisoners." *New York Times,* June 8, 1998, D5.

Nacci, Peter. U.S. Department of Justice Office of Justice Programs, National Institute of Justice. "Telemedicine." March 1999. http://www.ncjrs.gov/telemedicine/toc.html (accessed April 26, 2011).

Naditz, Alan. "Medical Connectivity: New Frontiers: Telehealth Innovations of 2010." December 2010. *Telemedicine and e-Health* 16, no. 10 (2010). http://www.himss.org/content/files/Code%20491_New%20Frontiers_Telehealth%20Innovations%20of%202010.pdf (accessed April 26, 2011).

Nelson, E. L., M. Barnard, and S. Cain. "Treating Childhood Depression over Videoconferencing." *Telemedicine Journal and e-Health Spring* 9, no. 1 (2003): 49–55. http://ebook-browse.com/treating-childhood-depression-over-videoconferencing-pdf-d41415583 (accessed April 26, 2011).

"NeuroCall Conducts 400th Teleconsultation in El Paso, TX." February 8, 2011. http://www.neurocall.com/press.html (accessed April 9, 2011).

"New Mobile Can Check Pulse, Send Ambulance." February 17, 2011. http://www.physorg.com/print217169458.html (accessed March 2, 2011).

Ng, C. H., and J. F. Yeo. "The Role of Internet and Personal Digital Assistant in Oral and Maxillofacial Pathology." July 2004. http://annals.edu.sg/pdf200409/V33N4p50S.pdf (accessed April 26, 2011).

"NLM National Telemedicine Initiative Summaries of Awards Announced October 1996." October 1996. http://www.nlm.nih.gov/research/initprojsum.html (accessed April 26, 2011).

Office of Health and the Information Highway, Health Canada. "How Canadian eHealth Initiatives Are Changing the Face of Healthcare: Success Stories." August 2002. http://www.hc-sc.gc.ca/hcs-sss/pubs/ehealth-esante/2002-succes/index_e.html (accessed April 26, 2011).

Office of Telemedicine. "Department of Corrections Brief History." http://www.vadoc.virginia.gov/about/history.shtm (accessed April 26, 2011).

Ohio Department of Rehabilitation and Correction. "Telemedicine." March 13, 2006. http://www.drc.state.oh.us/web/telemed.htm (accessed April 26, 2011).

Ong, C. A. "Telemedicine and Wound Care." [Abstract] 2008. http://www.ncbi.nlm.nih.gov/pubmed/18305332 (accessed March 3, 2011).

"Outsourcing Radiology Services to India." 2011. http://www.outsource2india.com/services/radiology.asp (accessed April 9, 2011).

Paar, David. "Telemedicine in Practice: Texas Department of Criminal Justice." UTMB Correctional Managed Care. May 2000. http://www.aegis.com/pubs/hepp/2000/HEPP2000-0501.html (accessed April 26, 2011).

Patel, Amit. "Lexi-Complete Clinical Reference Medical App Reviewed for the iPhone and iPad: Worth the Cost?" February 8, 2011. http://www.imedicalapps.com/2011/02/lexi-comp-app-review-iphone-medical/ (accessed February 16, 2011).

Patterson, V., J. Humphreys, and R. Chua. "Teleneurology by Email." *Journal of Telemedicine and Telecare* 9, no. 2 (2003): S42–3. http://www.ncbi.nlm.nih.gov/sites/entrez?

cmd=Retrieve&db=PubMed&list_uids=14728758&dopt=
AbstractPlus (accessed April 26, 2011).

Patterson, Victor, and Richard Wooten. "How Can Teleneurology
Improve Patient Care?" July 17, 2006. http://www.medscape.
com/viewarticle/540191 (accessed April 26, 2011).

Purc-Stephenson, Rebecca J., and Christine Thrasher.
"Telenurses Struggle with Patient Care and Available
Services: Nurses' Experiences with Telephone Triage and
Advice: A Meta-Ethnography." *Journal of Advanced Nursing*
66, no. 3 (2010): 482–494. http://ts-si.org/healthcare/23129-
telenurses-struggle-with-patient-care-and-available-ser
vices.html (accessed March 9, 2011).

Pyke, Bob. "Research, Training, and Practical Applications:
A Look at Developing Programs at the University of Texas
Medical Branch at Galveston." Interview with Vincent E.
Friedewald, 2003. http://my.opera.com/OceanStarz/blog/
index.dml/tag/RESEARCH%20TRAINING%20
PRACTICAL%20APPLICATIONS%20LOOK%20
AT%20D (accessed April 26, 2011).

Ramo, Joshua Cooper. "Doc in a Box." *Time,* Fall 1996, 55–57.

"Remote Telemedicine for Epilepsy." 2011. https://www.epi-
lepsy.com/epilepsy/telemedicine (accessed April 9, 2011).

Romanow, K., and J. A. Brannon. "Telepractice Reimbursement
Is Still Limited." November 2, 2010. *The ASHA Leader.*
http://www.asha.org/Publications/leader/2010/101102/
Bottom-Line-101102/ (accessed April 26, 2011).

Sarasohn-Kahn, Jane. "The Connected Patient: Charting the
Vital Signs of Remote Health Monitoring." February 2022.
http://www.chcf.org/publications/2011/02/the-connected-
patient (accessed April 9, 2011).

Sarasohn-Kahn, Jane. "How Smartphones Are Changing
Healthcare for Consumers and Providers." April 2010. http://
www.chcf.org/publications/2010/04/how-smartphones-
are-changing-health-care-for-consumers-and-providers
(accessed February 16, 2011).

"Secretary Shalala Announces National Telemedicine
Initiative." 1996. http://www.nih.gov/news/pr/oct96/nlm-08.
htm (accessed April 26, 2011).

Shepard, Scott. "Telemedicine Brings Memphis Healing to
Third-World Patients." January 17, 2003. http://memphis.
bizjournals.com/memphis/stories/2003/01/20/story4.html
(accessed April 26, 2011).

"'Smart' Fabrics to Keep Patients Healthy." March 16, 2005.
http://www.medicalnewstoday.com/articles/21338.php
(accessed April 26, 2011).

"Smartphone Apps for Health." December 6, 2010. http://thistime
thisspace.com/2010/12/06/smartphone-apps-for-health/
(accessed February 16, 2011).

Stout, Hilary. "Technologies Help Adult Children Monitor Aging
Parents." July 28, 2010. http://www.nytimes.com/2010/07/
29/garden/29parents.html (accessed February 16, 2011).

Struber, Janet C. "An Introduction to Telemedicine and Email
Consultations." July 2004. http://ijahsp.nova.edu/articles/Vol2
number3/telemedicine_Struber.htm (accessed April 26, 2011).

"Telecardiology." *Telemedicine Today.* 2002. http://www2.
telemedtoday.com/articles/telecardiology.shtml (accessed
April 26, 2011).

"Telemedicine." June 30, 2010. http://searchhealthit.techtar-
get.com/definition/telemedicine (accessed April 25, 2011).

"Telemedicine and Telehealth." August 23, 2010. http://www.
cms.gov/Telehealth/ (accessed November 12, 2010).

"Telemedicine Can Help Address Mental Health Needs of
Elderly Homebound Individuals." October 2010. http://
www.news-medical.net/news/20101004/Telemedicine-can-
help-address-mental-health-needs-of-elderly-homebound-
individuals.aspx (accessed February 18, 2011).

"Telemedicine Defined." 2010. http://www.americantelemed.
org/i4a/pages/index.cfm?pageID=3333 (accessed April 25,
2011).

"Telemedicine for Psychiatry." June 9, 2006. http://medgadget.
com/archives/2006/06/telemedicine_fo_1.html (accessed
April 26, 2011).

"Telemedicine Report to Congress." January 31, 1997. http://
www.ntia.doc.gov/reports/telemed/intro.htm (accessed April
26, 2011).

"Telemedicine Trends and Technologies." February 8, 2010.
http://www.impact-advisors.com/UserFiles/file/IA%20
Telemedicine%20Overview%2020100208.pdf (accessed
February 18, 2011).

"Telepathology Page." http://www.hoslink.com/telepathology.
htm (accessed August 22, 2006).

"Telepsychiatry Helps Address Mental Health Worker Shortage."
September 10, 2008. http://www.ihealthbeat.org/articles/
2008/9/10/Telepsychiatry-Helps-Address-Mental-Health-
Worker-Shortage.aspx?topicID=60 (accessed February 16,
2011).

Thielst, Christina Beach. "Health Information Exchange
and Telehealth Netweoks: Opportunities for Leveraging
Resources." 2010. http://www.himss.org/ASP/topics_News_
item.asp?cid=75399&tid=33 (accessed March 9, 2011).

"Top 10 Medical Innovations for 2011: #6 Telehealth
Monitoring for Individuals with Heart Failure/Implanted
Wireless Cardiac Device for Monitoring Heart Failure." 2010.
http://www.clevelandclinic.org/innovations/summit2010/
topten11/six.html (February 28, 2011).

Tufts University Department of Medicine. "Massachusetts
Telehealth Access Program." 2001. http://www.ntia.doc.
gov/otiahome/top/research/exemplary/tufts.htm (accessed
April 26, 2011).

Turisco, Fran, and F. Jane Metzger. "Technology Use in
Rural Health Care: California Survey Results." April 2003.

http://www.chcf.org/documents/hospitals/RuralHealth CareSurvey.pdf (accessed April 26, 2011).

Turner, Jeanine. "Telepsychiatry as a Case Study of Presence: Do You Know What You Are Missing?" *Journal of Computer-Mediated Communication* 6, no. 4 (2001). http://jcmc.indiana.edu/vol6/issue4/turner.html (accessed April 26, 2011).

Tye, Larry. "A High-Tech Link to Boston Aids Vineyard Stroke Victims." July 10, 2001. http://www.highbeam.com/doc/1P2-8663847.html (accessed April 26, 2011).

"USDA to Award Grants for Telehealth Programs in Rural US Locations." January 25, 2011. http://www.ihealthbeat.org/articles/2011/1/25/usda-to-award-grants-for-telehealth-programs-in-rural-us-locations.aspx (accessed April 9, 2011).

"VA Announces Budget Request for 2012." February 14, 2011. http://www.va.gov/opa/pressrel/pressrelease.cfm?id=2054 (accessed March 26, 2011).

VA Technology Assessment Program Short Report. "Physiologic Telemonitoring in CHF." January 2001. http://www.va.gov/VATAP/docs/PhysiologicMontioringCHF2001tm.pdf (accessed April 26, 2011).

"Virtual Colonoscopy and Teleradiology Bring Colorectal Cancer Screening to Patients in Rural Areas." October 21, 2010. http://esciencenews.com/articles/2010/10/21/virtual.colonoscopy.and.teleradiology.bring.colorectal.cancer.screening.patients.rural.areas (accessed March 2, 2011).

Wachter, Glenn W. "HIPAA's Privacy Rule Summarized: What Does It Mean for Telemedicine?" February 23, 2001. http://www.connected-health.org/policy/federal-and-state/external-resources/hipaa's-privacy-rule-summarized-what-does-it-mean-for-telemedicine.aspx (accessed April 26, 2011).

White, Martha C. "With the iPad, Apple May Just Revolutionize Health Care." April 11, 2010. http://www.washingtonpost.com/wp-dyn/content/article/2010/04/09/AR2010040906341.html (accessed February 16, 2011).

"Wound Care Solutions Telemedicine." 2011. http://wound-caresolutions-telemedicine.co.uk (accessed March 3, 2011).

Wpodajo, Felasfa. "Scutsheet Aims to Help Students Replace Their Note Cards with iPads to Better Track Their Inpatients." February 9, 2011. http://www.imedicalapps.com/2011/02/scutsheet-aims-to-help-students-and-residents-replace-their-note-cards-with-ipads-to-better-track-their-inpatients/ (accessed February 16, 2011).

"X-Rays Outsourced to India." 2011. http://health.indiatimes.com/articleshow/1435209.cms (accessed April 25, 2011).

# Related Web Sites

The American Telemedicine Association (http://www.atmeda.org) is a nonprofit association "promoting greater access to medical care via telecommunications technology." It provides almost unlimited information on the latest developments in telemedicine.

Arent Fox (http://www.arentfox.com) is an excellent source of information on legislative matters relating to telemedicine.

The National Library of Medicine (http://www.nlm.nih.gov) can provide you with access to a great deal of information, including bibliographies.

*Telemedicine and Telehealth Networks: The Newsmagazine of Distance Healthcare* (http://www.telemedmag.com) is a journal covering the field. Online access to past issues is free.

PEARSON
**myhealthprofessionskit**

Go to www.myhealthprofessionskit.com to access the Companion Web site created for this textbook. Simply select "Basic Health Science" from the choice of disciplines. Find this book and register to access self-assessment quizzes, flashcards, and more.

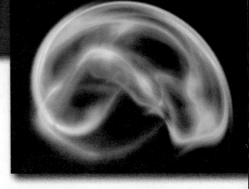

# Information Technology in Public Health

- Chapter Summary
- Key Terms
- Review Exercises
- Notes
- Additional Resources
- Related Web Sites

## LEARNING OBJECTIVES

Upon completion of this chapter, the reader will be able to:

- Define the field of public health and public health informatics.
- Discuss the impact of inequality on health.
- Discuss the use of computers in the study of disease.
- Define epidemics and pandemics, and the role of computers and statistics in their study.
- Define computer modeling of disease.
- Define global warming and its effects.
- Discuss Hurricane Katrina (2005); the Deepwater Horizon oil spill (2010); and the earthquake, tsunami, and radiation disaster in Japan (2011) as public health issues.

## INTRODUCTION

### Definition

**Public health** has many definitions. John M. Barry, writing on the flu pandemic of 1918–1919, states that public health "is where the largest numbers of lives are saved, usually by understanding the epidemiology of a disease—its patterns, where and how it emerges and spreads—and attacking it at its weak points. This can lead to prevention by means of public health measures like better sanitation, or providing cleaner water. It can also lead to the development and widespread distribution of vaccinations."[1] **Epidemiology** refers to "the study of diseases in populations by collecting and analyzing statistical data."[2] The collection of data on infectious diseases and their spatial and temporal patterns is crucial to public health. National Institutes of Health researchers attempt to do this with pocket personal computers (PCs) and Global Positioning Systems (GPS). The data (geographical location, symptoms, digital images, and class status) are automatically sent to a database.[3]

Even simple measures like advising people to wash their hands, not to share eating utensils and dishes, and to cover their mouths when they cough can have an effect on the spread of some diseases. The effects of quarantine have been questionable in some instances and effective in others.[4] Public measures like decent sanitation can also affect the spread of disease. In 2010, researchers reported that, worldwide, 7 percent of disease can be traced to "unsafe sanitation and drinking water, together with poor hygiene." Two million child deaths per year could be prevented by "improv[ing] hygiene, sanitation, and water supply." This is mostly a problem of rural areas in poor developing countries.[5]

The field of public health is very broad. It includes the care of the environment (water, earth, and air). **Public health informatics** supports public health practice and research with information technology. *The New York Times* reported in 2006 that "10 million people [were] at risk from pollution." Those living in the 10 most polluted cities in the world (Chernobyl, Ukraine; Dzerzhinsk, Russia; Haina, Dominican Republic; Kabwe, Zambia; La Oroya, Peru; Linfen, China; Maiuu Suu, Kyrgyzstan; Norilsk, Russia; Ranipet, India; and Rudnaya Pristan/Dalnegorsk, Russia) are at risk from "poisoning . . . cancers, lung infections, [and] mental retardation." In the Russian city of Dzerzhinsk, which was a center of chemical weapons manufacture, the population (300,000) has a life expectancy of 42 years for men and 47 years for women.[6] An extensive study issued in 2010 focused on six pollutants worldwide (lead, mercury, chromium, arsenic, pesticides, and radionuclides) that impact on health. In developing countries, "the health of roughly 100 million people is at risk." These six pollutants pose specific risks to both physical and mental health. They can cause "organ dysfunction, neurological disorders, developmental problems for . . . fetuses and children, cancers, and . . . death." They can also cause the immune system to deteriorate, leaving people susceptible respiratory infections, gastrointestinal problems, tuberculosis, and other disorders. These pollutants can be cleaned up, according to the report.[7]

Public health includes the health issue of tobacco use, planning for natural disaster, protecting food supply, and the identification and prevention or containment of epidemics. We have chosen to focus on just a few of these areas: using computers to study disease and to model disease; global warming; new diseases that challenge public health systems; and the public health response to Hurricane Katrina (2005), and the Deepwater Horizon oil spill (2010), and the earthquake, tsunami, and radiation disaster (2011) in Japan. It should also be noted that 100,000 Americans per year are killed by infections they have acquired during hospital stays because of hospital errors—a huge public health concern.[8] A 2011 study found that only about 10 percent of errors causing injuries are reported.[9]

## Social Inequality, Poverty, and Health

Some definitions of public health stress that public health involves the health of the whole community, even the whole world, not only the medical treatment of individuals. Because social inequality and absolute poverty are important determinants of health, the field of public health goes far beyond the scope of this text. That is, a poor country with a more equal distribution of wealth and income may have a healthier population than a rich country with an unequal distribution

of wealth. For example, the United States, which is ranked first in health spending, has a health system that is ranked 37th in the world by the **World Health Organization (WHO)**, which is the directing and coordinating authority for health within the United Nations system (2000).[10] In terms of longevity and infant mortality, statistics show that the United States is not among the top 20 nations in the world.[11] Therefore, to effectively address questions on the health of a local community, a nation, or the international community, one has to minimize or at least decrease social inequality by, for example, providing universal health care, day care, and subsidies to bring people above the poverty line, and using the tax system to reduce inequality (rather than redistributing income to the top as we have been doing). In the United States, economic and social inequalities have been increasing since 1967. This means that the distribution of income and wealth has been increasingly unequal and the opportunity for social mobility has decreased.[12]

The fact that health depends more on social class and relative inequality than on the availability of medical treatment was recognized in 1975 by Theodore Cooper, then U.S. Assistant Secretary for Health; he stated, "It is one of the great and sobering truths of our profession that modern health care probably has less impact on the population than economic status, education, housing, nutrition and sanitation. Yet we have fostered the idea that abundant, readily available high quality health care would be some kind of panacea for the ills of society and the individual. This is a fiction, a hoax."[13] It has been hypothesized that the constant stress on poor people in a highly stratified society may account for higher rates of illness and death. These questions are beyond the scope of this text but need to be mentioned in any honest discussion of public health. (See discussion of Hurricane Katrina later in this chapter.)

According to data from the Congressional Budget Office, inequality continues to grow. Between 1979 and 2007, in the United States, the income gap between the top 1 percent and the middle and poorest fifths of the population tripled. In 2007, "the share of after-tax income going to the top 1 percent hit its highest level (17.1 percent) since 1979, while the share going to the middle fifth of Americans shrank to its lowest level during this period (14.1 percent)." Adjusted for inflation, during the same period, after-tax incomes for the top 1 percent rose by 281 percent (about a $973,100 increase per household) compared to 25 percent ($11,200) for the middle fifth and 16 percent ($2,400) for the bottom fifth. The average household at the top had an income of $1.3 million (up $88,000 in one year). The average middle-income household earned $55,300, and the average bottom fifth income was $17.700 (Figure 5.1▶).[14]

The gap between the top 1 percent and the poorest fifth grew from 22.7 times higher in 1979 to 74.6 times higher in 2007, "more than tripling the income gap" in less than 30 years; the average after-tax income of the top 1 percent nearly quadrupled, while that of the bottom fifth grew by only 16 percent.[15] The incomes at the very top (in the 99.99th percentile) have soared from about $2 million in the 1970s to about $10 million in 2009.[16]

As the incomes at the top continue to grow, the number of people living in poverty and the percentage of the population living in poverty also continue to grow. According to the Census Bureau, in 2008, there were 39.8 million people living in poverty (13.2 percent); in 2009, 43.6 million people

(14.3 percent) were living below the poverty line ($21,954 for a family of four). Statistics on poverty have been kept for 51 years. In 2009, more people were poor than in any previous year for which data are available.[17]

In 2011, the U.S. Centers for Disease Control and Prevention (CDC) published a report on health disparities and inequality. "A health disparity is a particular type of health difference that is closely linked with social, economic, and/or environmental disadvantage," according to the Department of Health and Human Services (DHHS). The CDC found that "the data pertaining to inequalities in income, morbidity, mortality, and self-reported healthy days highlight the considerable and persistent gaps between the healthiest persons and states and the least healthy." The CDC also found that "the correlation between poor health and . . . inequality at the state level holds at all levels of income." They found inequality in infant mortality between African Americans and whites and inequality in death from stroke and heart disease between African Americans and whites. Minorities are less likely to get preventive care and, when sick, less likely to receive quality health care. As incomes get lower, rates of preventable hospitalizations rise.[18]

On April 8, 2011, the DHHS announced that it was "launch[ing] two strategic plans aimed at

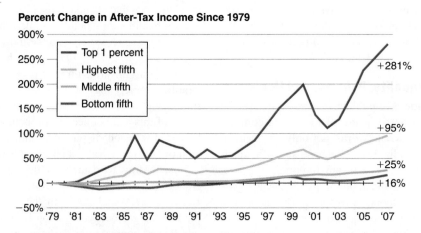

▶ **Figure 5.1**   After-tax income gains, 1979–2007.
*Source:* Courtesy of the Center on Budget and Policy Priorities.

reduc[ing] health disparities among racial and ethnic minorities." Among the steps to be taken are increasing access and expanding insurance coverage; recruiting personnel from underserved areas for careers in public health and training community health workers; efforts to target cardiovascular disease, childhood obesity, smoking, maternal and child health, and flu and asthma; improving health data collection and outcomes research; and evaluating the progress made toward meeting these goals.[19]

Not only has income inequality continued to grow, but according to the U.S. Census Bureau, in 2010, "the number of people with health insurance dropped for the first time in 23 years." The percentage of people (16.7 percent) without private insurance also increased. The number of people covered by government insurance (like Medicare and Medicaid) rose from 87.4 million in 2008 to 93.2 million in 2009. The rise of the uninsured occurred in every group except children. The loss of insurance "is mostly attributed to the loss of employer-provided insurance." Most of the uninsured have incomes of less than $25,000. However, one-half of the newly uninsured have incomes above $50,000. The provisions of the Patient Protection and Affordable Care Act that would allow or require them to buy coverage do not take effect until 2014.[20]

# USING COMPUTERS TO STUDY DISEASE

Information technology (IT) can play a significant role in helping infection control practitioners (ICPs) in their "never-ending whirlwind of surveillance tasks, outbreak monitoring . . . and reporting." According to Dr. Gary A. Noskin (Northwestern University Feinberg School of Medicine), IT "can allow for real-time surveillance. . . . If you have targeted organisms, you might not know if there is a patient . . . [with] that organism . . . " but with computerization, the lab can identify and alert you. IT can also identify trends.[21]

Preventing and controlling epidemics is based on accurate statistics. To answer the question

"Is there an epidemic?" statisticians need to define the normal distribution of a disease and the extra, unexpected cases. Models of a disease and how it is transmitted need to be created. Computers are perfect for these tasks.

Computers can create **what-if scenarios** or **simulations** of what would happen to an infectious disease if something else happened (e.g., if air travel increased or decreased, if the temperature rose or fell, if there was an adequate supply of antiviral drugs, or if a vaccine existed or did not exist). Computers can also do a what-if simulation to predict the growth of tobacco use as a public health issue. According to the Cancer Atlas, if tobacco use continues to grow as it is growing now, "tobacco will kill a billion people this century, ten times the toll it took in the twentieth century, public health officials said. [It] accounts for one in five cancer deaths, or 1.4 million deaths worldwide each year, according to two new reference guides that chart global tobacco use and cancer." According to the Massachusetts Department of Health, between 2000 and 2006, the level of nicotine in many brands of cigarettes rose by 10 percent. This means it is easier to become addicted and more difficult to stop smoking.[22] The World Health Organization (WHO) predicts that 500 million people will die from diseases related to tobacco use.[23] In 2011, the brain mechanism that leads to nicotine addiction was identified.[24] Apparently unrelated to this is the development of a vaccine that shows some promise in early trials.[25]

Computational models are the programs that create the simulations. All of these what-ifs are plugged into a model. Models can be built to answer all sorts of different questions about epidemics. "The experiments consist of computer simulations—representations of actual communities based on demographic and transportation information. . . . [T]he researchers can introduce an infectious agent . . . and watch it spread. . . . [T]he scientists start with assumptions about how people interact and how infectious agents spread." Anyone in the community can contract or transmit the disease through contact with other people. Scientists are using a model to see how a person gets infected and then how he or she spreads the disease. They can change variables to yield different results and answer different questions. Two of these variables are the size of the community and the virulence of the infection. Using very powerful computers, the models may produce millions of possible outcomes, none of which may develop. Computer simulations or models may help public health officials prepare for outbreaks in states, in nations, and globally. The **Models of Infectious Disease Agent Study (MIDAS)** is modeling the flu and asking whether we can contain it at the source. Using models, public health officials test such measures as vaccination, the distribution of antiviral medications, the closing of schools, and the quarantining of neighborhoods or infected people. They also study what could happen if the flu spreads, for example in the Unites States, given the amount that people travel.[26] In 2010, simulation modeling of the H1N1 flu, some of which used patterns followed by the Great Flu Pandemic of 1918, predicted that the rapid development and delivery of vaccines would have "a disproportionately large impact" in reducing rates of infection.[27]

## STATISTICS AND EPIDEMICS: A HISTORICAL OVERVIEW

An **epidemic** is "an excess in the number of cases of a given health problem. . . . To determine what constitutes an excess implies knowing what is normal or to be expected." Thus the very definition of epidemic is based on statistics. The study of epidemics is one of the important areas of the field of public health. Simple spreadsheet software (such as Microsoft Office Excel) can be used to calculate expected rates for past and present epidemics.[28]

The field of public health has been successful in controlling and containing many diseases. "Science had first contained smallpox, then cholera, then plague, then yellow fever, all through large scale public health measures, everything from filtering water to testing and killing rats, to vaccination."[29]

Before modern science, before any understanding of disease and its causes, there were at least two instances of conferring immunity to smallpox. In China, in the 10th century, "physicians . . . induced immunity by having patients inhale the dust from a pulverized scab taken from a smallpox lesion." In Constantinople, in the 1500s, peasant women were inserting needles that had been infected with smallpox into veins to prevent smallpox.[30]

The use of vaccinations to confer immunity works on the following principle: Antibodies that help white cells destroy disease are produced naturally by a healthy immune system about 2 weeks after the start of the infection. The next time that those bacteria attack, the antibodies immediately destroy them. "A vaccine is a weakened, killed, or incomplete form of a microorganism that cannot cause disease, but will result in the production of antibodies when it is injected into the body."[31] Vaccinations are not effective against all bacteria or viruses. Although Edward Jenner is referred to as the "father of smallpox vaccination," there were several earlier successful attempts by others to confer immunity. A smallpox vaccine to immunize people was used in 1774 in England (predating Jenner by more than 20 years). It was developed by Benjamin Jesty and was based on folk wisdom and observation; he had no knowledge of bacteria or understanding of disease and immunity. It was common folk wisdom in rural areas that people who developed cowpox (a relatively mild disease) did not contract smallpox. Jesty "reasoned that if dairymaids who caught cowpox accidentally were immune to smallpox, then someone who caught cowpox deliberately should be equally immune. He . . . infect[ed] his family. . . . He took infected pus from the udder of a cow. . . . He scratched his wife's arm." He also vaccinated his two sons. They all caught cowpox and recovered. His neighbors expected the whole family to turn into cows. They of course did not, and there is evidence that Jesty went on to vaccinate other people.[32] Jenner's vaccine was first given in 1796.

Today, vaccines are used against such diseases as tetanus, measles, polio, diphtheria, mumps, rubella, and hepatitis. However, the rising cost and number of vaccines has led to a situation in which insurers may refuse to reimburse doctors. This could possibly mean that childhood diseases long held in check would recur.[33] Some vaccinations do not confer lifetime immunity, but most adults do not get revaccinated. Between January and September of 2010, 11,500 cases of whooping cough were reported in the United States; nine people died. Some of these cases might have been prevented if adults had been vaccinated.[34] Where there are concentrations of unvaccinated people, diseases such as measles and pertussis occur.[35] Since February 2011, measles has been spreading in Minneapolis among unvaccinated populations fearful of the false and discredited alleged connection between vaccinations and autism.[36] Another outbreak occurred in Boston.[37]

Antivaccination movements are not new in the United States. During a smallpox epidemic in 1900, public health officials enforced compulsory, universal vaccinations using "club-wielding police."[38] Today, some parents are concerned about an alleged but false connection between autism and the measles–mumps–rubella (MMR) vaccine because of an article published in *The Lancet* in the late 1990s. According to Dr. Andrew Kroger of the CDC Immunization Service, "That study was . . . seriously flawed." *The Lancet* printed a retraction. A U.S. Federal court ruled in 2009 that the MMR vaccine did not cause autism. Some parents are concerned that too many vaccines are required. The small risks of vaccines are far outweighed by the risks of childhood diseases. In the United States, it is not too difficult to avoid vaccination. Nineteen states allow exemption for nonreligious reasons. More and more children are not receiving all of the recommended vaccinations. Although the national percentage of parents who choose not to have their children vaccinated is only 3 percent, these parents tend to be concentrated geographically in affluent communities. For example, although the statewide exemption rate in California is only 1.5 percent, in some kindergartens, 10 to 19 percent of children have not been vaccinated. Because nonvaccinated children are concentrated in certain areas, "public health officials [are] worried because high enough rates of non-vaccination can lead to a resurgence of vaccine-preventable diseases." For highly contagious diseases such as measles, if vaccination rates fall below 90 to 95 percent, "the disease [could] become endemic again."

The risks of vaccines pale against the risks of some childhood diseases; for example, the death rate from diphtheria for children under 5 is up to 20 percent, and for tetanus, it is 10 percent. Before the measles vaccine, 3 million people caught measles and 400 to 500 people died in the United States from the disease each year. Complications (which may affect up to 20 percent of cases) include pneumonia, bronchitis, encephalitis, and low platelet count. Measles was declared to be eliminated from the United States in 2000. However, after 2007, the number of people with measles rose. In 2000 to 2007, there were 63 cases per year. In 2008, there were 126 cases.[39] The failure to vaccinate children against preventable diseases can become a public health problem.

Statistics and mapping of a disease progression were used to contain an epidemic for the first time in the 19th century. An early example of public health in action involves the London cholera epidemic of 1854. Dr. John Snow (one of the few scientists who hypothesized that cholera was spread through contaminated water) noticed a large cluster (500 deaths in 10 days) of cholera in one neighborhood. He plotted the cases on a map. The neighborhood got its water from one pump. Snow reasoned that this was the source of the outbreak. The pump handle was removed and the epidemic contained.[40]

By the beginning of the 20th century, public health measures had successfully contained some epidemic diseases. Vaccination could prevent smallpox. The eradication of mosquitoes could stop yellow fever. Clean water could stop cholera. Then in the early 20th century, epidemic polio struck in New York for the first time. It defied explanation: Although, "[f]ilth, poverty, and overcrowding had successfully predicted other infectious infant disease," polio appeared more frequently in suburban and rural areas than in urban slums. This might suggest a relationship between cleanliness and polio; but epidemiologists did not see this.[41] It took the next 50 years to develop a thorough understanding of the virus that causes polio, to see how it was transmitted, and to develop a vaccine. In early 2000, polio cases began to reappear in "21 previously polio-free countries" such as Kenya.[42] In 2010 and 2011, **polio** has reappeared in 19 countries, including the Republic of Congo, the Democratic Republic of Congo, Angola, Tajikistan, and the Ivory Coast. There are only four countries where polio remains endemic (where polio's "spread has never been interrupted"): India, Pakistan, Afghanistan, and Nigeria. In response to the reappearance of polio, the WHO is conducting mass vaccination campaigns.[43]

When diseases are airborne and when people from many neighborhoods, states, and nations with different immunities are brought together in close contact, diseases spread quickly. The flu pandemic of 1918–1919 killed anywhere from 20 million to 100 million people worldwide. A **pandemic** is a global disease outbreak to which everyone is susceptible. The flu pandemic killed strong young people fast and spread throughout the world. How did this happen? War brings people of all areas into close contact with each other. World War I was no exception. The new flu virus apparently was first seen in Kansas in 1918. It spread to a Kansas army base, which housed 56,000 soldiers from across the United States; then with the soldiers, it spread to Europe, later returning to North America, from where it spread to Europe, Asia, Africa, and the Pacific islands. At the time that the flu first appeared, it was not seen as a public health concern.[44] It was not the killer it would become in the second wave of the disease. During the War, the U.S. government controlled the dissemination of information.[45] The government's focus was on winning the war, not spreading information about the flu. Doctors and nurses worked for the army. Civilian populations lacked medical care.[46]

In Europe and the United States, public health measures were taken to combat spread of the flu. In the United States, the measures varied from state-to-state and city-to-city. Most of the measures grew out of then-current scientific understanding of disease and how it spread. Most of these measures were ineffective. The attempt was to put in place measures that would "prevent those infected from sharing the same air as the uninfected."

Patients in hospitals were separated by sheets and slept head to foot. The authorities attempted to limit public meetings and recommended good ventilation. Some schools were closed, as were movie theatres, bars, and dance halls. Churches were open, but public funerals banned. In New York and Illinois, those with the flu were isolated and quarantined. Of course, troop trains and ships were still effectively spreading the disease. The American Public Health Association (APHA) believed that contamination of the hands by sputum and the sharing of dishes and utensils spread the disease. They attempted to teach the public to be careful when coughing or sneezing and to wash their hands often. They recommended frequent disinfection in hospitals and that hospital personnel not wear work clothes outside the hospital. In hospitals and among the general public, masks were worn that were believed to prevent the spread of the disease. In San Diego, they observed "a rapid decline" in new cases. However, in the Great Lakes, a study of hospital personnel found that "8 percent who used the mask developed the infection [whereas] 7.75 percent of non-mask wearers did." Gargling with antiseptics was believed to prevent the disease; the APHA thought that because this attacked the mucus barrier to infection, it was of no value.[47] The epidemic ran its course.

## THE EMERGENCE OF DISEASES IN THE LATE 20TH AND EARLY 21ST CENTURIES

### AIDS

By the last quarter of the 20th century, humanity had apparently conquered infectious disease, by medical and public health measures, at least in the developed countries. However, since 1973, "30 new pathogens, including Ebola and HIV, have appeared."[48] Today, infectious diseases are an international public health concern. For the latest information on epidemic and pandemic alert and response, the WHO maintains a Web page at http://www.who.int/csr/don/en/. The WHO now requires the reporting of any disease that could cross an international border.

No one was thinking "about new plagues in the 1970s because it was widely assumed that vaccination, sanitation and antibiotics were making infections obsolete. The retroviruses . . . were . . . of academic interest only."[49] Then the first cases of a new syndrome started appearing in New York City, Los Angeles, and San Francisco in June of 1981.[50] It was named **acquired immune deficiency syndrome (AIDS)** at a meeting of the CDC in 1982.[51] AIDS attacked the immune system, leading to susceptibility to opportunistic infection and eventually to death. After years of study, it was found that people were infected through body fluids, not casual contact. **Human immunodeficiency virus (HIV)**, the virus that causes AIDS, was identified in 1984. However, more than 30 years after the first cases were identified, although there are effective treatments to lengthen life, there is no cure for or vaccination against AIDS. In addition, the treatments are too expensive for most AIDS sufferers. By 2005, over 40 million people were living with AIDS, and the AIDS pandemic had left 13 million children orphans. In 2004, five million new cases of HIV occurred, and more than three million people died. In the United States alone, the CDC estimated that between 1981 and 2003, 1.6 million people were infected with HIV, of whom more than 500,000 died. The rates of new infection in the United States and death due to AIDS have declined since the 1980s, and the AIDS surveillance system is one of the best in the country. However AIDS continues to spread in epidemic fashion in much of the rest of the world.[52]

Currently, IT allows researchers to look at "all the genes and proteins in the virus and the human genome, as well as . . . every . . . piece of DNA." (See Chapter 8 on IT in pharmacy.) Supercomputers can investigate vaccine development and analyze health and population statistics. Several nations are using supercomputers and bioinformatics to help in developing an effective vaccine. Biomedical informatics integrates "health-related data on all levels, such as molecule, cell, tissue, organ, people, and the entire population." Modeling and simulations by supercomputers can contribute to knowledge on prevention and help in designing effective medications.[53]

AIDS in 2006 is not as simple as it was 25 years ago when it was untreatable. Some who are infected with HIV do not get sick. Some get sick and die quickly. Although there are effective treatments for many, some patients do not respond, and many cannot afford the treatments. There are patients who cannot tolerate the drugs' effects. For others, the drugs simply stop working after a time. However, as the death rate due to AIDS (in the United States at least) declines, the number of people living with AIDS increases.[54] In 2010 (using 2006 statistics), the CDC estimated that out of the U.S. population of 309 million people, about 1,206,400 people are living with HIV. Of these, 79 percent know they have HIV. The number of people with HIV has increased, whereas the number of new cases each year (56,300) is stable—down from 130,000 in 1985. The transmission of HIV from mother to child has declined dramatically, as has transmission among drug users. Still, each year, more than 18,000 people with AIDS die. CDC's work with HIV/AIDS includes behavioral interventions; making sure people know how to prevent HIV transmission and that they are motivated to reduce their risk; testing for HIV; and getting people treatment.[55]

AIDS has not only left millions dead and dying, but also has made some important contributions to society and medicine. AIDS is a factor in the push for living wills and health care proxies, do-not-resuscitate orders, and hospice care. AIDS helped create a social movement that not only changed the drug approval process, but also introduced patients who sometimes had as much information as scientists and doctors into scientific meetings.[56]

## SARS

**Severe acute respiratory syndrome (SARS)** is a form of pneumonia. It is caused by a virus that was identified in 2003. The infection leads to difficulty in breathing; it can cause death. It spread quickly around the world. However, the public health response stopped it from becoming a pandemic. "Within 6 weeks of its discovery, it had infected thousands of people around the world, including people in Asia, Australia, Europe, Africa, and

North and South America. . . . The WHO had identified SARS as a global health threat, and issued an unprecedented travel advisory. Daily WHO updates tracked the spread of SARS seven days a week." Although SARS did not become a pandemic, it is still present.[57]

### West Nile Virus

**West Nile virus** first appeared in the 1930s. It is a form of encephalitis or brain inflammation. It cycles between mosquitoes and birds. Infected birds will infect mosquitoes. Mosquitoes can spread the disease to humans. It can be diagnosed by magnetic resonance imaging. There is no treatment or vaccine. Most people do not become very sick (only about 1 in 150). About four-fifths of people with West Nile virus will have no symptoms. However, it can be very serious. "The severe symptoms can include high fever, headache, neck stiffness, stupor, disorientation, coma, tremors, convulsions, muscle weakness, vision loss, numbness and paralysis. These symptoms may last several weeks, and neurological effects may be permanent." It has become a seasonal epidemic in North America.[58]

### Antibiotic Resistance

The introduction of antibiotics in the 20th century led to a decline in the death rate in the United States by 220 per 100,000, a great advance in public health. However, currently, the development of antibiotic-resistant strains of bacteria poses a grave threat to health. Bacterial resistance happens even without antibiotics, but the use and abuse of these drugs exacerbates the resistance and leads to the development of **superbugs**.[59] Governments in the United States and Europe recognize the public health problem and are attempting to take action, establishing the Transatlantic Task Force on Antibiotic Resistance. The CDC is trying to educate people on the appropriate use of antibiotics. Drug companies of late have not been developing new antibiotics to treat the superbugs.[60] However, researchers at IBM are attempting to develop a new type of drug—one that uses nanoparticles to poke holes in bacteria. Clinical trials have not been promising.[61] According to

scientists from the Infectious Diseases Society of America, **antibiotic resistance** is a "dire issue." They call for measures to spur the development of new antibiotics; without them, resistant bacteria can "increasingly claim the lives of healthy people."[62]

MRSA **MRSA (methicillin-resistant *Staphylococcus aureus*)** is a staphylococcal infection resistant to many antibiotics. It appeared in Europe in the 1960s, which coincides with the first widespread use of antibiotics. A recent study "confirm[s] that the evolution of resistant strains and their spread are primarily driven by antibiotic use." Although "MRSA is . . . related to exposures to healthcare delivery . . ." rates of MRSA are rising in athletes and among other populations. In 2005 in the United States, there were more than 15,000 deaths from MRSA. A 2007 report stated that there were more than 94,000 cases and about 18,000 deaths. In 2010 by using a new way of sequencing DNA, small genetic changes can be pinpointed. This allows researchers to trace the spread of MRSA around the world and even within one hospital. This might lead to ways of controlling the spread of MRSA. Some hospitals are attempting to use flashing ultraviolet light to kill the bacteria that cause MRSA.[63] A study published in *Science* analyzed the mutations of MRSA, directly "pinpoint[ing] antibiotics and their overuse as the primary culprit."[64]

In April 2011, two studies on MRSA were published in the *New England Journal of Medicine*. The first reviewed an evaluation of a 4-year program at Veterans Affairs (VA) hospitals to combat MRSA. "The study of 153 Veterans Affairs hospitals . . . found a 62 percent drop in the rate of infections caused by . . . MRSA" over an almost 3-year period in intensive care units. Other units experienced a 45 percent drop. The VA cut the infection rate with a group of measures including screening patients with nasal swabs and isolating those with MRSA. The VA required staff to wear gloves and gowns when treating patients with MRSA and to wash their hands. These measures could be instituted in all hospitals. However, the second study questions the necessity and cost effectiveness of screening every patient in the intensive care unit when admitted and discharged.[65]

It should be noted that 1.5 percent of the population carries MRSA. Most of these people will not get sick unless their immune systems are compromised and the bacteria invade the bloodstream. In 2011, MRSA and other antibiotic-resistant bacteria were found in meat and bed bugs.[66] However, scientists see no cause for alarm, yet.[67]

CRKP **CRKP (carbapenem-resistant** *Klebsiella pneumoniae*) is a deadly bacterium. Carbapenems have been the "antibiotic of last resort," working when no other antibiotic could. This is no longer true. As CRKP spread, it became more and more resistant to antibiotics, even carbapenem. CRKP can cause pneumonia, bloodstream infections, and infections in wounds and surgical sites. It appears in hospitals and other healthcare settings. It was diagnosed in Israeli hospitals in 2006. It has also been seen in New York and North Carolina. It is now becoming a problem worldwide. It is appearing in hospitals in southern California. In a 7-month period, more than 350 people in Los Angeles became infected. It has been reported in 36 states. There are no drugs to cure it. About 40 percent of people who get it will die.[68] One way to control its spread is by handwashing.[69]

CRKP, like MRSA, is related to the overuse of antibiotics, both by patients and by farmers for cattle. In 2010, *Science* published a study that contended that "superbugs appear to be the direct descendents of mutated bacteria created as a result of . . . antibiotic drugs."[70] When people take antibiotics to cure a bacterial infection, they need to take the whole prescription. If they fail to, some bacteria remain and grow stronger. People also overuse antibiotics by using them for colds and viruses—illnesses not affected by antibiotics. Industrial farms feed healthy animals antibiotics to speed their growth. "Seventy percent of all antibiotics sold in the US are given to healthy food animals." According to the American Medical Association, the American Academy of Pediatrics, the American Public Health Association, and the Infectious Diseases Society of America "the

routine use of antibiotics in food animals presents a serious and growing threat to human health because it creates new strains of dangerous antibiotic-resistant bacteria."[71]

NDM-1 **NDM-1 (New Delhi metallo-beta-lactamase-1)** is an enzyme that makes bacteria resistant to antibiotics. It first appeared in hospitals in India. Four percent of water from public taps contained antibiotic-resistant bacteria. Thirty percent of water from waste seepage sites contained them. Patients from the United Kingdom and Europe were found to carry NDM-1 even though they had not been in hospitals in India. It has also appeared in the United States, Netherlands, Australia, and Canada. The leader of a study of NDM-1, Professor Tim Walsh, called this "an urgent matter of public health . . . [which is] international" in scope.[72]

### Vector-borne Diseases

A **vector-borne disease** is a disease transmitted to a human or animal host by a tic, mosquito, or other arthropod that carries the bacteria or virus. According to the CDC, vector-borne diseases are emerging and re-emerging. Vector-borne diseases are affected by climate. Some examples of vector-borne diseases are malaria and, in the 19th century, yellow fever. With global warming, patterns of insect migration have changed, leading scientists to predict an increase in vector-borne disease in the United States. Cases of dengue fever have appeared in Florida for the first time.[73]

## USING INFORMATION TECHNOLOGY TO TRACK AND COMBAT A 21ST-CENTURY EPIDEMIC: CHOLERA

In October 2010, an epidemic of cholera in Haiti began drawing the attention of public health workers. Originating in northern Haiti, the epidemic spread across the country in what the CDC called a "highly susceptible" population. Epidemic cholera was new to Haiti. By the beginning of December, 93,000 people had caught the disease and 2,100 were dead. Through DNA analysis, the origin of the bacteria was traced to its likely origin: South Asia. Efforts are being made to rehydrate patients and to prevent the spread of the disease by providing clean food and water. However, IT is playing a big part in trying to combat the epidemic. Public health officials are using text messages and radio to warn the population of health risks. Cell phones are being used to track the spread of the disease. Because cell phones can be used to monitor a person's movements, for example, from areas with cholera to areas without, predictions of new outbreaks are possible. When people with disease travel, disease travels with them. People are contacted via text message with information about the epidemic and the disease. "Working with the country's biggest cell phone carrier . . . [they are] tracking cell phone owners who live in northern epidemic areas—people who carry the disease without knowing it." The knowledge helps public health workers know where to send medical personnel. The people are contacted via text message and told where to call for information. By February 2011, the number of new cases was dropping.[74]

## INFORMATION TECHNOLOGY— COLLECTION, MODELING, AND SURVEILLANCE OF DISEASE AGENTS

The United States recognizes the importance of public health. The fourth goal of the Office of the National Coordinator for Health Information Technology (ONCHIT) is the improvement of the "health of the entire nation." It proposes the following: "unifying public health surveillance systems" to safeguard against epidemics and unsafe foods. To achieve this, it proposes a national interoperable network of health care institutions and public health agencies to gather and disseminate information in a timely manner. A fully interoperable system would connect telehealth activities and the electronic health record.[75] ONCHIT also recommends "standards for quality of care." Research information needs to be disseminated quickly. IT

can speed up U.S. Food and Drug Administration (FDA) review of clinical trials.[76]

Registries exist that are organized "system[s] for the collection, storage, retrieval, analysis, and dissemination of information" on people with a disease, a predisposition toward a disease, and exposure to anything thought to cause ill health. The information in registries can help define a problem and its size and examine trends over time. A registry may focus on one disease, a group of diseases, or exposure to toxins. Data on individuals can come from doctors and hospital reports, pathology reports, vital statistics, and hospital discharge records. Registries are operated by the federal and state governments, universities, hospitals, nonprofit organizations, or private groups.[77]

Public health also includes the modeling of disease agents—best done by computers. One approach to containing infectious disease that is being explored is called **syndromic surveillance**, which uses "health-related data that precede diagnosis and signal a sufficient probability of a case or an outbreak."[78] Syndromic surveillance can be used, for example, in shelters where there are no medical personnel; people can look out for signs and symptoms (for instance diarrhea) and report them. New York City's syndromic surveillance program "looks for unusual patterns of disease in . . . emergency rooms." The federal government uses "biosensor detectors" in cities to "draw in air and analyze it for . . . pathogens" to guard against bioterrorism.[79]

Public health encompasses the distribution of information; the protection of clean air and water, of the earth, and of a healthy food supply; and the creation of vaccines for prevention of and medication for treatment of disease. Computers are involved in all of these tasks.

Today, with "neighborhoods" worldwide, easy air travel, and hence the easy spread of infectious disease, one person cannot possibly gather all the statistics on a disease. Computers—from supercomputers to handheld personal digital assistants (PDAs)—are used for this purpose. In the developing countries of Asia and Africa, **SATELLIFE** PDAs are used for the collection and dissemination of information, warnings, education, and so on. SATELLIFE can bring information to health workers where there are no land lines, electricity, or Internet. It increases access to current information via e-mail.[80] Great Britain has established cancer registries that use new computer systems to generate and collect data.[81] Some U.S. counties are attempting to institute disease-tracking systems.[82] We do have national registries for some diseases such as amyotrophic lateral sclerosis (ALS) (a disease of the nerve cells in the brain and spinal cord) and kidney disease.[83] However, we are far from having an effective national registry for disease.

The **National Electronic Disease Surveillance System (NEDSS)** (a part of the public health information network) will promote "integrated surveillance systems that can transfer . . . public health, laboratory and clinical data . . . over the Internet." This will be a national electronic surveillance system that will allow epidemics to be identified quickly. Eventually it will automatically collect data in real time.[84]

There are several epidemiologic software tools used to map and predict the spread of diseases. The Joint United Nations Programme on HIV/AIDS (UNAIDS) describes several such tools. Between 2011 and 2015, UNAIDS aims to "to advance global progress in achieving country set targets for universal access to HIV prevention, treatment, care and support and to halt and reverse the spread of HIV."[85] The estimation and projection package (EPP) is used "to estimate and project adult HIV prevalence from surveillance data." The data can be used by SPECTRUM, which calculates the numbers infected, new infections, orphans, treatment needs, and deaths from AIDS.[86] The modes of transmission (MoT) spreadsheets predict the number of new infections based on the current infection data and risk patterns. SPECTRUM combines several models.

On May 23, 2005, the WHO approved new rules to control the global spread of disease. The rules went into effect in 2007. They "require member countries to . . . develop . . . capabilities to identify and respond to public health emergencies of international concern and to take routine preventive measures at ports, airports, and border

stations." It provides a list of reportable diseases including smallpox, AIDS, and polio. Its objectives are to establish global disease surveillance systems and to overcome technical, political, resource, and legal obstacles.[87]

The obstacles confronting an effective global response to a new pandemic are daunting. By definition, a pandemic is a *global* outbreak of disease to which every individual in the world is susceptible. Much of the world's population will need medical care, which most nations including our own cannot provide. We are lacking in staff, medication (antiviral drugs), and hospital beds. Our health care system lacks surge capacity (the ability to expand rapidly beyond normal services). There may or may not be a vaccine, at least in the beginning of the pandemic. Economic and social disruption is likely to result from business and school closings, travel bans, and fear of contagion.

Fighting infectious disease was recognized as an international task at the Group of Eight (G8) Summit, which focused on public health in July 2006. They called for increased international cooperation on surveillance and pledged to support programs that fight HIV/AIDS, tuberculosis, malaria, and polio.[88]

## COMPUTER MODELING OF DISEASE: HEALTH STATISTICS AND INFECTIOUS DISEASE

### Models of Infectious Disease Agent Study (MIDAS)

In 2004, the United States funded a plan for researchers to use computers to model diseases; this plan is called MIDAS. The researchers seek "to develop computational models of the interactions between infectious agents and their hosts, disease spread, prediction systems and response strategies."[89] The goal of the project is to develop statistical tools to identify and monitor infectious disease. If successful, it will use electronic health information. The researchers are supposed to simulate the effects of outbreaks and responses on communities of various sizes. They will also evaluate the effectiveness of preventive measures, such as vaccination, and containment strategies, such as quarantine. The effect of social networks on the spread of disease will be examined, as will outbreaks of disease. Eventually, these models will help guide policy.[90] The models will focus on how many people normally use health care facilities and services and on detection models that notify the public of potential outbreaks. Models will be evaluated using historical information on real outbreaks and "simulated data based on infectious disease models."

Once the models are created, they will enable public health officials to make more meaningful use of health statistics. Newly gathered statistics will simply be entered into the model. **WHONET** is a microbiology information system developed at Brigham and Women's Hospital in Massachusetts. It is used to monitor antibacterial resistance. MIDAS will take its microbiology data from WHONET (an information system developed to support the WHO's goal of global surveillance of bacterial resistance to antimicrobial agents).[91]

There is an international attempt to model what would happen if the bird flu (avian flu, common in birds, but rarely passed to people) began to pass easily between people (not just from birds and animals to people). In the United States, computer experts who use MIDAS and scientists in the flu branch of the CDC are working together to develop simulations that should help to control outbreaks if certain conditions are met, including early identification, sufficient supplies of antiviral drugs and the means to get them to those who need them, the ability to enforce quarantine, international cooperation including restricting travel, and sharing antiviral drugs.[92]

As soon as cases of H1N1 appeared in April 2009, MIDAS started to create models of the possible spread of the disease; they built on models they had earlier created for bird flu and information from the Great Flu Pandemic of 1918. The model includes the world population and information about immunity. It predicted the severity of the outbreak by sampling flu patients in two cities. A simulation was also created to evaluate interventions such as vaccination of children. In this model, various variables were changed, such as the type of vaccine, how contagious the virus was, and how many children were vaccinated. The economic value of vaccinating employees was also evaluated. The cost per vaccine was $35, and the potential savings were $15 to $1,494 per worker.[93]

## CLIMATE CHANGE: GLOBAL WARMING

"According to the Union of Concerned Scientists: *The scientific consensus is in.* Our planet is warming, and we are helping to make it happen by adding more heat-trapping gases, primarily carbon dioxide ($CO_2$), to the atmosphere. The burning of fossil fuel (oil, coal, and natural gas) alone accounts for about 75 percent of annual $CO_2$ emissions from human activities. Deforestation, the cutting and burning of forests that trap and store carbon, accounts for about another 20 percent" (emphasis added).[94] The consensus among the scientific community continues to build. In a letter signed by 20 heads of scientific organizations, the following was stated in 2009:

> Observations throughout the world make it clear that climate change is occurring, and rigorous scientific research demonstrates that the greenhouse gases emitted by human activities are the primary driver. These conclusions are based on multiple independent lines of evidence, and contrary assertions are inconsistent with an objective assessment of the vast body of peer-reviewed science.[95]

In 2011, Dr. Georges Benjamin, head of the American Public Health Association, stated, "The science is unequivocal that global warming is occurring and that human activity is the cause of it." According to the head of the American Medical Association, extreme winter conditions and summer heat waves are both dangerous to health. There has been an increase in insect-borne diseases (e.g., dengue fever in Florida) and in air pollution; over 30 years, the asthma and allergy season has been extended by 20 days.[96]

A study by the University of New Hampshire has shown that "the northeastern United States has warmed over the past hundred years, and that the rate of this warming is increasing over the past thirty years."[97] According to the American Geophysical Union, which represents 41,000 scientists "Human activities are increasingly altering the Earth's climate . . . add[ing] to natural influences."[98]

**Global warming** is already having a devastating effect on the earth and on human health: More intense heat waves lead to more heat-related deaths. Asthma and eczema in children have been linked to global warming.[99] More intense storms (e.g., Hurricane Katrina in 2005 in New Orleans) and flooding of major rivers are increasing. A study by the National Academy of Science in 2004 predicted a doubling of heat waves.[100] More intense storms also cause increasing run-off that may pollute water supplies.[101] California depends on the Sierra Nevada snow pack for water. Global warming could cut the snow pack by 29 percent in the next 100 years.[102] Droughts may increase. When sea levels rise, coastal areas may disappear. Global warming has also contributed to forest fires in California.[103]

In Alaska in 2011, permafrost is thawing, causing mudslides on roads used by sightseers. Glaciers are receding. The average temperature in Alaska is rising three times faster than the average temperature in the lower 48 states. The risk of floods is increasing. Erosion is threatening some parks. In the summers of 2009 and 2010, floods closed the road to one of a park's popular attractions. What used to be ice-covered hills are melting into "cascades of mud." In some parks, the temperature is rising to above freezing.[104]

In the developing world, global warming is having a devastating effect. Drought has destroyed crops. Rising sea levels could threaten 70 million people with floods by 2080. "More than a quarter of the habitats for African wildlife risked destruction."[105]

One of the concrete steps that could be taken to slow global warming is cutting $CO_2$ emissions. In November 2009, President Obama announced his goal to "cut greenhouse gas emissions by 17 percent by 2020." However, emissions from U.S. businesses continue to grow. There is an annual increase by the S&P 100 of 0.36 percent, instead of a decrease of 1.05 percent per year needed to meet the goal. Ninety percent of the emissions come from four sectors of the economy: utilities, industrials, energy, and materials.[106] There is some disagreement over whether the Environmental Protection Agency (EPA) has the authority to curb greenhouse gas emissions. As of 2011, the EPA was threatened with both a one-third budget cut and a Congressional resolution that would prohibit the EPA from enacting a new greenhouse emissions law.[107]

## THE PUBLIC HEALTH RESPONSE TO HURRICANE KATRINA

Hurricane Katrina "slammed into the Gulf Coast on 29 August [2005]. . . . [S]everal levees protecting New Orleans failed the following day, and the city, about 80% of which is below sea level, filled with water"[108] (Figure 5.2, A and B▶).

The storm damage can be classified as both a natural disaster (a category 5 hurricane: winds above 175 miles per hour) and a human-made disaster. (In the words of a scientist who studied hurricanes, "We've had plenty of knowledge to know this was a disaster waiting to happen.") Katrina flooded New Orleans both because it was a "monster hurricane" and because the levees failed; this should not have been surprising. Computers are used to model various hurricanes and their paths and effects. In 2004, "in an exercise simulating a direct hit by a slow-moving category three hurricane [using two different models], both models showed that the levees would not prevent flooding in New Orleans." A report published in May 2006 found that "the levees in New Orleans failed . . . not because the storm was so big, but because of problems in the way they were designed, built, and maintained."[109]

With this knowledge in hand, an adequate public health plan could have been in place before the storm: evacuation plans; the designation of shelters provided with adequate food, clean water,

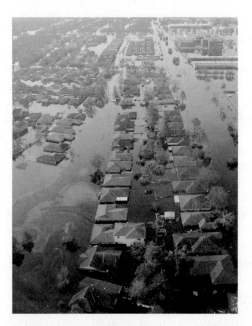

▶ **Figure 5.2** (A) New Orleans flooded by Hurricane Katrina.
*Source:* Caitlin Mirra/Shutterstock.com

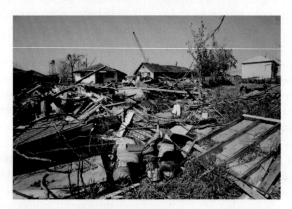

▶ **Figure 5.2** (B) Homes in the Ninth Ward of New Orleans after Katrina.
*Source:* Brian Nolan/Shutterstock.com

medications, and vaccinations; plans to get all the people to those shelters; and plans to clean up and rebuild the city. Apparently, adequate plans were not in place.

Katrina caused the most "massive displacement of a U.S. population" in our history, most of whom were poor, sick, and/or old. A statement on poverty, health, and Katrina that the National Association of County and City Health Officials issued on September 23, 2005, reports, "in New Orleans, areas with significant flooding had lower incomes, higher poverty rates and less education.

The overall poverty rate for New Orleans is 28 percent." Their health was significantly worse before the hurricane because "American disease and death rates are not arbitrary."[110] After the hurricane, many were "stranded without basic human necessities and exposed to human waste, toxins, and physical violence." Many shelters lacked electricity and air-conditioning.[111] The aftermath of Katrina brought on the possibility of a host of public health problems including sanitation, hygiene, unsafe water, infectious disease, surveillance of health problems, the need for immunization, and lack of access to health care. Shelters lacked basic needs: water, food, and space. This was a perfect situation for the spread of infectious disease. The standing water brought with it the possibility of vector-borne disease, especially viral encephalitis. Systematic syndromic surveillance is needed to identify possible disease. Because shelters do not include health professionals, simple questionnaires should be available to report symptoms; the efforts of the agencies that collect this information (Red Cross, local government, state health departments, or the federal CDC) need to be coordinated. It is necessary to immunize people who have not been vaccinated against preventable disease. Information on immunization could be gathered when people register for a shelter. People with chronic diseases or whose health depends on continual medical care (dialysis; medications for heart disease, HIV, or tuberculosis) are particularly vulnerable. The hurricane disproportionately affected "the economically disadvantaged . . . largely black population of New Orleans whose access to health care was limited before Katrina. . . . In the long run, the destruction of the public health and medical care infrastructure . . . [can be] . . . more devastating to the health of the population than the event itself."[112]

Months after the hurricane, according to a federal mental health agency, conditions such as depression had increased. The agency and the Federal Emergency Management Agency (FEMA) have funded counseling centers and a hotline.[113] The number of attempted suicides rose after Katrina.[114] Because people were forced to use gasoline-powered generators, the number of carbon monoxide poisonings rose.[115]

Eleven months after the hurricane, most New Orleans residents were still living with mold and debris. Almost every empty piece of land, including parks and medians, had been turned into trailer parks (with FEMA providing the trailers). The rebuilding of some of the 125,000 structures damaged or destroyed only began being federally funded in July of 2006.[116] Only three of its 11 hospitals were open. Many residents got their mail by visiting the post office every 10 days. In many neighborhoods, there were no dry cleaners, supermarkets, banks, or churches. Garbage that had been attracting rats was just starting to be cleared. Government agencies removed 17.6 million pounds of garbage. In some neighborhoods, "Electricity [was] erratic or nonexistent. . . . Water [was] not safe." Bodies were still turning up. Unemployment insurance benefits were running out, ensuring greater poverty. Neighborhoods were gone, and families were split up around the country. Most public housing was still closed, and many units were going to be demolished under a federal plan. The population was down from a pre-Katrina 450,000 to 225,000. Revitalization had begun, but it did not begin to address the needs of the poor residents. Thanksgiving 2006 saw three times as many Katrina victims in FEMA trailers (99,000) than Thanksgiving 2005.[117] This was a result of the lack of public health preparedness and planning.

Years after Katrina, the population of New Orleans was 29 percent smaller than it was in 2000 (343,829 in 2010, down from 484,674 in 2000). The percentage of the city that is white has grown by 30 percent, although the number of whites has shrunk by 24,000 people. Black residency is down by 118,000 people. New Orleans was once two-thirds black; it is now less than 60 percent black. The number of children dropped by over 40 percent. Rebuilding of housing, particularly rentals, has been slow. No one knows how many people want to return. However, "nonprofit rebuilding groups say their waiting lists are long."[118]

## THE BP DEEPWATER HORIZON OIL SPILL

On April 20, 2010, the BP Deepwater Horizon oil rig exploded in the Gulf of Mexico immediately killing 11 human beings. Among the first effects was the spill of tens of thousands of barrels of oil a day into the Gulf, effectively polluting the water, damaging the shoreline, and killing wildlife (Figure 5.3▶). A total of 4.9 million barrels were spilled by the time the well was capped in July. The **Deepwater Horizon oil spill** was not stopped for 85 days. According to the *Journal of the American Medical Association*, "The oil spill in the Gulf of Mexico poses direct threats to human health from inhalation or dermal contact with the oil and dispersant chemicals, and indirect threats to seafood safety and mental health." Exposure causes headaches, chest pain, and respiratory problems. To assess the public health effects of the spill, researchers from the Public Policy Research Lab at Louisiana State University started a telephone survey in which 900 interviews were conducted. They were started fewer than 60 days after the explosion. Their findings include a doubling of self-rated stress; 60 percent of participants felt worried constantly during the week of the interview; and over 80 percent worried about how they and those they knew would earn a living, causing 70 percent to consider moving out of the area even though the majority had lived there all their lives. As a result of the stress, 40 percent of participants had stomachaches some or all the time, 38 percent had headaches some or all the time, and 34 percent had aches and pains all or some of the time. Over 40 percent had trouble sleeping, taking care of their families, and focusing on work.[119]

The National Oceanic and Atmospheric Administration (NOAA) used computer models to predict what coastal regions would be affected by the oil spill. The model used computer programs of "historical weather and water current patterns." The probability of the oil hitting certain regions was as follows: the Mississippi-Alabama-Florida panhandle coast, 81 to 100 percent; the Florida Keys, Miami, and Fort Lauderdale, 60 to 80 percent; the Texas coast, 1 to 40 percent; and the

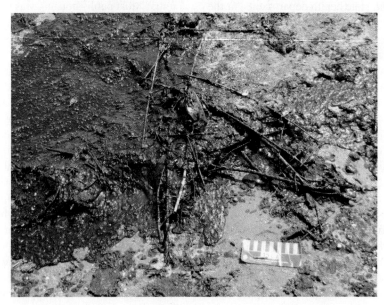

▶ **Figure 5.3** A close up of weathered, emulsified oil located in an intertidal area on Grand Isle, Louisiana.
*Source:* Courtesy of NOAA, http://oceanservice.noaa.gov/deepwaterhorizon/images.html#151.

northern Atlantic coast, 1 to 20 percent. NOAA monitored the slick and updated its projections every 72 hours.[120]

Scientists recommended a response involving government at all levels, nongovernmental organizations, and residents of the area, and the creation of "science-based models of how oil could affect the Gulf." At a conference sponsored by the Institute of Medicine in June 2010, Dr. Lynn Goldman, a Professor of Public Health at Johns Hopkins said, "We have an unknown number of people exposed to an unknown danger. . . . There has not been preparedness in the public health community." No one knows what the long-term effects will be.[121]

The response of the Obama Administration has been inadequate. The National Commission on the BP Deepwater Horizon Oil Spill and Offshore Drilling (although appointed by the president) criticized the federal government. According to the National Commission, "By initially underestimating the amount of oil flow and then at the end of the summer, appearing to underestimate the amount of oil remaining in the Gulf, the federal government created the impression that it was either not fully competent to handle the spill or not fully candid with the American people." The Office of Management and Budget refused the NOAA permission to publicize its "worst-case models." The government, according to the National Commission, put too much faith in BP to control the situation; this might have slowed the necessary government response. The Obama Administration replied that they "pushed BP every step of the way." The government and common media interpretation of the National Incident Report released in August that only 25 percent of the oil remained is disputed by many scientists, who maintain that 10 percent is gone (either skimmed from the surface or burned) and 90 percent remains "dispersed . . ., dissolved, . . . [or] residual," and that it is dangerous in all of these forms.[122] The future health effects of exposure to the oil are not known nor are the effects of the slow governmental response.

# A NOTE ON THE EARTHQUAKE, TSUNAMI, AND RADIATION DISASTER IN JAPAN

As we write, an ongoing public health disaster is unfolding in Japan and may be spreading around the world. We have no idea of the outcome. On March 11, 2011, a 9.0-magnitude earthquake hit Japan followed by **tsunami** with 30-foot waves. NOAA used computer models to track the tsunami in real time. "The models predicted both the timing and intensity of the waves as they made their way to the west coasts of North and South America."[123] In March, the statistics (although incomplete) were frightening: more than 10,000 dead and almost 18,000 missing, 390,000 displaced and homeless, and 118,000 buildings damaged. The estimated cost is $200 billion. The damage and destruction has also had an effect on the world's economy. For example, 40 percent of electronic components come from Japanese factories. In 2010, 75 percent of AFLAC's sales were in Japan.[124]

The earthquake and tsunami destroyed the cooling systems of several nuclear reactors "triggering explosions and fires, releasing radiation and sparking global fears of a widening disaster." In Japan, people were evacuated first from a 12-mile radius; later, 19 miles was recommended. The United States recommended a 50-mile evacuation.[125] Drinking water and farms are contaminated. Radiation is in the Pacific Ocean. The radiation continues to rise from one day to the next. From March 26 to 27, the amount of iodine-131 a few hundred meters from the plant rose from 1,250 times the legal limit to 1,850 times the legal limit. On March 30, the levels in the sea near the plant were 3,355 times the legal limit. On April 12, the Japanese government raised the severity rating of the nuclear disaster to 7, which "means there has been a 'major' release of radioactive material and widespread health and environmental effects."[126] The change in status was based on computer models that showed the emissions of radioactive materials from March 14 to 16.[127]

By April 4, 2011, radiation was found in the water of more than a dozen U.S. cities, in air and rain on the West Coast, and in milk in Vermont, Phoenix, and Los Angeles. Most of the contamination is below EPA standards for exposure. There are several exceptions: In Chattanooga, Tennessee, the EPA says the level in the drinking water is high but not dangerous. In Phoenix and Los Angeles, iodine-131 levels were "roughly equal to the maximum contaminant level permitted by the EPA."[128] However, this is a continuing and worsening situation. On April 10, milk from Little Rock, Arkansas, contained three times the EPA's maximum contaminant level. According to the EPA, this poses no danger. Philadelphia's drinking water was also contaminated.[129] Other scientific experts disagree and maintain that any exposure may pose a health risk and that there is "no such thing as a safe dose of radiation."[130] Although we are exposed to relatively harmless background radiation and to necessary (and sometimes harmful) medical radiation, the kind of radiation emitted from a damaged nuclear plant is harmful and may lead to higher rates of certain cancers, birth defects, and infant death. Even after the Three Mile Island accident in Pennsylvania in 1979 (a much less serious incident), "in the five-year period . . . following the meltdown, the number of persons living within 10 miles of Three Mile Island who were diagnosed with cancer rose 64%."[131] After Chernobyl, a United Nations study predicted that about 4,000 people would eventually die of cancer from exposure to radiation.[132] The disaster continues to unfold, perhaps leading to global public health concerns.

By the beginning of 2012, 160,000 people in Japan had not yet returned to their homes although the economy had recovered. The cleanup effort is ongoing. Debris is still being detected on the coastline. Only 3 of Japan's 54 reactors are operating.[133]

## DISCUSSION

Public health involves the protection of the health of whole populations. As the world becomes "smaller" due to globalization and frequent air travel, public health becomes an international concern. It is clear that global warming requires a global response. Containment of possible epidemics (which can be transmitted across the globe) also requires cooperation between nations, with timely reporting of symptoms and diseases. Whether the report is via a PDA from Africa or a phone call from a small-town U.S. physician, every case needs to be counted and mapped. Computers can model disease (MIDAS), prevention, and containment strategies. Another example

# IN THE NEWS

In "Leprosy, Plague and Other Visitors to New York," by Anemona Hartcollis published on February 10, 2011, in *The New York Times*, the author contends that any illness that appears anywhere will find its way to New York City. Because of the ease of world travel, diseases such as leprosy and bubonic plague find their way to New York City every few years. New York has about one case of cholera per year.

Looking at emergency rooms, syndromic surveillance finds unusual diseases. New York City keeps a database (EpiQuery) of communicable diseases. Some of the diseases found include malaria (about 500 cases per year), Lyme disease, rabies (not one human case since 1944, although about 100 raccoons suffer from it), and cholera (usually about one case per year).

of the use of computer modeling and simulation, or what-if scenarios, of disease outbreak can be found on the following Web site: http://publications.nigms.nih.gov/computinglife/simsickness.htm. Here researchers and scientists have been able to create simulations of disease outbreaks to learn how to better prepare for and manage these situations.

Computers can also be used to model natural disasters. If the model points to strategies to minimize damage, perhaps it should be used by policymakers in a timely fashion. Adequate public health plans can be put into place to deal with the aftermath of a predicted disaster. Some "natural disasters" are not merely a product of nature, but also a product of human activity or the lack of it.

## Chapter Summary

This chapter introduced the reader to the field of public health.

- Public health focuses on the health of the whole community: epidemics, pandemics, natural disaster, human-made disaster, environmental health, and any other issue that affects the health of the community.

- Public health measures include education, prevention, vaccination, and any other necessary community health measure.

- Social inequality and absolute poverty are important determinants of health.

- Because statistics are needed to even define an epidemic, computers are vital to the study of public health.

- Computers are also needed to create models of a disease and the path it will take to spread.

- Computers can model global warming, which is already affecting us, and make predictions about future climate change.

- Public health officials still have to deal with unexpected disease outbreaks.

- Hurricane Katrina illustrates how a combination of factors (human-made and natural) can overwhelm a public health system, leading to major disasters.

- The Deepwater Horizon oil spill will have public health consequences for people and wildlife into the future.

- We cannot even speculate on the health outcomes of the ongoing disaster in Japan.

## Key Terms

acquired immune deficiency syndrome (AIDS)

antibiotic resistance

climate change

CRKP (carbapenem-resistant *Klebsiella pneumoniae*)

Deepwater Horizon oil spill

epidemic

epidemiology

global warming

human immunodeficiency virus (HIV)

Models of Infectious Disease Agent Study (MIDAS)

MRSA (methicillin-resistant *Staphylococcus aureus*)

National Electronic Disease Surveillance System (NEDSS)

NDM-1 (New Delhi metallo-beta-lactamase-1)

pandemic

polio

public health

public health informatics

SATELLIFE

severe acute respiratory syndrome (SARS)

simulations

superbugs

syndromic surveillance

tsunami

vector-borne diseases

West Nile virus

what-if scenarios

WHONET

World Health Organization (WHO)

# Review Exercises

## Multiple Choice

1. _____ is where the largest numbers of lives are saved, usually by understanding the epidemiology of a disease—its patterns, where and how it emerges and spreads—and attacking it at its weak points.
   a. Surgery
   b. Pharmacy
   c. Public health
   d. None of the above

2. One major focus of public health is the study of _____ .
   a. epidemics
   b. radiologic images
   c. All of the above
   d. None of the above

3. A/An _____ is a *global* outbreak of disease to which every individual in the world is susceptible.
   a. epidemic
   b. infectious disease
   c. pandemic
   d. None of the above

4. A/An _____ is "an excess in the number of cases of a given health problem."
   a. epidemic
   b. infectious disease
   c. natural disaster
   d. None of the above

5. In 2004, the United States funded a plan for researchers to use computers to model diseases, which was called _____ .
   a. MIDAS
   b. model informatics
   c. computational informatics
   d. None of the above

6. _____ is a microbiology information system developed at Brigham and Women's Hospital in Massachusetts. It is used to monitor antibacterial resistance.
   a. WHERENET
   b. WHYNET
   c. HOWNET
   d. WHONET

7. _____ are the programs that create the simulations.
   a. Computational models
   b. Syndromics
   c. Pandemic modems
   d. None of the above

8. _____ refers to "the study of diseases in populations by collecting and analyzing statistical data."
   a. Pandemiology
   b. Epidemiology
   c. A and B
   d. None of the above

9. Computers can create what-if scenarios or _____ .
   a. pictures
   b. graphics
   c. simulations
   d. None of the above

10. In developing countries in Asia and Africa, _____ PDAs are used for the collection and dissemination of information, warnings, and education.
    a. collection
    b. reporting
    c. epidemic control
    d. SATELLIFE

11. Today, some reportable diseases include _____ .
    a. smallpox
    b. polio
    c. AIDS
    d. All of the above

12. Data can be used by SPECTRUM, which calculates the numbers infected with and deaths from _____ .

a. smallpox
b. polio
c. AIDS
d. All of the above

13. In developing countries in Asia and Africa, SATELLIFE PDAs are used for _____ .
    a. the collection of information, warnings, and education
    b. the dissemination of information
    c. health-related education
    d. All of the above

14. Global warming is already having a devastating effect on the earth and on human health; its effects include which of the following?
    a. More intense heat waves
    b. More intense storms
    c. Flooding of major rivers
    d. All of the above

15. Bacteria resistant to antibiotics are known as _____ .
    a. superbugs
    b. *Streptococcus*
    c. A and B
    d. None of the above

## True/False

1. The northeastern United States has warmed over the past hundred years; the rate of this warming has been increasing over the past 30 years. _____

2. WHONET is a microbiology information system used to monitor antibacterial resistance. _____

3. An epidemic is a *global* outbreak of disease to which every individual in the world is susceptible. _____

4. MRSA (methicillin-resistant *Staphylococcus aureus*) is a staphylococcal infection resistant to many antibiotics. _____

5. Currently there are national standards for the collection of health statistics. _____

6. One goal of ONCHIT is the improvement of the "health of the entire nation." _____

7. The definition of an epidemic is based on statistics. _____

8. An epidemic is "an excess in the number of cases of a given health problem." _____

9. Social inequality and absolute poverty are important determinants of health. _____

10. Severe acute respiratory syndrome (SARS) is a form of pneumonia. _____

## Critical Thinking

1. What goals and procedures would you have in place in the event of a catastrophe such as a terrorist attack, a chemical accident, a pandemic, or an epidemic?

2. How would you make sure that first responders are able to communicate with each other and a command center?

3. In the event of a pandemic or epidemic, how would you ensure that sufficient supplies of vaccinations and antiviral drugs are produced and distributed to the general public? In your answer, discuss funding and what institutions would be involved (e.g., existing pharmaceutical companies, government, or perhaps a new institution you would set up).

4. List several effects of global warming.

5. How can we prevent another Katrina-like catastrophe? Deal with the aftermath (death, relocation, destruction, and the failure to rebuild infrastructure), as well as the pre-Katrina crumbling infrastructure (levees).

# Notes

1. John M. Barry, *The Great Influenza* (New York: Penguin, 2005).

2. "Mesothelioma and Asbestos: A Glossary of Related Terms and Definitions," March 24, 2011, http://internationalmesothelioma.net/?p=1097 (accessed May 15, 2011).

3. Brad Lobitz, "NIH Researchers Track Disease with Pocket PCs," July 2004, http://www.pocketpcmag.com/_archives/Jul04/NIHResearch.aspx (accessed April 27, 2011).

4. Howard Markel, *When Germs Travel* (New York: Vintage, 2005).

5. "Better Sanitation Could Save 2 Million Lives: Study," November 16, 2010, http://in.reuters.com/article/2010/11/16/idINIndia-52933820101116 (accessed February 10, 2011).

6. Tracee Herbaugh, "10 Million People at Risk from Pollution," October 19, 2006, http://www.blacksmithinstitute.org/top10/baltimoreexaminerarticle.pdf (accessed April 27, 2011).

7. "Top 6 Toxic Threats Revealed in New Report," November 3, 2010, http://worstpolluted.org/files/FileUpload/files/2010/WWPP-Report-2010-Top-Six-Toxic-Threats-Web.pdf (accessed April 9, 2011).

8. Robert Pear, "Medicare Says It Won't Cover Hospital Errors," August 19, 2007, http://www.nytimes.com/2007/08/19/washington/19hospital.html (accessed April 27, 2011).

9. Jeffrey Young, "Hospital Errors Occur 10 Times More Than Reported, Study Finds," April 7, 2011, http://www.businessweek.com/news/2011-04-07/hospital-errors-occur-10-times-more-than-reported-study-finds.html (accessed April 9, 2011).

10. James Lardner and David A. Smith, eds., *Inequality Matters* (New York: The New Press, 2005); Christopher J. L. Murray and Julio Frenk, "Ranking 37th — Measuring the Performance of the U.S. Health Care System," January 6, 2010, *New England Journal of Medicine*, http://healthpolicyandreform.nejm.org/?p=2610 (accessed March 13, 2011).

11. Lardner and Smith, *Inequality Matters*.

12. Ibid.

13. Anita Pereira, "Live and Let Live: Healthcare Is a Fundamental Human Right," 2004, http://www.law.uconn.edu/system/files/private/pereira.pdf (accessed April 27, 2011).

14. Arloc Sherman and Chad Stone, "Income Gaps between the Very Rich and Everyone Else More Than Tripled in Last Three Decades, New Data Show," June 25, 2010, http://www.cbpp.org/cms/index.cfm?fa=view&id=3220 (accessed March 11, 2011).

15. Ibid.

16. David Leonhardt, "Income Inequality," January 18, 2011, http://topics.nytimes.com/top/reference/timestopics/subjects/i/income/income_inequality/index.html (accessed February 18, 2011).

17. "Income, Poverty and Health Insurance Coverage in the United States: 2009," February 2, 2011, http://www.census.gov/prod/2010pubs/p60-238.pdf (accessed February 20, 2011).

18. "CDC Health Disparities and Inequalities Report – United States, 2011," January 13, 2011, http://www.nesri.org/news/2011/01/cdc-health-disparities-and-inequalities-report-united-states-2011 (accessed March 11, 2011); "HHS Announces Plan to Reduce Health Disparities," April 8, 2011, http://www.hhs.gov/news/press/2011pres/04/20110408a.html (accessed April 8, 2011).

19. "HHS Announces Plan to Reduce Health Disparities"; "HHS Action Plan to Reduce Racial and Ethnic Health Disparities," April 8, 2011, http://www.hhs.gov/news/press/2011pres/04/04hdplan04082011.html (accessed April 8, 2011).

20. "Census Bureau: Recession Fuels Record Number of Uninsured Americans," September 17, 2010, http://www.kaiserhealthnews.org/Daily-Reports/2010/September/16/uninsured-census-statistics.aspx (accessed February 20, 2011).

21. Jennifer Schraag, "Eliminating the Paper Chase: How Informatics Helps the ICP," January 1, 2006, http://www.infectioncontroltoday.com/articles/611feat4.html (accessed April 27, 2011).

22. "Nicotine Levels Rose 10 Percent in Last Six Years, Report Says," August 31, 2006, http://www.nytimes.com/2006/08/31/health/31nicotine.html (accessed April 27, 2011).

23. Jon Gertner, "Incendiary Device," *The New York Times*, June 12, 2005.

24. "Key Mechanism Governing Nicotine Addiction Discovered," January 31, 2011, http://www.sciencedaily.com/releases/2010/01/110130194139.htm (accessed March 14, 2011).

25. Chris Rangel, "Nicotine Vaccine to Treat Tobacco and Nicotine Addiction," January 25, 2011, http://www.kevinmd.com/blog/2011/01/nicotine-vaccine-treat-tobacco-abuse-nicotine-addiction.html (accessed March 14, 2011).

26. "Modeling Infectious Diseases Fact Sheet: Using Computers to prepare for Disease Outbreaks," February 2010, http://www.nigms.nih.gov/Research/FeaturedPrograms/MIDAS/Background/Factsheet.htm (accessed April 27, 2011).

27. "H1N1 Influenza Pandemic Modeling for Public Health Action," http://www.sciencedaily.com/releases/2009/07/090720134227.htm (accessed November 12, 2010); "H1N1 Simulation Modeling Shows Rapid Vaccine Rollout Effective in Reducing Infection Rates," http://www.sciencedaily.com/releases/2009/10/091013112526.htm (accessed November 12, 2010).

28. Marcelo Bortman, "Establishing Endemic Levels or Ranges with Computer Spreadsheets," [Abstract] January 1999, http://www.ncbi.nlm.nih.gov/pubmed/10050608 (accessed April 27, 2011).

29. Barry, *The Great Influenza*.

30. Michael T. Kennedy, *A Brief History of Disease, Science & Medicine* (Portland, OR: Asklepiad Press, 2004).

31. T. M. Wassenaar, "Vaccination (Immunization)," January 6, 2009, http://www.bacteriamuseum.org/cms/How-We-Fight-Bacteria/vaccination-immunization.html (accessed April 27, 2011).

32. "The First Recorded Smallpox Vaccination," 2000, http://www.thedorsetpage.com/history/smallpox/smallpox.htm (accessed April 27, 2011).

33. Andrew Pollack, "Pediatricians Voice Anger over Costs of Vaccines," March 23, 2007, http://www.nytimes.com/2007/03/24/business/24vaccine.html?_r=1&oref=slogin (accessed April 27, 2011).

34. Lesley Alterman, "Cost and Lack of Awareness Hamper Adult Vaccination Efforts," September 24, 2010, http://www.nytimes.com/2010/09/25/health/25patient.html (accessed September 27, 2010).

35. "Pertussis Outbreak in an Amish Community—Kent County, Delaware, September 2004–February 2005," August 4, 2006, http://www.cdc.gov/mmwr/preview/mmwrhtml/mm5530a1.htm (accessed March 15, 2011); Kim Mulholland. "Measles in the United States, 2006," *The New England Journal of Medicine* 355 (2006): 440–3, http://www.nejm.org/doi/full/10.1056/NEJMp068149 (accessed March 14, 2011).

36. Steve Karnowski, "Vaccine Fears Complicate Measles Outbreak in Minn," *The Star-Ledger,* April 3, 2011, 3.

37. Deborah Huso, "Boston Measles Outbreak Points to Importance of Vaccination," March 3, 2011, http://www.aolhealth.com/2011/03/03/boston-measles-outbreak-vaccination/ (accessed April 27, 2011).

38. Michael Willrich, *Pox: An American History* (New York: Penguin Press, 2011).

39. Lisa Farino, "The Risks of Skipping Kids' Vaccines," 2011, http://health.msn.com/health-topics/vaccinations/articlepage.aspx?cp-documentid=100213272 (accessed April 12, 2011); "Measles," June 2, 2009, http://www.mayoclinic.com/health/measles/DS00331 (accessed April 12, 2011).

40. Steven Johnson, *The Ghost Map* (New York: Riverhead Books, 2006).

41. Naomi Rogers, *Dirt and Disease* (New Brunswick, NJ: Rutgers University Press, 1996).

42. Yael Waknine, "Highlights from MMWR: Minimizing Polio Spread in Polio-Free Countries and More," February 17, 2006, http://www.medscape.com/viewarticle/523891 (April 27, 2011).

43. "Kenya: First Case of Polio in Decades," October 18, 2006. http://query.nytimes.com/gst/fullpage.html?res=9B03E0DE1F30F93BA25753C1A9609C8B63&fta=y (accessed April 27 2011); "Ivory Coast Polio Outbreak Could Spread Abroad: WHO," April 21, 2011, http://www.reuters.com/article/2011/04/21/us-polio-outbreak-idUSTRE73K4XF20110421 (accessed April 27, 2011); Stephanie Nebehay, "Acute Polio Outbreak Kills Nearly 100 in Congo: WHO," November 11, 2010, http://www.reuters.com/article/2010/11/11/us-polio-idUSTRE6AA3F720101111 (accessed April 27, 2011).

44. Barry, *The Great Influenza.*

45. Ibid.

46. Ibid.

47. "The Public Health Response," http://virus.stanford.edu/uda/fluresponse.html (accessed April 27, 2011).

48. Andy Ho, "Why Epidemics Still Surprise Us," April 1, 2003, http://www.nytimes.com/2003/04/01/opinion/01ANHO.html (accessed April 27, 2011).

49. Abigail Zuger, "What Did We Learn from AIDS?" November 11, 2003, http://www.nytimes.com/2003/11/11/science/what-did-we-learn-from-aids.html (accessed April 27, 2011).

50. Sarah Abrams, "The Gathering Storm," July 25, 2006, http://www.hsph.harvard.edu/review/the_gathering.shtml (accessed April 27, 2011).

51. Elizabeth Fee and Daniel M. Fox, eds., *AIDS: The Making of a Chronic Disease* (Berkeley, CA: University of California Press, 1991); Jennifer Kates, "HIV Testing in the United States," June 2005, http://www.kff.org/hivaids/upload/Updated-Fact-Sheet-HIV-Testing-in-the-United-States.pdf (accessed April 27, 2011); Jennifer Kates, "The HIV/AIDS Epidemic in the United States," July 2007, http://www.kff.org/hivaids/upload/3029-071.pdf (accessed April 27, 2011).

52. Lawrence K. Altman, "Report Shows AIDS Epidemic Slowdown in 2005," May 31, 2006, http://www.nytimes.com/2006/05/31/world/31aids.html (accessed April 27, 2011).

53. Nicola Mawson, "Supercomputers Accelerate the Search for HIV/AIDS Cure," January 23, 2006, http://www.meraka.org.za/news/Supercomputers_hiv_cure.htm (accessed April 27, 2011).

54. Abigail Zuger, "AIDS, at 25, Offers No Easy Answers," June 6, 2006, http://www.nytimes.com/2006/06/06/health/06aids.html (accessed April 27, 2011).

55. "CDC's HIV Prevention Progress in the United States," July 2010, http://www.cdc.gov/hiv/resources/factsheets/cdcprev.htm (accessed March 15, 2011); "CDC Responds to HIV/AIDS," July 2010, http://www.cdc.gov/hiv/aboutDHAP.htm (accessed March 15, 2011); "HIV in the United States," July 2010, http://www.cdc.gov/hiv/resources/factsheets/us.htm (accessed March 15, 2011).

56. Zuger, "What Did We Learn from AIDS?"

57. "Severe Acute Respiratory Syndrome (SARS)," May 21, 2011, http://health.nytimes.com/health/guides/disease/severe-acute-respiratory-syndrome-sars/news-and-features.html?page=2 (accessed May 21, 2011).

58. "West Nile Virus: What You Need to Know, CDC Fact Sheet," April 18, 2011, http://www.cdc.gov/ncidod/dvbid/westnile/wnv_factsheet.htm (accessed May 21, 2011).

59. John G. Bartlett, "The Rapidly Evolving Field of Infectious Disease," January 5, 2011, http://www.medscape.com/ (accessed April 9, 2011).

60. Ibid.

61. Katherine Bourzac, "New Type of Drug Kills Antibiotic-Resistant Bacteria," April 5, 2011, http://www.technologyreview.com/biomedicine/37268/ (accessed April 13, 2011).

62. Kathleen Blanchard, "Battling Superbugs No Longer Possible without New Antibiotics." http://www.emax

health.com/1020/battling-superbugs-no-longer-possible-without-new-antibiotics (accessed April 27, 2011).

63. Steven Reinberg, "Genetics Used to Track Transmission of MRSA Bacteria," January 21, 2010, http://www.business-week.com/lifestyle/content/healthday/635225.html (accessed February 10, 2011); "Researchers Show How MRSA Transmission Can Be Tracked in Hospital Settings," January 22, 2010, http://www.news-medical.net/news/20100122/Researchers-show-how-MRSA-transmission-can-be-tracked-in-hospital-settings.aspx (accessed February 10, 2011); "MRSA Tracked with DNA Mapping," January 22, 2010, http://www.nursingtimes.net/specialist-news/infection-control-news/mrsa-tracked-with-dna-mapping/5010700.article (accessed February 10, 2011); "Preventing Infection with Technology: CDH Disinfects with Flashing UV Light," February 3, 2011, http://www.medicalnewstoday.com/articles/215504.php (accessed March 12. 2011).

64. Jonathan Benson, "Deadly New 'Superbug' Sweeps Southern California Hospitals, Nursing Homes," March 27, 2011, http://www.naturalnews.com/031859_superbug_nursing_homes.html (accessed April 12, 2011).

65. Kevin Sack, "Study Finds Drop in Deadly V.A. Hospital Infections," April 13, 2011, http://www.nytimes.com/2011/04/14/health/14infections.html (accessed May 3, 2011).

66. Marissa Cevallos, "MRSA in Bedbugs and Meat--An Expert Weighs In," May 13, 2011, http://articles.latimes.com/2011/may/13/news/la-heb-mrsa-bedbugs-meat-20110513 (accessed May 14, 2011).

67. Vincent Iannelli, "Bed Bugs and MRSA," May 12, 2011, http://pediatrics.about.com/b/2011/05/12/bed-bugs-and-mrsa.htm (accessed May 14, 2011).

68. Benson, "Deadly New 'Superbug' Sweeps Southern California Hospitals, Nursing Homes"; "Carbapenem-Resistant Klebsiella Pneumonia," 2011, http://publichealth.lacounty.gov (accessed April 12, 2011); "Q&A with a Superbug Expert: How Dangerous Is CRKP," March 3, 2011, http://healthland.time.com/2011/03/30/qa-with-a-superbug-expert-how-dangerous-is-crkp/ (accessed April 12, 2011).

69. Andrea Parrish, "CRKP Superbug in California Can Be Easily Controlled," March 25, 2011, http://www.newsytype.com/5127-crkp-superbug-california/ (accessed April 12, 2011).

70. Benson, "Deadly New 'Superbug' Sweeps Southern California Hospitals, Nursing Homes."

71. "Human Health and Industrial Farming," http://saveantibiotics.org/ (accessed April 12, 2011); "Pew Urges End to Overuse of Antibiotics in Food Animal Production," July 14, 2010, http://www.pewtrusts.org/news_room_detail.aspx?id=59990 (accessed April 12, 2011).

72. Tim Walsh, "New antibiotic-Resistant Bacteria Discovery," April 8, 2011, http://medicine.cardiff.ac.uk/en/news/antibiotic-resistant-bacteria/ (Accessed April 13, 2011).

73. Steven Reinberg, "Medical Groups Warn of Climate Change's Potential Impact on Health," February 24, 2011, http://www.businessweek.com/lifestyle/content/health-day/635225.html (accessed March 14, 2011).

74. Christopher Joyce, "Text Messages, Radio Alert Haitians to Cholera Risks," October 29, 2010, http://www.wbez.org/story/cholera-haiti/text-messages-radio-alert-haitians-cholera-risks (accessed February 1, 2011); "Cholera Outbreak—Haiti," October 28, 2010, http://www.cdc.gov/mmwr/preview/mmwrhtml/mm5945a1.htm (accessed March 13, 2011); "Scientists Trace Origin of Recent Cholera Epidemic in Haiti," December 10, 2010, http://www.hhmi.org/news/waldor20101209.html (accessed February 10, 2011); "NEWS SCAN: HUS Treatment Patented; Cholera in Haiti; Bloodstream Infections; Polio in Pakistan, DR-Congo; Hand Washing in Schools," February 28, 2011, http://www.cidrap.umn.edu/cidrap/content/fs/food-disease/news/mar0111newsscan.html (accessed March 13, 2011).

75. "Integration of Telehealth Activities and Electronic Patient Records Systems Imperative for Telemedicine Market Growth," July 6, 2005, http://www.highbeam.com/doc/1G1-133803521.html, (accessed April 27, 2011).

76. Office of the National Coordinator for Health Information Technology, "Goals of Strategic Framework," December 10, 2004, http://www.hhs.gov/healthit/goals.html (accessed April 27, 2011).

77. "FAQ on Public Health Registries," May 23, 2007, http://www.ncvhs.hhs.gov/9701138b.htm (accessed April 27, 2011).

78. "Tulsa Health Department FAQs," 2011, http://www.tulsabiowatch.com/pages.aspx?pageid=9 (accessed April 27, 2011).

79. Anemona Hartocollis, "Leprosy, Plague and Other Visitors to New York," February 10, 2011, http://www.nytimes.com/2011/02/11/nyregion/11diseases.html (accessed March 14. 2011).

80. Andrew Sideman, "Handheld Computers Used to Address Critical Health Needs in Rural Africa and Asia," August 21, 2005, http://www.medicalnewstoday.com/articles/29443.php (accessed April 27, 2011); "Moving Information into the Hands of Those Who Heal," May 21, 2009, http://www.satellife.org/ict (accessed April 12, 2011).

81. Phil Elliott, "Computing Aids to Track Cancer," July 4, 2005, http://news.bbc.co.uk/2/hi/technology/4648475.stm (accessed April 27, 2011).

82. Tony Saavedra, "County System Would Track Disease," December 20, 2005, http://www.ocregister.com/ocregister/news/local/article_904817.php (accessed April 27, 2011).

83. "For Immediate Release: ATSDR Launches National ALS Registry," October 20, 2010, http://www.cdc.gov/media/pressrel/2010/r101020.html (accessed April 13, 2011); "US Renal Data System," No date, http://www.usrds.org/faq.htm (accessed April 13, 2011).

84. West Virginia Bureau of Public Health, "Office of Epidemiology and Prevention Services," 2011, http://www.wvsdc.org/SpecialProjects/WVDESS/tabid/1627/Default.aspx (accessed April 26, 2011); "Background on Public Health Surveillance," http://www.cdc.gov/nedss/About/purpose.htm (accessed April 26, 2011); "An Overview of the NEDSS Initiative," http://www.cdc.gov/nedss/About/overview.html (accessed March 15, 2011); "CDC NEDSS – Vitalnet Health Statistics," 2011, http://www.ehdp.com/vitalnet/nedss.htm (accessed April 12, 2011).

85. UNAIDS, 2010, http://www.unaids.org/en/ (accessed April 12, 2011).

86. "Global Report," 2010, http://www.unaids.org/documents/20101115_GR2010_methodology.pdf (accessed April 12, 2011).

87. "WHO Updates Rules to Prevent the Spread of Disease," May 25, 2005, http://www.cidrap.umn.edu/cidrap/content/influenza/avianflu/news/may2405regs.html (accessed April 26, 2011); Michael G. Baker and David P. Fidler, "Global Public Health Surveillance under New International Health Regulations," July 10, 2006, http://cdc.gov/ncidod/eid/vol12 no07/05-1497.htm (accessed April 26, 2011).

88. "G8 Commitments to Infectious Disease Can Improve Global Health Security," July 18, 2006, http://www.who.int/mediacentre/news/statements/2006/s11/en/index.html (accessed April 26, 2011).

89. "Models of Infectious Disease Agent Study," January 24, 2011, http://www.nigms.nih.gov/Initiatives/MIDAS/ (accessed April 12, 2011).

90. "NIH Funds Computer Modeling of Disease Outbreaks, Responses," May 7, 2004, http://www.cidrap.umn.edu/cidrap/content/bt/bioprep/news/may0704modeling.html (accessed April 27, 2011); "Computers Combat Disease: New Modeling Grants Target Epidemics, Bioterror," May 4, 2004, http://www.nigms.nih.gov/News/Results/MIDAS.htm, http://www.nih.gov/news/pr/may 2004/nigms-04.htm (accessed April 27, 2011).

91. "Mathematics and Statistics Combat Epidemics and Bioterror," February 2, 2006, http://www.terradaily.com/reports/Mathematics_And_Statistics_Combat_Epidemics_And_Bioterror.html (accessed April 27, 2011).

92. Mayo Clinic, "Threat of Avian Influenza Pandemic Grows, but People Can Take Precautions," December 6, 2005, http://www.sciencedaily.com/releases/ 2005/12/051206084029.htm (accessed April 27, 2011); "UCI Joins International Effort to Model Influenza Outbreaks," February 1, 2006, http://today.uci.edu/news/release_detail.asp?key=1427 (accessed April 27, 2011); "Researchers Model Avian Flu Outbreak, Impact of Interventions," August 3, 2005, http://www.nigms.nih.gov/News/Results/ 08032005.htm (accessed April 27, 2011).

93. "NIH Study Models H1N1 Flu Spread," September 21, 2010, http://www.nih.gov/news/health/sep2010/nigms-21.htm (accessed March 12, 2011).

94. Union of Concerned Scientists, "Common Sense on Climate Change: Practical Solutions to Global Warming," May 2006, http://ucsusa.org/ (accessed April 27, 2011).

95. "The conclusions in this paragraph reflect the scientific consensus represented by, for example, the Intergovernmental Panel on Climate Change and U.S. Global Change Research Program. Many scientific societies have endorsed these findings in their own statements, including the American Association for the Advancement of Science, American Chemical Society, American Geophysical Union, American Meteorological Society, and American Statistical Association." Quoted from a letter to a Senator, October 21, 2009, http://www.ucsusa.org/assets/documents/ ssi/climate-change-statement-from.pdf (accessed March 14, 2011).

96. Reinberg, "Medical Groups Warn of Climate Change's Potential Impact on Health."

97. Cameron Wake, "Indicators of Climate Change in the Northeast over the Past 100 Years," July 17, 2006, http://www.climateandfarming.org/pdfs/FactSheets/I.2Indicators.pdf (accessed April 27, 2011).

98. "Climate Change," 2006, http://worldwildlife.org/climate/ (accessed April 27, 2011).

99. "Experts Link Asthma to Global Warming," http://news.scotsman.com/health/Experts-link-asthma-to-global.2539193.jp, June 22, 2004, http://healthandenergy.com/asthma_&_global_warming.htm (accessed April 27, 2011).

100. Felicity Barringer, "Officials Reach California Deal to Cut Emissions," August 31, 2006, http://www.nytimes.com/2006/08/31/washington/31warming.html (accessed April 27, 2011).

101. Anthony DePalma, "New York's Water Supply May Need Filtering," July 20, 2006, http://www.nytimes.com/2006/07/20/nyregion/20water.html (accessed April 27, 2011).

102. Barringer, "Officials Reach California Deal to Cut Emissions."

103. "Global Warming Linked to Increase in Western U.S. Wildfires," July 12, 2006, http://www.ens-newswire.com/ens/jul2006/2006-07-12-04.asp (accessed April 27, 2011).

104. Yereth Rosen, "Climate Change Keenly Felt in Alaska's National Parks," February 12, 2011, http://www.reuters.com/article/2011/02/12/us-alaska-climate-idUSTRE71B23320110212 (accessed March 14, 2011).

105. Gerard Wynn and Daniel Wallis, "Global Warming Major Threat to Humanity: Kenya," November 6, 2006, http://www.climateark.org/shared/reader/welcome.aspx?linkid=63324 (accessed April 27, 2011).

106. Joanna Lee, "Bad News: U.S. Business Emissions Growing, Not Slowing," April 23, 2010, http://www.greenbiz.com/blog/2010/04/23/us-business-emissions-growing-not-slowing (accessed March 14, 2011).

107. Reinberg, "Medical Groups Warn of Climate Change's Potential Impact on Health."

108. John Travis, "Hurricane Katrina: Scientists' Fears Come True as Hurricane Floods New Orleans," *Science* 309, no. 5741 (September 9, 2005): 1656–9, http://www.science

mag.org/cgi/content/full/309/5741/1656 (accessed April 27, 2011).

109. "Are the Levees Ready?" June 14, 2006, http://katrinareader.org/are-levees-ready (accessed April 27, 2011).

110. Statement of the National Association of County and City Health Officials, "Health Disparities in the Gulf Coast Before and After Katrina: The Public Health Response," September 23, 2005, http://www.umaryland.edu/health-security/mtf_conference/Documents/Additional%20 Reading/Session%203/Health%20Disparities%20in%20 the%20Gulf%20Coast%20Before%20and%20After%20 Katrina.pdf (accessed April 27, 2011).

111. P. Gregg Greenough and Thomas D. Kirsch, "Public Health Response—Assessing Needs," *The New England Journal of Medicine* 353, no. 15 (2005): 1544–6.

112. Ibid.

113. Cheryl Corley, "Emotional Scars Still Haunt Katrina Survivors," npr.org, June 14, 2006, http://www.npr.org/templates/story/story.php?storyId=5485268 (accessed April 27, 2011).

114. Alix Spiegel, "Suicide Attempts Increase in Katrina's Aftermath," November 16, 2005, http://www.npr.org/templates/story/story.php?storyId=5014682 (accessed April 27, 2011).

115. "Carbon Monoxide Poisoning after Hurricane Katrina— Alabama, Louisiana, and Mississippi, August— September 2005," *MMWR Weekly*, October 7, 2005, http://www.cdc.gov/mmwR/preview/mmwrhtml/ mm5439a7.htm (accessed April 27, 2011).

116. Ann M. Simmons, "New Orleans Endures the 'New Normal,'" July 15, 2006, http://articles.latimes.com/2006/jul/15/nation/na-neworleans15 (accessed April 27, 2011).

117. National Public Radio, "The Morning Edition," November 23, 2006, http://minnesota.publicradio.org/features/npr.php?id=6529452 (accessed April 27, 2011).

118. Campbell Robertson, "Smaller New Orleans after Katrina, Census Shows," February 4, 2011, http://www.nytimes. com/2011/02/04/us/04census.html?page wanted=all (accessed March 13, 2011).

119. Matthew R. Lee and Tony C. Blanchard, "Health Impacts of the Deepwater Horizon Oil Disaster on Coastal Louisiana Residents," July 2010, http://www.lsu. edu/pa/mediacenter/tipsheets/spill/pub lichealthreport_2.pdf (accessed March 14, 2011).

120. Alice Lipowicz, "NOAA Computer Models Predict Coastal Areas to Be Hit by Oil Spill," July 2, 2010, http://fcw. com/articles/2010/07/02/noaa-computer-models-predict-coastal-areas-to-be-hit-by-oil-spill.aspx (accessed March 14, 2011).

121. Gina Solomon and Sarah Janssen, "Health Effects of Gulf Oil Spill," 2010, *Journal of the American Medical Association*, http://jama.ama-assn.org/content/304/10/1118. extract (accessed November 12, 2011); Mark Schleifstein, "Scientists Wary of BP Oil Spill's Long-Term Effects on Species," November 10, 2010, http://www.reefrelieffounders.

com/drilling/2010/11/13/nola-com-scientists-wary-of-bp-oil-spills-long-term-effects-on-species/ (accessed November 12, 2010); "BP Oil Spill Leads to Gulf Region Public Health Disaster," November 12, 2010, http://lecanadian. com/2010/11/12/bp-oil-spill-leads-to-gulf-region-public-health-disaster/ (accessed November 12, 2010); "A Look Back at Last Month's Events and the Spill's Impact to Date," May 20, 2010, http://www.nwf.org/News-and-Magazines/ Media-Center/News-by-Topic/Wildlife/2010/05-20-10-Oil-Spill-One-Month.aspx (accessed November 12, 2010); "Miss. DEQ Seek Help in Assessing Oil Spill Damage," 2010, http://www.worlddisaster.info/klfy-tv-10-acadianas-local-news-weather-and-sports-leader-miss-deq-seek-help-in-assessing-oil-spill-damage (accessed November 12, 2010); Mike Orcutt, "How Will the Gulf Oil Spill Effect Public Health?" August 15, 2010, http://www.popularmechanics.com/science/health/med-tech/gulf-oil-spill-health-effects (accessed November 12, 2010); Harlan Kirgan, "Draft Report from State Oil Spill Panel Due Soon," November 12, 2010, http://blog.gulflive.com/mississippi-press-news/2010/11/draft_report_from_state_oil_sp.html (accessed November 12, 2010); Bryan Walsh, "Assessing the Health Effects of the Oil Spill," June 25, 2010, http:// www.time.com/time/health/article/0,8599,1999479,00. html (accessed November 12, 2010); Christopher Weber, "Commission Report Slams Government's Oil Spill Response," 2010, http://www.politicsdaily.com/2010/10/06/ commission-report-slams-governments-oil-spill-response/ print/ (accessed November 12, 2010).

122. Solomon and Janssen, "Health Effects of Gulf Oil Spill"; Schleifstein, "Scientists Wary of BP Oil Spill's Long-Term Effects on Species"; "BP Oil Spill Leads to Gulf Region Public Health Disaster"; "A Look Back at Last Month's Events and the Spill's Impact to Date"; "Miss. DEQ Seek Help in Assessing Oil Spill Damage"; Orcutt, "How Will the Gulf Oil Spill Effect Public Health?"; Kirgan, "Draft Report from State Oil Spill Panel Due Soon"; Walsh, "Assessing the Health Effects of the Oil Spill"; Weber, "Commission Report Slams Government's Oil Spill Response"; John R. Broder, "Report Slams Administration for Underestimating Gulf Spill," October 6, 2010, http://www.nytimes.com/2010/10/07/science/ earth/07spill.html (accessed March 13, 2011); Chuck Hopklinson, "Outcome/Guidance from Georgia Sea Spill Grant Program: Current Status of BP Oil Spill," August 17, 2010, http://oilspill.uga.edu/wp-content/uploads/ Georgia-Sea-Grant-Oil-Spill-Report-20100816.pdf (accessed March 14, 2011).

123. Michael Feldman, "Computer Simulations Illustrate Scope of Japanese Disaster," March 16, 2011, http:// www.hpcwire.com/hpcwire/2011-03-16/computer_ simulations_illustrate_scope_of_japanese_disaster.html (accessed April 13, 2011).

124. Derek Thompson, "By the Numbers: The Japanese Disaster and the Nuclear Crisis," March 2011, http:// www.theatlantic.com/business/archive/2011/03/by-the-numbers-the-japanese-disaster-and-the-nuclear-crisis/72729/ (accessed April 13, 2011).

125. David Jolly, Hiroko Tabuchi, and Keith Bradsher, "Japan Encourages a Wider Evacuation from Reactor Area," March 26, 2011, http://www.nytimes.com/2011/03/26/world/asia/26japan.html?pagewanted=all (accessed April 13, 2011). Read more at: http://www.ndtv.com/article/world/japan-encourages-a-wider-evacuation-from-reactor-area-94229?cp.

126. "Radiation Levels Soar Near Fukushima Nuclear Plant," March 30, 2011, http://www.dailytelegraph.com.au/news/breaking-news/radiation-levels-soar-near-fukushima-nuclear-plant/story-e6freuz9-1226030854699 (accessed April 13, 2011); Bloomberg, "Japan Raises Highest Alert Amid Increased Radiation," April 13, 2011, http://www.manilastandardtoday.com/insideNews.htm?f=2011/april/13/news2.isx&d=2011/april/13 (accessed April 13, 2011).

127. Keith Bradsher, Hiroko Tabuchi, and Andrew Pollack. "Japanese Officials on Defensive as Nuclear Alert Level Rises." April 12, 2011. http://www.nytimes.com/2011/04/13/world/asia/13japan.html?pagewanted=all (accessed April 13, 2011).

128. Jeff McMahon, "Radiation Detected in Drinking Water in 13 More US Cities, Cesium-137 in Vermont Milk," April 9, 2011, http://www.forbes.com/sites/jeff mcmahon/2011/04/09/radiation-detected-in-drinking-water-in-13-more-us-cities-cesium-137-in-vermont-milk/ (accessed April 13, 2011).

129. Jeff McMahon, "EPA: New Radiation Highs in Little Rock Milk, Philadelphia Drinking Water," April 10, 2011, http://www.forbes.com/sites/jeffmcmahon/2011/04/10/epa-new-radiation-highs-in-little-rock-milk-philadelphia-drinking-water/ (accessed April 13, 2011).

130. "No Such Thing as a Safe Dose of Radiation," No date, http://www.nirs.org/factsheets/nosafedose.pdf (accessed April 13, 2011).

131. Lindsay Goldwert, "How Harmful Is Radiation Exposure? Nuclear Disaster in Japan Sparks Chernobyl-Type Cancer Fears," March 15, 2011, http://articles.nydailynews.com/2011-03-15/entertainment/29149226_1_radiation-exposure-nuclear-waste-public-health-project/2 (accessed April 13, 2011).

132. George Johnson, "Radiation's Enduring Afterglow," March 26, 2011, http://www.nytimes.com/2011/03/27/weekinreview/27johnson.html?pagewanted=all (accessed April 13, 2011).

133. *New York Times*, "Japan — Earthquake, Tsunami and Nuclear Crisis (2011)," February 16, 2012, nyt.com (accessed February 18, 2012.

# Additional Resources

"A Look Back at Last Month's Events and the Spill's Impact to Date." May 20, 2010. http://www.nwf.org/News-and-Magazines/Media-Center/News-by-Topic/Wildlife/2010/05-20-10-Oil-Spill-One-Month.aspx (accessed November 12, 2010).

Abrams, Sarah. "The Gathering Storm." July 25, 2006. http://www.hsph.harvard.edu/review/the_gathering.shtml (accessed April 27, 2011).

Alterman, Lesley. "Cost and Lack of Awareness Hamper Adult Vaccination Efforts." September 24, 2010. http://www.nytimes.com/2010/09/25/health/25patient.html (accessed September 27, 2010).

Altman, Lawrence K. "Report Shows AIDS Epidemic Slowdown in 2005." May 31, 2006. http://www.nytimes.com/2006/05/31/world/31aids.html (accessed April 27, 2011).

"An Overview of the NEDSS Initiative." http://www.cdc.gov/nedss/About/overview.html (accessed March 15, 2011).

"Are the Levees Ready?" June 14, 2006. http://katrinareader.org/are-levees-ready (accessed April 27, 2011).

"Background on Public Health Surveillance." http://www.cdc.gov/nedss/About/purpose.htm (accessed April 26, 2011).

Baker, Michael G., and David P. Fidler. "Global Public Health Surveillance Under New International Health Regulations." July 10, 2006. http://cdc.gov/ncidod/eid/vol12no07/05-1497.htm (accessed April 26, 2011).

Barringer, Felicity. "Officials Reach California Deal to Cut Emissions." August 31, 2006. http://www.nytimes.com/2006/08/31/washington/31warming.html (accessed April 27, 2011).

Barry, John M. *The Great Influenza*. New York: Penguin, 2005.

Bartlett, John G. "The Rapidly Evolving Field of Infectious Disease." January 5, 2011. http://www.medscape.com/ (accessed April 9, 2011).

Benson, Jonathan. "Deadly New 'Superbug' Sweeps Southern California Hospitals, Nursing Homes." March 27, 2011. http://www.naturalnews.com/031859_superbug_nursing_homes.html (accessed April 12, 2011).

"Better Sanitation Could Save 2 Million Lives: Study." November 16, 2010. http://in.reuters.com/article/2010/11/16/idINIndia-52933820101116 (accessed February 10, 2011).

Blanchard, Kathleen. "Battling Superbugs No Longer Possible Without New Antibiotics." http://www.emaxhealth.com/1020/battling-superbugs-no-longer-possible-without-new-antibiotics (accessed April 27, 2011).

Bloomberg. "Japan Raises Highest Alert Amid Increased Radiation." April 13, 2011. http://www.manilastandard-today.com/insideNews.htm?f=2011/april/13/news2.isx&d=2011/april/13 (accessed April 13, 2011).

Bortman, Marcelo. "Establishing Endemic Levels or Ranges with Computer Spreadsheets." [Abstract] January 1999.

http://www.ncbi.nlm.nih.gov/pubmed/10050608 (accessed April 27, 2011).

Bourzac, Katherine. "New Type of Drug Kills Antibiotic-Resistant Bacteria." April 5, 2011. http://www.technologyreview.com/biomedicine/37268/ (accessed April 13, 2011).

"BP Oil Spill Leads to Gulf Region Public Health Disaster." November 12, 2010. http://lecanadian.com/2010/11/12/bp-oil-spill-leads-to-gulf-region-public-health-disaster/ (accessed November 12, 2010).

Bradsher, Keith, Hiroko Tabuchi, and Andrew Pollack. "Japanese Officials on Defensive as Nuclear Alert Level Rises." April 12, 2011. http://www.nytimes.com/2011/04/13/world/asia/13japan.html?pagewanted=all (accessed April 13, 2011).

Campbell, Carl Ann. "Medicare Ends Coverage of Hospital Errors." *The Sunday Star-Ledger*, August 12, 2007, 1, 11.

"Carbapenem-Resistant Klesiella Pneumonia." 2011. http://publichealth.lacounty.gov (accessed April 12, 2011).

"Carbon Monoxide Poisoning After Hurricane Katrina—Alabama, Louisiana, and Mississippi, August—September 2005." *MMWR Weekly*. October 7, 2005. http://www.cdc.gov/mmwR/preview/mmwrhtml/mm5439a7.htm (accessed April 27, 2011).

"CDC Health Disparities and Inequalties Report – United States, 2011." January 13, 2011. http://www.nesri.org/news/2011/01/cdc-health-disparities-and-inequalities-report-united-states-2011 (accessed March 11, 2011).

"CDC NEDSS – Vitalnet Health Statistics." 2011. http://www.ehdp.com/vitalnet/nedss.htm (accessed April 12, 2011).

"CDC Responds to HIV/AIDS." July 2010. http://www.cdc.gov/hiv/aboutDHAP.htm (accessed March 15, 2011).

"CDC's HIV Prevention Progress in the United States." July 2010. http://www.cdc.gov/hiv/resources/factsheets/cdcprev.htm (accessed March 15, 2011).

"Census Bureau: Recession Fuels Record Number of Uninsured Americans." September 17, 2010. http://www.kaiserhealthnews.org/Daily-Reports/2010/September/16/uninsured-census-statistics.aspx (accessed February 20, 2011).

"Cholera Outbreak—Haiti." October 28, 2010. http://www.cdc.gov/mmwr/preview/mmwrhtml/mm5945a1.htm (accessed March 13, 2011).

"Climate Change." 2006. http://worldwildlife.org/climate/ (accessed April 27, 2011).

"Computers Combat Disease: New Modeling Grants Target Epidemics, Bioterror." May 4, 2004. http://www.nih.gov/news/pr/may2004/nigms-04.htm (accessed April 27, 2011).

Corley, Cheryl, "Emotional Scars Still Haunt Katrina Survivors." June 14, 2006. http://www.npr.org/templates/story/story.php?storyId=5485268 (accessed April 27, 2011).

DePalma, Anthony . "New York's Water Supply May Need Filtering." July 20, 2006. http://www.nytimes.com/2006/07/20/nyregion/20water.html (accessed April 27, 2011).

Elliott, Phil. "Computing Aids to Track Cancer." July 4, 2005. http://news.bbc.co.uk/2/hi/technology/4648475.stm (accessed April 27, 2011).

"Experts Link Asthma to Global Warming." June 22, 2004. http://news.scotsman.com/health/Experts-link-asthma-to-global.2539193.jp (accessed April 27, 2011).

"FAQ on Public Health Registries." May 23, 2007. http://www.ncvhs.hhs.gov/9701138b.htm (accessed April 27, 2011).

Farino, Lisa. "The Risks of Skipping Kids' Vaccines." 2011. http://health.msn.com/health-topics/vaccinations/articlepage.aspx?cp-documentid=100213272 (accessed April 12, 2011).

Fee, Elizabeth, and Daniel M. Fox, eds. *AIDS: The Making of a Chronic Disease*. Berkeley, CA: University of California Press, 1991.

Feldman, Michael. "Computer Simulations Illustrate Scope of Japanese Disaster." March 16, 2011. http://www.hpcwire.com/hpcwire/2011-03-16/computer_simulations_illustrate_scope_of_japanese_disaster.html (accessed April 13, 2011).

"For Immediate Release: ATSDR Launches National ALS Registry." October 20, 2010. http://www.cdc.gov/media/pressrel/2010/r101020.html (accesses April 13, 2011).

"G8 Commitments to Infectious Disease Can Improve Global Health Security." July 18, 2006. http://www.who.int/mediacentre/news/statements/2006/s11/en/index.html (accessed April 26, 2011).

Gertner, Jon. "Incendiary Device." *The New York Times*, June 12, 2005.

"Global Report," 2010. http://www.unaids.org/documents/20101115_GR2010_methodology.pdf (accessed April 12, 2011).

"Global Warming Linked to Increase in Western U.S. Wildfires." July 12, 2006. http://www.ens-newswire.com/ens/jul2006/2006-07-12-04.asp (accessed April 27, 2011).

Goldwert, Lindsay. "How Harmful Is Radiation Exposure? Nuclear Disaster in Japan Sparks Chernobyl-Type Cancer Fears." March 15, 2011. http://articles.nydailynews.com/2011-03-15/entertainment/29149226_1_radiation-exposure-nuclear-waste-public-health-project/2 (accessed April 13, 2011).

Greenough, P. Gregg, and Thomas D. Kirsch. "Public Health Response—Assessing Need." *The New England Journal of Medicine* 353, no. 15 (2005): 1544–6.

"H1N1 Influenza Pandemic Modeling for Public Health Action." http://www.sciencedaily.com/releases/2009/07/090720134227.htm (accessed November 12, 2010).

"H1N1 Simulation Modeling Shows Rapid Vaccine Rollout Effective in Reducing Infection Rates." http://www.sciencedaily.com/releases/2009/10/091013112526.htm (accessed November 12, 2010).

Hartocollis, Anemona. "Leprosy, Plague and Other Visitors to New York." February 10, 2011. http://www.nytimes.com/2011/02/11/nyregion/11diseases.html (accessed March 14. 2011).

Herbaugh, Tracee. "10 Million People at Risk from Pollution." October 19, 2006. http://www.blacksmithinstitute.org/top10/baltimoreexaminerarticle.pdf (accessed April 27, 2011).

"HHS Action Plan to Reduce Racial and Ethnic Health Disparities." April 8, 2011. http://www.hhs.gov/news/press/2011pres/04/04hdplan04082011.html (accessed April 8, 2011).

"HHS Announces Plan to Reduce Health Disparities." April 8, 2011. http://www.hhs.gov/news/press/2011pres/04/20110408a.html (accessed April 8, 2011).

"HIV in the United States." July 2010. http://www.cdc.gov/hiv/resources/factsheets/us.htm (accessed March 15, 2011).

Ho, Andy. "Why Epidemics Still Surprise Us." April 1, 2003. http://www.nytimes.com/2003/04/01/opinion/01ANHO.html (accessed April 27, 2011).

"Human Health and Industrial Farming." http://saveantibiotics.org/ (accessed April 12, 2011).

Huso, Deborah. "Boston Measles Outbreak Points to Importance of Vaccination." March 3, 2011. http://www.aolhealth.com/2011/03/03/boston-measles-outbreak-vaccination/ (accessed April 27, 2011).

"Income, Poverty and Health Insurance Coverage in the United States: 2009." February 2, 2011. http://www.census.gov/prod/2010pubs/p60-238.pdf (accessed February 20, 2011).

"Integration of Telehealth Activities and Electronic Patient Records Systems Imperative for Telemedicine Market Growth." July 6, 2005. http://www.highbeam.com/doc/1G1-133803521.html (accessed April 27, 2011).

"Ivory Coast Polio Outbreak Could Spread Abroad: WHO." April 21, 2011. http://www.reuters.com/article/2011/04/21/us-polio-outbreak-idUSTRE73K4XF20110421 (accessed April 27, 2011).

Johnson, George. "Radiation's Enduring Afterglow." March 26, 2011. http://www.nytimes.com/2011/03/27/weekinreview/27johnson.html?pagewanted=all (accessed April 13, 2011).

Johnson, Steven. *The Ghost Map*. New York: Riverhead Books, 2006.

Jolly, David, Hiroko Tabuchi, and Keith Bradsher. "Japan Encourages a Wider Evacuation from Reactor Area." March 26, 2011. http://www.nytimes.com/2011/03/26/world/asia/26japan.html?pagewanted=all (accessed April 13, 2011).

Joyce, Christopher. "Text Messages, Radio Alert Haitians to Cholera Risks." October 29, 2010. http://www.wbez.org/story/cholera-haiti/text-messages-radio-alert-haitians-cholera-risks (accessed February 1, 2011).

Karnowski, Steve. "Vaccine Fears Complicate Measles Outbreak in Minn." *The Star-Ledger,* April 3, 2011.

Kates, Jennifer. "HIV Testing in the United States." June 2005. http://www.kff.org/hivaids/upload/Updated-Fact-Sheet-HIV-Testing-in-the-United-States.pdf (accessed April 27, 2011).

Kates, Jennifer. "The HIV/AIDS Epidemic in the United States." July 2007. http://www.kff.org/hivaids/upload/3029-071.pdf (accessed April 27, 2011).

Kennedy, Michael T. *A Brief History of Disease, Science and Medicine*. Portland, OR: Asklepiad Press, 2004.

"Kenya: First Case of Polio in Decades." October 18, 2006. http://query.nytimes.com/gst/fullpage.html?res=9B03E0DE1F30F93BA25753C1A9609C8B63&fta=y (accessed April 27, 2011).

"Key Mechanism Governing Nicotine Addiction Discovered." January 31, 2011. http://www.sciencedaily.com/releases/2010/01/110130194139.htm (accessed March 14, 2011).

Kirgan, Harlan. "Draft Report from State Oil Spill Panel Due Soon." November 12, 2010. http://blog.gulflive.com/mississippi-press-news/2010/11/draft_report_from_state_oil_sp.html (accessed November 12, 2010).

Lardner, James, and David A. Smith, eds. *Inequality Matters*. New York: The New Press, 2005.

Lee, Joanna. "Bad News: U.S. Business Emissions Growing, Not Slowing." April 23, 2010. http://www.greenbiz.com/blog/2010/04/23/us-business-emissions-growing-not-slowing (accessed March 14, 2011).

Lee, Matthew R., and Tony C. Blanchard. "Health Impacts of the Deewater Horizon Oil Disaster on Coastal Louisiana Residents." July 2010. http://www.lsu.edu/pa/mediacenter/tipsheets/spill/publichealthreport_2.pdf (accessed March 14, 2011).

Leonhardt, David. "Income Inequality." January 18, 2011. http://topics.nytimes.com/top/reference/timestopics/subjects/i/income/income_inequality/index.html (accessed February 18, 2011).

Lipowicz, Alice. "NOAA Computer Models Predict Coastal Areas to Be Hit by Oil Spill." July 2, 2010. http://fcw.com/articles/2010/07/02/noaa-computer-models-predict-coastal-areas-to-be-hit-by-oil-spill.aspx (accessed March 14, 2011).

Lobitz, Brad. "NIH Researchers Track Disease with Pocket PCs." July 2004. http://www.pocketpcmag.com/_archives/Jul04/NIHResearch.aspx (accessed December 26, 2007).

Markel, Howard. *When Germs Travel*. New York: Vintage, 2005.

"Mathematics and Statistics Combat Epidemics and Bioterror." February 2, 2006. http://www.terradaily.com/reports/Mathematics_And_Statistics_Combat_Epidemics_And_Bioterror.html (accessed April 27, 2011).

Mawson, Nicola. "Supercomputers Accelerate the Search for HIV/AIDS Cure." January 23, 2006. http://www.meraka.org.za/news/Supercomputers_hiv_cure.htm (accessed April 27, 2011).

Mayo Clinic. "Threat of Avian Influenza Pandemic Grows, but People Can Take Precautions." December 6, 2005. http://www.sciencedaily.com/releases/2005/12/051206084029.htm (accessed April 27, 2011).

McMahon, Jeff. "EPA: New Radiation Highs in Little Rock Milk, Philadelphia Drinking Water." April 10, 2011. http://www.forbes.com/sites/jeffmcmahon/2011/04/10/epa-new-radiation-highs-in-little-rock-milk-philadelphia-drinking-water/ (accessed April 13, 2011).

McMahon, Jeff. "Radiation Detected in Drinking Water in 13 More US Cities, Cesium-137 in Vermont Milk." April 9, 2011. http://www.forbes.com/sites/jeffmcmahon/2011/04/09/radiation-detected-in-drinking-water-in-13-more-us-cities-cesium-137-in-vermont-milk/ (accessed April 13, 2011).

"Measles." June 2, 2009. http://www.mayoclinic.com/health/measles/DS00331 (accessed April 12, 2011).

"Mesothelioma and Asbestos: A Glossary of Related Terms and Definitions." March 24, 2011. http://www.articles-base.com/cancer-articles/mesothelioma-and-asbestos-a-glossary-of-related-terms-and-definitions-407421.html (accessed April 27, 2011).

"Modeling Infectious Diseases Fact Sheet: Using Computers to Prepare for Disease Outbreaks." February 2010. http://www.nigms.nih.gov/Research/FeaturedPrograms/MIDAS/Background/Factsheet.htm (Accessed April 27, 2011).

"Models of Infectious Disease Agent Study." January 24, 2011. http://www.nigms.nih.gov/Initiatives/MIDAS/ (accessed April 12, 2011).

"Moving Information into the Hands of Those Who Heal." May 21, 2009. http://www.satellife.org/ict (accessed April 12, 2011).

"Miss. DEQ Seek Help in Assessing Oil Spill Damage." 2010. http://www.worlddisaster.info/klfy-tv-10-acadianas-local-news-weather-and-sports-leader-miss-deq-seek-help-in-assessing-oil-spill-damage/ (accessed November 12, 2010).

"MRSA Tracked with DNA Mapping." January 22, 2010. http://www.nursingtimes.net/specialist-news/infection-con-trol-news/mrsa-tracked-with-dna-mapping/5010700.article (accessed February 10, 2011).

Mulholland, Kim. "Measles in the United States, 2006." *The New England Journal of Medicine* 355 (2006): 440–3. http://www.nejm.org/doi/full/10.1056/NEJMp068149 (accessed March 14, 2011).

Murray, Christopher J. L., and Julio Frenk. "Ranking 37th — Measuring the Performance of the U.S. Health Care System." January 6, 2010. *New England Journal of Medicine.* http://healthpolicyandreform.nejm.org/?p=2610 (accessed March 13, 2011).

National Public Radio. "The Morning Edition." November 23, 2006. http://minnesota.publicradio.org/features/npr.php?id=6529452 (accessed April 27, 2011).

Nebehay, Stephanie. "Acute Polio Outbreak Kills Nearly 100 in Congo: WHO." November 11, 2010. http://www.reuters.com/article/2010/11/11/us-polio-idUS-TRE6AA3F720101111 (accessed April 27, 2011).

*New York Times.* "Japan — Earthquake, Tsunami and Nuclear Crisis (2011)." February 16, 2012, nyt.com (accessed February 18, 2012).

"NEWS SCAN: HUS Treatment Patented; Cholera in Haiti; Bloodstream Infections; Polio in Pakistan, DR-Congo; Hand Washing in Schools." February 28, 2011. http://www.cidrap.umn.edu/cidrap/content/fs/food-disease/news/mar0111newsscan.html (accessed March 13, 2011).

"Nicotine Levels Rose 10 Percent in Last Six Years, Report Says." August 31, 2006. http://www.nytimes.com/2006/08/31/health/31nicotine.html (accessed April 27, 2011).

"NIH Funds Computer Modeling Of Disease Outbreaks, Responses." May 7, 2004. http://www.cidrap.umn.edu/cidrap/content/bt/bioprep/news/may0704modeling.html (accessed April 27, 2011).

"NIH Study Models H1N1 Flu Spread." September 21, 2010. http://www.nih.gov/news/health/sep2010/nigms-21.htm (accessed March 12, 2011).

"No Such Thing as a Safe Dose of Radiation." http://www.nirs.org/factsheets/nosafedose.pdf (accessed April 13, 2011).

Office of the National Coordinator for Health Information Technology. "Goals of Strategic Framework." December 10, 2004. http://www.hhs.gov/healthit/goals.html (accessed April 27, 2011).

Orcutt, Mike. "How Will the Gulf Oil Spill Effect Public Health?" August 15, 2010. http://www.popularmechanics.com/science/health/med-tech/gulf-oil-spill-health-effects (accessed November 12, 2010).

Parrish, Andrea. "CRKP Superbug in California Can Be Easily Controlled." March 25, 2011. http://www.newsytype.com/5127-crkp-superbug-california/ (accessed April 12, 2011).

Pereira, Anita. "Live and Let Live: Healthcare Is a Fundamental Human Right." 2004. http://www.law.uconn.edu/system/files/private/pereira.pdf (accessed April 27, 2011).

Pérez-Peña, Richard. "City Tackles Meningitis in Brooklyn." June 29, 2006. http://www.nytimes.com/2006/06/29/nyregion/29meningitis.html (accessed April 27, 2011).

"Pertussis Outbreak in an Amish Community—Kent County, Delaware, September 2004–February 2005." August 4, 2006. http://www.cdc.gov/mmwr/preview/mmwrhtml/mm5530a1.htm (accessed March 15, 2011).

"Pew Urges End to Overuse of Antibiotics in Food Animal Production." July 14, 2010. http://www.pewtrusts.org/news_room_detail.aspx?id=59990 (accessed April 12, 2011).

Pollack, Andrew. "Pediatricians Voice Anger over Costs of Vaccines." March 23, 2007. http://www.nytimes.com/2007/03/24/business/24vaccine.html?_r=1&oref=slogin (accessed April 27, 2011).

"Preventing Infection with Technology: CDH Disinfects with Flashing UV Light." February 3, 2011. http://www.medical-newstoday.com/articles/215504.php (accessed March 12, 2011).

"Radiation Levels Soar Near Fukushima Nuclear Plant." March 30, 2011. http://www.dailytelegraph.com.au/news/breaking-news/radiation-levels-soar-near-fukushima-nuclear-plant/story-e6freuz9-1226030854699 (accessed April 13, 2011).

Rangel, Chris. "Nicotine Vaccine to Treat Tobacco and Nicotine Addiction." January 2010. http://www.kevinmd.com/blog/2011/01/nicotine-vaccine-treat-tobacco-abuse-nicotine-addiction.html (accessed March 14, 2011).

Reinberg, Steven. "Genetics Used to Track Transmission of MRSA Bacteria." January 21, 2010. http://www.businessweek.com/lifestyle/content/healthday/635225.html (accessed February 10, 2011).

Reinberg, Steven. "Medical Groups Warn of Climate Change's Potential Impact on Health." February 24, 2011. http://news.yahoo.com/medical-groups-warn-climate-changes-potential-impact-health-20110224-140606-991.html (accessed March 14, 2011).

"Researchers Model Avian Flu Outbreak, Impact of Interventions." August 3, 2005. http://www.nigms.nih.gov/News/Results/08032005.htm (accessed April 27, 2011).

"Researchers Show How MRSA Transmission Can Be Tracked in Hospital Settings." January 22, 2010. http://www.news-medical.net/news/20100122/Researchers-show-how-MRSA-transmission-can-be-tracked-in-hospital-settings.aspx (accessed February 10, 2011).

Robertson, Campbell. "Smaller New Orleans after Katrina, Census Shows." February 4, 2011. http://www.nytimes.com/2011/02/04/us/04census.html?pagewanted=all (accessed March 13, 2011).

Rogers, Naomi. *Dirt and Disease*. New Brunswick, NJ: Rutgers University Press, 1996.

Rosen, Yereth. "Climate Change Keenly Felt in Alaska's National Parks." February 12, 2011. http://www.reuters.com/article/2011/02/12/us-alaska-climate-idUSTRE71B23320110212 (March 14, 2011).

Saavedra, Tony. "County System Would Track Disease." December 20, 2005. http://www.ocregister.com/ocregister/news/local/article_904817.php (accessed April 27, 2011).

Sack, Kevin. "Study Finds Drop in Deadly V.A. Hospital Infections." April 13, 2011. http://www.nytimes.com/2011/04/14/health/14infections.html (accessed May 3, 2011).

Schleifstein, Mark. "Scientists Wary of BP Oil Spill's Long-Term Effects on Species." November 10, 2010. http://www.reefrelieffounders.com/drilling/2010/11/13/nola-com-scientists-wary-of-bp-oil-spills-long-term-effects-on-species/ (accessed November 12, 2010).

Schraag, Jennifer. "Eliminating the Paper Chase: How Informatics Helps the ICP." January 1, 2006. http://www.infectioncontroltoday.com/articles/611feat4.html (accessed April 27, 2011).

"Scientists Trace Origin of Recent Cholera Epidemic in Haiti." December 10, 2010. http://www.hhmi.org/news/waldor20101209.html (accessed February 10, 2011).

Sherman, Arloc, and Chad Stone. "Income Gaps Between the Very Rich and Everyone Else More Than Tripled in Last Three Decades, New Data Show." June 25, 2010. http://www.cbpp.org/cms/index.cfm?fa=view&id=3220 (accessed March 11, 2011).

Sideman, Andrew. "Handheld Computers Used to Address Critical Health Needs in Rural Africa and Asia." August 21, 2005. http://www.medicalnewstoday.com/articles/29443.php (accessed April 27, 2011).

Simmons, Ann M. "New Orleans Endures the 'New Normal.'" July 15, 2006. http://articles.latimes.com/2006/jul/15/nation/na-neworleans15 (accessed April 27, 2011).

Solomon, Gina, and Sarah Janssen. "Health Effects of Gulf Oil Spill." 2010. *Journal of the American Medical Association.* http://jama.ama-assn.org/content/304/10/1118.extract (accessed November 12, 2011).

Spiegel, Alix. "Suicide Attempts Increase in Katrina's Aftermath." November 16, 2005. http://www.npr.org/templates/story/story.php?storyId=5014682 (accessed April 27, 2011).

Statement of the National Association of County & City Health Officials. "Health Disparities in the Gulf Coast before and after Katrina: The Public Health Response." September 23, 2005. http://www.umaryland.edu/healthsecurity/mtf_conference/Documents/Additional%20Reading/Session%203/Health%20Disparities%20in%20the%20Gulf%20Coast%20Before%20and%20After%20Katrina.pdf (accessed April 27, 2011).

"The First Recorded Smallpox Vaccination." 2000. http://www.thedorsetpage.com/history/smallpox/smallpox.htm (accessed April 27, 2011).

"The Public Health Response." http://virus.stanford.edu/uda/fluresponse.html (accessed April 27, 2011).

Thompson, Derek. "By the Numbers: The Japanese Disaster and the Nuclear Crisis." March 2011. http://www.theatlantic.com/business/archive/2011/03/by-the-numbers-the-japanese-disaster-and-the-nuclear-crisis/72729/ (accessed April 13, 2011).

"Top 6 Toxic Threats Revealed in New Report." November 3, 2010. http://worstpolluted.org/files/FileUpload/files/2010/

WWPP-Report-2010-Top-Six-Toxic-Threats-Web.pdf (accessed April 9, 2011).

Travis, John. "Hurricane Katrina: Scientists' Fears Come True as Hurricane Floods New Orleans." *Science* 309, no. 5741 (September 9, 2005): 1656–9. http://www.sciencemag.org/cgi/content/full/309/5741/1656 (accessed April 27, 2011).

"Tulsa Health Department FAQs." 2011. http://www.tulsabiowatch.com/pages.aspx?pageid=9 (accessed April 27, 2011).

"UCI Joins International Effort to Model Influenza Outbreaks." February 1, 2006. http://today.uci.edu/news/release_detail.asp?key=1427 (accessed April 27, 2011).

UNAIDS. 2010. http://www.unaids.org/en/ (accessed April 12, 2011).

Union of Concerned Scientists. "Common Sense on Climate Change: Practical Solutions to Global Warming." May 2006. http://www.ucsusa.org/global_warming/solutions/big_picture_solutions/common-sense-on-climate-5.html (accessed April 27, 2011).

"US Renal Data System." No date. http://www.usrds.org/faq.htm (accessed April 13, 2011).

Wake, Cameron, "Indicators of Climate Change in the Northeast over the Past 100 Years." July 17, 2006. http://www.climateandfarming.org/pdfs/FactSheets/I.2Indicators.pdf (accessed April 27, 2011).

Waknine, Yael. "Highlights from MMWR: Minimizing Polio Spread in Polio-Free Countries and More." February 17, 2006. http://www.medscape.com/viewarticle/523891 (accessed April 27, 2011).

Walsh, Bryan. "Assessing the Health Effects of the Oil Spill." June 25, 2010. http://www.time.com/time/health/article/0,8599,1999479,00.html (accessed November 12, 2010).

Walsh, Tim. "New Antibiotic-Resistant Bacteria Discovery." April 8, 2011. http://medicine.cardiff.ac.uk/en/news/antibiotic-resistant-bacteria/ (Accessed April 13, 2011).

Wassenaar, T. M. "Vaccination (Immunization)." January 6, 2009. http://www.bacteriamuseum.org/cms/How-We-Fight-Bacteria/vaccination-immunization.html (accessed April 27, 2011).

Weber, Christopher. "Commission Report Slams Government's Oil Spill Response." 2010. http://www.politicsdaily.com/2010/10/06/commission-report-slams-governments-oil-spill-response/print/ (accessed November 12, 2010).

West Virginia Bureau of Public Health. "Office of Epidemiology and Prevention Services." 2011. http://www.wvsdc.org/SpecialProjects/WVDESS/tabid/1627/Default.aspx (accessed April 26, 2011).

"WHO Updates Rules to Prevent the Spread of Disease." May 24, 2005. http://www.cidrap.umn.edu/cidrap/content/influenza/avianflu/news/may2405regs.html (accessed April 26, 2011).

Willrich, Michael. *Pox: An American History*. New York: Penguin Press, 2011.

Wynn, Gerard, and Daniel Wallis. "Global Warming Major Threat to Humanity: Kenya." November 6, 2006. http://www.climateark.org/shared/reader/welcome.aspx?linkid=63324 (accessed April 27, 2011).

Young, Jeffrey. "Hospital Errors Occur 10 Times More Than Reported, Study Finds." April 7, 2011. http://www.businessweek.com/news/2011-04-07/hospital-errors-occur-10-times-more-than-reported-study-finds.html (accessed April 9, 2011).

Zuger, Abigail. "AIDS, at 25, Offers No Easy Answers." June 6, 2006. http://www.nytimes.com/2006/06/06/health/06aids.html (accessed April 27, 2011).

# Related Web Sites

"Indicators of Climate Change in the Northeast 2005." http://www.cleanair-coolplanet.org/information/pdf/indicators.pdf

PEARSON
**myhealthprofessionskit**™

Go to www.myhealthprofessionskit.com to access the Companion Web site created for this textbook. Simply select "Basic Health Science" from the choice of disciplines. Find this book and register to access self-assessment quizzes, flashcards, and more.

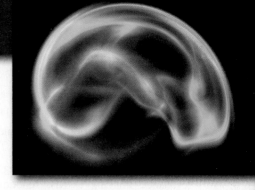

# Information Technology in Radiology

## LEARNING OBJECTIVES

Upon completion of this chapter, the reader will be able to:

- Describe the contributions of digital technology to imaging techniques.
- List the uses of traditional X-rays and the advantages of digital X-rays.
- Define the uses of ultrasound.
- Discuss the newer digital imaging techniques of computed tomography (CT) scans, magnetic resonance imaging (MRI), functional MRI, positron emission tomography (PET) scans, and single-photon emission computed tomography (SPECT) scans, and their uses, advantages, and disadvantages.
- Define nanotechnology.
- Describe computer-aided detection.
- Discuss the dangers of medical radiation.
- Define picture archiving and communications systems (PACS).
- Describe interventional radiology techniques of bloodless surgery.

## INTRODUCTION

The purpose of this chapter is to give students in the health care fields an idea of the extent and impact of information technology in the field of radiology—the branch of medicine that uses imaging techniques to diagnose and radio waves to treat disease. This chapter focuses on digital imaging techniques.

The new imaging techniques use computers to generate pictures of internal organs of the body. A digital image is an image in a form computers can process and store, that is, in binary digits. Computers can make pictures out of mathematical information. The technical methods used by computers to generate the mathematical information are very complex and beyond the scope of this text. The beginning of this chapter presents a short survey of the older imaging techniques like **X-ray** and **ultrasound** and the newer technologies that use computer technology, including **computed tomography (CT) scan**, **magnetic resonance imaging (MRI)**, **single-photon emission computed tomography (SPECT)** scan, and **positron emission tomography (PET)** scan. Some of these scans can now use computer-aided detection to automatically read the scan immediately, before the radiologist sees it. The use of nanoparticles as contrast agents may make images more precise.

Although the focus of the chapter is on digital imaging techniques, radiology is also increasingly concerned with treatment. Interventional radiologists treat disease without surgery; they are now able to open blocked blood vessels and do other procedures. The line between radiology and surgery is changing as bloodless surgery and gamma knife surgery (which does not involve cutting) become more and more widely used. As images become more and more accurate and complete, as they have during the past 20 years, the field of radiology becomes increasingly involved with treatment as well as diagnosis. Interventional radiologists currently treat aneurysms and arthrosclerosis and perform bloodless surgeries on tumors. These issues will be touched on briefly in this chapter.

Precise, detailed images and image-guided therapies are slowly replacing invasive procedures such as cystoscopies and, perhaps in the future, colonoscopies. Radiological screening for diseases has decreased the need for exploratory surgeries, leading to more timely diagnosis and treatment. Research continues into more and more sophisticated imaging techniques, which promise to change some aspects of clinical medicine.[1] In 2011, the U.S. Food and Drug administration (FDA) approved a mobile radiology viewer and a smartphone ultrasound probe. Images can now be viewed on smartphones and tablet computers.[2]

With all the benefits of the extensive use of radiological images to study and diagnose disease and the growing use of interventional radiology to treat disease, there are dangers. Although most people who are treated with radiation are helped or cured, accidents, including massive overdoses, happen. They may be devastating to the patient.

## X-RAYS

Digital technology is radically transforming the field of radiology. Not only are newer imaging techniques (CT scans, MRIs, and PET scans) available, but also older procedures like X-rays and ultrasound are making use of the new technology. A traditional X-ray uses high-energy electromagnetic waves to produce a two-dimensional picture on film. If the X-ray encounters bone, which it cannot penetrate, this appears white on the film. Whatever organ the X-ray passes through appears black on the film. Some soft tissue appears gray. Contrast agents can improve the clarity of the images, but X-rays do not produce good images of all organs and cannot see behind bones at all (Figure 6.1 ▶)

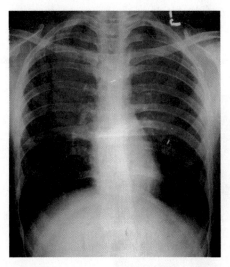

▶ **Figure 6.1** X-ray of human chest. A traditional X-ray uses high-energy electromagnetic waves to create a picture on film.
*Source:* jaimaa/Shutterstock.com

Digital images have several advantages over images on film. Digital X-rays do not have to be developed but are immediately available and can be viewed directly on a computer screen, making them accessible to more than one person at a time, that is, to anyone on a computer network. They are more flexible: Areas can be enhanced, emphasized, and highlighted, and made larger or smaller. The quality of a copy of a digital X-ray is as good as the quality of the original. They can be immediately transmitted over telephone lines for a second opinion. In the future, it is hoped that by taking more than one picture, the X-ray image can be three-dimensional.

X-rays still dominate in several areas. If a broken bone is suspected, an X-ray is likely. Many dentists still depend on traditional X-rays, although digital imaging is becoming more widely used. Digital X-rays use less radiation than conventional X-rays. For a digital X-ray, a highly sensitive sensor containing a microchip is put into the patient's mouth. Because it is so sensitive, less radiation can be used. The data are sent to the computer, which displays an image on the monitor within a few seconds. The image can be manipulated, highlighted, enlarged, and shared on a network. The quality of the image is no better than a traditional X-ray, but it does expose patients to less radiation. However, the equipment that is required is still quite expensive.

At the present time, a major imaging area dominated by traditional X-rays is mammography, although this may be changing. In 2000, the FDA approved the first digital mammography system. In 2011, the FDA approved the first three-dimensional digital mammography system that gives a clearer view of breast tissue.[3] Ultrasound, which can distinguish between harmless cysts and tumors, may be used with a mammogram. Other digital imaging techniques may also be used if an abnormality is spotted by a mammogram. But even with the traditional X-ray, computers can play a part: Computer software has been developed that can be used to reexamine mammogram films, perhaps decreasing the percentage of women whose mammograms are read by radiologists as cancer free, but who do in fact have malignant tumors. An FDA-approved scanner can further evaluate breast abnormalities found by a mammogram. It is connected to a computer, which displays an image of the breast based on differences in the flow of electricity in normal versus malignant tissue. Currently, although digital mammography is not done as a matter of course, it can pinpoint tumors; radiation doses can be adjusted by tracking the tumor. Digital imaging saves the cost of printing, storing, maintaining, and mailing film X-rays.

## ULTRASOUND

Ultrasound technology predates computers by many years. However, it now makes use of computers to create dynamic images. Unlike X-rays, ultrasound uses no radiation. It uses very high-frequency sound waves and the echoes they produce when they hit an object. This information is used by a computer to generate an image, producing a two-dimensional moving picture on a screen. Ultrasound is most closely identified with examining a moving fetus (Figure 6.2 ▶).

It is also used to study blood flow and to diagnose gallstones and prostate disease. Ultrasound, like other imaging techniques, is being used to decrease the need for surgical biopsies. Ultrasound has been approved for the treatment of prostate disease.

In 2002, an 11 × 6.5 inch, 3-pound handheld ultrasound scanner was developed. The traditional ultrasound is 200 to 300 pounds. The handheld scanner has a small liquid crystal display. It is easy to use in a doctor's office or emergency room and can be taken to battlefields and accident scenes.[4] In 2008, an even smaller (pocket-size) ultrasound was developed.[5]

In March 2006, ultrasound was found useful in diagnosing cancer in pregnant women. A study of 23 pregnant women with breast cancer found that mammograms detected the cancer in 90 percent of the cases and ultrasound in 100 percent of the cases.[6] Ultrasound is also being used to diagnose breast cancer in women with dense breast tissue.[7] Elastography ultrasound is also being used to eliminate unnecessary breast biopsies by distinguishing between soft and firm tissue. The latter is more likely to be cancerous. Elastography (which involves no radiation) correctly diagnosed a lesion in 58 out of 59 cases in one study and 54 out of 69 cases in another study.[8]

A three-dimensional ultrasonic endoscope has been developed for use in minimally invasive surgery. It gives surgeons doing endoscopic surgery (see Chapter 7) a three- instead of a two-dimensional view of the inside of the body and might lead to more precise surgeries.[9]

A tiny ultrasound device was cleared by the FDA in March 2006. The device is about the size

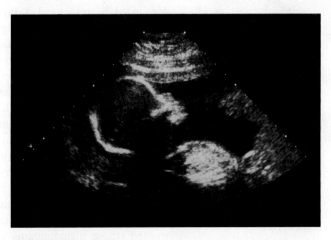

▶ **Figure 6.2** An ultrasound image of a 4-month-old human fetus.
*Source:* Christophe Testi/Shutterstock.com

of a silver dollar. It is being used to monitor fetal heart rate.[10]

## DIGITAL IMAGING TECHNIQUES

Sophisticated imaging machinery uses computers to reduce massive amounts of mathematical data, generated in various ways, to pictures. The pictures that the computer constructs are clearer than traditional X-rays. In addition, the increased use of digital technology has produced kinds of images that were not possible with traditional X-rays, including three-dimensional representations; pictures that clearly distinguish soft tissue within the body; images of function, change, and movement; and images of the electrical and chemical processes in the brain.

The machinery needed to produce CT scans, MRIs, and PET scans is very expensive compared to the machines needed for X-rays and ultrasound. However, by providing a clearer, more detailed, and more accurate picture of the inside of the body, sophisticated diagnostic imaging is reducing the need for exploratory surgery, reducing cost and hospital stays, along with pain. When surgery is necessary, it may be less traumatic, because it is guided by precise, accurate images. By allowing a view of the activity in the brain, digital imaging techniques are also improving the understanding of the chemical and physical bases of mental illness and aiding in the development of effective medications. Another form of digital imaging is the SPECT scan. It, like the PET scan, shows movement. However, SPECT scans are less precise. SPECT is sometimes used because it is less expensive than PET. Both SPECT and PET scans are classified under nuclear medicine.

### Computed Tomography

CT scans use X-rays and digital technology to produce a cross-sectional image of the body. CT scans use radiation passing a series of X-rays through the patient's body at different angles. It is now possible for CT exams to contain thousands of images.[11] The computer then creates cross-sectional images from these X-rays. Soft tissue can be distinguished because it absorbs the X-ray differently (Figure 6.3 ▶). A CT scan produces a more useful image than a traditional X-ray. In addition, CT scans can be used to locate nerve centers, thus helping in the reduction of pain. In enhanced CT scans, a dye is used. Enhanced CT scans are used to show brain tumors: Compounds cannot cross normal blood vessels in the brain; abnormal vessels let substances through—including the dye. This can be

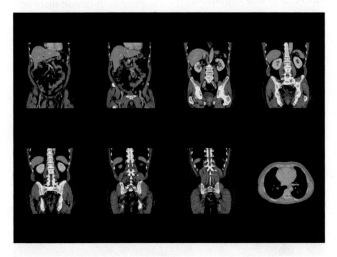

▶ **Figure 6.3** CT scans of human chest and abdomen.
*Source:* Skyhawk/Shutterstock.com

seen on a CT scan. CT scans help diagnose other conditions, including severe acute respiratory syndrome (SARS). In 2003, a virtual cystoscopy using CT scans was developed to screen for bladder tumors. A traditional cystoscopy is invasive and involves inserting a probe into the bladder, but this does not allow a complete examination. In a virtual cystoscopy, a CT scan of the bladder, an expert uses an image-processing algorithm for help in locating tumors.[12] CT scans are also being used to perform virtual colonoscopies; however, the results still need to be compared to the results of real colonoscopies.

According to a government study done in 2010, annual lung CT scans could save lives among heavy smokers. The study focused on "53,000 current and former heavy smokers, aged 55 to 74, who had smoked for at least 30 pack-years"—30 years at one pack a day or 15 years at two packs a day. In the test, half of the participants were given both X-rays and CT scans. It was found that annual CT scans can save 1 out of 300 heavy smokers. However, it must be noted that these scans should not be given to others because they would expose them to excess radiation.[13] A variation of the traditional CT scan, called the **ultrafast CT** scan, may be used in place of coronary angiograms to examine coronary artery blockages. Compared to a coronary angiogram, the ultrafast CT is painless, less dangerous, noninvasive, and less expensive.[14]

## Magnetic Resonance Imaging

MRI machines use computer technology to produce images of soft tissue within the body that cannot be pictured by traditional X-rays. Unlike CT scans, MRIs can produce images of the insides of bones. Using a technique called **scientific visualization**, MRI machines use computers and a very strong magnetic field and radio waves to produce pictures. The images are constructed from mathematical data generated by the interaction of radio waves and the protons inside the nuclei of hydrogen atoms in the water and fatty tissue in the human body. The MRI machine creates a magnetic field many times stronger than the earth's; it then generates radio waves. The response of the body's cells is measured by a computer, which uses these data to create an image (Figures 6.4 and 6.5 ▶). MRI can produce accurate and detailed pictures of the structures of the body and the brain and can distinguish between normal and abnormal tissue. MRI is more accurate than other imaging methods for detecting cancer that has spread to the bone, although PET/CT scans find cancer of the lungs more accurately. MRIs may be used for diagnosis and for the treatment of certain conditions that used to require surgery. For example, using MRI, radiologists can now clean or close off arteries without surgery.[15]

MRIs do not use radiation and are noninvasive. MRIs are used to image brain tumors and in helping to diagnose disorders of the nervous system

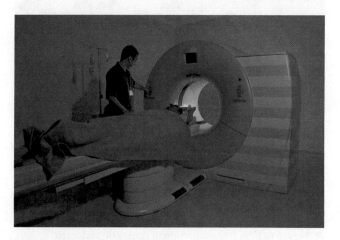

▶ **Figure 6.4** An MRI machine.
*Source:* Levent Konuk/Shutterstock.com

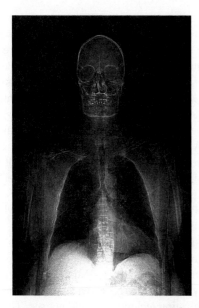

▶ **Figure 6.5**  An MRI of the head,
shoulders, chest, arms, and heart
of a man.
*Source:* Carolina K. Smith, M. D./
Shutterstock.com

such as multiple sclerosis (MS). MRIs also detect stroke at an earlier stage than other tests. MRIs can help find brain abnormalities in patients suffering from dementia.[16] It is particularly useful with brain disorders because it can distinguish among different types of nerve tissue. In 2003, MRIs were used to study comatose patients and were able to detect normal brain activity.[17] MRIs can now be used to image asthma. If patients inhale helium-3 gas before an MRI, doctors can see blocked airways.[18] A new technique will attempt to use MRIs in combination with lasers for instant bloodless high-resolution biopsies. High-powered, pulsed lasers are focused on cells. This gives the cells the ability to glow. Computer software is then used to create a picture of the location of the beam and fluorescence of the cells. Any change in the cell is seen. Because this technique cannot see far into the body, MRIs must be used for a complete picture.

In 2010, a study was done to measure the survival in women at high risk for breast cancer either because of family history or genetic mutations. Women with a family history of breast cancer have a lifetime risk of breast cancer of 15 to 50 percent; women with genetic mutations have a lifetime risk of 50 to 85 percent; an average woman has a lifetime risk of 12.2 percent. The women at high risk were given yearly MRI scans along with yearly mammograms. After 6 years, all of the women with a family history of breast cancer were alive. Ninety-three percent of the women with genetic mutations were alive, compared with 74 percent of women at 5 years in earlier studies. For women at high risk for breast cancer, yearly MRIs and mammograms appear to save some lives. MRIs are not recommended for average women because of too many false positives.[19] Breast tomosynthesis combines three-dimensional ultrasound and MRIs to create three-dimensional breast images. It can find tumors that are hidden.[20]

**Functional MRIs (fMRIs)** measure small metabolic changes in an active part of the brain. fMRIs can identify brain activity by changes in blood oxygen. fMRIs can be used to identify brain area by function in the operating room and help the surgeon avoid damaging areas such as those that are associated with speech. Strokes, brain tumors, or injuries can change the areas of the brain where functions such as speech, sensation, and memory occur. fMRIs can help locate these areas and can then be used to help develop treatment plans. They can also help in the treatment of brain tumors and assess the effects of stroke, injury, or other disease on brain function. fMRIs can be used to predict who will develop early dementia (identical to Alzheimer's) because of a genetic mutation. fMRIs can find biomarkers in people as young as 18. This might lead to early intervention.[21] fMRIs are being used to study conditioned response in people—what the brain does when learning to associate a stimulus, such as a bell or an image, with food. They are also being used, along with PET scans, to study schizophrenia.[22]

Another technique modifies the conventional MRI. It is called dynamic contrast-enhanced MRI. This technology is being studied in research institutions. It can take 1,000 images of a tumor before a dye is introduced and during and after its introduction. Software analyzes the images. It can reveal new tiny blood vessels and how permeable they are. (Blood vessels that feed tumors are full of holes.) This technique will be able to show the growth of new blood vessels that feed cancerous tumors at an early stage and thus give scientists more information to help develop drugs to inhibit the growth of those blood vessels.[23]

A new MRI-related imaging technique is called **diffusion tensor imaging (DTI)**; it can aid in neurosurgery. It shows the white matter of the brain, the connections between parts of the brain, so that these parts are not damaged during surgery. It has improved brain surgery outcomes, according to the director of neuroradiology at Johns Hopkins in Baltimore.[24] It may also help prove that brain injuries exist.[25] DTI is also used to show brain dysfunction in stroke, MS, dyslexia, and schizophrenia.[26]

## Positron Emission Tomography

PET scans use radioisotope technology to create a picture of the body in action. PET scans use computers to construct images from the emission of positive electrons (positrons) by radioactive substances administered to the patient. PET scans—unlike traditional X-rays and CT scans—produce images of how the body works, not just how it looks. PET scans may help detect changes in cell function (disease) before changes in structure can be seen by other imaging techniques.[27] PET scans create representations of the functioning of the body and the mind. They are used to study Alzheimer's disease, Parkinson's disease, epilepsy, learning disabilities, moral reasoning, bipolar disorder, and cancer. PET scans are also used to diagnose arterial obstructions. They are accurate and can avoid invasive catheterization.[28]

In a recent study, PET scans were compared with more common diagnostic tests for breast cancer. The two techniques disagreed in 25 percent of the cases; PET scans provided the correct diagnosis 80 percent of the time as compared with 12 percent using conventional imaging techniques. "PET scans found 6 'true positives' that were not found with conventional imaging tests. As a result those women began more aggressive treatment. Otherwise they would not have received treatment at that particular time."[29] A study published in 2006 concluded that whole-body PET scans could help determine whether breast cancer had spread before surgery.[30]

A recent study has found that PET scans can measure an esophageal cancer patient's response to chemotherapy and radiation therapy before surgery. PET scans can detect metastases that other imaging techniques could not see. They can be used to predict survival rates.[31]

Additionally, PET scans can show the functioning of the brain by measuring cerebral blood flow (Figure 6.6 ▶). PET scans produce a picture of activity and of function. A person is administered a small amount of radioactive glucose. The area of the brain that is active uses the glucose more quickly, and this is reflected in the image that the computer constructs. Neuroimaging techniques using PET can present a picture of brain activity associated with cognitive processes like memory and the use of language.

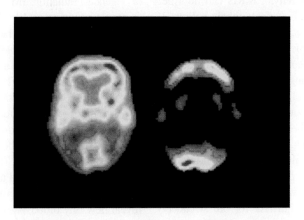

▶ **Figure 6.6** A PET scan of the human brain.
*Source:* Science Source

PET scans are used to study the chemical and physiological processes that take place in the brain when a person speaks correctly or stutters. PET can show the specific brain activity associated with schizophrenia, manic depression, posttraumatic stress disorder, and obsessive-compulsive disorder. PET scans have shown the precise area of the brain that malfunctions in certain mental illnesses and the effects of both drugs, such as Prozac, and traditional talking therapy on nerve cells. With PET, a picture of a drug's effect on brain function can be developed. PET scans can now predict which patient will be helped by which medication. Because these pictures are anatomically and physiologically exact, they should help in the development of new psychiatric drugs.

In a study in 2002, Dr. Lewis Baker compared the effects of psychotropic medications and talk therapy on patients with obsessive-compulsive disorder. Using PET scans of the brain, he found that the two very different treatments produce similar effects on brain function.[32]

PET scans have even been used to shed light on an issue that philosophers have been concerned with for centuries: moral reasoning. In 2002, a study surveyed the areas of the brain involved in solving moral dilemmas. When a group of people were asked if they would throw a switch that would kill one person to save five others, most said yes. But when asked if they would personally push one person to his death to save five others, most said no. PET scans showed that depending on how the question was phrased, different areas of the brain were brought into action. The first question was stated impersonally, and the reasoning part of the brain was engaged. The second question was asked personally, and the emotional part of the brain was engaged.[33]

Software packages help researchers study the effects of drugs by combining PET and MRI, allowing them to correlate the functional information from PET scan images of brain activity with the anatomical details acquired by MRIs. Studies of the effects of certain drugs (including alcohol and cocaine) on the brain may make use of the precise image of brain structure that MRI produces and the picture of the functioning of the brain that PET can give us.

Brain imaging techniques, including both PET scans and fMRIs, are aiding in the comprehension of schizophrenia. People with schizophrenia are tormented by auditory hallucinations; their suffering is so great that sometimes it results in suicide. Until now, some psychiatrists ignored the voices and the content of the messages. In 2003, scientists began using fMRIs to correlate the hallucinations to the activity of specific areas of the brain. They found increased activity in areas involved in hearing, speech, emotion, and memory. This has led to a discussion of new theories about schizophrenia. One new treatment has been developed. The treatment involves sending low-frequency magnetic pulses to areas of the brain identified by MRIs as active during hallucinations. It gives temporary relief to patients who do not respond to standard medications.[34]

In 2011, an FDA advisory panel recommended conditional approval of a dye (florbetapir) that would make the plaques associated with Alzheimer's disease visible on an amyloid PET scan. Until now, the plaques associated with Alzheimer's could only be studied after the death of the patient. The new test could help in *ruling out* Alzheimer's as a diagnosis and in testing the effectiveness of medications for Alzheimer's. Radiologists would have to learn how to interpret the scans. Definitions would have to be developed to determine how much plaque means the patient has Alzheimer's disease.[35]

The Given Diagnostic Imaging System does not fit into any of our categories. It is a capsule with a video camera, lights, transmitter, and batteries. The patient swallows the capsule, which takes pictures of the small intestine, sending them to a small recorder on the patient's belt. After 8 to 72 hours, the capsule passes out of the digestive track, and the health care provider analyzes the pictures. This device cannot be used on anyone wearing an implantable medical device like a pacemaker.

In pediatric patients, surgery has been needed to find the cause of bleeding between the stomach and colon. Now an imaging device called "video capsule endoscopy" produces high-resolution images of the small intestine. The child swallows a capsule containing a camera; it is wireless and weighs one-seventh of an ounce. It takes 50,000 pictures. They are transmitted to a "small data recorder that is worn around the waist." The pictures are later downloaded to a computer. The device was approved by the FDA for adults in 2001 and for children in 2005. It can show more abnormalities than traditional imaging. It can diagnose Crohn's disease, celiac disease, tumors, and injuries. It can also show the effects of medications.[36]

### Single-Photon Emission Computed Tomography Scans

Like PET scans, SPECT scans are a part of nuclear medicine. However, the machinery needed is much cheaper and available at hospitals that lack the technology for PET scans. Whereas PET injects the patient with radioactive glucose and measures the response, SPECT depends on gamma radiation. SPECT images are not as good as those from PET. SPECT can be used to study blood flow, stress fractures, infection, and tumors. SPECT is used in a majority of heart imaging and some bone scanning.[37] One study found that in patients who went to an emergency room, SPECT scans resulted in a 10 percent reduction in unnecessary admissions.[38]

CT scans (which show anatomy) are being combined with both PET and SPECT scans, and the result is better diagnostic accuracy. For example, in heart imaging, CT scans show only anatomy. SPECT or PET scans show blood flow and can pinpoint the defective artery.[39]

### Bone Density Tests

Osteoporosis is a condition of weak bones. Bones lose mineral content or density. Osteoporosis increases the risk of hip and spine fractures. Some bone loss is a normal accompaniment of aging. Several kinds of tests can be done to diagnose this condition. A bone density scan or **dual X-ray absorptiometry (DEXA) scan** is a special kind of low-radiation X-ray that shows changes in the rays' intensity after passing through bone. Doctors can see small changes in bone density from the amount of change in the X-ray. Quantitative CT creates a three-dimensional image of a skeleton. CT scans are used to measure the amount by which beams of radiation lose power (attenuate) as they pass through matter. This measures the mineral content of bones. Quantitative ultrasound is used but is not as accurate a test.

## OTHER IMAGING TECHNOLOGY

Two imaging systems have recently been approved by the FDA. In March 2006, the FDA approved the **LUMA Cervical Imaging System** to help detect cervical cancer. It will be used with colposcopy, which magnifies the cervix of women who have had abnormal Pap tests. Colposcopy can detect many precancerous lesions. LUMA shines a light on the cervix and analyzes how it responds. It creates a color-coded map for the doctor. The map may help identify more suspicious areas to biopsy.[40]

In March 2006, the FDA also approved a digital flat-panel biplane imaging system (Innova). According to General Electric (GE), which makes **Innova**, it is "capable of imaging the finest vessels and cardiovascular anatomy [and producing] three-dimensional images of the vascular system, bone and soft tissue." The system is capable of imaging "the full size of the patient's lateral and frontal anatomy simultaneously" and can be used for many interventional, image-guided procedures.[41]

**SoftScanR**, which "has the potential to improve diagnosis and effective treatment of breast cancer," is now used in clinical trials. It is meant to be a diagnostic tool that will complement mammography. SoftScanR "provides functional or physiological information about a lesion, such as tissue perfusion, blood oxygen and water content, and that allows a lesion to be characterized as benign or malignant."[42]

## NANOTECHNOLOGY

**Nanotechnology** works with matter on an almost molecular or cellular scale.[43] Nanoparticles can be used as contrast agents. They can help detect cellular processes.[44] Nanoparticles called quantum dots, or qdots, are under development (2011). They are nanocrystals of 1 to 10 nanometers.

When light is focused on a qdot, it emits its own light; different size qdots emit different light. They are also brighter than other dyes.[45]

The qdots attach themselves to some cancer cells. "[I]njected into animal models, qdots produce high-resolution multicolored molecules" in the animals' cells. This makes it possible to track them over time. Eventually, they may be used to "generate a kind of optical barcode reflecting the levels of various tumor markers . . . indicat[ing] tumor type and stage."[46]

Different kinds of nanoparticles are used with different imaging techniques. Suffice it to say that nanoparticles of different kinds can be used as contrast agents in MRI scans, PET scans, and CT scans.[47]

## COMPUTER-AIDED DETECTION

**Computer-aided detection** uses software to help radiologists interpret images, whether mammograms, CT scans, or MRIs. Although there is debate over its efficacy (one study in 2007 found that it *decreased* the accuracy of mammograms), its use is increasing. It is even "becoming standard practice in breast diagnosis."[48]

Computer-aided detection is also being developed at the Mayo Clinic and IBM to find brain aneurisms early—before brain hemorrhage occurs or neurological damage is done. As soon as the images are taken, they are automatically analyzed by the software that can spot and mark even small potential aneurisms. Radiologists can then analyze the image. The software has been used to analyze more than 15 million images from thousands of patients. The most recent trial of the software "showed a sensitivity rate of as high as 95% when analyzing MR angiography images from a historic set of known patient cases . . . compared to a 70% sensitivity that doctors exhibited when analyzing the same images." The Mayo Clinic plans to use similar software to diagnose cancer.[49]

Software that automatically identifies polyps has been approved by the FDA for reading virtual or CT colonoscopies. An early clinical trial showed that "more than two-thirds of the CAD-enabled CT colonoscopy readers were more accurate than non-assisted readers. CAD-assisted colonoscopies also were 5 percent more likely to detect polyps 6 millimeters or more in size." The company (iCAD) that produces this software also sells CAD equipment for breast and prostate cancer.[50] CAD is also being used to find "potential nodules in the lungs."[51]

Iterative Reconstruction in Image Space (IRIS) reconstructs CT images. In a study published in March 2010, it was found that CT images of the abdomen reconstructed with IRIS were better at detecting lesions than images reconstructed by the standard method. Radiation doses may be reduced by one-third without compromising the images.[52]

In 2010, software was developed that "for the first time provides neuroradiologists with current information about the status of the brain tissue during minimally invasive procedures." Speed is crucial in the treatment of stroke. The new software shortens the time between diagnosis and treatment. The information is available in 40 seconds.[53]

In 2011, neurologists developed new software that "detects subtle brain lesions in MRI scans" in epileptic patients. It did well compared to expert radiologists, identifying abnormal areas in 92 percent of the scans that had already been identified by expert radiologists.[54]

## PICTURE ARCHIVING AND COMMUNICATIONS SYSTEMS

The transformation of radiology from a discipline working with chemicals and film to one working with computers and monitors has also made images available almost instantaneously. A **picture archiving and communications system (PACS)** "is an electronic and ideally filmless information system for acquiring, sorting, transporting, storing, and electronically displaying medical images." PACS is a server. The standard communication protocols of imaging devices are called **digital imaging and communications in medicine (DICOM)**.[55] The use of PACS to transmit and store digital images offers new speed in the transmission of digital images. The "copy" is available as soon as the original. There is no need to move patients to a facility that has better imaging equipment. PACS moves the images and makes the images available to any authorized physician. It also reduces hospital stays by speeding up diagnosis.[56] In 2010, PACS can combine two-dimensional, three-dimensional, and four-dimensional diagnostic reporting.[57] In 2011, health care providers want PACS that are integrated with radiology information systems (RIS) (see Chapter 2).[58]

PACS, however, is not yet integrated into surgery. Computer-assisted surgery is largely image directed. Ideally the development of a surgery PACS (S-PACS) "would focus on intraoperative imaging, with real-time and multidimensional visualization."[59]

## INTERVENTIONAL RADIOLOGY: BLOODLESS SURGERY

The effects of digital technology on the practice of medicine cannot be overestimated. As images become more precise, they can guide surgeons better, and thus operations are less invasive. In addition, conditions that once required surgery may be amenable to treatment by interventional radiology. Some biopsies can now be done with a needle instead of surgically. Stereotactic breast biopsies make use of digital X-rays to locate the abnormality and use a needle to extract tissue. They are less invasive than surgical biopsies but not as accurate and cannot be used with all patients.

Among the developments in radiology is radiosurgery. On the borderline between radiology and surgery, **stereotactic radiosurgery (gamma knife surgery)** is a noninvasive technique that is currently used to treat brain tumors in a 1-day session. The use of the gamma knife for brain surgery has grown exponentially over the last few years. It is appropriate for brain tumors because the head can be immobilized. It may be used to treat other parts of the body in a different form called fractionated stereotactic radiosurgery; this is delivered over weeks of treatment.[60] Radiosurgery

can be performed by a modified linear accelerator, which rotates around the patient's head and delivers blasts of radiation to the tumor, or by a gamma knife. Called a painless, bloodless surgical device, the gamma knife works by delivering focused beams of radiation directly at the tumor. This kills the tumor and spares the surrounding tissue. The procedure makes use of three-dimensional imaging that locates the tumor in the body and uses computerized targeting to make sure that the center of the tumor gets the most radiation (Figure 6.7 ▶). One published review of 55 patients found radiosurgery to be quite effective.

Interventional radiography equipment allows nonsurgical repair of some thoracic abnormalities. The gamma knife is appropriate for some benign brain tumors and all malignant brain tumors. It is also being used to treat neuralgia, intractable pain, Parkinson's disease, and epilepsy. Some of the advantages of gamma knife surgery are its relatively low cost, the lack of pain to the patient, the elimination of the risks of hemorrhage and infection, and

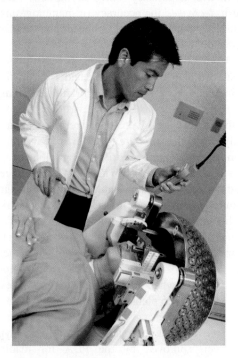

▶ **Figure 6.7** Patient undergoing radiosurgery.
*Source:* Zorik Galstyan/Shutterstock.com

short hospital stay. Patients are able to resume daily activities immediately. However, as the procedure grows in popularity, some doctors are questioning its safety and efficacy. What will the effects of high doses of radiation be in the long run? Although it is recognized as effective in treating some brain tumors, they question its widespread use.[61] The newer **cyber knife**, because it compensates for patient movement, can be used to treat brain and spinal tumors with radiosurgery. In 2011, research at the University of Pittsburgh found that if a first gamma knife radiosurgery failed, a repeat radiosurgery is likely to be effective.[62]

Research is being done on the effects of ultrasound on malignancies. **Focused ultrasound surgery** does not involve cutting, but does involve the use of sound waves. Studies of focused ultrasound surgery used ultrasound to stop massive bleeding and to treat cancer. In Europe, it has been approved for the treatment of pain from bone cancer and for uterine fibroids. It is in clinical trials for the treatment of breast cancer. An MRI identifies the target in the body. The treatment "concentrates up to 1000 intersecting beams of ultrasound energy" on the target, heating and destroying tissue. Focused ultrasound surgery is in an early stage of development.[63]

The uses of **interventional radiology** continue to expand. A procedure called radiofrequency ablation (RFA) has been used on non-small cell lung cancers in their early stages since 2000. An ablation needle is inserted into the tumor. An electric current heats the tumor and kills it. Small studies have reported its safety and efficacy. However, there have been no long-term clinical studies of its effects. In chemoembolization, a catheter is used to deliver drugs into a liver tumor. Stronger chemotherapy can be used with fewer side effects, because there is less circulation of drugs in the blood. It is used to treat liver cancer.[64]

At the 31st Annual Meeting of the Society of Interventional Radiology in March and April, 2006, research into many new uses of interventional radiology was presented, including the use of treating blocked carotid arteries in patients who do not exhibit stroke symptoms and the use of an improved embolization procedure to treat and reverse male infertility. Lasers are being used to treat children with painful vascular malformations. Interventional radiology is being tested as a treatment for uterine fibroids. In a study of complications after the surgical versus nonsurgical treatment of uterine fibroids, interventional radiology was shown to be effective and to have a low rate of complications. Nonsurgical techniques can be used to treat painful cancerous chest tumors by heating or freezing the cells, killing both the cells and the nerve endings.[65]

**Cone beam CT (CBCT)** can be used to more precisely focus a beam of radiation on a tumor. It can be attached to the machine delivering radiation, creating three-dimensional images so that doctors can compare the latest images with the earlier images they used to plan the treatment. They can then adjust the patient's position. Traditionally a patient's skin was marked for radiation treatment based on earlier tests; now the CBCT can adjust the treatment in real time.[66]

Some of the findings of interventional radiologists include the following: Stenting of the carotid artery improves memory and thinking ability; and interventional radiology (embolization) can be successfully used to treat fibroid tumors in 92 percent of postmenopausal women.[67]

# THE DANGERS OF MEDICAL RADIATION

In the United States, "the average lifetime dose of diagnostic radiation has increased sevenfold since 1980, and more than half of all cancer patients receive radiation therapy." With the increased use of radiation have come increases in severe injury and death. Between 2000 and 2010, there were 1,000 reports filed of injuries and deaths involving radiotherapy equipment. A study in *The New York Times* traces many mistakes to "software flaws, faulty programming, poor safety procedures or inadequate staffing and training." It is very difficult to find adequate information on these injuries because of underreporting and the fact that no one agency oversees medical radiation. Some who have studied radiation injuries estimate that half of the accidents remain hidden. In 2010, at one hospital, 90 cancer patients received an incorrect dose; the hospital did not report it. In 2005, at another hospital, 77 patients received an overdose of radiation because "linear accelerators had been programmed incorrectly for nearly a year." The number and seriousness of radiation injuries are not known because of underreporting and the fact that some injuries from radiation may take years to develop. However, in 2009, 3,000 serious radiation injuries were treated by a large U.S. wound care company. *The New York Times* analyzed records in New York State, which is ahead of much of the country in overseeing radiation therapy. Under the law, many accidents are confidential. However, between 2001 and 2008, there were 621 mistakes; "on 133 occasions, devices used to shape . . . radiation beams . . . were left out, wrongly positioned or otherwise misused." Radiation missed its intended target 284 times. Many of these accidents result in minor injuries. Some are devastating, painful, and deadly.[68]

Between 2000 and 2010, linear accelerators that attack cancer cells continued to be developed. Each allows doctors to use more radiation. **Intensity-modulated radiation therapy (IMRT)** is the latest; IMRT "shapes and varies the intensity of radiation beams." However, these machines have caused serious injuries. Some injuries are due to miscalibrations of the machines, some to software errors, and some to lack of adequately trained personnel. The results of overdoses may not be evident for months. "The popularity of IMRT exploded before there were national standards." The FDA has not thoroughly reviewed these machines "on the grounds that they just extended existing technology." There are no national standards for machine-generated radiation; states vary in their standards.[69]

The increasing use of CT scans is exposing patients to risky and unnecessary radiation, according to two government experts. One CT scan is equivalent in radiation to 400 chest X-rays. "An estimated 70 million CT . . . scans are performed in the United States every year, up from 3 million in the early 1980s, and as many as 14,000 people may die every year of radiation-induced cancers as a result." CT scans that are being used as a diagnostic tool for healthy patients (e.g., virtual colonoscopy) are especially controversial, because they may cause as well as detect cancer."[70]

Children are particularly susceptible to radiation. Yet, dentists continue to use X-rays, and many still use film X-rays that require more radiation. Specialists have adopted a new form of CT scan called the cone beam CT scanner, which "provides brilliant 3-D images of teeth, roots, jaw and even skull." Although many dentists insist on the safety of this new device, much of the research on it has been underwritten by its manufacturers. There is little independent testing of the device, which may be both harmful and unnecessary.[71] Children are also being exposed to more radiation in the emergency room. Between 1995 and 2008, the number of CT scans on children in emergency rooms has increased from 330,000 to 1.65 million, an increase of 500 percent. The scans may improve diagnosis, but they also expose children to radiation that might be related to developing cancer in the future.[72]

Many patients (400 so far) who receive a test for stroke called a CT brain perfusion scan are being overdosed with radiation. Some overdoses are due to technician error and lack of adequate training, whereas others are due to software design. None of the overdoses were caused by scanner malfunction. One hospital used higher doses of radiation to get clearer images; the "hospital said no mistakes were made," so no investigation was made. Patients reported hair loss, headaches, memory loss, and confusion; in the future, they are at higher risk of brain damage and cancer. There are no "hard standards" for radiation, and the requirements for reporting are loose. Even though patients reported hair loss where they had been radiated, for over a year, doctors and hospitals did not find overdoses.[73]

There is a feature on the machines that can automatically adjust the dose according to the patient, which is supposed to reduce the radiation dose. However, if the automatic setting is used with certain other settings, it *raises* the dose. Some patients received eight times the radiation necessary. There is no warning or automatic shutoff to prevent a dangerous overdose. Some states investigated the overdoses; others did not.

# IN THE NEWS

According to "X-Rays and Unshielded Infants" by Walt Bogdanich and Kristina Rebelo, published on February 27, 2011, in *The New York Times*, in some hospitals, infants are given full-body X-rays or babygrams, even though they expose the baby to high levels of radiation.

Radiation technologists are not regulated in 15 states. Many mistakes occur: For example, in 2010, in Michigan, several cancer patients were burned when their healthy tissue was given radiation treatments. According to Christine Lung, the technologist association's vice president of government relations, "It's amazing to us, knowing the complexity of medical imaging, that there are states that require massage therapists and hairdressers to be licensed, but they have no standards in place for exposing patients to ionizing radiation."

In 2007, a New York hospital (Downstate) brought in an expert, Dr. Amodio, to evaluate their radiology practices, particularly with children. Dr Amodio found that incorrect settings were used with babies. According to Dr. Amodio, "Excessively irradiating children is something we must have zero tolerance about." According to Downstate, "We are working with the New York State Department of Health to re-evaluate the issues raised by our Department of Radiology in 2007, and to ensure that we are in compliance with national and state standards."

A bill in Congress, CARE, would require radiologists to keep up with changes in the field. It has not yet been passed.

The FDA depended on state reports, but some states, such as Alabama, do not define an acceptable radiation dose; therefore, in Alabama, there is no such thing as an overdose! Even after the FDA issued an alert, overdosing continued. Some patients have not been told of the overdoses. One hospital did not record radiation dose until 2009.[74] After reviewing hundreds of overdoses from a CT brain perfusion scan, the FDA recommended better training for those who perform the scans and that machines automatically issue a warning that an overdose is about to be given.[75]

## Chapter Summary

- During the past 20 years, imaging techniques have become more precise and accurate because of computer technology. X-rays, which image bones, and ultrasound, which shows moving images, have been supplemented by computer-based techniques.

- The CT scan takes many images and combines them in a two- or three-dimensional slice.

- MRI uses magnetism to image soft tissue. Functional MRIs can see small metabolic changes in the brain and can be used to map brain function.

- The PET scan images function. PET can allow the radiologist to see the difference between normal and cancerous cells and can be used to study brain function in normal and mentally ill patients. PET can watch the brain think and judge.

- The SPECT scan is used for most heart imaging.
- The combination of PET with CT and SPECT with CT improves diagnosis.
- The use of these detailed and accurate images has made diagnosis more accurate and made exploratory surgery rare.
- Nanotechnology can help by creating contrast agents.
- Special software programs can read various images.
- Information technology in the form of the PACS system has made accurate digital images available anywhere.

- Radiology has moved from diagnosis to treatment, using radiosurgery to treat brain tumors and focused ultrasound to treat other kinds of tumors. Interventional radiology is a growing discipline, treating many conditions including cancers, pain, and male infertility.
- Fibroid tumors can now be treated by interventional radiologists using an embolization technique, instead of surgery.
- When used inappropriately, medical radiation can lead to devastating human consequences.

# Key Terms

computed tomography (CT)

computer-aided detection

cone beam CT (CBCT)

cyber knife

diffusion tensor imaging (DTI)

digital imaging and communications in medicine (DICOM)

dual X-ray absorptiometry (DEXA) scan

focused ultrasound surgery

functional MRIs (fMRIs)

gamma knife surgery

Innova

intensity-modulated radiation therapy (IMRT)

interventional radiology

LUMA Cervical Imaging System

magnetic resonance imaging (MRI)

nanotechnology

picture archiving and

communications system (PACS)

positron emission tomography (PET)

scientific visualization

single-photon emission computed tomography (SPECT)

SoftScanR

stereotactic radiosurgery

ultrafast CT

ultrasound

X-ray

# Review Exercises

## Multiple Choice

1. Which of the following uses sound waves and the echoes they produce when they encounter an object to create an image?
   a. X-rays
   b. Ultrasound
   c. Positron emission tomography
   d. Magnetic resonance imaging

2. _____ study(ies) brain function by sensing small changes in oxygen levels.

   a. X-rays
   b. CT scans
   c. Ultrasound
   d. Functional magnetic resonance imaging

3. _____ uses small amounts of radioactive materials to create a picture of the body in action.
   a. X-ray
   b. Ultrasound
   c. Positron emission tomography
   d. Magnetic resonance imaging

4. _____ take a series of X-rays at different angles. A computer then creates a cross-sectional image.
   a. X-rays
   b. CT scans
   c. PETs
   d. MRIs

5. _____ can be used to show the functioning of the brain.
   a. X-rays
   b. CT scans
   c. Positron emission tomography
   d. All of the above

6. _____ can image soft tissue and the inside of bones.
   a. X-rays
   b. CT scans
   c. Positron emission tomography
   d. Magnetic resonance imaging

7. An advantage of digital X-rays over traditional film X-rays is _____ .
   a. a digital X-ray is available immediately
   b. a digital X-ray can be enhanced
   c. digital X-rays use less radiation
   d. All of the above

8. _____ creates images from data generated by the interaction of radio waves and the protons in hydrogen atoms in the water in the human body.
   a. X-ray
   b. CT scan
   c. Positron emission tomography
   d. Magnetic resonance imaging

9. If you wanted to study the effect of Prozac on the brain you would use _____ .
   a. X-rays
   b. CT scans
   c. positron emission tomography
   d. None of the above

10. _____ is used to picture a moving fetus.
    a. X-ray
    b. Ultrasound
    c. Positron emission tomography
    d. Magnetic resonance imaging

11. _____ scanning is used to image the heart in a majority of cases.
    a. SPECT
    b. Ultrasound
    c. Positron emission tomography
    d. Magnetic resonance imaging

12. _____ can be used to diagnose breast cancer in pregnant women.
    a. X-rays
    b. Ultrasound
    c. Positron emission tomography
    d. Magnetic resonance imaging

13. _____ transmits, stores, retrieves, and displays digital images and communicates the information over a network.
    a. SPECT
    b. MEDCIN
    c. DICOM
    d. PACS

14. The overexposure to X-rays can cause _____.
    a. obesity
    b. cancer
    c. A and B
    d. None of the above

15. Interventional radiology (embolization) can be successfully used to treat _____ in a majority of postmenopausal women.
    a. early liver cancer
    b. fibroid tumors
    c. appendicitis
    d. All of the above

## True/False

1. PET scans can show the different activity in the brain when a person speaks correctly versus when he or she stutters. _____

2. Ultrasound uses radiation to create an image. _____

3. Images can now be viewed on smartphones and tablet computers. _____

4. Nanotechnology works with matter on an almost molecular or cellular scale. _____

5. PET scans are usually used for broken bones. _____

6. Interventional radiology is concerned with the treatment of disease. _____

7. Stereotactic radiosurgery involves removing tumors surgically. _____

8. A gamma knife is used to make incisions. _____

9. Dentists still use X-rays, which may be traditional or digital. _____

10. SPECT scans, like PET scans, show the body in motion. _____

## Critical Thinking

1. Using MRIs and PET scans, researchers are studying the functioning of the brain. Comment on the possible positive and negative ramifications this could have on developing more effective psychotropic medications to control the mind.

2. Advances in radiology are changing the boundary between radiology and surgery so that, at times, it is difficult to distinguish between the fields. Bloodless surgery (gamma knife surgery) is now used to treat certain tumors. What other uses can you imagine?

3. What are the advantages and disadvantages of using digital X-rays in dentistry?

4. When a mammogram is done, it can be read by a technician, checked by special software, and scanned by a computerized scanner. If the image is misread, who is responsible—the technician, the software publisher, and/or the hardware manufacturer?

5. Digital imaging equipment is becoming more affordable so that more medical institutions can acquire it. Discuss the advantages and disadvantages of each method (CT scans, MRIs, SPECT, and PET scans).

# Notes

1. Clare Tempany and Barbara McNeil, "Advances in Biomedical Imaging," *Journal of the American Medical Association* 285, no. 5 (2001): 562–7.
2. Iltifat Husain, "A Key Milestone in Mobile Imaging: FDA Approves Mobile Radiology Viewer and Smartphone Ultrasound Probe," February 9, 2011, http://www.imedicalapps.com/2011/02/fda-approves-diagnostic-radiology-viewer-smartphone-ultrasound-probe/# (accessed February 16, 2011).
3. "First FDA-Approved 3D Digital Mammography Available at Albany Med," February 15, 2011, http://www.amc.edu/PR/PressRelease/02_15_11_T.html (accessed April 29, 2011).
4. Michel Marriott, "A Palm-Size Ultrasound Scans Safely in a Flash," October 10, 2002, http://query.nytimes.com/gst/fullpage.html?res=9906E1D91F3BF933A25753C1A9649C8B63 (accessed April 28, 2011).
5. "The World's Smallest Ultrasound Device," January 10, 2008, http://www.siemens.com/press/en/presspicture/?press=/en/presspicture/pictures-photonews/2008/pn200802.php (accessed March 16, 2011).
6. Kenneth F. Trofatter, Jr., "Breast Cancer Diagnosis during Pregnancy," October 8, 2006, http://www.healthline.com/blogs/pregnancy_childbirth/2006/10/breast-cancer-diagnosis-during.html (accessed April 28, 2011).
7. "European Congress of Radiology 2010: Siemens Introduces Innovations for Imaging and Diagnostics," March 5, 2010, http://www.siemens.com/press/en/events/healthcare/2010-03-ecr.php (accessed November 12, 2010).
8. Fran Lowry, "Elastography Imaging during Breast Ultrasound Reduces Unnecessary Biopsy Rate," December 1, 2009, http://www.medscape.com (accessed April 16, 2010).
9. "3D Ultrasound Device Poised to Advance Minimally Invasive Surgery," March 30, 2006, http://www.sciencedaily.com/releases/2006/03/060330161609.htm (accessed April 28, 2011); Jingkuang Chen, Xiaoyand Cheng, I-Ming Shen, Jing-Hung Liu, Pai-Chi Li, and Mengli Wang, "A Monolithic Three-Dimensional Ultrasonic Transducer Array for Medical Imaging," October 1, 2001, http://ieeexplore.ieee.org/xpl/freeabs_all.jsp?arnumber=4337780 (accessed April 28, 2011).
10. "Analogic OK'd on Fetal Ultrasound Device," March 29, 2006, http://www.upi.com/Health_Business/Analysis/2006/03/29/analogic_okd_on_fetal_ultrasound_device/2684/ (accessed April 28, 2011); "Analogic Corporation Receives 510(k) FDA Clearance for Wide-Beam Fetal Ultrasound Transducer," March 29, 2006, http://www.analogic.com/387531/news-and-events-press-releases-detail.htm (accessed April 28, 2011).

11. Guido Vaccari and Claudio Saccavini, "Radiology Informatics and Work Flow Redesign," *PsychNology Journal* 4, no. 1 (2006): 87–101, http://www.psychnology. org/File/PNJ4(1)/PSYCHNOLOGY_JOURNAL_4_1_ VACCARI.pdf (accessed April 28, 2011).

12. Jaume Sylvain, Matthieu Ferrant, Benoît Macq, Lennox Hoyte, Julia R. Fielding, Andreas Schreyer, Ron Kikinis, and Simon K. Warfield, "Tumor Detection in the Bladder Wall with a Measurement of Abnormal Thickness in CT Scans," March 2003, http://people.csail.mit.edu/ sylvain/jaume-ieee-tbme03.pdf (accessed April 28, 2011).

13. Tara Parker-Pope and Stuart Bradford, "The Downside of a Study Extolling CT Scans," November 15, 2010, http:// well.blogs.nytimes.com/2010/11/15/the-downside-of- a-cancer-study-extolling-ct-scans/ (accessed November 16, 2010).

16. "Ultrafast CT Scan," https://www.stjosephsatlanta.org/ HealthLibrary/content.aspx?pageid=P01281 (accessed February 17, 2012).

15. Heather Babiar, "New Cardiac MRI Pinpoints Closed Arteries without Surgery," June 27, 2006, http://www. eurekalert.org/pub_releases/2006-06/rson-ncm062006.php (accessed April 28, 2011).

16. "MRI of the Head," 2003, http://www.radiologyinfo.org/en/ info.cfm?pg=headmr (accessed April 28, 2011).

17. Carl Zimmer, "What if There Is Something Going on in There," September 28, 2003, http://www.nytimes. com/2003/09/28/magazine/what-if-there-is-something- going-on-in-there.html (accessed April 28, 2011).

18. "Detecting Asthma: Radiologists Develop Asthma Imaging Method," January 1, 2009, http://www.sciencedaily. com/videos/2009/0106-detecting_asthma.htm (accessed November 12, 2010).

19. Denise Grady, "M.R.I.'s Help Fight High Risk of Cancer," November 15, 2010, http://www.nytimes.com/2010/11/16/ health/16cancer.html (accessed March 16, 2011).

20. "European Congress of Radiology 2010: Siemens Introduces Innovations for Imaging and Diagnostics."

21. Pam Belluck, "For Edge on Alzheimer's, Testing Early Treatments," November 8, 2010, http://www.nytimes. com/ref/health/healthguide/alzheimers_ess.html (accessed November 12, 2010).

22. P. J. Johnston, W. Stojanov, H. Devir, and U. Schall, "Functional MRI of Facial Emotion Recognition Deficits in Schizophrenia and Their Electro physiological Correlates," [Abstract] February 2005, http://onlineli- brary.wiley.com/doi/ 10.1111/j.1460-9568.2005.04294.x/ full (accessed April 28, 2011).

23. Anne Eisenberg, "What's Next: A Budding Tumor Unmasked by the Vessels That Feed It," July 24, 2003, http://query.nytimes.com/gst/fullpage.html?res=9E0CE1 D7153FF937A15754C0A9659C8B63 (accessed April 28, 2011); F. L. Giesel, H. Bischoff, H. von Tengg-Kobligk, M.-A. Weber, C. M. Zechmann, H.-U. Kauczor, and M. V. Knopp, "Dynamic Contrast-Enhanced MRI of Malignant Pleural Mesothelioma: A Feasibility Study of Noninvasive Assessment, Therapeutic Follow-up, and Possible Predictor of Improved Outcome," June 2006, http://www.

mesotheliomamedical.com/modules.php?name=News&fi le=print&sid=1677 (accessed April 28, 2011).

24. Angela Stewart, "Seeing into the Brain," *The Star Ledger,* March 14, 2006, 33.

25. Peter Vieth, "New Imaging Techniques May Help Prove, or Disprove, Brain Injuries," January 3, 2011, http://tgblaw.blogspot.com/2011/01/new-imaging- techniques-may-help-prove.html (accessed March 17, 2011).

26. Avneesh Chhabra, "Diffusion Tensor Imaging," December 10, 2008, http://emedicine.medscape.com/article/345561- overview (accessed April 28, 2011).

27. "Heart PET Scan," March 28, 2011, http://www.nlm.nih. gov/medlineplus/ency/article/007343.htm (accessed April 28, 2011); "PET Scan," 2010, http://www.betterhealth.vic. gov.au/BHCV2/bhcarticles.nsf/pages/PET_scan?Open (accessed April 28, 2011).

28. "Heart PET Scan"; "Nuclear Medicine," 2011, https://www. asrt.org/content/The Public/AboutRadiologicProcedures/ Nuclear_Medicine.aspx (accessed April 28, 2011).

29. "Do PET Scans Help Cancer Patients Live Longer?" November 14, 2007, http://www.ivanhoe.com/channels/p_ channelstory.cfm?storyid=17501 (accessed April 28, 2011).

30. "Imaging Technique Helps Predict Breast Cancer Spread before Surgery," August 23, 2006, http://www.snm.org/ index.cfm? PageID=5484 (accessed April 28, 2011).

31. "PET Scans Promising for Assessing Treatment Response in Esophageal Cancer," 2006, http://demo.cancerconsultants. com/Content.aspx?Section=cance-rnews&DocumentID= 34881 (accessed April 28, 2011).

32. Richard A. Friedman, "Like Drugs, Talk Therapy Can Change Brain Chemistry," August 27, 2002, http://www. nytimes.com/2002/08/27/health/behavior-like-drugs-talk- therapy-can-change-brain-chemistry.html (accessed April 28, 2011).

33. Sandra Blakeslee, "Watching How the Brain Works as It Weighs a Moral Dilemma," September 25, 2001, http:// www.nytimes.com/2001/09/25/science/watching-how- the-brain-works-as-it-weighs-a-moral-dilemma.html (accessed April 28, 2011).

34. Erica Goode, "Experts See Mind's Voices in New Light," May 6, 2003, http://www.nytimes.com/2003/05/06/science/ experts-see-mind-s-voices-in-new-light.html (accessed April 28, 2011).

35. Gina Kolata, "FDA Sees Promise in Alzheimer's Imaging Drug," January 20, 2011, http://www.nytimes. com/2011/01/21/health/21alzheimers.html (accessed February 10, 2011); "Alzheimer's Association Statement on Florbetapir PET Amyloid Imaging," January 24, 2011, http://www.alz.org/news_and_events_pet_amyloid_imag- ing.asp (accessed February 16, 2011); "Top 10 Medical Innovations for 2011: #1 New Molecular Imaging Biomarker for Early Detection, Prevention and Treatment of Alzheimer's Disease," 2010, http://www.cleveland- clinic.org/innovations/summit2011/topten11/one.html (accessed February 28, 2011).

36. "Top 10 Medical Innovations for 2011: #10 Capsule Endoscopy for Diagnosis of Pediatric GI Disorders," 2010,

http://www.clevelandclinic.org/innovations/summit2011/topten11/ten.html (accessed February 28, 2011).

37. Mark Dye, "PET and SPECT: Happy Together," June 2005, http://www.medicalimagingmag.com/issues/articles/2005-06_01.asp (accessed April 28, 2011); Susan Spinasanta, "Nuclear Imaging: PET and SPECT Scans," December 8, 2004, http://www.spineuniverse.com/displayarticle.php/article231.html (accessed April 28, 2011).

38. Urmilla R. Parlikar, "Heart Imaging Procedure Helps Physicians Evaluate Patients Suspected of Having a Heart Attack," http://johnbbassettdmd.com/PATIENTS/HEALTHLIBRARY/tabid/606/contentid/28792/Default.aspx (accessed April 28, 2011).

39. "Going beyond CT Angiography—SPECT/CT Heart Study Is SNM's Image of the Year," June 5, 2006, http://interactive.snm.org/index.cfm?PageID=5210 (accessed April 28, 2011).

40. "LUMA™ Cervical Imaging System- P040028," July 8, 2009, http://www.fda.gov/MedicalDevices/Productsand MedicalProcedures/DeviceApprovalsandClearances/Recently-ApprovedDevices/ucm078285.htm (accessed April 22, 2011).

41. Barbara Kram, "FDA Clears GE Healthcare's New Innova Digital Flat Panel Biplane Imaging System," October 30, 2006, http://www.dotmed.com/news/story/2748/ (accessed April 28, 2011); "Interventional X-Ray: Innova 3100 IQ for Cardiology," 2010, http://www3.gehealthcare.com/en/Products/Categories/Interventional_Image_Guided_Systems/Interventional_X-ray_for_Cardiology/Innova_3100-IQ_Optima_Edition (accessed April 22, 2011).

42. "ART Advanced Research Technologies Inc.," 2011, http://www.art.ca/en/clinical/index.php (accessed April 28, 2011); "ART Initiates Clinical Trials of the SoftScan 'R' System at the University of California-San Diego as Part of Its North American Pivotal Study," March 29, 2006, http://www.marketwire.com/press-release/art-initiates-clinical-trials-softscanr-system-university-california-san-diego-as part-tsx-ara-586633.htm (accessed April 28, 2011).

43. National Organic Standards Board Materials Committee, "Nanotechnology in Organic Production, Processing, and Packaging Request for Information for Developing a Usable Definition of the Term in Organics," February 25, 2010, http://www.ams.usda.gov/AMSv1.0/getfile?dDocN ame=STELPRDC5083223 (accessed March 17, 2011).

44. David P. Cormode, Torjus Skajaa, Zahi Fayad, and Willem J. M. Mulder, "Nanotechnology in Medical Imaging: Probe Designs and Applications," December 4, 2008, http://www.ncbi.nlm.nih.gov/pmc/articles/PMC2844987/ (accessed March 17, 2011).

45. L. A. Bentolila, X. Michalet, F. F. Pinaud, J. M. Tsay, S. Doose, J. J. Li, G. Sundaresan, A. M. Wu, S. S. Gambhir, and S. Weiss, "Quantum Dots for Molecular Imaging and Cancer Medicine," July 25, 2009, http://www.discovery-medicine.com/L-A-Bentolila/2009/07/25/quantum-dots-for-molecular-imaging-and-cancer-medicine/ (accessed March 17, 2011).

46. "Nanotechnology Diagnostics," 2011, http://cancer.stanford.edu/research/imaging/nanotechnology.html (accessed February 16, 2011).

47. Cormode, Skajaa, Fayad, and Mulder, "Nanotechnology in Medical Imaging: Probe Designs and Applications."

48. "Computer-Aided Detection Is Increasingly Being Used in Screening and Diagnostic Mammography," October 1, 2010, ttp://www.sciencedaily.com/releases/2010/10/101001163335.htm (accessed March 16, 2011); "Computer-Aided Detection Reduces the Accuracy of Mammograms," April 2001, http://www.cancer.gov/newscenter/pressreleases/2007/cadmammographyrelease (accessed March 16, 2011).

49. Joel Streed, "Mayo Clinic and IBM Advance Early Detection of Brain Aneurysms," January 22, 2010, http://www.mayoclinic.org/news2010-rst/5600.html (accessed March 16, 2011). "Computer Aided Detection May Be Better Than Doctors at Spotting Aneurysms," January 25, 2010, http://medgadget.com/2010/01/computer_aided_detection_may_be_better_than_doctors_at_spotting_aneurysms.html (accessed March 16, 2011).

50. "iCad Wins FDA Nod for Computer-Aided Detection in Virtual Colonoscopies," August 5, 2010, http://www.massdevice.com/news/icad-wins-fda-nod-computer-aided-detection-virtual-colonoscopies (accessed March 16, 2011).

51. "European Congress of Radiology 2010: Siemens Introduces Innovations for Imaging and Diagnostics."

52. Sameer Tipnis, Ashok Ramachandra, Walter Huda, Andrew Hardie, Joseph Schoepf, Philip Costello, Thomas Flohr, and Martin Sedlmair, "Iterative Reconstruction in Image Space (IRIS) and Lesion Detection in Abdominal CT," [Abstract] March 2010, http://adsabs.harvard.edu/abs/2010SPIE.7622E..89T (accessed March 16, 2011).

53. "New Functional Imaging for Interventional Neuroradiology— Syngo Neuro PBV IR Displays Cerebral Blood Flow during Interventional Procedures," February 9, 2010, http://www.siemens.com/press/en/presspicture/?press=/en/presspicture/2010/imaging_it/him201002023-01.htm (accessed March 16, 2011).

54. "Neurologists Develop Software Application to Help Identify Subtle Epileptic Lesions," February 17, 2011, http://www.redorbit.com/news/technology/1997860/neurologists_develop_software_application_to_help_identify_subtle_epileptic_lesions/ (accessed February 17, 2011).

55. S. H. Becker and R. L. Arenson, "Costs and Benefits of Picture Archiving and Communication Systems," *Journal of the American Medical Informatics Association* 1, no. 5 (1994): 361–71, http://www.ncbi.nlm.nih.gov/pmc/articles/PMC116218/ (accessed April 28 2011).

56. "Picture Archiving and Communications System (PACS)," January 29, 2007, http://webarchive.nationalarchives.gov.uk/20070129145236/ (accessed April 28, 2011); "Memphis Hospital Implements Latest Advances in Radiology System," January 23, 2006, http://www.methodisthealth.org/methodist/About+Us/Newsroom/News+Archive/Memphis+Hospital+System+Implements+Major+Techno-logy+Advances (accessed April 28, 2011).

57. "European Congress of Radiology 2010: Siemens Introduces Innovations for Imaging and Diagnostics."

58. Nicole Lewis, "Healthcare Providers Prize PACS-RIS Integration, Clinicians Want Seamless Integration Between Picture Archiving and Communication Systems

and Radiology Information Systems and Will Sacrifice Some Functionality to Achieve It, According to a KLAS Survey," April 22, 2011, http://www.informationweek.com/news/healthcare/interoperability/229402057 (accessed April 22, 2011).

59. Paula Gould and John C. Hayes, "Informatics Integration Drives Intraoperative Planning," CARS/EuroPACS 2005 Conference Reporter, October 5, 2005, http://www.diagnosticimaging.com/pacsweb/features/showArticle.jhtml?articleID=171202282 (accessed April 28, 2011).

60. "Stereotactic Radiosurgery," 2003, http://www.surgeryencyclopedia.com/St-Wr/Stereotactic-Radiosurgery.html (accessed April 28, 2011).

61. Laurie Tarkan, "Brain Surgery, without Knife or Blood, Gains Favor," April 29, 2003, http://www.nytimes.com/2003/04/29/health/brain-surgery-without-knife-or-blood-gains-favor.html (accessed April 28, 2011).

62. Daniel M. Keller, "Repeat Gamma Knife Radiosurgery Fixes Most Brain AVMs," April 20, 2011, http://www.medscape.com (accessed April 22, 2011).

63. "Focused Ultrasound Is a Revolutionary Technology That Could Help Treat Diseases That Affect Virtually Everyone," April 11, 2011, http://www.fusfoundation.org/MRgFUS-Overview/about-focused-ultrasound-surgery (accessed April 28, 2011); "Focused Ultrasound Surgery for Uterine Fibroids," March 31, 2011, http://www.mayoclinic.com/health/focused-ultrasound-surgery/MY00503/METHOD=print (accessed April 28, 2011).

64. Terrance T. Healey and Damian Dupuy, "Radiofrequency Ablation: A Safe and Effective Treatment in Nonoperative Patients with Early-Stage Lung Cancer," January–February 2011, http://journals.lww.com/journalppo/Abstract/2011/01000/Radiofrequency_Ablation__A_Safe_and_Effective.7.aspx (accessed April 28, 2011); "Chemoembolization," No date, http://www.hopkinsmedicine.org/vascular/procedures/chemoembolization/ (accessed April 28, 2011).

65. "Research Shows Laser Effectively Treats Children's Painful Vascular Malformations," April 3, 2006, http://www.sirweb.org/news/newsPDF/Burrows_Pediatrics_Malformations.pdf (accessed April 28, 2011); "Non-Surgical Embolization Treats Male Infertility and Pain, and Chronic Pelvic Pain in Women Caused by Enlarged Veins," March 31, 2001, http://www.sirweb.org/news/newsPDF/male_infertility.pdf (accessed April 28, 2011); "Non-Surgical Management of Uterine Fibroids," 2008, http://humupd.oxfordjournals.org/content/14/3/259.abstract (accessed April 28, 2011).

66. "Radiation Oncologists Use 'Cone Beam' CT to Improve Treatment Accuracy," September 6, 2006, http:// www.sciencedaily.com/releases/2006/08/060830214759.htm (accessed March 23, 2011).

67. "Study Shows Carotid Stenting Improves Memory and Thinking Ability in Patients Classified as 'Asymptomatic,'" March 31, 2006, http://www.sirweb.org/news/newsPDF/carotid_stenting_cognitive_function.pdf (accessed April 29, 2011); "Interventional Radiologists Provide Hope in Delaying Growth, Spread of Breast Cancer—Keeping Cancer Dormant: Researchers Target Tumor Metabolism by Blocking Energy Production Required for Malignant Cancer Growth," March 29, 2011, http://www.sirweb.org/news/newsPDF/8_Breast_cancer_final.pdf (accessed April 29, 2011); "First Study of Uterine Fibroid Embolization Post-Menopause," April 3, 2006, http://www.health.am/gyneco/more/first_study_of_uterine_fibroid_embolization_post_menopause/ (accessed April 29, 2011).

68. Walt Bogdanich, "The Radiation Boom, Radiation Offers New Cures, and Ways to Do Harm," January 23, 2010, http://www.nytimes.com/2010/01/24/health/24radiation.html?pagewanted=all (accessed November 24, 2010); Tara Parker-Pope, "More Protection for Radiation Patients," April 9, 2010, http://well.blogs.nytimes.com/2010/04/09/more-protection-for-radiation-patients/ (accessed February 16, 2011).`

69. Walt Bogdanich, "As Technology Surges, Radiation Safeguards Lag," January 26, 2010, http://www.nytimes.com/2010/01/27/us/27radiation.html (accessed February 16, 2011).

70. Gardiner Harris, "Scientists Say FDA Ignored Radiation Warnings," March 28, 2010, http://www.nytimes.com/2010/03/29/health/policy/29fda.html (accessed February 16, 2011).

71. Parker-Pope, "More Protection for Radiation Patients."

72. Roni Caryn Rabin, "Hazards: For Children in E.R., a Big Increase in CT Scans," April 7, 2011, http://www.nytimes.com/2011/04/12/health/research/12scan.html (accessed April 8, 2011).

73. Walt Bogdanich, "After Stroke Scans, Patients Face Serious Health Risks," July 31, 2010, http://www.nytimes.com/2010/08/01/health/01radiation.html (accessed February 16, 2011).

74. Ibid.

75. Walt Bogdanich, "FDA Urges Two Steps for Safer CT Scans," November 9, 2010, http://www.nytimes.com/2010/11/09/health/policy/09scan.html (accessed February 16, 2011).

# Additional Resources

"Alzheimer's Association Statement on Florbetapir PET Amyloid Imaging." January 24, 2011. http://www.alz.org/news_and_events_pet_amyloid_imaging.asp (accessed February 16, 2011).

ART Advanced Research Technologies Inc. 2011. http://www.art.ca/en/clinical/index.php (April 22, 2011).

Babiar, Heather. "New Cardiac MRI Pinpoints Closed Arteries Without Surgery." June 27, 2006. http://www.eurekalert.org/pub_releases/2006-06/rson-ncm062006.php (accessed April 28, 2011).

Beardsey, Tim. "Putting Alzheimer's to the Tests." *Scientific American,* February 1995, 12–13.

Belluck, Pam. "For Edge on Alzheimer's, Testing Early Treatments." November 8, 2010. http://www.nytimes.com/ref/health/healthguide/alzheimers_ess.html (accessed November 12, 2010).

Bentolila, L. A., X. Michalet, F. F. Pinaud, J. M. Tsay, S. Doose, J. J. Li, G. Sundaresan, A. M. Wu, S. S. Gambhir, and S. Weiss. "Quantum Dots for Molecular Imaging and Cancer Medicine." July 25, 2009. http://www.discoverymedicine.com/L-A-Bentolila/2009/07/25/quantum-dots-for-molecular-imaging-and-cancer-medicine/ (accessed March 17, 2011).

Blakeslee, Sandra. "Watching How the Brain Works as It Weighs a Moral Dilemma." September 25, 2001. http://www.nytimes.com/2001/09/25/science/watching-how-the-brain-works-as-it-weighs-a-moral-dilemma.html (accessed April 28, 2011).

Bogdanich, Walt. "After Stroke Scans, Patients Face Serious Health Risks." July 31, 2010. http://www.nytimes.com/2010/08/01/health/01radiation.html (accessed February 16, 2011).

Bogdanich, Walt. "As Technology Surges, Radiation Safeguards Lag." January 26, 2010. http://www.nytimes.com/2010/01/27/us/27radiation.html (accessed February 16, 2011).

Bogdanich, Walt. "FDA Urges Two Steps for Safer CT Scans." November 9, 2010. http://www.nytimes.com/2010/11/09/health/policy/09scan.html (accessed February 16, 2011).

Bogdanich, Walt. "The Radiation Boom, Radiation Offers New Cures, and Ways to Do Harm." January 23, 2010. http://www.nytimes.com/2010/01/24/health/24radiation.html?pagewanted=all (accessed November 24, 2010).

Chen, Jingkuang, Xiaoyand Cheng, I-Ming Shen, Jing-Hung Liu, Pai-Chi Li, and Mengli Wang. "A Monolithic Three-Dimensional Ultrasonic Transducer Array for Medical Imaging." October 1, 2001. http://ieeexplore.ieee.org/xpl/freeabs_all.jsp?arnumber=4337780 (accessed April 28, 2011).

Chhabra, Avneesh. "Diffusion Tensor Imaging." December 10, 2008. http://emedicine.medscape.com/article/345561-overview (accessed April 28, 2011).

Cluett, Jonathan. "Do I Need a Bone Density Test?" http://orthopedics.about.com/cs/osteoporosis/a/bonedensitytest.htm#b (accessed April 29, 2011).

"Computer-Aided Detection Is Increasingly Being Used in Screening and Diagnostic Mammography." October 1, 2010. http://www.sciencedaily.com/releases/2010/10/101001163335.htm (accessed March 16, 2011).

"Computer-Aided Detection May Be Better Than Doctors at Spotting Aneurysms." January 25, 2010. http://medgadget.com/2010/01/computer_aided_detection_may_be_better_than_doctors_at_spotting_aneurysms.html (accessed March 16, 2011).

"Computer-Aided Detection Reduces the Accuracy of Mammograms." April 2001. http://www.cancer.gov/newscenter/pressreleases/2007/cadmammographyrelease (accessed March 16, 2011).

"Computerized Scanner Double-Checks Suspicious Mammograms." August 1999. http://www.highbeam.com/doc/1G1-55182958.html (accessed April 29, 2011).

Cormode, David P., Torjus Skajaa, Zahi Fayad, and Willem J. M. Mulder. "Nanotechnology in Medical Imaging: Probe Designs and Applications." December 4, 2008. http://www.ncbi.nlm.nih.gov/pmc/articles/PMC2844987/ (accessed March 17, 2011).

"Detecting Asthma: Radiologists Develop Asthma Imaging Method." January 1, 2009. http://www.sciencedaily.com/videos/2009/0106-detecting_asthma.htm (accessed November 12, 2010).

Dye, Mark. "PET and SPECT: Happy Together." June 2005. http://www.medicalimagingmag.com/issues/articles/2005-06_01.asp (accessed April 28, 2011).

Eisenberg, Anne. "What's Next; a Budding Tumor Unmasked by the Vessels That Feed It." July 24, 2003. http://query.nytimes.com/gst/fullpage.html?res=9E0CE1D7153FF937A15754C0A9659C8B63 (accessed April 28, 2011).

Eisenberg, Anne. "What's Next; Lasers Set Cells Aglow for a Biopsy without the Knife." June 26, 2003. http://www.nytimes.com/2003/06/26/technology/what-s-next-lasers-set-cells-aglow-for-a-biopsy-without-the-knife.html (accessed April 29, 2011).

"Esophageal Cancer." 2006. http://www.cancer.org/downloads/PRO/EsophagealCancer.pdf (accessed April 29, 2011).

"European Congress of Radiology 2010: Siemens Introduces Innovations for Imaging and Diagnostics." March 5, 2010. http://www.siemens.com/press/en/events/healthcare/2010-03-ecr.php (accessed November 12, 2010).

"First FDA-Approved 3D Digital Mammography Available at Albany Med." February 15, 2011. http://www.amc.edu/PR/PressRelease/02_15_11_T.html (accessed April 29, 2011).

"Focused Ultrasound Is a Revolutionary Technology That Could Help Treat Diseases That Affect Virtually Everyone." April 11, 2011. http://www.fusfoundation.org/MRgFUS-Overview/about-focused-ultrasound-surgery (accessed April 28, 2011).

"Focused Ultrasound Surgery for Uterine Fibroids." March 31, 2011. http://www.mayoclinic.com/health/focused-ultrasound-surgery/MY00503/METHOD=print (accessed April 28, 2011).

Foreman, Judy. "Brain Scanning and OCD." June 3, 2003. http://judyforeman.com/columns/brain-scanning-and-ocd (accessed April 29, 2011))

Fox, Peter T., Roger J. Ingham, Janis C. Ingham, Traci B. Hirsch, J. Hunter Downs, Charles Martin, Paul Jerabek, Thomas Glass, and Jack L. Lancaster. "A PET Study of the Neural Systems of Stuttering." *Nature* 382, no. 6587 (1996): 158–62.

Friedman, Richard A. "Like Drugs, Talk Therapy Can Change Brain Chemistry." August 27, 2002. http://www.forensic-psych.com/articles/artNYTTalkTherapy8.27.02.html (accessed April 28, 2011).

"Functional MR Imaging (fMRI) – Brain." February 10, 2010. http://www.radiologyinfo.org/en/info.cfm?pg=fmribrain&bhcp=1 (accessed April 29, 2011).

"Gamma Knife Surgery." 2006. http://www.irsa.org/gamma_knife.html (accessed April 29, 2011).

Giesel, F. L., H. Bischoff, H. von Tengg-Kobligk, M.-A. Weber, C. M. Zechmann, H.-U. Kauczor, and M. V. Knopp. "Dynamic Contrast-Enhanced MRI of Malignant Pleural Mesothelioma: A Feasibility Study of Noninvasive Assessment, Therapeutic Follow-up, and Possible Predictor of Improved Outcome." June 2006. http://chestjournal.chestpubs.org/content/129/6/1570.full (accessed April 28, 2011).

Giger, Maryellen, and Charles A. Pelizzari. "Advances in Tumor Imaging." *Scientific American,* September 1996, 110–2.

"Given Diagnostic Imaging System – K010312." June 30, 2009. http://www.fda.gov/MedicalDevices/ProductsandMedical Procedures/DeviceApprovalsandClearances/Recently-ApprovedDevices/ucm085396.htm (accessed April 29, 2011).

Goode, Erica. "Experts See Mind's Voices in New Light." May 6, 2003. http://www.nytimes.com/2003/05/06/science/experts-see-mind-s-voices-in-new-light.html (accessed April 28, 2011).

Goode, Erica. "Studying Modern-Day Pavlov's Dogs, of the Human Variety." August 26, 2003. http://www.hnl.bcm.tmc.edu/articles/Studying%20Modern-Day%20Pavlov's%20Dogs,%20of%20the%20Human%20Variety.htm (accessed April 29, 2011).

Grady, Denise. "M.R.I.'s Help Fight High Risk of Cancer." November 15, 2010. http://www.nytimes.com/2010/11/16/health/16cancer.html (accessed April 28, 2011).

Harris, Gardiner. "Scientists Say F.D.A. Ignored Radiation Warnings." March 28, 2010. http://www.nytimes.com/2010/03/29/health/policy/29fda.html (accessed February 16, 2011).

Healey, Terrance T., and Damian Dupuy. "Radiofrequency Ablation: A Safe and Effective Treatment in Nonoperative Patients with Early-Stage Lung Cancer." January–February 2011. http://journals.lww.com/journalppo/Abstract/2011/01000/Radiofrequency_Ablation__A_Safe_and_Effective.7.aspx (accessed April 28, 2011).

Heiken, Jay P., Christine M. Peterson, and Christine O. Menias. "Virtual Colonoscopy for Colorectal Cancer Screening: Current Status." July 9, 2006. http://2006.confex.com/uicc/uicc/techprogram/P10382.HTM (accessed April 29, 2011).

Hooper, Judith. "Targeting the Brain." *Time,* Special Issue, Fall 1996, 46–50.

Husain, Iltifat. "A Key Milestone in Mobile Imaging: FDA Approves Mobile Radiology Viewer and Smartphone Ultrasound Probe." February 9, 2011. http://www.imedicalapps.com/2011/02/fda-approves-diagnostic-radiology-viewer-smartphone-ultrasound-probe/# (accessed February 16, 2011).

"iCad Wins FDA Nod for Computer-Aided Detection in Virtual Colonoscopies." August 5, 2010. http://www.massdevice.com/news/icad-wins-fda-nod-computer-aided-detection-virtual-colonoscopies (accessed March 16, 2011).

"Interventional X-Ray: Innova 3100 IQ for Cardiology." 2010. http://www3.gehealthcare.com/en/Products/Categories/Interventional_Image_Guided_Systems/Interventional_X-ray_for_Cardiology/Innova_3100-IQ_Optima_Edition (accessed April 22, 2011).

Keller, Daniel M. "Repeat Gamma Knife Radiosurgery Fixes Most Brain AVMs." April 20, 2011. http://www.medscape.com (accessed April 22, 2011).

Kevles, Bettyanne Holtzmann. "Body Imaging." *Newsweek,* Winter 1997–98, 74–76.

Kevles, Bettyanne Holtzmann. *Naked to the Bone: Medical Imaging in the Twentieth Century.* New Brunswick, NJ: Rutgers University Press, 1997.

Khafagi, Frederick A., and S. Patrick Butler. "Nuclear Medicine." *The Medical Journal of Australia* 176, no. 1 (2002): 27. http://www.mja.com.au/public/issues/176_01_070102/kha10734_fm.html (accessed April 29, 2011).

Kolata, Gina. "FDA Sees Promise in Alzheimer's Imaging Drug." January 20, 2011. http://www.nytimes.com/2011/01/21/health/21alzheimers.html (accessed February 10, 2011),

Lewis, Nicole. "Healthcare Providers Prize PACS-RIS Integration, Clinicians Want Seamless Integration between Picture Archiving and Communication Systems and Radiology Information Systems and Will Sacrifice Some Functionality to Achieve It, According to a KLAS Survey." April 22, 2011. http://www.informationweek.com/news/healthcare/interoperability/229402057 (accessed April 22, 2011).

Lowry, Fran. "Elastography Imaging during Breast Ultrasound Reduces Unnecessary Biopsy Rate." December 1, 2009. http://www.medscape.com (accessed April 16, 2010).

"LUMA™ Cervical Imaging System—P040028." July 8, 2009. http://www.fda.gov/MedicalDevices/ProductsandMedical Procedures/DeviceApprovalsandClearances/Recently-ApprovedDevices/ucm078285.htm (accessed April 22, 2011).

Marriott, Michel. "A Palm-Size Ultrasound Scans Safely in a Flash." October 10, 2002. http://query.nytimes.com/gst/fullpage.html?res=9906E1D91F3BF933A25753C1A9649C8B63 (accessed April 28, 2011).

Motluk, Alison. "Cutting Out Stuttering." *New Scientist,* February 1, 1997, 32–5.

"Nanotechnology Diagnostics." 2011. http://cancer.stanford.edu/research/imaging/nanotechnology.html (accessed February 16, 2011).

National Organic Standards Board Materials Committee. "Nanotechnology in Organic Production, Processing, and Packaging Request for Information for Developing a Usable Definition of the Term in Organics." February 25, 2010. http://www.ams.usda.gov/AMSv1.0/getfile?dDocName=ST ELPRDC5083223 (accessed March 17, 2011).

"Neurologists Develop Software Application to Help Identify Subtle Epileptic Lesions." February 17, 2011. http://www. redorbit.com/news/technology/1997860/neurologists_ develop_software_application_to_help_identify_subtle_ epileptic_lesions/ (accessed February 17, 2011).

"New Functional Imaging for Interventional Neuroradiology— Syngo Neuro PBV IR Displays Cerebral Blood Flow during Interventional Procedures." February 9, 2010. http:// www.siemens.com/press/en/presspicture/?press=/en/ presspicture/2010/imaging_it/him201002023-01.htm (accessed March 16, 2011).

"Osteoporosis: A Guide to Prevention and Treatment." 2010. http://www.health.harvard.edu/special_health_reports/ Osteoporosis.htm (accessed April 29, 2011).

Parker-Pope, Tara. "More Protection for Radiation Patients." April 9, 2010. http://well.blogs.nytimes.com/2010/04/09/more-pro tection-for-radiation-patients/ (accessed February 16, 2011).

Parker-Pope, Tara, and Stuart Bradford. "The Downside of a Cancer Study Extolling CT Scans." November 15, 2010. http://well.blogs.nytimes.com/2010/11/15/the-downside- of-a-cancer-study-extolling-ct-scans/ (accessed November 16, 2010).

Parlikar, Urmilla R. "Heart Imaging Procedure Helps Physicians Evaluate Patients Suspected of Having a Heart Attack." http:// johnbbassettdmd.com/PATIENTS/HEALTHLIBRARY/ tabid/606/contentid/28792/Default.aspx (accessed April 28, 2011).

"PET Scans Detect Therapy Responses in Esophageal Cancer Patients." 2010. http://demo.cancerconsultants.com/Content. aspx?Section=cancernews&DocumentID=34881 (accessed April 29, 2011).

Rabin, Roni Caryn. "Hazards: For Children in E.R., a Big Increase in CT Scans." April 7, 2011. http://www.nytimes. com/2011/04/12/health/research/12scan.html (accessed April 8, 2011).

"Radiation Oncologists Use 'Cone Beam' CT to Improve Treatment Accuracy." September 6, 2006. http://www. sciencedaily.com/releases/2006/08/060830214759.htm (accessed March 23, 2011).

Raichle, Marcus E. "Visualizing the Mind." *Scientific American,* April 1994, 58–64.

Spinasanta, Susan. "Nuclear Imaging: PET and SPECT Scans." December 8, 2004. http://www.spineuniverse.com/ displayarticle.php/article231.html (accessed April 28, 2011).

Streed, Joel. "Mayo Clinic and IBM Advance Early Detection of Brain Aneurysms." January 22, 2010. http:// www.mayoclinic.org/news2010-rst/5600.html (accessed March 16, 2011).

Tipnis, Sameer, Ashok Ramachandra, Walter Huda, Andrew Hardie, Joseph Schoepf, Philip Costello, Thomas Flohr, and Martin Sedlmair. "Iterative Reconstruction in Image Space (IRIS) and Lesion Detection in Abdominal CT." [Abstract] March 2010. http://adsabs.harvard.edu/abs/2010 SPIE.7622E..89T (accessed March 16, 2011).

"Top 10 Medical Innovations for 2011: #1 New Molecular Imaging Biomarker for Early Detection, Prevention and Treatment of Alzheimer's Disease." 2010. http://www.clevel andclinic.org/innovations/summit2011/topten11/one.html (accessed February 28, 2011).

"Top 10 Medical Innovations for 2011: #10 Capsule Endoscopy for Diagnosis of Pediatric GI Disorders." 2010. http://www.clevelandclinic.org/innovations/summit2011/ topten11/ten.html (accessed February 28, 2011).

Trofatter, Kenneth F., Jr. "Breast Cancer Diagnosis during Pregnancy." October 8, 2006. http://www.healthline.com/ blogs/pregnancy_childbirth/2006/10/breast-cancer-diagno- sis-during.html (accessed April 28, 2011).

Vaccari, Guido, and Claudio Saccavini. "Radiology Informatics and Work Flow Redesign." *PsychNology Journal* 4, no. 1 (2006): 87–101. http://www.psychology. org/File/PNJ4(1)/PSYCHNOLOGY_JOURNAL_4_1_ VACCARI.pdf (accessed April 28, 2011).

Vieth, Peter. "New Imaging Techniques May Help Prove, or Disprove, Brain Injuries." January 3, 2011. http://tgblaw. blogspot.com/2011/01/new-imaging-techniques-may-help- prove.html (accessed March 17, 2011).

Wang, Gene-Jack. "Study Reveals Biochemical Signature of Cocaine Craving in Humans." June 13, 2006. http://www. bnl.gov/bnlweb/pubaf/pr/PR_display.asp?prID=06-74 (accessed April 29, 2011).

Wu, D., and S. S. Gambhir. "Positron Emission Tomography in Diagnosis and Management of Invasive Breast Cancer: Current Status and Future Perspectives." [Abstract] April 2003. http://www.ncbi.nlm.nih.gov/pubmed/12756080 (accessed April 29, 2011).

Zimmer, Carl. "What if There Is Something Going on in There?" September 28, 2003. http://www.nytimes. com/2003/09/28/magazine/what-if-there-is-something- going-on-in-there.html (accessed April 28, 2011).

# Related Web Sites

American College of Physicians. http://www.acponline.org/running_practice/technology/

American College of Physicians. http://www.acponline.org/running_practice/technology/

PEARSON
**myhealthprofessionskit**™

Go to www.myhealthprofessionskit.com to access the Companion Web site created for this textbook. Simply select "Basic Health Science" from the choice of disciplines. Find this book and register to access self-assessment quizzes, flashcards, and more.

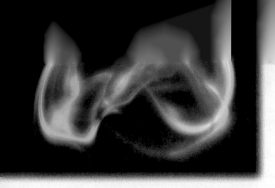

## CHAPTER 7

# Information Technology in Surgery—The Cutting Edge

## LEARNING OBJECTIVES

Upon completion of this chapter, the reader will be able to:

- List some of the uses of computers in surgery.
- Describe the role of computers in surgical planning.

- Define robotic surgery, endoscopic surgery, minimally invasive surgery, augmented reality, and telepresence surgery, and be aware of the Socrates system, which allows long-distance mentoring of surgeons in real time.
- Describe NASA Extreme Environment Mission Operation (NEEMO).
- Describe the Operating Room of the Future.
- List some of the robots used in surgery including ROBODOC, AESOP, ZEUS, and da Vinci.
- Describe some of the advantages and disadvantages of computer-assisted surgery.
- Describe the use of lasers in surgery.

## OVERVIEW

Information technology has entered the 21st century with profound challenges and extraordinary techniques in the field of surgery. Hardware and software are being developed that help in the planning and carrying out of surgical procedures. Sophisticated simulation software and speech recognition systems, in addition to **robots** equipped with **artificial intelligence**—programmed to "hear," "see," and "respond" to their environments—are already helping to perform certain operations. Special system software is used to network all the computerized devices in an operating room.

Health care personnel can use a combination of computer-generated images, virtual and augmented reality, and robotic devices to assist before and during operations. Currently, computer-generated graphics assist in planning surgery, in guiding operations, and in training surgeons and other health care professionals. Enhanced images and precision instruments have made the development of the field of **minimally invasive surgery (MIS)** possible. MIS is surgery performed through small incisions. Most minimally invasive procedures are done using an **endoscope**—a thin tube that can be connected to a minuscule camera. It projects an image of the surgical site onto a monitor. The surgeon does not look at the patient; instead, she or he looks at a monitor on which is projected an *image* of the patient. Thus, much of **computer-assisted surgery** is said to be **image-directed**. **Distance (or telepresence) surgery** performed by robotic devices controlled by surgeons at another site has been successfully performed. It is conceivable that a robot controlled only by a computer program could perform surgery.

## COMPUTER-ASSISTED SURGERY

### Computer-Assisted Surgical Planning

Computer-assisted surgical planning involves the use of **virtual environment** technology to provide surgeons with realistic accurate models on which to teach surgery and to plan and practice operations. With **virtual reality (VR)** technology, the computer can create an environment that seems real, but is not. VR simulations were first used in the 1940s to train pilots. Currently, these lifelike simulations are used in the health care field. The models created by VR technology can look, sound, and feel real. They can respond to pressure, by changing shape, and to being cut, by leaking. A model such as this, which is interactive, allows surgeons not only to plan surgeries more precisely, but also to practice operations without touching a patient. Some models include a predictive element that shows the results of the doctor's actions. For example, plastic surgeons can practice on a model of a face and see the results of their work. The Netra system allows planning of biopsies, tumor resections, surgical implants, and surgery for motor disorders. The Compass system allows surgeons to plan operations for brain tumors by providing a three-dimensional model from computed tomography (CT) scans and magnetic resonance imaging (MRI). The image is also used as a guide during the operation.

## Minimally Invasive Surgery

MIS, using an endoscope or a laparoscope, performs procedures through small incisions that involve a minimum of damage to healthy tissue (Figure 7.1 ▶).

However, some laparoscopic surgeries involve electronic cutting tools, posing some risk for the patient. Still, there is less bleeding and pain, and a shorter recovery time. This means a shorter hospital stay and lower costs. You will recall that an endoscope projects an image of the surgical field onto a monitor.

Recognizing that a picture on a monitor is not the same as viewing the surgical field, some doctors are attempting to improve the picture by connecting endoscopes to high-definition televisions. Gall bladder disease has been treated with minimally invasive techniques for many years.

One form of minimally invasive robotic surgery is called **endoluminal surgery**. Endoluminal

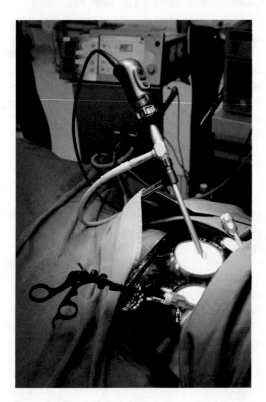

▶ **Figure 7.1** A demonstration of minimally invasive surgery.
*Source:* Norman Chan/Shutterstock.com

surgery does not require incisions. It is also called natural orifice surgery. For example, devices recently approved by the U.S. Food and Drug Administration (FDA) give the surgeon access to the stomach through the patient's mouth. Endoluminal surgery is being used in the relief of gastroesophageal reflux disease (GERD).[1] "An untethered miniature robot . . . inserted through the mouth would . . . be able to enter the abdominal cavity."[2]

Minimally invasive heart surgery is now (2011) in clinical trials at 40 sites in the United States. Traditionally, surgery to replace a heart valve required the surgeon to split the breastbone and put the patient on a heart-and-lung machine. In minimally invasive heart surgery for valve replacement, "a catheter [is] inserted into the femoral artery. Then a device called a CoreValve – made of a special alloy and heart material from a pig – [is] threaded through the blood vessels to the aortic valve using X-ray guidance. Once implanted, it expand[s] and becomes an entirely new gateway." This procedure, if approved by the FDA, would help people with aortic stenosis (where the aortic valve does not open correctly) who are too sick for the traditional open heart surgery. In Europe, the **CoreValve** has been approved; 15,000 people have had the surgery.[3]

## COMPUTER-ASSISTED SURGERY AND ROBOTICS

Computer-assisted surgery makes use of robotics and computer-generated images such as CT scans and MRIs. The robots are under the control of software and the surgeon. Through a combination of hardware and software, a robot may be able to "see" via video devices and to "hear" through microphones using speech recognition software.

Robots, unlike humans, can hold endoscopes and other instruments without becoming tired or shaky. Robots are also used to scale down the surgeon's motions. Some surgeons report that this makes their hands "rock steady," making surgery on small delicate areas such as the eye safer.

Feedback mechanisms allow the robot to determine the proper pressure and tension needed to manipulate a particular object. Robots are able to compare tissue density and thus "decide" whether tissue is normal or a tumor by remembering its "pressure signature."

Currently, doctors are trying to give robots a delicate sense of touch; the robots will also be able to palpate tissue. To restore the sense of touch to surgeons, a chip containing 64 sensors will be inside the patient's body; it will scan the patient. When it encounters a lump, the pressure in a sensor will rise. Outside the patient, the doctor's finger rests on motorized pins that rise or fall according to the sensors. Through the pins, the doctor will feel the object inside the patient's body.

Currently, robotics and MIS are being used in complex surgeries. New computer-controlled systems are making it possible to perform trauma surgery (such as femoral fracture fixation) through quarter-inch incisions; one such system has received FDA clearance. Minimally invasive knee and hip replacements are also a possibility. FDA-approved hardware and software will make hip replacement through a tiny incision possible; the software allows the surgeon to have more information by keeping track of the implant and the instruments and their relation to the patient. The information is given to the surgeon in real time.

New instruments are being developed to make surgery even less invasive. Laprotek is developing flexible, computer-controlled catheters; the surgeon can control them inside the patient. The catheters can carry out suturing. European clinical trials began in May 2003.

One program, eXpert Trainer, attempts to teach the special skills that are needed to perform MIS. The skills include working with long instruments, learning "eye-hand disassociation" to work on a patient while looking at a monitor, working in a three-dimensional field while looking at a two-dimensional screen, and learning to reverse right and left motions and images. (See Figure 7.2 ▶).

## ROBODOC, AESOP, ZEUS, da Vinci, MINERVA, NeuroArm, and Other Robotic Devices

The earliest use of a robot in surgery was in hip replacement operations. Integrated Surgical Systems' **ROBODOC** (which was approved

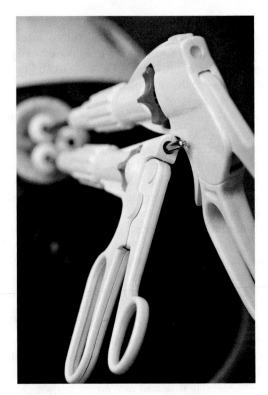

▶ **Figure 7.2**  Instruments of minimally invasive surgery.
*Source*: iStockphoto.com/Michael Miller

by the FDA in 2008) is a computer-controlled, image-directed robot that performed its first hip replacement in 1992. It can be used only with cementless implants, which constitute about one-third of implants done each year. It has been used in thousands of hip replacement operations worldwide. Because ROBODOC actually cuts into a patient's femur, there have to be strict built-in safeguards. They come from the program that controls the robot and physical limitations on how much ROBODOC can move. Before the operation, the hip navigation system helps surgeons align implants. The surgeon inserts three pins into the patient's hip. ROBODOC will use these as guides for locating the point to start drilling. Currently, some hip replacements are being performed without pins, and studies are being carried out to compare the two methods. ROBODOC works with ORTHODOC, which using CT scans creates a three-dimensional image of the hip. The doctor plans the surgery using the image. The plan is translated into drilling instructions for ROBODOC, which drills a perfect opening for the implant. ROBODOC is up to 10 times more accurate than a human being.

In a report of U.S. multicenter trials comparing outcomes of hip replacement done with ROBODOC to those performed by hand, it was found that at 24 months there were no differences in complications between the two groups; however, the group undergoing ROBODOC surgery had no intraoperative fractures, but blood loss and surgical time were greater. The most significant findings were that ROBODOC did "improve implant size, selection, position, and accuracy." One of the advantages of ROBODOC is that it forces surgeons to plan carefully, thus avoiding the wrong-sized implant and reaming defects. The study predicts better long-term performance with ROBODOC. A German study focused on safety. It found that an operation had never had to be stopped for safety reasons with ROBODOC and that the robot itself would stop the surgery if it sensed any errors in data. The surgery could then be completed by hand.

**Automated endoscopic system for optimal positioning (AESOP)**, which was introduced in 1994 by Computer Motion Inc., is the first FDA-cleared surgical robot. Originally developed for the space program, AESOP is now used as an assistant in endoscopic procedures. It holds and moves the endoscope under the direction of the surgeon. AESOP was first developed to be controlled by foot pedals. However, currently it responds to voice commands such as "AESOP move left" or "AESOP stop." "AESOP move right" causes a continuous movement for 2.5 seconds. The surgeon can tell AESOP to save a position and later to return to it. Any surgeon who uses AESOP trains the robot to recognize his or her voice. If it fails to recognize the surgeon's voice or command during an operation, a backup system of manual controls can be relied on. Unlike a human assistant, AESOP does not become tired or shaky. It has been used in a wide variety of procedures including appendectomy, splenectomy, and relief of intestinal obstruction.

In May 1998, in France, heart surgeries were performed on six patients using computers and robots. The incisions were small. The surgeon touched only the console located at a distance of several yards from the patient; she or he could see inside the heart via a three-dimensional camera inside the patient; the robot actually performed the surgery directed by the surgeon. More and more cardiac surgeries are being performed as minimally invasive surgeries.

**ZEUS** is a robotic surgical system that will make minimally invasive microsurgery possible. ZEUS has three interactive robotic arms, one of which holds the endoscope, while the other two manipulate the surgical instruments. The surgeon, sitting at a console, controls the arms. The endoscope is controlled by voice commands. The surgeon manipulates instruments, which resemble surgical tools, while looking at a monitor; the surgeon's manipulations control the robotic arms, which are actually doing the surgery. ZEUS includes a feedback system so that the surgeon "feels" the tissue. The computer-controlled robotic arms also scale down the surgeon's movements, filtering out any hand tremor. This means that a 1-inch movement by the surgeon becomes a one-tenth of an inch movement of the robot's surgical instrument. By eliminating the hand's vibrations, ZEUS makes delicate procedures safer. Thus, ZEUS can increase the surgeon's dexterity. Computer Motion Inc., which manufactures ZEUS, states that it will be able to perform heart bypass surgery endoscopically through incisions the diameter of a pencil instead of the traditional 30-cm splitting of the breast bone. ZEUS may be approved for use in coronary bypass, mitral valve replacement, and laparoscopic and thoracic surgery.

Similar to ZEUS, the **da Vinci** robot (Figures 7.3, 7.4, 7.5, and 7.6 ▶) was first cleared for assisting in surgery in 1997, for performing some surgeries in 2000, and for performing cardiac surgery such as mitral valve repair in November 2002. A small study in December 2000 found that patients undergoing minimally invasive mitral valve repair have less pain and shorter hospital stays than those who undergo conventional surgery, and these patients returned to work 50 percent faster. Minimally invasive heart surgeries

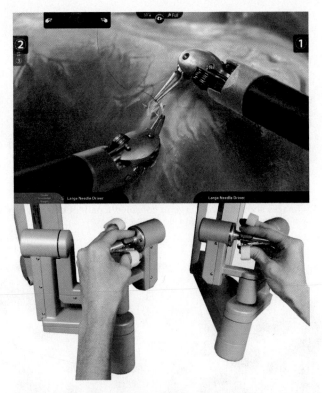

▶ **Figure 7.3**   Images showing hands on the master controls
of the surgeon console and the operative screen.
*Source:* Courtesy of Intuitive Surgical (©2011 Intuitive Surgical, Inc.).

are performed through three tiny incisions: one for the endoscope that projects the surgical field on to a monitor, and the other two for surgical instruments. The instruments are held by a robot. Its wrists can move 180 degrees (a greater range of motion than humans have) and follow the surgeon's hand motions; the surgeon's hands are attached to controls. The surgeon watches the surgery on a screen in three-dimensional, high-resolution images and can see any part of the surgical field. One advantage of da Vinci is that it mimics the surgeon's hand motions. To control other laparoscopic instruments, the surgeon has to move the opposite way; for instance, to move the instrument right, the surgeon must move left, up is down, and so on. On January 17, 2002, the first endoscopic cardiac bypass surgery was performed in the United States. However, the FDA has not yet approved this for widespread use. da Vinci

is also used to repair an inborn condition called atrial septal defect (ASD). Patients born with ASD have an opening between the two upper chambers of the heart, which untreated can result in congestive heart failure, hypertension, and increased risk of stroke. It should be noted that at least one person has died in a robot-aided surgery. da Vinci was being used to remove a cancerous kidney. However, the patient's aorta was accidentally cut during the surgery, and he died 2 days later. The hospital denied that the robot was to blame. Several other people have been injured, some seriously, in robot-assisted surgeries.[4]

In 2005, da Vinci was approved for gynecological procedures. It can be used to perform hysterectomies, to remove fibroid tumors, and in all urologic procedures. Cleared for heart surgery in 2004, da Vinci has been used in over 2,000 heart and chest surgeries.

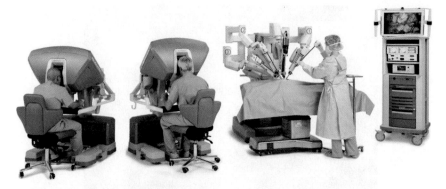

▶ **Figure 7.4**  Images showing two surgeon consoles, a patient cart, and a vision cart.
*Source:* Courtesy of Intuitive Surgical (©2011 Intuitive Surgical, Inc.).

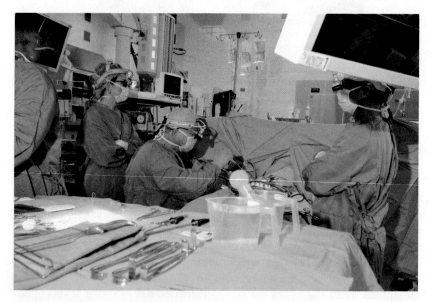

▶ **Figure 7.5**  Dr. Renata Bastos Ford (left), Dr. W. Randolph Chitwood (center), and Dr. Chayanin Vatcharasiritham in the operating room.
*Source:* Courtesy of the East Carolina Heart Institute at East Carolina University.

da Vinci can be used in mitral valve repairs and coronary bypass procedures. It is also used in prostate surgery (the most common robotic surgery) and gynecological and infertility surgeries. The use of da Vinci has increased from 1,500 procedures in 2000 to 20,000 in 2004.[5] It continues to grow; in 2009, in the United States, 86 percent of prostate surgeries were performed using da Vinci. According to Intuitive Surgical, da Vinci "leads to less tissue trauma, requires fewer surgical assistants, and is less physically taxing for the surgeon." In 2011, da Vinci performed a hysterectomy. According to a study of Medicare patients, it did lead to fewer complications in the hospital "but had worse results for impotence and incontinence." Adding haptic feedback and training on a new Simulated Surgical System may help with these problems.[6]

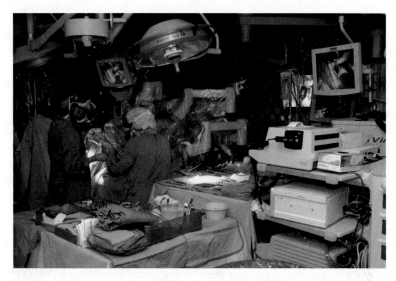

▶ **Figure 7.6**   Dr. W. Randolph Chitwood (not pictured) performing a robotic mitral valve repair in the operating room.
*Source:* Courtesy of the East Carolina Heart Institute at East Carolina University.

In October 2010, da Vinci performed the first all-robotic surgery in Canada. With the help of its anesthetist, McSleepy, da Vinci removed a prostate. Human surgeons controlled the operation from a monitor on which three-dimensional images were projected.[7]

Researchers at Columbia University College of Physicians and Surgeons in New York are currently conducting clinical trials on Evalve Cardiovascular Valve Repair System. Evalve is being used for the treatment of mitral valve regurgitation. Untreated, this condition can lead to arrhythmias and congestive heart failure. The valve repair procedure is non-surgical. Guided by images, a catheter is inserted into the vascular system to the mitral valve where it places a clip to repair the leaky valve.[8]

**MINERVA** is a robot developed to perform stereotactic neurosurgical procedures. Used to treat some brain tumors, the stereotactic method involves fixing a metal frame, similar to a cage, on the patient's head. The surgeon uses an MRI or CT scan to calculate how to reach the tumor with a minimum of trauma to surrounding tissue. The surgeon does not see the surgical site and must rely on the CT scan to avoid damaging vital parts of the brain. For successful robot-assisted surgery,

the robot must be highly accurate. MINERVA operates inside the CT scan. This enables the surgeon to follow the position of the instruments. The doctor selects the target. MINERVA makes the calculations, and responding to the doctor's commands, performs the procedure. NeuroMate was developed in France for neurosurgical applications and is FDA approved. It has performed over 1,000 tumor biopsies. It collects data from images of the patient and, with special software, plans the path to the tumor. This information is transferred to a control workstation. The surgeon uses all the information, including X-rays, to command the robot to insert a guide. The guide is then used to introduce a surgical instrument. Stereotactic radiosurgery or gamma knife surgery (see Chapter 6) is less invasive than robot-assisted stereotactic neurosurgery; it does not involve cutting, but uses radiation to shrink certain brain tumors, which then may not need to be surgically removed. The newer cyber knife, because it compensates for patient movement, can be used to treat brain and spinal tumors with radiosurgery.

Other robots have been developed. Using **ARTEMIS**, a surgical system that works with the simulation software **KISMET**, a surgeon can perform MIS while viewing three screens, which show the view presented by the endoscope and simulations. ARTEMIS can also perform minimally invasive breast biopsies.

Robots can assist in needle placement in the insertion of nerve blocks for back pain and minimally invasive kidney procedures (percutaneous access of the kidney/remote center of motion [PAKY/RCM]). ACROBAT, or active constraint robot, is used for total knee replacement. PROBOT helps in prostate surgery. Steady-hand robot was developed for microsurgery where smaller than human movements of the hand are needed. A robot is being developed in Germany that reduces the risks of extremely delicate spinal surgery; it would make it possible to monitor the surgery in real time, possibly diminishing risks such as paralysis.

System software is required to connect the operating room hardware into a network that a surgeon can control with voice commands. **HERMES** is an FDA-cleared operating system that performs these tasks, allowing the surgeon to use his or her voice to control all the electronic equipment in the operating room, coordinating the endoscope and robotic devices. It also allows the surgeon to adjust lighting with a voice command. The surgeon can use HERMES to take and print pictures and access the patient's electronic medical record including images and other information.

The **NeuroArm Robot** was developed at the University of Calgary in Canada. It has two arms. It is controlled by a surgeon sitting at a console. Unlike other surgical robots, it can operate in an MRI. According to NeuroArm's Web site, it can operate "inside the bore of the magnet with near real-time image guidance." Its arms can be moved 50 microns at a time—a microscopic scale. These tiny steady movements make it safer to operate on the human brain.[9]

**SpineAssist** is a robot that can be clamped on a patient's back. Doctors take a picture of where the spine surgery will take place, and a computer plans the robot's path. The robot creates a three-dimensional map of a patient's spine. This makes it possible for the surgeons to plan "exactly where to place pins or make incisions." Following the path, SpineAssist actually drills into the patient's vertebrae. According to one recent paper in *Spine*, "SpineAssist raises spine implant accuracy to 98 percent." One report stated that it reduces hospital stays by one-third. SpineAssist has successfully completed 2,000 surgeries.[10]

A major problem with surgical robots is their size. In 2006, doctors and engineers at Purdue University were attempting to create "less expensive, portable, and versatile surgical robots," and they planned to include sensors so that surgeons would be able to feel tissue. The sensors would communicate with the computer, which would create a color-coded "tactile map." Surgical robots currently cost around $1 million. The portable robot would cost about $250,000.[11]

## Augmented Reality

Because much computer-assisted surgery is **image-guided surgery**, software has been developed that enhances what the surgeon sees. This kind of surgery is called **augmented reality** surgery. It makes use of computer-generated imagery to provide the surgeon with information that otherwise would be unavailable. The computer-generated images may either be fused with the image on the monitor or projected directly onto the patient's body during the operation, allowing the doctor to virtually see inside the patient. However, an image on a monitor is two-dimensional. A head-mounted display that combines the computer-generated images and the image of the patient allows the surgeon to see a three-dimensional field and see different views by simply turning her or his head instead of adjusting the endoscope, making it more like traditional open surgery. The image and the reality must of course be perfectly aligned (registered) with each other. One use of augmented reality is in using an ultrasound to allow the technician to see an image of the fetus on the abdomen of the patient. Another is in image-guided breast biopsies. It is also used in brain surgery, where an MRI or CT scan may be projected on the patient's head, so that the surgeon can see a tumor, which would otherwise be invisible.

A new four-dimensional model of the human body called CAVEman has been developed in Canada. It can be used to plan surgery and to educate patients. "[T]he larger-than-life computer image encompasses more than 3,000 distinct body parts, all viewed in a booth that gives the image height, width and depth. . . . It also plots the passage of time [the 4th dimension]." The model looks like it is floating just out of reach. High-resolution computer-generated images can be projected onto CAVEman giving a view of the inside of a particular patient. There is only one finished CAVEman in the world today. Researchers plan to use the model to study the genetic components of several diseases including cancer, diabetes, multiple sclerosis, and Alzheimer's disease. It will make it possible to "merge patients' diagnostic results, . . . internal images and blood tests—in one place." CAVEman can be viewed using three-dimensional glasses and its parts moved by a joystick.[12]

## Telepresence Surgery

**Telepresence surgery (distance surgery)** is at the cutting edge of telemedicine. The National Aeronautics and Space Administration (NASA) first sought to develop telepresence surgery for space flight medical emergencies. Actual surgeries have been performed with the patient and surgeon at a distance and have been successful. Distance surgery thus has the potential of making surgical expertise available on battlefields, space stations, and in remote rural areas. Several research groups are working on telesurgical systems. Some of this work is funded by the Advanced Research Projects Agency (ARPA) of the U.S. Department of Defense, which first conceived of robotic surgery and still sees remote surgery as a way of saving lives on the battlefield and protecting surgeons from dangerous environments. One of the systems that has been developed is the Green Telepresence Surgical System in which surgeons wearing three-dimensional glasses can view the operating room and patient. The system has been used to practice suturing. It has demonstrated its precision by slicing a grape

into 1-mm slices. Distance operations were first performed on animals.

In telepresence surgery, as in MIS, the doctor looks at an image of the patient, not the actual patient. The instruments in the surgeon's hands feel real, but in fact, they only direct the robot at a distant site (theoretically hundreds of miles away) that is performing the surgery.

In September 2001, a woman in France had her gall bladder removed by doctors in New York. She spent 2 days in the hospital. Technically, the surgery made use of high-speed fiber optics, so that time delay was minimal. Much of the system is not yet FDA approved. "It was amazing for the doctors . . . to see the surgical tools suddenly start moving themselves and doing the operation, without any surgeon in the room guiding them," according to one of the doctors on the French team.[13] In this computer-assisted laparoscopic procedure, patient and doctor never touch; the surgeon controls the robot through hand signals. Successful prostate cancer surgery was performed in April 2002 between Germany and Virginia. Using the Socrates system, the American doctor was able to see and hear as if he were in the operating room in Berlin; he also controlled AESOP, while the German surgeon performed the surgery. Using Socrates, the remote doctor can teleconnect to the operating room, see and hear, and control devices networked by HERMES. **Socrates** is basically a mentoring system, allowing a surgeon in one place to give expert advice in real-time to a distant surgeon. In 2001, the Socrates system was cleared by the FDA, which at the same time created a new classification of device: Robotic Telemedicine Device.

In March 2003, ZEUS was used to perform distance surgery in Canada to correct a patient's acid reflux disease. At one hospital, endoscopic instruments were inserted into the patient's stomach. At another hospital 400 kilometers away, a surgeon used ZEUS to perform the successful surgery. ZEUS's sensors took the information from the surgeon's hand movements and sent it to the distant instruments. The Canadian federal government sees distance surgery as a way of serving its northern population.

## NASA Extreme Environment Mission Operation

The NASA Extreme Environment Mission Operation (**NEEMO**) is a series of NASA missions in which groups of scientists live in Aquarius. The major purpose of these projects is to enable astronauts to be operated on in space from earth using wireless technology and robotics. **Aquarius** is the only undersea lab in the world. Aquarius is now 67 feet under the ocean's surface off the Florida Keys. It is 13 feet wide and 45 feet long with approximately 400 square feet of space for living and laboratory activities.[14]

Early NEEMO missions tested living and building in an extreme environment, similar to outer space. NEEMO 7 and 9 included doctors, but no surgeons. One of NEEMO 7's goals was to see whether doctors with no training in surgical techniques could successfully perform surgery with the help of telementoring and telerobotics. According to one of the family practitioners on board, the techniques were "very new for us." The projects used telemedicine techniques to perform gall bladder surgery and suturing on a simulated patient. The project used wireless communications. According to the commander Bob Thirsk, the suturing was not successful. "My perception is that some special skills may be necessary." There were some problems on NEEMO 7 regarding the size of the robotic surgeon (a modified ZEUS) and communication delays. "If a signal is delayed more than 0.7 seconds, a surgeon will begin to have problems controlling the robot."[15] NEEMO 9 succeeded in assembling a surgical robot, and completed surgeries controlled by a doctor in Canada.[16]

The NASA NEEMO 12 crew conducted advanced medical experiments using robotic telesurgery (Figure 7.7 ▶). Their purpose was to improve future care for astronauts, in part by "overcome[ing] interplanetary lag time." They practiced several emergency procedures on simulated patients. **Raven**, a 50-pound, mobile surgical robot was used on NEEMO 12 (Figure 7.7).[17]

NEEMO 14 (completed in May 2011) did not include surgeries but did "simulate the transfer of an incapacitated astronaut from the ocean floor to

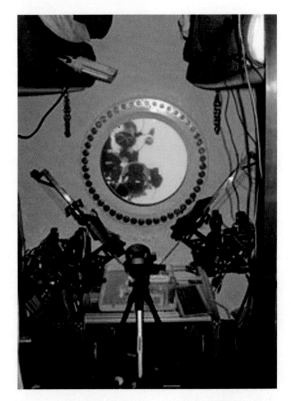

▶ **Figure 7.7** A two-armed remotely controlled robot named RAVEN set up in the operating room of NEEMO 12.
*Source:* Courtesy of NASA.

the deck of the craft," a maneuver that might need to accompany surgery in the future.[18]

An independent study completed in 2004 that investigated the feasibility of using "real-time or simultaneous surgical consultation and education to students in distant locations, . . . [reported] the successful integration of robotics, video-teleconferencing, and intranet transmission using currently available hardware and Internet capabilities." Ninety percent of those viewing anatomical structures telemedically were able to correctly identify them.[19]

## THE OPERATING ROOM OF THE FUTURE

Until very recently, picture archiving and communication systems (PACS), the systems used to organize and display digital images, could not interact with the operating room. This meant that real-time images were not available to surgeons. Because most computer-assisted surgeries are image directed, this was a serious problem. Integration of systems is a current focus of medical informatics.

In the Operating Room of the Future, images from all sources will be integrated and available to surgeons and other personnel. "Multiple image display processors integrate OR video cameras, laparoscopic and endoscopic cameras, MRI, CT, and PET imagery, PACS images, fluoroscopic imaging, ultrasound, patient monitoring data, hemodynamic activity, and patient history on a single, centralized screen for viewing by the surgical team." Information displayed includes a patient's vital statistics, allergies, and the whereabouts of operating room (OR) personnel. Eventually the equipment will be identified and tracked also. The display on four screens (called the wall of knowledge) shows integrated patient information in an easy-to-understand format, in one location.[20] By 2006, 21 ORs of the future were in operation in Memorial Sloan-Kettering alone. The purpose of this was to enhance patient safety and improve efficiency by providing real-time, integrated information.[21]

In some ORs of the future, all personnel including doctors are identified and their movements tracked by **radio frequency identification (RFID) tags**. (See Chapter 1.) A list of staff for an operation is displayed, and when the doctor or nurse enters the OR, that person's name is brightly lit.[22] RFID-tagged sponges have been created "to help prevent the deadly problem of surgeons accidentally leaving them inside patients." After the surgery, a wand is waved over the patient to check for tags. Because it is so new, no one knows what effect leaving an RFID tag inside a patient would have.[23]

## LASERS IN SURGERY

**Laser** stands for light amplification by the stimulated emission of radiation. A laser beam can be narrowed to the size of a few cells. Lasers can be used in surgery to cut, vaporize tumors, and seal small blood vessels to prevent blood loss. They can also be used to slow the spread of tumors

by closing lymph vessels, to reduce pain by closing nerve endings, to remove some brain and liver tumors, and for many kinds of skin surgery. Lasers can be used in minimally invasive back surgery. They can be used after strokes to eliminate the clot. This takes a much shorter time than a clot-dissolving drug. They can also be used to dissolve plaque in arteries. A relatively new use for laser surgery is in cancer of the mouth and throat. An early diagnosis is essential if laser surgery is to be used. At early stages, laser surgery can cure these cancers and leave the patient's voice intact.[24] Lasers are also used in gynecology; orthopedics; urology; ear, nose, and throat; gastroenterology; and cardiovascular medicine[25] (Figure 7.8 ▶).

**LASIK** is an eye surgery that uses lasers to correct vision by changing the shape of the cornea (Figure 7.9 ▶). In the LASIK procedure, a laser is used to create a flap in the cornea. The flap is folded out of the way, and the surgeon uses an excimer laser to remove tissue from the cornea.

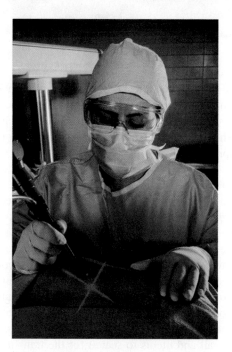

▶ **Figure 7.8**   Lasers in surgery can cut, vaporize tumors, and seal small blood vessels.
*Source:* Larry Mulvehill/Corbis

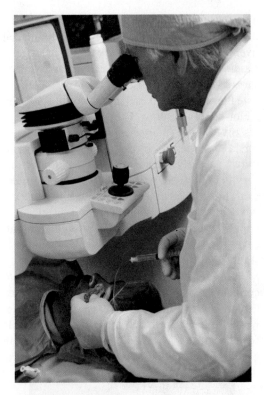

▶ **Figure 7.9** A doctor performing laser eye surgery.
*Source:* Monkey Business Images/Shutterstock.com

The excimer laser reshapes the cornea by using a cool ultraviolet light beam. After the cornea is reshaped, the flap is replaced. LASIK can help both nearsighted and farsighted people. Vision is improved almost immediately.[26]

Ten to 15 percent of identical twins who share a placenta in utero may develop twin-to-twin transfusion syndrome. An artery incorrectly sends nutrients and oxygen to the wrong twin. One twin is losing nutrients and cannot grow; the other twin can develop heart failure. If untreated, 70 to 80 percent of these twins die. Endoscopic laser surgery can be used to treat this condition in utero. "The target is the twin receiving too much blood. The surgeon uses a small fiberoptic scope/camera inserted through the mother's abdominal wall and uterus to search for the transfusion site. Once identified . . . [the surgeon] severs the connecting vessel with a laser attached to the scope."[27]

## DISCUSSION AND FUTURE DIRECTIONS

Computer-assisted surgery encompasses everything from the well-established use of a robotic assistant in an endoscopic procedure to telepresence surgery. It is an evolving field. New robotic devices, nanotechnology, new software, new techniques, and new applications are being developed. Thus, this cannot be an exhaustive survey of the uses of robotics, augmented reality techniques, or MIS procedures. Currently, computer-generated images help make surgery more precise. Making three-dimensional real-time images available in surgery (linking PACS with the OR) would certainly help. MIS results in smaller incisions, less trauma, and therefore less pain and shorter recovery time. This leads to some economic benefits including shorter hospitals stays and less time lost from work. Even though the equipment is quite expensive, it may be less expensive in the long run to use a robot than a human assistant to hold an endoscope in the OR. However, there are substantial difficulties involved in using MIS. The workspace is small. The doctor is looking at a monitor, not a patient while *indirectly* manipulating surgical instruments. This may cause the surgeon to be less dexterous and have less eye–hand coordination. Research is currently being done to help solve these problems. MIS procedures continue to be developed and improved.

### Nanotechnology

**Nanotechnology** is an emerging field of medicine. Nanotechnology works with objects "on the scale of atoms and molecules. . . . A nanometer is one-billionth of a meter." That is, 1/75,000 of a human hair. Nanotechnology holds promise in regenerative medicine. Injected into mice with spinal cord injuries, "the nanofibers . . . are the key to not only preventing the formation of harmful scar tissue that inhibits spinal cord healing, but to stimulating the body into regenerating lost or damaged cells." The mice walked![28] Nanotechnology has the potential of helping people with Parkinson's disease, Alzheimer's disease, diabetes, and spinal cord injuries. It has also regenerated heart cells after a heart attack. The National Research Council warns that along with new possibilities may come new safety hazards.[29]

The world's lightest carbon material ("multiwalled carbon nanotube [MCNT] aerogel") has been created. This spongy substance, one of the lightest solids or aerogels, nicknamed "frozen smoke," could be used to improve robotic surgery. Carbon nanotubes are tiny; thousands can fit on one hair. They can detect the smallest change in pressure. "Strips of . . . [the] aerogel could be used in robotic fingers and hands to make them super sensitive."[30]

In the future, nanotechnology may help in cancer surgeries. In a National Cancer Institute study funded in 2010, "researchers will be merging nanotechnology and cancer surgery." Nanoparticles that can bind to cancer cells are injected into the body. Special scanning equipment can be used to identify every cell involved in the cancer, which can then be removed.[31] Research is also being done on the use of nanomaterials in orthopedic surgery in enhancing "the cell response selectively for biological tissue integration or increas[ing] the strength and wear resistance of current orthopedic materials."[32] Researchers in Germany have found that certain types of lasers "are capable of reaching pulse energies that will allow modifications of living cells, e.g. making accurately controlled incisions in cell structures." In other words, a laser could be used as a scalpel to operate on one cell.[33] In 2011, researchers at the University of Michigan found ways of using nanofibers to help cells grow tissue in order to heal wounds more quickly.[34]

## CONCLUSION

Computer-assisted surgery holds great promise. The use of augmented images to teach surgeons and plan and guide operations can reduce unnecessary cutting and make operations more precise

# IN THE NEWS

According to "Hospitals with Robots Do More Prostate Cancer Surgery," by Tara Parker-Pope, published on March 11, 2011, in *The New York Times*, the surgical treatment of men's prostate cancer has increased by an average of 29 operations a year per hospital. The prevalence of prostate surgeries may be occurring due to enhanced robotic surgical techniques and the vested interests of the hospitals.

According to a study published in *Medical Care* and done by New York University researchers, which looked at robots bought at 554 hospitals and treatments for more than 30,000 men with prostate cancer, men at hospitals with the robots are more likely to have surgery for treatment than before the robots were acquired. According to the author of the study, Dr. Danil V. Makarov, assistant professor of urology at New York University's Langone Medical Center, "If you have the technology, it will get used." Although robotic surgery costs more, there is no evidence that patients do better.

Hospitals market robotic surgery. According to Dr. David Penson, a study co-author and director of the Center for Surgical Quality and Outcomes Research at Vanderbilt University, "If you're a hospital and you get a robot, clearly you want to use it." "There are some real pressures here that have nothing to do with science," he said. "We have this interplay of patients' fascination with technology coupled with business interests on the part of the hospital and device makers, pushing people to try a new technology perhaps before it's been fully tested."

Another recent study found that patients are opting for intensity-modulated radiotherapy (IMRT) and that they are sometimes referred to IMRT by doctors with a financial interest in IMRT.

and less invasive. This chapter highlights many of the benefits of minimally invasive procedures and the use of robots. However, it should be remembered that aside from a few established procedures such as cementless hip replacement and gall bladder removal, this field is in its early stages. It is also important to keep in mind the dangers and disadvantages. Looking at a monitor is never quite as good as looking at a live patient; feeling via sensory feedback mechanisms is not the same as actually having one's hands on living tissue. MIS is more difficult to learn and requires more training than traditional surgery. Further, doctors trained in traditional open surgery methods will be understandably reluctant to learn the new methods.

The most experimental area of computer-assisted surgery is telepresence or distance surgery. High-bandwidth channels are required for transmitting endoscopy, and networks must be 100 percent reliable because any delay or failure could result in the death of a patient. At the present time, the Canadian federal government is working with doctors to promote the use of distance surgery to treat rural populations. In addition, NASA has conducted experiments in telemedicine in their undersea missions (NEEMO).

Another experimental technology is nanotechnology, which holds promise of the most precise, minimal surgery possible for the regeneration of cells, tissues, and organs, leading the body to heal itself. It may ultimately relieve the symptoms of diabetes, spinal cord injuries, Parkinson's disease, heart disease, and cancer, among many other conditions.

## Chapter Summary

This chapter introduces the student to some of the uses of information technology in surgery.

- Computer-assisted surgery involves the use of computer technology in the planning and/or performance of operations.
- Computer-generated images make planning operations more precise and allow surgeons to practice on realistic models.
- In the operating room, robotic devices that can "see," "hear," and respond are used as surgical assistants.
  - Robotic devices are used in minimally invasive surgery, much of which involves the use of an endoscope, a viewing device that can project an image of the surgical site onto a monitor. The image is used to guide the surgeon.
  - ROBODOC, AESOP, ZEUS, da Vinci, and MINERVA are robots used in minimally invasive endoscopic procedures.
  - In MIS, three-dimensional, computer-generated images may be fused with the image of the surgical site or actually projected onto the patient to enhance or augment reality.
  - The surgeon's manipulations guide the robotic arms, which operate on the patient. Voice commands control the arm that holds the endoscope.
- Telepresence surgery, in which the surgeon is at one site and the patient is at another site, is being performed. The Socrates system allows a surgeon to mentor another surgeon at a distant location in real time.
  - NEEMO 7 and 9 attempted to demonstrate distance surgery from Canada to the Aquarius off the Florida Keys. NEEMO 12 attempted telesurgery on simulated patients.
- In the Operating Room of the Future, all information systems will be integrated and available to surgeons.
- Lasers are being used to perform several kinds of surgery.
- Nanotechnology, using regenerative medicine, may lead to the body healing itself.

# Key Terms

Aquarius
ARTEMIS
artificial intelligence
augmented reality
automated endoscopic system for optimal positioning (AESOP)
computer-assisted surgery
CoreValve
da Vinci
distance (or telepresence) surgery
endoluminal surgery

endoscope
GERD
HERMES
image-guided surgery
KISMET
laser
LASIK
MINERVA
minimally invasive surgery (MIS)
nanotechnology
NEEMO
NeuroArm Robot

radio frequency identification (RFID) tags
Raven
ROBODOC
robots
telepresence surgery (distance surgery)
Socrates
SpineAssist
virtual environment
virtual reality (VR)
ZEUS

# Review Exercises

## Multiple Choice

1. In the _____ procedure, a laser is used to create a flap in the cornea.
   a. endoscopic
   b. arthroscopic
   c. LASIK
   d. None of the above

2. _____ may be used to help train surgeons and to allow realistic practice operations.
   a. Virtual environment technology
   b. Endoscopes
   c. Robots
   d. ZEUS

3. _____ is a robotic device used in some hip replacement operations.
   a. ROBODOC
   b. AESOP
   c. ZEUS
   d. HERMES

4. An endoscope is _____ .
   a. a surgical instrument that cuts into the patient
   b. only used to produce the image the surgeon sees
   c. a thin tube with a light source
   d. B and C

5. Surgery that makes use of computer-generated images to enhance what the surgeon sees is called _____ .
   a. virtual reality
   b. augmented reality
   c. telepresence surgery
   d. None of the above

6. Among the benefits of MIS could be _____ .
   a. smaller scars
   b. shorter recovery time
   c. less trauma to healthy tissue
   d. All of the above

7. The most frequently done laparoscopic procedure is _____ .
   a. gall bladder removal
   b. open heart surgery
   c. brain surgery
   d. knee replacement

8. The first FDA-cleared surgical robot was _____ .
   a. ZEUS
   b. HERMES
   c. AESOP
   d. HARRY

9. Computer technology may be involved in
   _____ .
   a. planning operations
   b. assisting in the operating room
   c. training surgeons
   d. All of the above

10. A robot developed to assist in stereotactic
    neurosurgery is _____ .
    a. ZEUS
    b. HERMES
    c. AESOP
    d. MINERVA

## True/False

1. The high-bandwidth communications lines
   needed for distance surgery are in place.
   _____

2. Computer-generated graphics can give a surgeon virtual X-ray vision. _____

3. One of the advantages of MIS is that the surgeon
   looks at a monitor not at the patient. _____

4. A robotic device can "decide" whether what
   it is touching is a tumor or normal tissue.
   _____

5. Telepresence surgery was first conceived of
   by the U.S. Department of Defense. _____

6. A disadvantage of MIS is longer hospital
   stays. _____

7. Virtual reality technology creates environments that seem real but are not. _____

8. Surgeons make use of computer models to
   plan operations. _____

9. Some surgical robots were originally developed for the space program. _____

10. Hip replacement operations using ROBODOC
    cannot possibly be as good as those with
    human surgeons only. _____

## Critical Thinking

1. Many challenging issues arise from the
   innovative uses of computer-assisted surgery
   and the use of robots in the operating room.
   • Discuss how these developments might
     affect the patient and the surgeon.
   • What do you consider the responsibilities
     of the hardware manufacturer?
   • What do you consider the responsibilities
     of the software publisher?

2. Discuss the advantages and disadvantages of
   robotic surgery to the patient and the surgeon.

3. Given that computers are playing a more
   active role in surgery, what steps would you
   recommend be taken to protect patients from
   the effects of computer viruses, electrical
   malfunctions, and software bugs?

4. "Imagine you're having a hip replacement. . . .
   As you're wheeled into the operating room,
   you notice the nurses and anesthetist prepar-
   ing for your surgery. But wait, someone's
   missing. Your surgeon. You look around the
   room and finally spot the surgeon, off in the
   corner keying information into a computer
   terminal. And there, next to the doctor and
   computer is a five hundred pound, seven
   foot-high, jointed steel arm, with a tiny drill
   attached to one end. It's Robodoc. And it's
   going to assist in your surgery."[35] How do
   you feel about being operated on by a robot
   as opposed to a human being?

# Notes

1. T. Martinez-Serna and C. J. Filipi, "Endoluminal Surgery," *World Journal of Surgery* 23, no. 4 (1999): 368–77, http://www.ncbi.nlm.nih.gov/sites/entrez?db=pubmed&uid=10030860&cmd=showdetailview (accessed April 30, 2011); P. R. Schauer, Bruce D. Schirmer, and Stacy A. Brethauer, *Minimally Invasive Bariatric Surgery* (New York: Springer, 2007), http://books.google.com/books-?id=jzMofJBxLw8C&pg=PA395&lpg=PA395&dq=endoluminal+surgery+and+the+fda&source=bl&ots=3AYvPw StOm&sig=AeWzrpAd8pjru8huLOw-kpRJxhg&hl=en&ei=Ne67Tb61DMWltweoxKy0BQ&sa=X&oi=book_result&ct=result&resnum=1&ved=0CBYQ6AEwAA#v=onepage&q=endoluminal%20surgery%20and%20the%20fda&f=false (accessed April 30, 2011).

2. Mark E. Rentschler, Jason Dumpert, Stephen E. Platt, Shane M. Farritor, and Dmitry Oleynikov, "Natural Orifice Surgery with an Endoluminal Mobile Robot" (presented at

the 2006 SAGES Meeting), http://www.springerlink.com/content/kv85t13066v61072/ (accessed April 30, 2011).

3. Seth Augenstein, "New Heart Valves without Surgery," *The Star-Ledger*, March 25, 2011, 12.

6. Jim Dodson, "Examining Surgical Robots. More Harm Than Good? Florida Medical Negligence Lawyer," June 1, 2010, http://www.jwdodsonlaw.com/blog/examining-surgical-robots-more-harm-than-good-florida-medical-negligence-lawyer.cfm (accessed April 30, 2011).

5. Michelle Meadows, "Computer-Assisted Surgery: An Update," July–August 2005, http://findarticles.com/p/articles/ mi_m1370/is_4_39/ai_n27869166/ (accessed April 30, 2011); Carol Marie Cropper, "The Robot Is in—and Ready to Operate," *Business Week*, March 14, 2005; David Samadi, "Prostate Cancer Treatment—da Vinci Robotic Surgery," http://roboticoncology.com/Da-Vinci-Robotic-Prostatectomy.php (accessed April 30, 2011).

6. Steven Wasick, "Robot Surgery, Thy Name Is DaVinci," March 16, 2010, http://singularityhub.com/2010/03/16/robot-surgery-thy-name-is-davinci/ (accessed March 4, 2011); "Robots in the Operating Room," April 20, 2011, http://www.alegent.com/body.cfm?id=5465&action=detail&parent=2002&ref=9 (accessed April 30, 2011).

7. Joseph L. Flatley, "First All-Robot Surgery Performed at McGill University," October 21, 2010, http://www.engadget.com/2010/10/21/first-all-robot-surgery-performed-at-mcgill-university/ (accessed March 4. 2011).

8. "Heart Surgery without the Surgeon: Researchers Test Evalve for Noninvasive Mitral Valve Repair," August 23, 2006, http://www.columbiasurgery.org/pat/cardiac/news_evalve.html (accessed April 30, 2011).

9. Conrad Clymer, "Surgical Robotics: neuroArm Robot Performs Brain Surgery—A World First," August 22, 2010, http://medtechiq.ning.com/video/2140535:Video:2514 (accessed February 20, 2011).

10. "Mazor Robotics' SpineAssist Successfully Completes 2,000th Surgery," April 7, 2011, http://www.healthcaretechnologyonline.com/article.mvc/Mazor-Robotics-SpineAssist-Successfully-0001 (accessed April 22, 2011).

11. Leslie Versweyveld, "Lower Cost, Portable Surgical Robots Could Be Smooth Operators," March 2, 2006, http://news.uns.purdue.edu/html4ever/2006/ 060302.Peine.robots.html (accessed April 30, 2011).

12. Jeffrey Jones, "Virtual Human Puts Doctors Inside Patients," May 23, 2007, http://www.reuters.com/article/2007/05/24/us-virtual-human-idUSN2325171220070524 (accessed April 30, 2011).

13. Erica Klarreich, "Is There a Doctor on the Planet?" September 20, 2001. http://www.nature.com/news/1998/010920/full/news010920-9.html (accessed April 30, 2011).

14. Bill Todd, "NASA Space Simulation and Training Project: NEEMO 12," May 7–18, 2007, http://www.spaceref.com/news/viewsr.html?pid=24106 (accessed April 30, 2011).

15. Duncan Graham Rowe, "Scrubbing Up for Robotic Surgery in Space," October 11, 2004, http://www.newscientist.com/article/dn6512-scrubbing-up-for-robotic-surgery-in-space.html (accessed April 30, 2011); Michael Schirber, "NEEMO's Undersea Operations: Making Telemedicine a Long Distance Reality," October 19, 2004, http://www.space.com/451-neemo-undersea-operations-making-telemedicine-long-distance-reality.html (accessed April 30, 2011).

16. Tariq Malik, "NASA's NEEMO 9: Remote Surgery and Mock Moonwalks on the Sea Floor," April 19, 2006, http://www.space.com/2311-nasa-neemo-9-remote-surgery-mock-moonwalks-sea-floor.html (accessed April 30, 2011).

17. NASA, "NEEMO 12 Mission Journal," May 9, 2007, http://www.nasa.gov/mission_pages/NEEMO/ NEEMO12/mission_journal_3.html (accessed April 30, 2011); "NASA Undersea Mission Planned for May," *Science Daily*, February 27, 2007.

18. "NASA Announces Next Undersea Exploration Mission Dates and Crew," May 4, 2010, http://www.nasa.gov/home/hqnews/2010/may/HQ_10-104_NEEMO_Mission.html (accessed March 3, 2011); "NEEMO 14 Mission," July 14, 2010, http://www.nasa.gov/mission_pages/NEEMO/NEEMO14/index.html (accessed March 3, 2011).

19. Azhar Rafiq, James A. Moore, Xiaoming Zhao, Charles R. Doarn, and Ronald C. Merrell, "Digital Video Capture and Synchronous Consultation in Open Surgery," *Annals of Surgery* 239, no. 4 (2004): 567–73, http://www.ncbi.nlm.nih.gov/pmc/articles/PMC1356263/ (accessed April 20, 2011).

20. Stefanie Olsen, "Tomorrow's Operating Room to Harness Net, RFID," October 19, 2005, http://news.cnet.com/Tomorrows-operating-room-to-harness-Net,-RFID/2100-1008_3-5900990.html (accessed April 30, 2011); "Operating Room of the Future," 2011, http://www.cimit.org/programs-operatingroom.html (accessed April 22, 2011).

21. "Memorial Sloan-Kettering Cancer Center Using LiveData's OR-Dashboard: 'Wall of Knowledge' Deployed to 21 New Operating Rooms," June 19, 2006, http://www.livedata.com/ (accessed April 30, 2011); "Integrated Operating Room Systems Look to Become OR of the Future," 2006, http://www.medcompare.com/ (accessed April 30, 2011).

22. Olsen, "Tomorrow's Operating Room to Harness Net, RFID."

23. "Tagged Surgical Sponges Help Prevent Deadly Problem," July 18, 2006, http://www.medicalnewstoday.com/articles/47583.php (accessed April 30, 2011).

24. "Laser Surgery for Throat Cancer," *The Times of India*, February 5, 2011, http://articles.timesofindia.indiatimes.com/2011-02-05/mangalore/28362634_1_laser-surgery-voice-box-throat-cancer (Accessed February 11, 2011).

25. "Laser Surgery," 2011, http://www.ehow.com/facts_5957700_endoscopic-surgery-twin_to_twin-transfusion-syndrome.html (Accessed February 15, 2011); Molly Edmonds, "What Is Laser Clot Busting?" 2011, http://health.howstuffworks.com/medicine/modern-technology/

laser-clot-busting.htm (accessed February 15, 2011); Carol Wiley, "Endoscopic Laser Spine Surgery Recovery," January 27, 2010, http://www.ehow.com/facts_5920 636_endoscopic-laser-spine-surgery-recovery.html (accessed February 19, 2011).

26. Liz Segre, "The LASIK Procedure: A Complete Guide," April 2010, http://www.allaboutvision.com/visionsurgery/lasik.htm (accessed February 21, 2011); "LASIK," February 4, 2011, http://www.fda.gov/MedicalDevices/ProductsandMedicalProcedures/SurgeryandLifeSupport/LASIK/default.htm (accessed February 11, 2011).

27. Sarah Ketterman, "Endoscopic Laser Surgery for Twin-to-Twin Transfusion Syndrome," February 6, 2010, http://www.ehow.com/facts_5957700_endoscopic-surgery-twin_to_twin-transfusion-syndrome.html (accessed February 15, 2011).

28. "Nanotechnology Offers Hope for Treating Spinal Cord Injuries, Diabetes, and Parkinson's Disease," *Science Daily*, April 23, 2007, http://www.physorg.com/news96542517.html (accessed April 30, 2011).

29. Barnaby Feder, "Study Says U.S. Has Lead in Nanotechnology," September 26, 2006, http://www.nytimes.com/2006/09/26/technology/26nano.html (accessed April 30, 2011).

30. "Nanotechnology: New 'Frozen Smoke' May Improve Robotic Surgery, Energy Storage," March 1, 2011, http://www.sciencedaily.com/releases/2011/03/110301111457.htm (accessed March 3, 2011).

31. "Future Surgery: Removing Cancer with Aid of Nanotechnology," February 6, 2010, http://www.newhealthidea.com/2010/11/future-surgery-removing-cancer-with-aid-of-nanotechnology/ (accessed March 3, 2011).

32. Samir Mehta and Javad Parvizi, "Nanotechnology in Orthopaedic Surgery," 2009, http://www.touchmusculoskeletal.com/articles/nanotechnology-orthopaedic-surgery?mini=calendar%2F2012-01 (accessed March 3, 2011).

33. "Quantum-Dot Lasers May Lead to Practical Nanosurgery," April 16, 2010, http://medgadget.com/2010/04/quantumdot_lasers_may_lead_to_practical_nanosurgery.html (accessed March 4, 2011).

34. "Nanotech for Tissue Regeneration," April 18, 2011, http://www.kurzweilai.net/nanotech-for-wound-and-tissue-regeneration (accessed April 22, 2011).

35. "Robotic Surgery: Robots in the Operating Room," *FDA Consumer*, July/August, 1993, reprinted in 2002, http://www.fda.gov/bbs/topics/CONSUMER/CON00242.html (accessed April 30, 2011).

## Additional Resources

"Artemis Medical Receives 510K Clearance on New Image Guided Biopsy Device." April 22, 2002. http://goliath.ecnext.com/coms2/summary_0199-1664257_ITM (accessed April 30, 2011).

Augenstein, Seth. "New Heart Valves without Surgery." *The Star-Ledger*, March 25, 2011, 12.

Clymer, Conrad. "Surgical Robotics: neuroArm Robot Performs Brain Surgery—A World First." August 22, 2010. http://medtechiq.ning.com/video/2140535:Video:2514 (accessed February 20, 2011).

Christensen, Bill. "NEEMO 7: NASA's Undersea Robotic Telemedicine Experiment." October 15, 2004. http://www.livescience.com/32-neemo-7-nasa-undersea-robotic-telemedicine-experiment.html (accessed April 30, 2011).

Dodson, Jim. "Examining Surgical Robots. More Harm Than Good? Florida Medical Negligence Lawyer." June 1, 2010. http://www.jwdodsonlaw.com/blog/examining-surgical-robots-more-harm-than-good-florida-medical-negligence-lawyer.cfm (accessed April 30, 2011).

Edmonds, Molly. "What Is Laser Clot Busting?" 2011. http://health.howstuffworks.com/medicine/modern-technology/laser-clot-busting.htm (accessed February 15, 2011).

Eisenberg, Anne. "What's Next: A Sharper Picture of What Ails the Body." January 24, 2002. http://www.nytimes.com/2002/01/24/technology/what-s-next-a-sharper-picture-of-what-ails-the-body.html (accessed April 30, 2011).

Eisenberg, Anne. "What's Next; Restoring the Human Touch to Remote-Controlled Surgery." May 30, 2002. http://www.nytimes.com/2002/05/30/technology/what-s-next-restoring-the-human-touch-to-remote-controlled-surgery.html (accessed April 30, 2011).

"FDA Clearance of da Vinci Surgical System for Intracardiac Surgery Now Encompasses 'ASD' Closure." 2005. http://www.highbeam.com/doc/1G1-97073329.html (accessed April 30, 2011).

Feder, Barnaby. "Study Says U.S. Has Lead in Nanotechnology." September 26, 2006. http://www.nytimes.com/2006/09/26/technology/26nano.html (accessed April 30, 2011).

Flatley, Joseph L. "First All-Robot Surgery Performed at McGill University." October 21, 2010. http://www.engadget.com/2010/10/21/first-all-robot-surgery-performed- at-mcgill-university/ (accessed March 4. 2011).

Fogoros, Richard. "Robotic Heart Surgery: A Status Report." 2006. http://heartdisease.about.com/library/weekly/aa060401a.htm (accessed April 30, 2011).

"Future Surgery: Removing Cancer with Aid of Nanotechnology." February 6, 2010. http://www.newhealthidea.com/2010/11/future-surgery-removing-cancer-with-aid-of-nanotechnology/ (March 3, 2011).

Humphries, Kelly, and Delores Beasley. "NASA Prepares for Space Exploration in Undersea Lab." March 28, 2006. http://www.nasa.gov/home/ (accessed April 30, 2011).

Jones, Jeffrey. "Virtual Human Puts Doctors Inside Patients." May 23, 2007. http://www.reuters.com/article/2007/05/24/us-virtual-human-idUSN2325171220070524 http://pune360.com/News/2007/05/27/virtual-human-puts-doctors-inside-patients/ (accessed April 30, 2011).

Ketterman, Sarah. "Endoscopic Laser Surgery for Twin-to-Twin Transfusion Syndrome." February 6, 2010. http://www.ehow.com/facts_5957700_endoscopic-surgery-twin_to_twin-transfusion-syndrome.html (accessed February 15, 2011).

"Laser Surgery." 2011. http://www.ehow.com/facts_5957700_endoscopic-surgery-twin_to_twin-transfusion-syndrome.html (accessed February 15, 2011).

"Laser Surgery for Throat Cancer." *The Times of India.* February 5, 2011. http://articles.timesofindia.indiatimes.com/2011-02-05/mangalore/28362634_1_laser-surgery-voice-box-throat-cancer (Accessed February 11, 2011).

"LASIK." February 4, 2011. http://www.fda.gov/MedicalDevices/ProductsandMedicalProcedures/SurgeryandLifeSupport/LASIK/default.htm (accessed February 11, 2011).

Mack, Michael J. "Minimally Invasive and Robotic Surgery." *Journal of the American Medical Association* 285, no. 5 (2001): 568–72.

Matthews, Melissa, Kelly Humphries, Nicole Gignac, and Fred Gorell. "Undersea Habitat Becomes Experimental Hospital for NEEMO 7." August 11, 2004. http://www.nasa.gov/home/hqnews/2004/aug/HQ_04264_neemo.html (accessed April 30, 2011).

"Mazor Robotics' SpineAssist Successfully Completes 2,000th Surgery." April 7, 2011. http://www.healthcaretechnologyonline.com/article.mvc/Mazor-Robotics-SpineAssist-Successfully-0001 (accessed April 22, 2011).

Mehta, Samir, and Javad Parvizi. "Nanotechnology in Orthopaedic Surgery." 2009. http://www.touchmusculoskeletal.com/articles/nanotechnology-orthopaedic-surgery?mini=calendar%2F2012-01 (accessed March 3, 2011).

"Nanotech for Tissue Regeneration." April 18, 2011. http://www.kurzweilai.net/nanotech-for-wound-and-tissue-regeneration (accessed April 22, 2011).

"Nanotechnology: New 'Frozen Smoke' May Improve Robotic Surgery, Energy Storage." March 1, 2011. http://www.sciencedaily.com/releases/2011/03/110301111457.htm (accessed March 3, 2011)

"NASA, NEEMO History." March 21, 2006. http://www.nasa.gov/mission_pages/NEEMO/history.html (accessed April 30, 2011).

"NASA Announces Next Undersea Exploration Mission Dates and Crew." May 4, 2010. http://www.nasa.gov/home/hqnews/2010/may/HQ_10-104_NEEMO_Mission.html (accessed March 3, 2011).

"NEEMO 14 Mission." July 14, 2010. http://www.nasa.gov/mission_pages/NEEMO/NEEMO14/index.html (accessed March 3, 2011).

Olsen, Stefanie. "Tomorrow's Operating Room to Harness Net, RFID." October 19, 2005. http://news.cnet.com/Tomorrows-operating-room-to-harness-Net,-RFID/2100-1008_3-5900990.html (accessed April 30, 2011).

"Operating Room of the Future." 2011. http://www.cimit.org/programs-operatingroom.html (accessed April 22, 2011).

"Quantum-Dot Lasers May Lead to Practical Nanosurgery." April 16, 2010. http://medgadget.com/2010/04/quantumdot_lasers_may_lead_to_practical_nanosurgery.html (accessed March 4, 2011).

Rafiq, Azhar, James A. Moore, Xiaoming Zhao, Charles R. Doarn, and Ronald C. Merrell. "Digital Video Capture and Synchronous Consultation in Open Surgery." *Annals of Surgery* 239, no. 4 (2004): 567–73. http://www.ncbi.nlm.nih.gov/pmc/articles/PMC1356263/ (accessed April 20, 2011).

"Revolutionizing Trauma Surgery." August 23, 2006. http://www.smithnephew.com/ca_en/Standard.asp?NodeId=3399 (accessed April 30, 2011).

"Robot Reduces Spinal Injury Risk." March 12, 2000. http://news.bbc.co.uk/2/hi/health/672815.stm (accessed April 30, 2011).

"Robotic Surgeon to Team Up with Doctors, Astronauts on NASA Mission." November 16, 2008. http://www.danshope.com/news/post/32/Robotic-Surgeon-To-Team-Up-With-Doctors-Astronauts-On-NASA-Mission (accessed April 30, 2011).

"Robots Make the Cut in Hospitals." July 6, 2009. http://www.convergemag.com/workforce/Robots-Make-The-Cut-in-Hospitals.html (accessed April 30, 2011).

Rowe, Duncan Graham. "Scrubbing Up for Robotic Surgery in Space." October 11, 2004. http://www.newscientist.com/article/dn6512-scrubbing-up-for-robotic-surgery-in-space.html (accessed April 30, 2011).

Schauer, P. R., Bruce D. Schirmer, and Stacy A. Brethauer. *Minimally Invasive Bariatric Surgery.* New York: Springer, 2007. http://books.google.com/books?id=jzMofJBxLw8C&pg=PA395&lpg=PA395&dq=endoluminal+surgery+and+the+fda&source=bl&ots=3AYvPwStOm&sig=AeWzrpAd8pjru8huLOw-kpRJxhg&hl=en&ei=Ne67Tb61DMWltweoxKy0BQ&sa=X&oi=book_result&ct=result&resnum=1&ved=0CBYQ6AEwAA#v=onepage&q=endoluminal%20surgery%20and%20the%20fda&f=false (accessed April 30, 2011) .

Segre, Liz. "The LASIK Procedure: A Complete Guide." April 2010. http://www.allaboutvision.com/visionsurgery/lasik.htm (accessed February 21, 2011).

Vaze, Ajit. "Robotic Laparoscopic Surgery: A Comparison of the da Vinci and Zeus Systems." [Abstract] 2001. http://www.ncbi.nlm.nih.gov/pubmed/11744453 (accessed April 30, 2011).

Versweyveld, Leslie. "Lower Cost, Portable Surgical Robots Could Be Smooth Operators." March 2, 2006. http://news.uns.purdue.edu/html4ever/2006/060302.Peine.robots.html (accessed April 30, 2011).

Wasick, Steven. "Robot Surgery, Thy Name Is Da Vinci." March 16, 2010. http://singularityhub.com/2010/03/16/robot-surgery-thy-name-is-davinci/ (accessed March 4, 2011).

Wiley, Carol. "Endoscopic Laser Spine Surgery Recovery." January 27, 2010. http://www.ehow.com/facts_5920636_endoscopic-laser-spine-surgery-recovery.html (accessed February 19, 2011).

## Related Web Site

University of Southern California, Cardiothoracic Surgery. http://www.cts.usc.edu/videos.html

PEARSON
**myhealthprofessionskit**™

Go to www.myhealthprofessionskit.com to access the Companion Web site created for this textbook. Simply select "Basic Health Science" from the choice of disciplines. Find this book and register to access self-assessment quizzes, flashcards, and more.

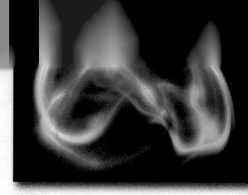

CHAPTER 8

# Information Technology in Pharmacy

## CHAPTER OUTLINE

## LEARNING OBJECTIVES

Upon completion of this chapter, the reader will be able to:

- Describe the Food and Drug Administration (FDA).
- Discuss uncertified medicines as a safety issue.
- Describe the contributions of information technology to the development and testing of drugs.
- Define biotechnology and rational drug design.
- Discuss the significance of the Human Genome Project (HGP) and its contribution to the understanding of genetic diseases.
- List the uses of computers in clinical drug trials.
- Discuss the relationship of the understanding of the molecular basis of a disease to real breakthroughs in treatment.
- List the uses of computer technology in pharmacies including:
  - The use of computers in the neighborhood drug store, from the printing of drug information for customers to the full automation of the process of filling prescriptions using robots and barcodes.
  - The use of computers in hospital pharmacies:
    - in centralized dispensing systems using robots and barcodes;
    - in decentralized point-of-use dispensing units;
    - in computerized IVs.
- Discuss telepharmacy—the linking of pharmacists via telecommunications lines to dispensing units in remote locations such as doctors' offices.
- Discuss the use of nanotechnology in drug design.
- Discuss the impact of information technology on pharmacy, as it affects pharmacists, patients, and hospital administrators.

## OVERVIEW

Information technology is transforming all aspects of pharmacy, from the design, testing, and approval of drugs, to the automation of drug stores in the community, to the automation of hospital pharmacies and drug delivery systems. Telepharmacy, or the linking of the prescribing doctor's office with the dispensing pharmacy via telecommunications lines, is expanding. Nanotechnology is in its early stages but could lead to effective treatments for cancer and bacterial infections among other conditions.

## THE FOOD AND DRUG ADMINISTRATION

In the United States, the **Food and Drug Administration (FDA)** is charged with overseeing the safety and efficacy of new medications:

The FDA is responsible for protecting the public health by assuring the safety, efficacy, and security of human and veterinary drugs, biological products, medical devices, our nation's food supply, cosmetics, and products that emit radiation. The FDA is also responsible for advancing the public health by helping to speed innovations that make medicines and foods more effective, safer, and more affordable; and helping the public get the accurate, science-based information they need to use medicines and foods to improve their health.[1]

Just as contributors to *The Journal of the American Medical Association (JAMA)* are required to disclose their financial ties,[2] likewise, we believe that everyone should be aware of the sources of funding of the FDA. Although much of its budget comes from Congress, since the 1992 passage of **PDUFA (Prescription**

**Drug User Fee Act renewed in 1997, 2002, and 2007**, referred to as PDUFA II, III, and IV), which requires drug companies to pay fees to support the drug review process and "companies [to] pay annual fees for each manufacturing establishment and for each prescription drug product marketed," user fees have steadily risen, until in 1992, 51 percent of the FDA's drug review budget came from the companies that the FDA regulates. Between 1996 and 2006, Congressional appropriations to the FDA stayed the same, whereas from 1998 to 2005, user fees doubled. In 2004, the $232 million in fees made up 53 percent of the FDA's new drug review budget. In 2006, $380 million came from drug user fees.[3]

> PDUFA authorized FDA to collect fees from companies that produce certain human drug and biological products. Any time a company wants the FDA to approve a new drug or biologic prior to marketing, it must submit an application along with a fee to support the review process. In addition, companies pay annual fees for each manufacturing establishment and for each prescription drug product marketed. Previously, taxpayers alone paid for product reviews through budgets provided by Congress. In the new program, industry provides the funding in exchange for FDA agreement to meet drug-review performance goals, which emphasize timeliness.

In addition to the business funding of FDA, since 1992, Congressional oversight has been sharply curtailed.[4]

PDUFA IV was due to expire in 2007 but was reauthorized by Congress and signed by President Bush on September 27, 2007. User fees to the FDA rose to $392.8 million, an increase of $87.4 million, by 2008.[5] However, Sean Hennessy and Brian Strom point out in their *The New England Journal of Medicine* article "PDUFA Reauthorization— Drug Safety's Golden Moment of Opportunity?" that, "A potentially thorny issue is that the large infusion of cash represented by user fees . . . might result in a conflict of interest for the FDA by creating competing allegiances to pharmaceutical manufacturers and the American People."[6]

PDUFA IV is now set to expire in 2012. In 2010, the FDA began the process of holding hearings to reauthorize PDUFA. PDUFA V will be presented to Congress in 2012. Among the areas that the FDA is interested in discussing are "ensur[ing] quality of patient-reported outcomes and other endpoint assessment tools" and "expanding the capacity for scientific advice to address complex manufacturing issues."[7] They appear to be ready to allow more consumer input in their decisions.[8] The FDA is in conflict with pharmaceutical companies over the FDA's proposal to lengthen review times because of the 2007 Congressional drug safety requirements.[9]

A consumer representative (the National Consumers League [NCL]) stated that the FDA should be funded out of the general treasury. However, it conceded that this would not be possible under current budget conditions. Congress has allowed "the regulated industries to dictate how the FDA allocates it resources. NCL believes there is too much at stake to allow this funding model." NCL advocates that the user fees be added to the FDA's budget, with no conditions.[10] However, the only financial issue that the FDA discussed was an inflation adjuster.[11]

The FDA wants more protection for human subjects in clinical trials. To this end, it wants to improve oversight. Industry wants "approaches that build in rigorous clinical trial oversight." The FDA and industry representatives are still discussing proposals.[12]

The FDA has many advisory panels. Some of their members have financial ties to the drug industry, and the FDA usually follows a panel's recommendations. A study by Public Citizen (a consumer advocacy group), reported in an article by Peter Lurie and colleagues, in *JAMA*, found that this "did not dramatically sway . . . outcomes." However, both Public Interest and some members of Congress are attempting to eliminate conflicts of interest. Representative Maurice Hinchey (Democrat, New York) stated that "allowing individuals with conflicts of interest to serve on advisory panels endangers the . . . American people . . . [because] pure objectivity is lost." Public Citizen could only study the members who reported conflicts of interest. According to Peter Lurie, ". . . these people . . . are honorable . . . , they would not allow themselves to be influenced. It's the unconscious we need to be afraid of."[13] The Center for Science in the Public Interest points to some FDA actions (or failures to act) including: (1) allowing five companies to market a laser treatment for smoking cessation, which has not been approved by the FDA, and (2) allowing drinks containing nicotine back on the market.[14]

Some of the dangerous side effects of a drug appear only years after the drug has been approved and is on the market. The FDA can now require new trials to assess the safety of approved drugs. The Institute of Medicine (IOM) recommended that for the trials to be ethical, they should only be conducted under the following conditions: if there is a question of public health; if there is not enough existing information and the information cannot be collected in any other way; if the trials are designed to study the efficacy and safety of the drug; and if the trials minimize the risk to participants.[15]

Even drugs that have been subject to clinical trials may pose hazards. Financial interest may get in the way of objectivity. Further, even though financial interest must be disclosed in individual drug trials, currently meta-analyses (studies of studies) of drug trials do not disclose conflicts of interest. These meta-analyses are published in research journals and may influence what doctors prescribe.[16]

## UNCERTIFIED MEDICINES

In June 2006, the FDA released information on drugs that are being sold without FDA review. According to Steven Galson, director of the FDA's Center for Drug Evaluation and Research, "We consider it a significant and serious drug safety issue . . . since these products may pose a risk to consumers." These products include both prescription and over-the-counter drugs. Although these drugs make up less than 2 percent of the market, they include "several thousand prescription medicines including cough remedies, painkillers and sedatives." Most doctors and pharmacists are not aware of this.[17]

Other problems exist besides uncertified medicines. According to the World Health Organization, there is a worldwide epidemic of fake drugs. Fake malaria medicines, tuberculosis and acquired immunodeficiency syndrome (AIDS) drugs, and meningitis vaccines are among the most common counterfeits. This epidemic has caused up to 200,000 deaths per year. It could also cause the development of drug-resistant strains of these diseases and others. These new strains could be spread and cause an epidemic or pandemic. Some have gone so far as to call selling fake drugs murder. At the present time, China is thought to be the biggest source for these drugs. People also buy fake drugs over the Internet. There is no effective regulation.[18]

Some actions have been taken to protect the U.S. public from uncertified medications. In October 2008, President Bush signed the Ryan Haight Online Pharmacy Consumer Protection Act. It prohibits the dispensing of controlled substances over the Internet unless the prescriber and patient have met at least once in person. In 2010, a Joint Strategic Plan was released by the U.S. Intellectual Property Enforcement Coordinator. It includes "several provisions aimed at curbing the online sale of counterfeit or substandard prescription medications."[19] In December of 2010, the Alliance for Safe Online Pharmacies estimated that 36 million Americans buy drugs online from any of 30,000 to 40,000 online pharmacies.[20] The Alliance was formed in 2010 and includes the American Pharmacists Association, Eli Lilly, and the National Chain Drug Store Association. Participant observers to the organization include the National Association of Boards of Pharmacy, National Health Council, and Partnership for Safe Medicines.[21] The group has been accused of being a front for Big Pharma by PharmacyChecker.com and of working to undermine access to safe and inexpensive medications by confusing the "problems of rogue online pharmacies and counterfeit drugs with buying safe and affordable medication from non-US pharmacies, such as many of those verified by PharmacyChecker.com."[22] PharmacyChecker.com was founded in 2003 by a physician to check online pharmacies all over the world and the medications they sell and to help consumers find inexpensive, safe medications.[23] One study did find "that prescription drugs ordered from online pharmacies verified by PharmacyChecker.com or the National Association of Boards of Pharmacy (NABP) result[ed] in the delivery of safe, genuine medication . . . . In contrast, the report found that some sites that are not verified by either of these two groups may sell fake medications."[24]

# BIOTECHNOLOGY AND THE HUMAN GENOME PROJECT

## Rational Drug Design

The technical details of drug design are beyond the scope of this text. However, computers are being used to help design and test new drugs. Genetic tests can be used to determine an individual's response to a specific medication. At St. Jude Hospital in Memphis, children with leukemia are being genetically tested so that medication can be tailored to each patient. This procedure is not covered by medical insurers, and pharmaceutical companies are not interested in manufacturing tailor-made medications.[25] In 2006, computer-aided drug design was being used to help combat human immunodeficiency virus (HIV)/AIDS, tuberculosis, malaria, and hepatitis C.[26] **Biotechnology** sees the human body as a collection of molecules and seeks to understand and treat disease in terms of these molecules. It attempts to identify the molecule causing a problem and then create another to correct it. Specific drugs are aimed at inhibiting the work of specific disease-causing agents. In order to be effective, the drug needs to bind to its target molecule. It needs to fit, something like a key in a lock. To achieve an exact fit, the precise structure of the target must be mapped. Powerful computers allow scientists to create graphical models. Before the availability of computer technology, many drugs were discovered by accident or trial and error. One way of developing drugs with the help of computers is called **rational drug design**. Developing drugs by design requires mapping the structure and creating a three-dimensional graphical model of the target molecule. Because this involves a huge number of mathematical calculations, without computers the process took many years; after the calculations

were completed, a wire model of the molecule had to be constructed. Now, supercomputers accurately do the calculations in a small fraction of the time, and graphical software produces the image on a computer screen. This is an example of the field of **scientific visualization**, which is defined by Donna Cox of the National Center for Supercomputing Applications as the process of graphically representing the results of numerical calculations. The model can be manipulated, rotated, and viewed from any angle. Specialized software is used to evaluate a drug's molecular structure, which can then be chemically synthesized. Of course, any compound developed this way still has to be tested in a *real* biological system. The modeling of the target molecule and development of the drug can be repeated several times until a chemical compound is found that satisfactorily inhibits or stimulates the activity of the target site's receptors. Drugs, which are used for Alzheimer's disease, hypertension, and AIDS, have been developed with the help of computers.

## Bioinformatics

The application of information technology to biology is called **bioinformatics**. Although this may be an oversimplification, the field of bioinformatics seeks to organize biological data into databases. The information is then available to researchers who can search through existing data and add new entries of their own. The **Human Genome Project (HGP)** (Figure 8.1▶) has contributed to making databases of biological information.

## The Human Genome Project

The development of new medications is becoming more dependent on knowledge of genes. The HGP, sponsored in the United States by the National Institutes of Health and the Department of Energy, began in 1990 and involved hundreds of scientists all over the world. It was "an . . . effort to understand the hereditary instructions that make each of us unique. The goal is to find the location of the 100,000 or so human genes and to read the entire genetic script, all three billion bits of information, by the year 2005" (Figure 8.2). One of the findings

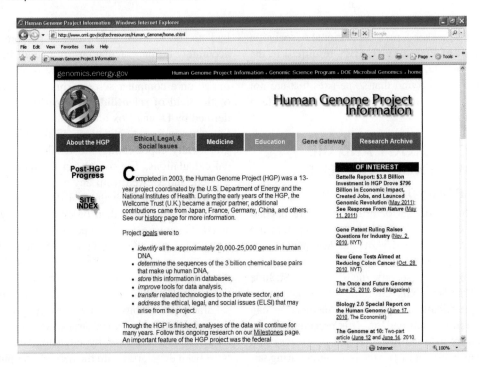

▶ **Figure 8.1** The Human Genome Project home page.
*Source:* Courtesy of Genomics.energy.gov.

of the HGP is that human beings have 21,000 protein-coding genes compared to 20,000 for the earthworm.[27] The project has succeeded in mapping the human genome. One of its goals is an attempt to understand the molecular bases of genetic diseases. This project would be inconceivable without computers and the Internet. Computers are used to keep track of the genes as they are identified; this prevents duplication of effort and ensures that no genes are overlooked. The Internet allows findings to be immediately communicated to scientists working on the project anywhere in the world. Three to four thousand diseases are caused by errors in genes. Altered genes also contribute to the development of other disorders such as cancer, heart disease, and diabetes. The HGP expects to be able to identify such genes, which might make prevention, early detection, and treatment possible.

The purpose of the **1000 Genomes Project** "is to provide a comprehensive public resource that supports researchers aiming to study . . . genetic variation that might cause human disease. [It seeks to] integrat[e] data on all types of variation that might cause human disease." Its samples come (with informed consent) from many different populations. There is no restriction on the free use of the data collected. In 2010, the 1000 Genomes Project published a map of genetic differences that may help to explain susceptibility to disease.[28] Once the gene is identified, drugs can be designed. Treatment may include gene therapy to replace the defective gene or the development of drugs. Ultimately, gene therapy may be tailored to specific patients. In 2006, the gene (Runx1) identified with chronic pain was found. It transmits external stimuli to the spinal cord. The finding could lead to the design of more effective pain therapies.[29] The identification of a disease-related gene is simply a starting point for research. For example, one of the genes related to stroke was identified in 2003, but according to Dr. Jonathan Rosand, a stroke specialist at Massachusetts General Hospital, it "is unlikely to yield new treatments any time soon."[30] And more than 20 years after the beginning of the HGP, this has proven true. Relatively few effective treatments have been associated with the findings of the HGP. The genetic link is only one small part of fully understanding and treating disease. For example, family history is a better predictor than genetics for heart disease.[31]

In July 2006, scientists made a major breakthrough in understanding the genetic makeup of the *Wolbachia* bacteria that infect mosquitoes and other insects that spread malaria.[32] In August 2006, researchers at the University of Pennsylvania "determined the structure of an important smallpox virus enzyme and how it binds to DNA" (Figure 8.2▶). This is very important in the creation of a drug to fight smallpox.[33] In August 2006, the genes that increase the risk of heart attack were identified.[34] Hypertension-susceptibility genes were identified in February 2006.[35] It should be noted that although genetic predisposition is important, other factors (such as lifestyle and environment and the extent of public health measures) play a major role in the development of disease.

More than 25 million Americans suffer from rare and genetic diseases. The Genetic and Rare Diseases Information Center, using information gathered by the HGP, provides health care consumers with reliable, immediate, and free information. The center receives thousands of requests for information.[36]

The HGP is the basis for new databases of biological information. Computers are being used to quickly screen tens of thousands of compounds a day, databases of genes, to find codes that could be useful in drug development. Then a model can be constructed and a drug rationally designed. It is a new form of trial and error, accelerated by computers, producing enormous amounts of information for researchers and computers to analyze.

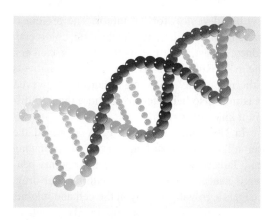

▶ **Figure 8.2**   An abstract of a DNA spiral.
*Source:* Allies Interactive Services Pvt Ltd/Shutterstock.com

## Developments in Biotechnology

Understanding the molecular basis of a disease can lead to medical advances. In September 1998, the U.S. FDA approved Herceptin as effective against certain types of metastatic breast cancer. Herceptin can work for patients who have too much of a specific gene in their tumor cells. The gene (HER-2/neu) produces a protein that engenders growth in the tumor cells. Herceptin binds to this protein and inhibits its work. According to Dr. Dennis Slamon who directed the research, the development of Herceptin "proves . . . that if we understand what is broken in the malignant cell, we may be able to fix it."[37] Herceptin may also be effective in fighting other cancers including gastric, endometrial, pancreatic, prostate, and colorectal cancers. Many other drugs are in the testing stages.

Lucentis was approved in June 2006 for the treatment of wet macular degeneration. Lucentis is an antibody that binds to a protein that is involved in the formation of blood vessels. In an early study, it was found that, on average, patients given Lucentis either maintained or gained vision, whereas the patients who did not take Lucentis, but received traditional treatments, experienced an average loss of vision.

In February 2004, the FDA approved Avastin, an antibody that inhibits the protein that plays a role in the maintenance and metastases of tumors. The protein, called vascular endothelial growth factor (VEGF), helps in the creation of new blood vessels for the tumor. The protein is active in cancers including metastatic, colorectal, kidney, breast, and nonsmall cell lung cancers. The most extensive trials have been with patients with metastatic colorectal cancer. However, Avastin is also being tested on more than 20 different kinds of tumors.

In November 2004, the FDA approved the use of Tarceva against lung cancer; the following year, Tarceva was approved for use against pancreatic cancer in combination with another drug. It targets a growth pathway in the cell and inhibits its activity, thus slowing or stopping the growth of the tumor in some patients.

In 2003, the FDA approved the use of Xolair as a treatment for asthma. Xolair binds to immunoglobulin E (IgE) antibodies in the blood, which may trigger asthmatic symptoms. This decreases the release of chemicals that lead to the symptoms.

In 2005, several new drugs were approved including:

| Arranon | To treat patients with certain cancers |
|---|---|
| Boostrix | Booster against tetanus, diphtheria, and pertussis |
| Byetta | To treat type II diabetes |
| Fluarix | A flu vaccine for adults |
| Fortical nasal spray | For osteoporosis |

*Source:* Approved Biotechnology Drugs (http://www.bio.org/speeches/pubs/er/approveddrugs.asp).

The following drugs have been approved as of 2006:

| Amitiza | For the treatment of chronic idiopathic constipation |
|---|---|
| Dacogen | For the treatment of myelodysplastic syndromes, formerly known as preleukemia |
| Eraxis | For the treatment of *Candida* fungal infections |
| Gardasil | For the prevention of cervical cancer caused by the human papillomavirus |

*Source:* Approved Biotechnology Drugs (http://www.bio.org/speeches/pubs/er/approveddrugs.asp).

In 2009, biotechnology drugs were the fastest growing part of drug development. Biotechnology companies predicted that by 2015, biotech drugs would comprise over one-half of drug approvals, and by 2025, 71 percent. The number of new biotech drugs approved is too great to list, but some approved in 2009 and 2010 are as follows[38]:

| Adcirca | For pulmonary arterial hypertension to improve exercise ability |
|---|---|
| Afinitor | For treatment of patients with advanced renal cell cancer |
| Agriflu | For immunization of adults against some flu |
| Azerra | For treatment of refractory chronic lymphocytic leukemia |
| Caldolor | For treatment of pain and fever |
| Extavior | For treatment of relapsing multiple sclerosis (MS) |
| Fanapt | For treatment of schizophrenia in adults |
| Lamictal ODT | For treatment of bipolar adults |
| Ampyra | For treatment of MS |

For a complete list, see Jennifer Van Brunt, "Biotech Drug Approvals: A Year of Firsts," February 9, 2010, http://www.recap.com/signalsmag.nsf/0/3DE9EAD5D34E5B8D88257 6C400810419.

**Antisense technology** is one experimental technology used to develop drugs to shut off disease-causing genes. Genasense, developed through antisense technology, promises to enhance chemotherapy in cancer patients by shutting off the gene producing Bcl-2, which helps cells stay alive. It is given before chemotherapy, radiation, and other cancer treatments to kill cells. Antisense technology is being used to develop treatments for breast cancer and Crohn's disease.[39]

Another new technology aimed at drug development is called **RNA interference (RNAi)**. RNAi is a natural process for gene silencing. RNA stands for **ribonucleic acid**. It is made in the nucleus of a cell but is not restricted to the nucleus. It is a long coiled-up molecule whose purpose is to take the blueprint from **deoxyribonucleic acid (DNA)** and build our actual proteins.

(DNA is a nucleic acid molecule containing genetic instructions for living things.) RNAi is a process that cells use to turn off genes. The attempt at developing drugs based on RNAi holds the promise of revolutionizing biotechnology.[40] In 2006, RNAi was used to shut off the effects of estrogen in "a specific part of the mouse brain," changing the behavior of the mouse. In another experiment attempting to cure hepatitis B, most of the mice died of liver poisoning. This could introduce a note of caution into the testing of RNAi on humans. This means that although RNAi may be used to help map out genes and neural networks, extreme care should be taken.[41] RNAi is currently (2011) being studied as a way of treating cancer and viruses in humans.[42]

In 2006, scientists at the University of Illinois "created a synthetic molecule which caused cancer cells to self-destruct." It may lead to new treatments for some cancer patients. However, it has not yet been tested for safety and effectiveness.[43] In 2010, research was done on using synthetic molecules to help treat prostate cancer.[44]

**Stem cells** are cells that can develop into different types of body cells; theoretically, they can repair the body. As a stem cell divides, the new cells can stay a stem cell or become another kind of cell.[45] It is possible that stem cell research may lead to regenerative or rehabilitative medicine. Stem cells are special in a number of ways:

> First, they are unspecialized cells that renew themselves for long periods through cell division. The second is that under certain physiologic or experimental conditions, they can be induced to become cells with special functions such as the beating cells of the heart muscle or the insulin-producing cells of the pancreas.[46]

Many scientists feel that stem cell research may hold the possibility of future cures, preventions, and therapies.[47] In November 2006, scientists succeeded in growing heart valves "using stem cells from the fluid that cushions babies in the womb." These valves might one day be used for babies born with heart defects.[48] In the past, scientists have either had to use embryonic stem cells or generate embryonic-like stem cells—a difficult process. But, in 2011, scientists at the Scripps Research Institute succeeded in "convert[ing] adult skin cells directly into beating heart cells." This technology might make possible new treatments for heart disease, Parkinson's disease, and Alzheimer's disease.[49]

## COMPUTER-ASSISTED DRUG TRIALS

Before a drug can be marketed, it has to undergo extensive clinical trials. Some last as long as 6 years and cost over $100 million. Now, however, software has been developed that allows companies to simulate clinical trials on a computer before the actual trials begin. A simulated drug trial uses information about the drug's effects from earlier trials, animal studies, or trials of similar drugs. By trying out many "what ifs" on computer models, the actual trials can be more precisely designed, making it more likely that they will be definitive. Critics maintain that the models are not precise enough because knowledge of the human body is incomplete. The **Physiome Project** is an international project seeking to create mathematical models of human organs—"digital models of every system and anatomical feature of the human body." It has created a virtual heart using mathematical equations to simulate the processes of the heart. It has been used in studies of irregular heartbeats. A draft of the lungs and skeletal system has been finished. The project is currently working on the digestive system and a database of cellular functions. In the future, the project hopes to model the nervous, endocrine, immune, sensory, skin, kidney–urinary, and reproductive systems. Utilizing these mathematical models, the project hopes to find treatments for conditions such as arthritis and other autoimmune disorders. These mathematical models will not only allow the testing of drugs, but "also enable medical engineers to fashion customized implants" and surgeons to perform "dry runs" of surgeries. The use of these models is still far from reality. Computer-assisted drug trials are not a replacement for actual clinical trials; they are a tool to make the trials more effective.[50] It is generally agreed that drugs submitted for clinical trials include computer simulations.[51]

The purpose of **computer-assisted trial design (CATD)** is to decrease the time and money spent on the trial phase of drug development.

## COMPUTER-ASSISTED DRUG REVIEW

After a new drug has been developed, the FDA reviews it. In 1995, the FDA began computerizing the drug review and approval process. This enables them to speed up the process by reviewing data online. According to the *FDA Consumer*, what used to take weeks can now be done in an instant. With FDA computers networked to a drug company's computer, data from clinical trials can be transferred instantly and reviewed more quickly than in the past. It is also easier to do comparisons with other drugs and spot possible problems. According to Roger Williams, associate director of the FDA's Center for Drug Evaluation, the drug review process makes use of giant electronic spreadsheets of perhaps 300 million cells for each review area for each drug. Computers make it possible to organize this massive amount of data.

## THE COMPUTERIZED PHARMACY

Computers were introduced in pharmacies more than 25 years ago. Initially, drug orders in hospitals could be entered into a computer. The computer system checked for adverse drug interactions and specific patient drug allergies. Today, computers can maintain complete medication profiles of all patients on databases and warn of drug interactions and allergies. This use of the database not only protects patients, but also makes information more easily available for national and international drug studies.

### Computers and Drug Errors

Computerizing any aspect of prescription entry, the filling of orders, and dispensing of medications appears to lead to a decrease in medication errors. Today, some medication errors in hospitals are caused by transcription errors and illegible handwriting. A **computerized physician order entry system (CPOE)** can lower prescription

errors.[52] Currently, computers are used in both hospital pharmacies and community drug stores. In any corner drug store, computers provide drug information for patients. According to *Quality Review: A Publication of the USP Practitioners Reporting Network*, by 1995, almost all pharmacies in the United States used computers to process prescriptions. Although the use of computers makes filling prescriptions faster and easier and streamlines record keeping, computers have also been the source of some errors. The errors can be caused by incorrect data entry, an incorrect choice from a computer list, or software error. Incorrect entry of a prescription or an incorrect choice from a list of medications is a human error that can happen whether or not computers are used. However, some errors stem directly from software. In one case, the programmer had used the same abbreviation (DOX100) to designate two different drugs. The incorrect medication lengthened one patient's hospital stay. Another program automatically printed "teaspoonful" when a liquid medication dose did not have a measure entered. This led to an infant being given an overdose of albuterol syrup. Other errors have occurred when software interpreted 1–2 (one to two) as 1/2.

However, errors in software can be corrected. Generally, all drug errors decline when computers are introduced. One study was done comparing drug errors before and after the introduction of a computerized physician order entry system in a large hospital. The study looked at errors in drug ordering, administration, and dispensing. Simply introducing a computerized order system cut errors at all three stages. Total errors fell by 55 percent. Errors in ordering fell by 19 percent, in transcription 84 percent, in dispensing 68 percent, and in administering 59 percent. When a menu-driven system was used, dosing errors decreased by 23 percent, and allergy errors decreased by 56 percent. Another study compared adverse drug events (ADEs) in a 726-bed hospital before and after the introduction of computerized drug ordering. It found 126 errors in the first phase of the study—which had not been caught—and caught 134 errors in the second phase of the study. From the first to the second phase of the study, transcription errors fell to five (84 percent).[53] The reduction in errors is partly due to making orders legible. Second, the computer checks dosage to make sure it is appropriate. It also checks for each patient's drug allergies and any possible drug interaction.

In a study published in the *American Journal of Health-System Pharmacy* in 2006, 7,000 medical errors caused by CPOE were analyzed. Dosing errors were most common. The study traced most errors to "faulty computer interface, miscommunication with other systems, and lack of adequate decision support."[54]

Computer warning systems can be used to prevent ADEs. Serious ADEs occur in about 7 percent of patients admitted to hospitals. Many of these are caused by a physician prescribing either the wrong drug or the wrong dosage, because of lack of knowledge of either the patient or the drug. In 1994, a computerized warning system was designed and put into place in one hospital. The hospital already had in place a database with patient information; the existing system warned of a patient's specific drug allergy and of adverse drug interactions. The new alert system added warnings of other likely ADEs. The warnings were printed out for the pharmacist, who could alert the prescribing physician if he or she believed it was necessary. Physicians reported that the computer-generated alerts made them aware of the potential danger in 44 percent of alerts. "The order changes in these patients were directly attributable to alert notification."[55]

According to the 1999 government report, "To Err Is Human," between 44,000 and 98,000 people die in U.S. hospitals each year as a result of medical errors. Seven thousand people die from medication errors both in and out of the hospital. Among the changes the report recommends to reduce medication errors is to "require that all hospitals and health care organizations *implement proven safety practices, such as the use of automated drug ordering systems*" (emphasis added).[56] Five years after the report, two of its authors noted that although there are "small improvements at the margins—fewer patients dying from accidental injection of potassium chloride, reduced infections in hospitals due to tightened infection control procedures—it is harder to see the overall,

national impact." They did note that at least there is a conversation about safety and efforts to change the way things are done in hospitals; this should lead to a safer healthcare environment.[57] In 2003, one doctor estimated that 16 percent of physicians scribble illegible prescriptions.[58] The Florida legislature even passed a bill in the spring of 2003 ordering doctors to improve their handwriting.[59] Several reports stressed that the use of computers to write prescriptions and check for errors in dosage is crucial in reducing ADEs. Handheld computers provide immediate access to drug databases and other information. They also make prescriptions legible.

In July 2006, "Preventing Medical Errors" stressed that medication errors are still a serious problem, harming 1.5 million people per year. Several thousand die each year. With the aging population, more medications are prescribed and more errors are made. Like the 1999 report, "To Err Is Human," the 2006 report recommends the use of e-prescribing and electronic health records (EHRs).[60] One report (October 2006) pointed to the 700,000 Americans who show up in emergency rooms with overdoses or allergic reactions to common prescription drugs including insulin, warfarin, and amoxicillin.[61] Whatever the cause of the error, many doctors would not inform the patient. With an error that the patient was unlikely to notice, 50 percent would tell the patient. Surgeons disclosed errors less frequently.[62]

In 2011, *Health Affairs* published a study using new methods of ranking hospital errors. The study found that almost one out of every three people admitted to a hospital is the subject of a medical mistake—10 times more than expected. In the past medical errors were measured by voluntary reporting and the Agency for Healthcare Research's indicator. The current study identified errors through medical claims data. "Among 795 patient records reviewed, voluntary reporting detected four problems, the Agency for Healthcare Research's quality indicator found thirty-five, and Healthcare Improvement's tool detected 354 events—10 times more than the AHR's method." Medical mistakes include everything from medication errors, to bed sores, to staph infections, and to objects left in the body during surgery. In response to this, the Obama Administration announced a "billion-dollar patient safety program . . . [called the Partnership for Patients Program] . . . aimed at reducing preventable . . . errors." The program aims at reducing errors by 40 percent and "preventable" readmissions by 20 percent. According to the Department of Health and Human Services, this could save as much as $35 billion. Some of the money will come from the Patient Protection and Affordable Care Act and will fund demonstration projects for 3 years.[63]

The adoption of EHRs and e-prescribing are important steps to decreasing medication errors and reconciliation errors. One study showed that CPOE could prevent 64.4 percent of prescribing errors. A 2008 retrospective review of 10 studies found that CPOE and **clinical decision support (CDS)** decreased ADEs in half of the studies. Under the American Recovery and Reinvestment Act of 2009 and the Medicare Improvements for Patients and Providers Act of 2008, incentives have been established for adopting certified EHRs and e-prescribing (see Chapter 2). The e-prescribing program provides monetary incentives from 2009 to 2013 (2 percent in 2009 and 2010, 1 percent in 2011 and 2012, and 0.5 percent in 2012) and penalties from 2012 and 2014 (1 percent in 2012, 1.5 percent in 2013, and 2 percent in 2014). This looks like an error, but the incentives and penalties seem to overlap. There are conflicts between these two incentive programs. The Centers for Medicare and Medicaid Services (CMS) is attempting to integrate the two programs.[64] In 2009, $148 million in incentive payments were paid by CMS. Unlike the EHR program, the e-prescribing program lacks certification.[65]

Health information technology (HIT) is important in preventing **medication reconciliation** errors. Medication reconciliation concerns identifying the most accurate list of a patient's medications. These errors typically occur when a patient changes status—that is, is admitted to, moved within, or released from a hospital. Between September 2004 and July 2005 in the United States, there were "2,022 reports of medication reconciliation errors. . . .

[T]wo-thirds . . . resulted from transfer within the facility, another 22% occurred at patient admission, and 12% . . . at discharge . . . . The Institute for Healthcare Improvement estimated that as much as 50% of medication errors and 20% of ADEs in hospitals result from mismanaged medication reconciliation. . . . EHRs . . . could make . . . reconciliation errors nearly nonexistent." CPOE integrated with EHR would make patient history available at all times and in all places. The records would also be legible.[66]

E-prescribing not only can prevent medication errors, but also has been found to be more efficient—using 26.6 percent less staff time (saving $0.97) for new prescriptions and 10.2 percent less time for refills (saving $0.37). However, some of the savings is offset by $0.22 or higher transaction fees for each claim.[67]

Pharmacists have been adopting HIT more quickly than physicians. The National Association of Chain Drug Stores estimates that, at the end of 2008, approximately 76 percent of community pharmacies and six of the largest mail order pharmacies could receive prescriptions electronically. In 2008, 46 percent of independent pharmacies were connected to a network for prescription routing; this is up from 27 percent in 2007.[68]

Although HIT can prevent many medication errors, it is crucial that its introduction be done carefully—that planning and training be adequate and clinicians be involved. Computer systems have to be maintained and upgraded carefully and in a timely fashion. Otherwise, errors can be caused by HIT. "The USP MEDMARX database for 2006 indicated that approximately 2% of the 176,409 medication errors . . . for the year involved . . . computer technology as part of the cause of the error." Barcodes were wrongly labeled and screens unclear. Some systems generate too many alerts, which eventually clinicians ignored.[69]

## The Automated Community Pharmacy

Although not yet in common use, fully automated pharmacy systems that can fill prescriptions do exist for community drug stores (Figure 8.3, A–E▶). Currently, the use of these systems is expanding with the successful use of robotic systems in Veterans Administration (VA) pharmacies and hospitals. A fully automated dispensing system involves the employment of a robot. In one such system, a prescription is entered into the pharmacy computer; the pharmacy computer, in turn, activates the pharmacy robot, which first determines what size vial is needed for the prescription—from the three available sizes. A robotic arm grips the correct size. One system has 200 cells, each containing a different drug. The arm is moved to the correct cell; the tablets or capsules are counted by a sensor and dropped into the vial. The computer prints a label and puts it on the vial, which is delivered via a conveyer belt to the pharmacist. The pharmacist uses a barcode reader to scan the barcode on the label; images of the medication and prescription information appear on the screen. The pharmacist puts the lid on and gives the customer the prescription. One robotic system can fill 60 prescriptions in an hour. Other robotic systems can fill prescriptions for liquid medications as well as tablets and capsules.

## Automating the Hospital Pharmacy

Hospitals are automating drug distribution systems. An automated hospital pharmacy presupposes the use of barcodes to identify drugs; it involves the use of robots in the hospital pharmacy to fill medication orders and/or the use of point-of-use dispensing units. A fully automated system may cost as much as $10 million and take several years to install.[70] Drugs are also being administered to patients by computerized infusion pumps. Automated dispensing systems can be centralized or decentralized. In a centralized system, robots are used in the hospital pharmacy to fill prescriptions. In a decentralized point-of-use dispensing system, drug cabinets, similar to ATM machines, are located throughout the hospital. Some hospitals use both robotics and automated point-of-use dispensing.

THE HOSPITAL PHARMACY—ROBOTS AND BAR-CODES In a hospital pharmacy system using a pharmacy robot, medication orders are either faxed to the pharmacy and the information entered into the computer system or entered at a terminal connected with the pharmacy computer. In 2006, only 15 percent of hospitals used a robotic system, up from 4.5 percent in 1999.[71] The information includes the name of the patient, his or her medication, and the dose. **Barcodes** identify each dose of medication, and each dose is kept in a bag. (Any medication that is not identified by a barcode has to be dispensed by hand.) Each patient has a bin into which the robot drops his or her medication. If a barcode is unclear, the robot rejects the dose. The dosages are checked by technicians. In 8 hours, one robot can do as much work as six or seven human technicians. The robot, its software, and 5 years of maintenance are extremely expensive. Hospital administrators maintain that a robot still costs less than hiring six or seven human technicians for 8 hours. Hospital managers, like managers in other businesses, see automation as a way to reduce costs, that is, staff, while maintaining service.

Each patient's medications are delivered to the nursing unit on a tray. As an added check on the accuracy of the computer, the barcodes on the patient's wristband and on the medication can be scanned. Dispensing errors are eliminated by using robots in the pharmacy. However, dispensing errors account for only 6 percent of medication errors. More than half occur at the prescribing stage and another third at the distribution stage.

The use of barcodes to identify medications and link them to patients also means that the robot is not only dispensing medication, but also keeping track of inventory. Additionally, it can automatically provide credit for medications, which are not used, and electronically order drugs when the supply is low. The use of barcodes became mandatory in 2004.[72]

A comprehensive new fully automated system is being introduced in 2011 in the medical centers of the University of California San Francisco (UCSF). Giant robots prepare all drug doses, including those for chemotherapy. According to UCSF, "Not a single error has occurred in the 350,000 doses of medication prepared during the system's recent phase in." The robots assemble

**(A)**

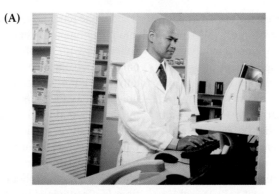

**(B)**

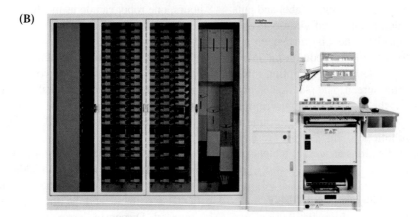

**(C)**

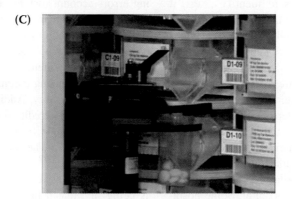

**(D)**

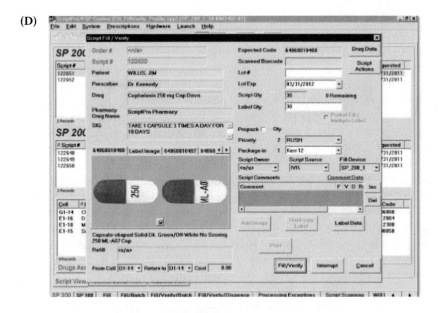

**(E)**

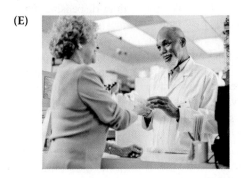

▶ **Figure 8.3**  ScriptPro SP 200 Robotic Prescription Dispensing System. The ScriptPro fully automated prescription dispensing process begins by (A) entering the prescription into the existing pharmacy computer system. © Corbis RF/Alamy (B) Via the interface, the pharmacy computer sends the fill command to the SP 200. (C) The SP 200 robotic arm then selects a standard vial. The vial is automatically transported to the correct drug cell, the cell barcode is scanned, and the robotic arm engages the cell. The medication is dispensed and counted directly into the vial. The standard prescription information (barcode and USP auxiliary labels) are printed and applied to the filled vial. The filled and labeled vial is then delivered on the conveyor to the pharmacist. The pharmacist scans the vial barcode and (D) verifies the prescription with an on-screen image of the medication and script information. (E) The pharmacist then delivers the prescription to the patient and completes the prescription process. © Corbis Super RF/Alamy
*Source:* Courtesy of ScriptPro.

and package all of each patient's medication for a 12-hour period. Intravenous (IV) syringes are filled. The system has both refrigerated and nonrefrigerated warehouses.[73]

POINT-OF-USE DRUG DISPENSING Some computerized hospital pharmacies are using point-of-use dispensing of drugs—a decentralized automated system. Adoption of this technology in healthcare started slowly, with only about 50 percent of hospitals using automated dispensing cabinets (ADCs) in 1999; but by 2005, close to 72 percent of acute care facilities had implemented these units, and by 2009, 80 percent of hospitals used ADCs.[74] A small computer attached to a large cabinet sits at the nursing unit. It is networked to the hospital pharmacy computer. A nurse types a password, and the unit displays a list of patients. The nurse selects the patient and enters the drug order, and the computer delivers it by opening the drawer containing the medication. The nurse enters the name of the drug and closes the drawer. The computer keeps track of all drug transactions, for billing and inventory purposes. It "counts, dispenses and tracks medications within the hospital." It can generate a variety of reports on patients, drug usage, and nurses. In 2003, the first automated drug-dispensing units located in patients' rooms were introduced. Doctors can use them to enter prescriptions. The bedside system will scan the nurse's badge, the patient's wristband, and the medication's barcode. It is linked to databases of information that will help avoid medication errors. It can also keep track of inventory.

Point-of-use dispensing has several advantages over traditional manual dispensing. It shortens the time between the order for a medication and its delivery to the patient. One study found that the waiting time for a first dose of medication went from 45 minutes to 1 minute! Automating drug distribution improves patient care in other ways too. Drugs are more likely to be administered on schedule, and significantly fewer doses are missed. Although apparently not reducing dispensing errors to zero like centralized robotic systems claim to do, one study found that a decentralized system decreased dispensing errors by

almost one-third. However, many studies disagree on the efficacy of point-of-use dispensing in reducing medical errors.[75]

Decentralized computerized drug delivery has a positive financial impact for the hospital, making it more likely that patients are charged for the medications used. It also decreases the time nurses spend on medication-related activities, such as counting controlled substances, charting, documentation, and billing; a survey of nurses in a surgery unit that had introduced decentralized dispensing found that 80 percent wanted to keep the new system. It also decreased the time that pharmacists spend on problem resolution. Automation (although requiring an initial investment) can save a hospital as much as $1 million over 5 years in personnel time savings.

Point-of-use dispensing is also being introduced in clinics and doctors' offices. An automated drug-dispensing unit (something like a vending machine) contains approximately 90 percent of routinely prescribed drugs. A prescription can be entered by a doctor (with a password) and the medication automatically dispensed. However, there are states in which a doctor is not allowed to give a patient prescription drugs without a pharmacist present.

COMPUTERIZED IVS AND BARCODES Included in the drug errors reported in "To Err Is Human" were intravenous (IV) administration errors. In 2005, the "smart pump" was introduced. It "contains several important new safety features including a barcode reader that enables medication verification for IV drugs at the point of care and patient-controlled analgesia (PCA)."[76] Two new safety technologies being introduced in 2006 are barcode medication administration (BCMA) and smart infusion systems with dose error reduction systems (DERS). BCMA uses barcodes to identify each patient and each medication, and according to clinical studies, it might prevent up to 58 percent of ADEs.[77] Integrating both systems involves barcoding infused medication. IV drugs tend to be higher risk drugs. IV drugs as well as oral drugs can be given to the wrong patient or in the wrong dose; however, the risk is far higher with IV drugs. "A nurse is unlikely to give a patient 10 or 100 pills, but all too easily can commit errors in programming a general-purpose infusion device—e.g., programming 603, instead of 6.3 mg/h—and inadvertently deliver a . . . massive overdose."[78] Using a built-in scanning device, this system links IV drug administration to an adverse drug alert monitor and sounds an alert if a mistake is made. The scanner identifies both the patient and the clinician. This system may avoid many IV medication errors.[79]

RADIO FREQUENCY IDENTIFICATION TAGS **Radio frequency identification (RFID) tags** include an antenna, a decoder to interpret data, and the tag that includes information. The antenna sends signals. When the tag detects the signal, it sends back information.[80] The tags can be used to keep track of anything, including medications. Unlike barcodes, RFIDs do not have to be scanned by hand; RFID readers can be embedded anywhere and automatically read the RFID tag. RFID tags are the size of a grain of rice and can contain more information than a barcode.[81] In 2004, the FDA approved implanting RFID tags in people; these tags would include medical information.

# TELEPHARMACY

**Telepharmacy** involves using a computer, a network connection, and a drug-dispensing unit to allow patients to obtain drugs outside of a traditional pharmacy, at, for example, a doctor's office or a clinic. It should not be confused with the unregulated sale of prescriptions and drugs over the Internet. However, once a patient has a prescription in hand, more and more patients are willing to fill it online "to save time and money," although they did express concerns about safety.[82] Traditional telepharmacy, however, links prescribing physicians with pharmacists via telecommunications lines. It may refer simply to the faxing of prescriptions from the prescribing doctor to the pharmacy for later pickup and to the use of computers to check for adverse drug interaction. However, in a fully computerized telepharmacy system, the physician's and pharmacy's computers are directly linked, and the

pharmacist remotely controls a drug cabinet at the physician's office. Once the pharmacist receives the prescription via a telecommunications link, a signal is sent to the remote drug cabinet to open a particular compartment. The dispensing cabinet (at the doctor's office) contains prepackaged drugs, each identified by a barcode. The software prints out a label and patient information and keeps track of inventory. A patient database includes the patient's age, allergies, drug use, diagnosis, and insurance provider. The software checks drug–drug interaction (DDI), drug–allergy interaction, and dosage, and it checks for duplicate prescriptions. Before the patient receives the medication, its barcode is scanned to make sure it is the right drug. The pharmacist and patient could then hold a video teleconsultation. Telepharmacy allows one pharmacist to serve a whole region.

There are several built-in safety checks. The barcode must be correct or the computer will not print a label, and, therefore, the patient will not get the drug. The computer also examines patient allergies, dangerous drug interactions, appropriate dosage, and expiration date; it immediately notifies the prescribing physician if there is a problem. The physician can, however, override the computer's warning. The cabinet in which the drugs are stored is secure and has alarms to guard against theft.

Although not yet in general use, telepharmacy promises to be especially helpful in rural areas and underserved urban neighborhoods where there is no accessible local pharmacy. Using a telepharmacy connection can mean that the patient walks out of the doctor's office with the medication in hand, having already teleconsulted with the pharmacist; neither patient nor pharmacist has to travel. It could prove to be particularly beneficial to populations who cannot travel easily. The elderly, for example, have a poor drug compliance record—due in part to their difficulty traveling. There are several other advantages to telepharmacy. A telepharmacy does not need to fill as many prescriptions as a conventional pharmacy to be cost-effective. Entering prescriptions directly into a computer may cut down on dispensing errors caused by illegible handwriting. Handwritten signatures are no longer necessary. Since the July 2000 law making the digital signature equivalent to the handwritten signature, a doctor can prescribe without faxes and paper signatures. Dispensing drugs at the doctor's office guarantees that the prescription is filled. Pharmaceutical counseling ensures that the patient understands how to take the medication.

Today, telepharmacy is slowly expanding in part because of a shortage of pharmacists. The expansion is also because of government interest in telepharmacy as a cost-saving device, largely because of the use of generic medications, but also reflecting the higher efficiency of the pharmacist. In 2002, the Department of Health and Human Services funded a telepharmacy project designed to serve 13,500 low-income and rural patients. A pharmacist at the central location receives faxes of prescriptions and then sends a signal to a remote "vending machine" where a technician labels the bottle and gives it to the patient. There are five remote locations within a 100-mile radius.[83] The VA, the U.S. Department of Defense (DOD), and the Immigration and Naturalization Service (INS) are also testing telepharmacy systems.[84] The telepharmacy technology can link to the DOD's computerized medical system and can automatically add prescriptions to a medical record. In a study begun in 2009 and not yet completed, the DOD is evaluating whether the Telepharmacy Robotic Medicine Delivery Unit (TRMDU) reduces costs and improves care.[85]

In 2010, the U.S. Navy began installing what may be the largest telepharmacy project yet, with 110 sites. Nonpharmacy staff will be able to dispense medications "with real-time remote monitoring and checks . . . by a licensed pharmacist" at a remote location. When a licensed pharmacist is needed, the staff "presses a call button that rings at all the other telepharmacy locations around the globe." A pharmacist answers and can see and hear the dispensing process by two-way audio and video. The U.S. Army is currently testing telepharmacy.[86]

There are problems with telepharmacy that could slow its expansion. Pharmacy has traditionally been subject to state regulation. Each state has different pharmacy regulations. The National Association of Boards of Pharmacy has model telepharmacy regulations, but only some states have adopted them.

## DRUG DELIVERY ON A CHIP

Some medications can currently be delivered on an implanted chip. This is the focus of a great deal of research. The drug is embedded in a chip, which is surgically implanted in the patient. The drug may be released by diffusion. It may be embedded in a biodegradable material that releases as it degrades. One drug, used to treat brain cancer, is a biodegradable implant placed directly on the site from which the tumor was removed. The newest chip to be announced (October 2003) can deliver several medications. It can also deliver specific doses at predetermined times. The chip is in the early stages of development. Medications are embedded in polymers (plastics) that have already been approved by the FDA for other uses in humans. Thus far, the chips have been tested only on animals. Some of its potential uses include delivering an entire course of medication over a period of months, delivering a series of vaccines at the correct time, and delivering medication that needs to be taken continuously, including painkillers and medications for chronic conditions. This "pharmacy on a chip" is completely biodegradable. One advantage of using chips to deliver medication is that because they bypass the stomach, they avoid stomach upsets.[87]

In 2006, research continued on a chip that "uses wireless signaling and [a] system of reservoirs that allow precise, efficient delivery of solids, liquids, or gels." It is the size of a stamp, includes 100 wells that can be filled with drugs, and will deliver substances that are very strong but have limited stability. Wireless technology can be used to deliver information. It will deliver the correct dose at the correct time. The devices also contain biosensors to deliver information, and the biosensors can be linked to the drug delivery system. The system will not be in human safety trials for a number of years.[88] At Rensselaer Polytechnic Institute, in 2011, researchers are developing electromagnetic liquid pistons that might in the future deliver drugs on an implanted chip that could release timed doses of medication.[89]

## NANOTECHNOLOGY AND PHARMACY

Nanotechnology, although still in the experimental stage, has the potential for treating many conditions. One area in which it shows promise is in the treatment of skin cancer. Tiny particles, nanoparticles (or tiny chemical robots), are made of polymers and proteins. When introduced into the bloodstream, "these nanoparticles are able to bind to the surface of skin cells and prevent the delivery of genetic codes delivered by RNA that would otherwise give instructions to make more cancer cells through . . . RNA interference."[90]

Research is being done on the combination of light and nanotechnology in the treatment of other cancers. Photodynamic therapy is used to treat skin cancer. "Infrared light can pass partway into the body . . . . [S]hining it on . . . nanoparticles sets off a chain of reactions, which release a reactive form of oxygen, which can kill . . . cancer cells."[91]

Nanoparticles carrying nitric oxide could kill bacteria and promote healing of methicillin-resistant *Staphylococcus aureus*. In the future, these nanoparticles could be incorporated into walls and floors, even into bandages. A "self-medicating bandage . . . laced with nanoparticles . . . [could] detect harmful bacteria in a wound and treat it."[92]

"Nanoemulsions made of soybean oil, alcohol, water, and detergent emulsified into droplets less than 400 nanometers in diameter are effective at killing bacteria, fungi, and viruses." Researchers believe that nanoemulsions can be used in the treatment of second-degree burns. Nanoemulsions have the benefit of being able to penetrate the skin. More laboratory studies need to be done before the treatment can be used for people. Nanoemulsions can also be used to treat cold sores (in clinical trials), toenail fungus, and cystic fibrosis infections.[93]

## THE IMPACT OF INFORMATION TECHNOLOGY ON PHARMACY

Information technology is having a great impact on the field of pharmacy—affecting doctors, patients, pharmacists, and hospital management in different ways. The increasing use of computers

# IN THE NEWS

According to "A Decade Later, Genetic Map Yields Few New Cures," by Nicholas Wade published on June 12, 2010, in *The New York Times*, although the Human Genome Project (HGP) has led to increased knowledge, it has not led to many cures. One of the major goals of the HGP was to find the genetic bases of diseases and therefore cures.

In a study of heart disease, family history was found to be a better predictor than genetics associated with heart disease. Although many disease-causing mutations have been found, they have not proved to be a major part in predicting risk. Some scientists suspect that the association is a "statistical illusion."

In the future, genetic research may lead to prediction and cures for disease, but at this time, there is no way to know how successful it will be.

requires doctors and pharmacists to be computer literate. The impact of automation on pharmacists is overwhelming. In both the hospital pharmacy and community drug store, robots can do what a human pharmacist has always done, that is, fill prescriptions. This allows pharmacists to be more involved in consulting with patients and physicians. In at least one hospital using a pharmacy robot, pharmacists now accompany doctors on rounds. However, hospitals using robots require fewer pharmacists; managers see this staff reduction as a benefit. It saves money, while maintaining services. It is unlikely that many pharmacists share this view.

The impact on patients appears to be beneficial. The HGP holds the promise of understanding the basis of diseases with a genetic link. This,

combined with rational drug design, may lead to the development of effective treatments and cures for many diseases. Automating drug dispensing in hospitals and drug stores has apparently reduced dispensing errors considerably.

Telepharmacy also affects patients, doctors, and pharmacists in different ways. Doctors can send a patient home with medication in hand, after teleconsulting with a pharmacist; patients do not need to travel long distances to fill prescriptions or to consult with a pharmacist. Pharmacists can serve a much wider geographic area and yet do not need to fill as many prescriptions to stay in business. Pharmacists need to achieve a high degree of computer literacy and familiarity with telecommunications and networks to be involved in telepharmacy.

# Chapter Summary

This chapter introduced the reader to the impact of information technology on the field of pharmacy.

- In the United States, the FDA is the agency charged with overseeing the safety and efficacy of drugs and medical devices. Much of its budget comes from drug manufacturers.

- There are a myriad of uncertified medications (prescription and over-the-counter) on the market.

- Computer technology is making a contribution to rational drug design. Because computers can do billions of calculations and then graphically represent the results, it is possible to create graphical models of a target molecule, for which a drug can be specifically designed.

- Bioinformatics is the application of information technology to biology.

- The Human Genome Project is leading to an understanding of the molecular bases of diseases that have a genetic link. This knowledge has led to the development of drugs that are currently in the testing stages. A genetic link

is only one part of the cause of a disease; treatments and cures are not being developed as quickly as originally expected.

- Drug trials can be simulated using computers, so that actual trials take less time and cost less and are more likely to be successful.

- Information technology is changing the way pharmacies do business.

  - Computers are used in the corner drug store to provide information for customers and pharmacists. Some drug stores are fully computerized, with robots filling the prescriptions.

  - In hospitals, two computerized pharmacy systems exist (and may co-exist).

    - A centralized system uses robots in the hospital pharmacy to fill drug orders typed in on terminals. The drugs are identified by barcodes. Each patient's medications are then delivered to the unit.

    - In a decentralized point-of-use dispensing system, computers attached to cabinets sit in various places in the hospital. A nurse may enter a password and type in a medication order; the drawer with the medication opens and the nurse can remove it.

- Both centralized and decentralized systems cut down on drug-dispensing errors and on the amount of time personnel spend on medication-related activity.

- Barcodes can be used to identify medications. RFID tags can also be used.

- Telepharmacy involves the linking of a pharmacist with a remote drug cabinet in a doctor's office via telecommunications lines.

- Nanotechnology is pioneering new treatments for a variety of conditions and diseases including cancer and cystic fibrosis.

- Information technology is affecting doctors, patients, pharmacists, and administrators in different ways.

# Key Terms

1000 Genomes Project

antisense technology

barcodes

bioinformatics

biotechnology

clinical decision support (CDS)

computer-assisted trial design (CATD)

computerized physician order

entry system (CPOE)

deoxyribonucleic acid (DNA)

Food and Drug Administration (FDA)

Human Genome Project (HGP)

medication reconciliation

PDUFA (Prescription Drug User Fee Act renewed in 1997, 2002, and 2007)

Physiome Project

radio frequency identification (RFID) tags

rational drug design

ribonucleic acid

RNA interference (RNAi)

scientific visualization

stem cells

# Review Exercises

## Multiple Choice

1. The creation of medications using computers to create a model of the target molecule and design a medication to inhibit or stimulate its work is called _____ .
   a. biotechnology
   b. rational drug design
   c. visualization
   d. None of the above

2. The _____ is a project attempting to understand the genetic makeup of the human being.
   a. International Genome Project
   b. National Institute of Health Project
   c. Genetic Script
   d. Human Genome Project

3. A centralized computerized hospital pharmacy system involves the use of _____ .
   a. barcodes to identify drugs
   b. robots
   c. A and B
   d. None of the above

4. Which of the following is true of decentralized point-of-use dispensing?
   a. It decreases the waiting time for the first dose of a drug.
   b. It increases the likelihood that drugs are administered on schedule.
   c. It decreases dispensing errors.
   d. All of the above

5. The linking of a drug cabinet in a doctor's office with a pharmacist via telecommunications lines is called _____ .
   a. telemedicine
   b. telepharmacy
   c. remote pharmacy
   d. robotic pharmacy

6. Information technology has made the Human Genome Project possible by _____ .
   a. enabling scientists to keep track of genes as they are identified and allowing findings to be immediately communicated via the Internet
   b. making pharmacy robots available internationally
   c. keeping track of new drugs as they enter clinical trials
   d. keeping records of the results of clinical drug trials

7. Telepharmacy raises certain legal problems associated with _____ .
   a. the prescribing of drugs that are not FDA approved
   b. interstate licensing of pharmacists
   c. a doctor prescribing medications
   d. None of the above

8. The genetic link is only one small part of fully understanding and treating disease. For example, _____ is a better predictor than genetics for heart disease.
   a. weight
   b. waist size
   c. family history
   d. None of the above

9. The use of computers to simulate drug trials _____ .
   a. means that we do not need actual clinical trials
   b. means actual clinical trials are more likely to succeed
   c. helps save both time and money
   d. B and C

10. DNA provides a blueprint of genetic information. _____ helps create the proteins.
    a. Biotechnology
    b. RNA
    c. TNA
    d. None of the above

## True/False

1. Errors in software can lead to errors in filling prescriptions. _____

2. Understanding the genetic basis of a disease can lead to the development of an effective drug. _____

3. Hospital pharmacy robots can dispense any drug with a barcode. _____

4. Decentralized hospital dispensing units reduce dispensing errors to zero. _____

5. Telepharmacy allows one pharmacist to serve a large geographical area. _____

6. Automation of pharmacy may lead to unemployment among pharmacists. _____

7. Antisense technology attempts to treat cancer by turning off a gene that keeps cells alive. _____

8. Biotechnology sees the human body as a collection of molecules. _____

9. Computers have helped in the development of drugs used to treat AIDS. _____

10. Computer-assisted trial design means that real clinical trials are not needed. _____

## Critical Thinking

1. Discuss the advantages and disadvantages of the introduction of computers in a local pharmacy:
   (a) from the pharmacist's point-of-view.
   (b) from the customer's point-of-view.

2. As the administrator of a small hospital, discuss the advantages and disadvantages of introducing a centralized computerized hospital pharmacy system using robots.

3. Telepharmacy could prove to be a benefit to elderly patients who have difficulty traveling. However, privacy, security, and legal issues may have to be settled before telepharmacy becomes an established part of health care. Discuss this statement. Consider licensing issues and the lack of security of networked communications in your answer.

4. How would you prevent pharmaceutical companies from influencing what medications doctors dispense to their patients?

# Notes

1. John R. Polito, "Senate Tobacco Bill Would Alter FDA's Mission," February 27, 2007, http://whyquit.com/pr/022707.html (accessed May 2, 2011).

2. "Medical Journal Says It Was Misled Again," July13, 2006, http://query.nytimes.com/gst/fullpage.html?res=9F04E1DE1E30F930A25754C0A9609C8B63 (accessed May 2, 2011).

3. Diedtra Henderson, "Drug Makers Lobby US to Hike FDA Funds: Firms Say Taxpayers Should Pay Bigger Part of Bill for Safety Tests," *The Boston Globe*, July 13, 2006, http://www.boston.com (accessed May 2, 2011).

4. Stanley M. Wolfe, "The 100th Anniversary of the FDA: The Sleeping Watchdog Whose Master Is Increasingly the Regulated Industries (HRG Publication #1776)," June 27, 2006, http://www.cspinet.org/new/pdf/statement_of_sidney_wolfe_md.pdf (accessed May 2, 2011); Gary W. Lawsen, "Impact of User Fees on Changes within the Food and Drug Administration," 2005, http://gradworks.umi.com/31/84/3184791.html (accessed May 2, 2011); Larry D. Sasich, "Testimony on Prescription Drug User Fee Act (PDUFA)," September 15, 2000, http://www.citizen.org/Page.aspx?pid=3476 (accessed May 2, 2011).

5. "FDA Proposes New Measures to Strengthen Drug Safety under PDUFA Reauthorized User Fee Program," January 11, 2007, http://www.pharmpro.com/Articles/2007/01/FDA-Proposes-New-Measures-to-Strengthen-Drug-Safety-Under-PDUFA-Reauthorized-User-Fee-Program/ (accessed May 2, 2011).

6. Sean Hennessy and Brian Strom, "PDUFA Reauthorization—Drug Safety's Golden Moment of Opportunity?" *New England Journal of Medicine*, April 26, 2007, http://healthpolicyandreform.nejm.org/?p=11579 (accessed May 3, 2011).

7. "FDA-Industry PDUFA V Reauthorization Meeting," January 10, 2011, http://www.fda.gov/downloads/ForIndustry/UserFees/PrescriptionDrugUserFee/UCM238732.pdf (accessed March 19, 2011).

8. "FDA to Make Big Change to Risk Benefit Equation Under PDUFA V," March 9, 2011, http://www.gekkowire.com/?p=7305 (accessed March 19, 2011).

9. Steve Usdin, "Sidebar: Elastic PDUFA Deadlines," November 6, 2010, http://www.biocentury.com/biotech-pharma-news/politics/2010-11-08/fda-bio-phrma-dickering-over-longer-review-times-in-pdufa-v-a17 (accessed March 19, 2011).

10. Sally Greenberg, "Examining the Prescription Drug User Fee Act," April 10, 2011, http://www.nclnet.org/health/106-prescription-drugs/390-examining-the-prescription-drug-user-fee-act (accessed March 18, 2011).

11. Thomas Sullivan, "FDA Receives Input on Prescription Drug User Fee Act Reauthorization 2012," January 11, 2011, http://www.policymed.com/2011/01/fda-receives-input-on-prescription-drug-user-fee-act-reauthorization-2012.html, (accessed March 19, 2011).

12. Sullivan, "FDA Receives Input on Prescription Drug User Fee Act Reauthorization 2012."

13. Diedtra Henderson, "Study Rebuts Conflict Fears around FDA Financial Ties of Panels," *The Boston Globe*, April 26, 2006, http://www.boston.com/business/globe/articles/2006/04/26/study_rebuts_conflict_fears_around_fda/ (accessed May 2, 2011).

14. "FDA Fails to Protect Americans from Dangerous Drugs and Unsafe Food, Watchdog Groups Say: Agency Captured by Industries It Should Be Regulating, According to Rep. Waxman, Public Citizen and CSPI," June 27, 2006, http://www.thenhf.com/article.php?id=1473 (accessed May 2, 2011).

15. "Ethical Issues in Studying the Safety of Approved Drugs," July 9, 2010, http://iom.edu/Reports/2010/Ethical-Issues-in-Studying-the-Safety-of-Approved-Drugs-Letter-Report.aspx (accessed February 21, 2011).

16. "Conflicts-of-Interest in Drug Studies Sneaking Back into Medical Journals, Say Investigators," March 11, 2010, http://www.sciencedaily.com/releases/2011/03/110308172830.htm (accessed April 22, 2011).

17. "Statement of Steven K. Galson, M.D., M.P.H., Regarding Unapproved Prescription Drugs—June 8, 2006," May 20, 2001, http://www.fda.gov/Drugs/GuidanceComplianceRegulatoryInformation/EnforcementActivitiesbyFDA/SelectedEnforcementActionsonUnapprovedDrugs/ucm153703.htm (accessed May 2, 2011).

18. Donald G. McNeil, Jr., "In the World of Life-Saving Drugs, a Growing Epidemic of Deadly Fakes," February 20, 2007, http://www.nytimes.com/2007/02/20/science/20coun.html?pagewanted=all (accessed May 2, 2011).

19. "Isn't There a New Federal Law to Address Online Pharmacy Drug Safety?" June 10, 2010, http://www.safeonlinerx.com/2010/06/isnt-there-a-new-federal-law-to-address-online-pharmacy-drug-safety-.html; "Safe Online Pharmacy Coalition Lauds New Intellectual Property Plan: Plan Recognizes the Problem of Illegal Online Drug Sellers," July 7, 2010, http://www.safeonlinerx.com/2010/07/safe-online-pharmacy-coalition-lauds-new-intellectual-property-plan-plan-recognizes-the-problem-of-i.html (accessed March 22, 2011).

20. "36 Million Americans Have Bought Medications Online without a Doctor's Prescription. Research about Dangerous Practice—and the 11 Internet Commerce Companies Partnering Together to Protect Patients—Announced as part of White House Forum," December 14, 2010, http://www.safeonlinerx.com/news/ (accessed March 22, 2011); "Cybercrime and Doing Time," December 12, 2010, http://garwarner.blogspot.com/2010/12/36-million-americans-buy-drugs-online.html (accessed March 22, 2011).

21. "Alliance for Safe Online Pharmacies Formed; Launches Website," May 19, 2010, http://legitscriptblog.com/2010/05/alliance-for-safe-online-pharmacies-formed-launches-website/ (accessed March 22, 2011).

22. Gabriel Levitt, "Alliance for Safe Online Pharmacies (safeonlinerx.com)–Really an "Alliance Against Safe and Affordable Online Pharmacies?" June 28, 2010, http://pharmacycheckerblog.com/alliance-for-safe-online-pharmacies-safeonlinerx-com-%E2%80%93-really-an-%E2%80%9Calliance-against-safe-and-affordable-online-pharmacies%E2%80%9D (accessed March 22, 2011).

23. "Find the Best Drug Prices from Verified Online Pharmacies," 2011, http://www.pharmacychecker.com/ (accessed March 22, 2011).

24. "New Study Shows Safety of Ordering Prescription Drugs from Foreign Pharmacy Websites Verified by Pharmacychecker.Com," August 13, 2010, http://pharmacychecker.com/news/internet_pharmacy_study_shows_strength_of_pharmacychecker_verification_program%20_081310.asp (accessed March 22, 2011).

25. Claudia Dreifus, "Saving Lives with Tailor-Made Medication," August 29, 2006, http://www.nytimes.com/2006/08/29/health/29conv.html (accessed May 2, 2011).

26. "Computer-Aided Drug Design," 2006, http://www.medfarm.uu.se/ (accessed December 20, 2007).

27. Nicholas Wade, "A Decade Later, Genetic Map Yields Few Clues," June 12, 2010, http://www.nytimes.com/2010/06/13/health/research/13genome.html (accessed February 21, 2011).

28. "1000 Genomes Project Publishes Analysis of Completed Pilot Phase: Produces Toolfor Research into Genetic Contributors to Human Disease," October 27, 2010, http://www.genome.gov/27541917 (accessed February 21, 2011).

29. "Master Genetic Switch Found for Chronic Pain," January 27, 2006, http://www.sciencedaily.com/releases/2006/01/060126195756.htm (accessed May 2, 2011).

30. Nicholas Wade, "Scientists in Iceland Discover First Gene Tied to Stroke," September 22, 2003, http://www.nytimes.com/2003/09/22/us/scientists-in-iceland-discover-first-gene-tied-to-stroke-risk.html (accessed May 2, 2011); "1000 Genomes Project Publishes Analysis of Completed Pilot Phase: Produces Tool for Research into Genetic Contributors to Human Disease."

31. Nicholas Wade, "A Decade Later, Genetic Map Yields Few Clues," June 12, 2010, http://www.nytimes.com/2010/06/13/health/research/13genome.html (accessed February 21, 2011).

32. "Gene Breakthrough Heralds Better Prospect for Malaria Solution," July 25, 2006, http://www.tonic.com/p/nanotechnology-breakthrough-cancer-treatment-rna-interference/ (accessed May 2, 2011).

33. "Penn Researchers Determine Structure of Smallpox Virus Protein Bound to DNA," University of Pennsylvania School of Medicine, August 7, 2006, http://www.sciencedaily.com/releases/2006/08/060805131526.htm (accessed May 2, 2011).

34. "Cardiologists Identify New Cardiac Arrest Gene," November 1, 2007, http://www.sciencedaily.com/releases/2007/10/071031114325.htm (accessed May 2, 2011).

35. A. Binder, "Identification of Genes for Complex Trait: Examples from Hypertension," *Current Pharmaceutical Biotechnology* 7, no. 1 (February 2006): 1–13.

36. The Genetic and Rare Diseases Information Center, March 27, 2011, http://www.genome.gov/10000409 (accessed May 2, 2011); "About the Genetic and Rare Diseases Information Center (GARD)," March 1, 2011, http://www.genome.gov/10000409 (accessed May 2, 2011).

37. David Tenenbaum. "Fighting breast cancer," September 11, 1998, http://whyfiles.org/shorties/herceptin.html. (accessed February 25, 2012).

38. Jennifer Van Brunt, "Biotech Drug Approvals: A Year of Firsts," February 9, 2010, http://www.signalsmag.com/signalsmag.nsf/0/3DE9EAD5D34E5B8D882576C400810419?Open (accessed March 20, 2011); Trista Morrison, "2010 FDA Approvals Could Lead to Launch of Eight Blockbuster Biotech Drugs," February 8, 2010, http://www.cbsnews.com/8301-505123_162-33746564/2010-fda-approvals-could-lead-to-launch-of-eight-blockbuster-biotech-drugs/ (accessed March 20, 2011); "Top 25 Biotech Drugs: The Next Biosimilars Targets?" October 19, 2009, http://www.gabionline.net/layout/set/print/content/view/full/306 (accessed March 20, 2011).

39. "Antisense Therapeutics," 2011, http://www.antisense.com (accessed May 2, 2011);"Antisense Technology," 2011, http://www.genta.com/Products_and_Pipeline/Genasense/Antisense_Technology.html (accessed May 2, 2011).

40. "Which Diseases Will RNAi Drugs Be Used to Treat and What Barriers Will RNAi Drugs Need to Overcome," July 25, 2006, http://www.highbeam.com/doc/1G1-148617066.html (accessed May 2, 2011).

41. Charles Choi, "RNAi: A New Targeted Silencer?" June 27, 2006, http://the-scientist.com (accessed May 2, 2011); Andrew Pollack, "Mice Deaths are Setback in Gene Tests," May 25, 2006, http://www.nytimes.com/1998/11/10/health/drug-testers-turn-to-virtual-patients-as-guinea-pigs.html (accessed May 2, 2011).

42. "RNA Interference Fact Sheet," March 21, 2011, http://www.nigms.nih.gov/News/Extras/RNAi/factsheet.htm (accessed April 22, 2011).

43. "Cancer Cell 'Executioner' Found," August 27, 2006, http://news.bbc.co.uk/2/hi/health/5284850.stm (accessed May 2, 2011).

44. Suzanne Taylor Muzzin, "Sticky Synthetic Molecules Aid Fight against Prostate Cancer," August 26, 2010, http://insciences.org/article.php?article_id=9451 (accessed April 22, 2011).

45. "Stem Cell Basics," April 28, 2009, http://stemcells.nih.gov/info/basics/basics1.asp (accessed May 2, 2011).

46. "Stem Cell Information," April 29, 2011, http://www.nih.gov (accessed May 2, 2011); "Stem Cell Basics: Introduction," April 28, 2009, http://stemcells.nih.gov/info/basics/basics1.asp (accessed May 2, 2011).

47. "Stem Cell Research," February 2006, http://www.news-batch.com (accessed November 21, 2007).

48. "Stem Cell Experiment Yields Heart Valves," November 18, 2006, http://www.nytimes.com/2006/11/18/health/18stem.html (accessed May 2, 2011); "Heart Valves Grown from Womb Fluid Cells," November 16, 2006, http://stemcell-cure.blogspot.com/2006_11_12_archive.html/ (accessed May 2, 2011).

49. "Adult Skin Cells Converted Directly to Beating Heart Cells," January 31, 2011, http://www.sciencedaily.com/releases/2011/01/110130213901.htm (accessed January 31, 2011).

50. Michael Behar, "The Doctor Will See Your Prototype Now: How Super-Accurate Sims Can Test the Effects of Drugs on Patients," February 2005, http://www.wired.com/ (accessed May 2, 2011).

51. American College of Physicians, "Improving FDA Regulation of Prescription Drug." Philadelphia: American College of Physicians; 2009, Policy Monograph, http://www.acponline.org/advocacy/where_we_stand/policy/fda.pdf. (accessed February 22, 2012).

52. "Computerized Doctors' Orders Reduce Medication Errors," June 27, 2007, http://www.sciencedaily.com/releases/2007/06/070627084702.htm (accessed May 2, 2011).

53. "Study: Computers Cut Mistakes in Doctors' Prescriptions," October 20, 1998, http://www.cnn.com/HEALTH/9810/20/drug.errors.ap./index.html (accessed December 3, 2007).

54. Chunliu Zhan, Rodney Hicks, Christopher Blanchette, Margaret A. Keyes, and Diane D. Cousins, "Potential Benefits and Problems with Computerized Prescriber Order Entry Analysis of a Voluntary Medication Error-Reporting Database," February 10, 2006, http://www.medscape.com/viewarticle/523006 (accessed May 2, 2010).

55. Robert A. Raschke, Bea Gollihare, Thomas A. Wunderlich, et al., "A Computer Alert System to Prevent Injury from Adverse Drug Events Development and Evaluation in a Community Teaching Hospital," *Journal of the American Medical Association* 280, no. 15 (1998): 1317–20, http://jama.ama-assn.org/cgi/content/full/15/1317 (accessed May 2, 2011).

56. Linda T. Kohn, Janet M. Corrigan, and Molla S. Donaldson, eds. "To Err Is Human: Building a Safer Health System," December 1, 1999, http://www.providersedge.com/ehdocs/ehr_articles/to_err_is_human_%20building_a_safer_health_system-exec_summary.pdf (accessed May 2, 2011).

57. Lucian L. Leape and Donald M. Berwick, "Five Years after 'To Err Is Human': What Have We Learned?" May 27, 2005, http://www.commonwealthfund.org/Content/Publications/In-the-Literature/2005/May/Five-Years-After–To-Err-Is-Human—What-Have-We-Learned.aspx (accessed May 2, 2011).

58. Bonnie Darves, "Seven Simple Steps to Prevent Outpatient Drug Errors," *American College of Physicians Observer*, June 2003, http://www.acponline.org/cgi-bin/htsearch (accessed May 2, 2011).

59. Damon Adams, "Florida Tells Doctors: Print Clearly or Else: Physicians Will Get a Grace Period to Adapt to the New Law, But After That, Violators Face Possible Discipline,"August 4, 2003, http://www.ama-assn.org/amednews/2003/08/04/prl20804.htm (accessed May 2, 2011).

60. Gardiner Harris, "Report Finds a Heavy Toll from Medication Errors," July 21, 2006, http://www.nytimes.com/2006/07/21/health/21drugerrors.html (accessed May 2, 2011).

61. "Study Finds a Widespread Risk of Reactions to Some Medicines," October 18, 2006, http://select.nytimes.com/gst/abstract.html?res=F70B12F735540C7B8DDDA90994DE404482 (accessed May 2, 2011).

62. Nicholas Bakalar, "Medical Errors? Patients May Be the Last to Know," August 29, 2006, http://www.nytimes.com/2006/08/29/health/29error.html (accessed May 2, 2011).

63. Jill Van Den Bos, Karan Rustagi, Travis Gray, Michael Halford, Eva Ziemkiewicz, and Jonathan Shreve, "The $17.1 Billion Problem: The Annual Cost of Measurable Medical Errors," [Abstract] April 2011, http://content.healthaffairs.org/content/30/4/596 (accessed May 3, 2011); "White House Launches Program to Target Medical Errors; New Billion-Dollar Patient Safety Initiative Will Lead to Introduction of Visual Healthcare Quality Assurance Technology," April 28, 2011, http://www.prnewswire.com/newsreleases/white-house-launches-program-to-target-medical-errors-new-billion-dollar-patient-safety-initiative-will-lead-to-introduction-of-visual-healthcare-quality-assurance-technology-120863869.html

(accessed May 3, 2011); G. Sink, "One in Three Patients Affected by Medical Mistakes, Study Says," April 07, 2011, http://www.injuryinsider.com/2011/04/07/one-in-three-patients-affected-by-medical-mistakes-study-says/ (accessed May 3, 2011); Ananya Mandal, "Obama's Next Target – Medical Error Reduction for Patient Safety," April 12, 2011, http://www.news-medical.net/news/20110412/Obamae28099s-next-target-medical-error-reduction-for-patient-safety.aspx (accessed May 3, 2011).

64. David Perera, "Two Health IT Programs Crosswise, Says GAO," February 23, 2011, http://www.fiercegovernmentit.com/story/two-health-it-programs-crosswise-says-gao/2011-02-23 (accessed March 28, 2011).

65. Mary Mosquera, "GAO: CMS Should Reconcile E-Prescribing, EHR Incentive Reporting," February 18, 2011, http://govhealthit.com/news/gao-cms-should-reconcile-e-prescribing-ehr-incentive-reporting (accessed March 5, 2011); Lisa Webster and Rachelle F. Spiro, "Health Information Technology: A New World for Pharmacy," February 2010, http://pharmacytoday.org/pdf/2010/CE/CE_Feb2010.pdf (accessed February 16, 2011).

66. Webster and Spiro, "Health Information Technology: A New World for Pharmacy."

67. Ibid.

68. Ibid.

69. Ibid.

70. Margie Manning, "Computers to Replace Docs' Scribbles at Barnes-Jewish: $10 Million System Will Place Orders for Drugs, Tests; Should Be in Place Within Three Years," March 4, 2002, http://www.bizjournals.com/stlouis/stories/2002/03/04/story8.html (accessed May 2, 2011).

71. Rebecca Logan, "Hospitals Turn to Robots, Bar Codes to Organize Pharmacies," March 3, 2006, http://www.bizjournals.com/baltimore/stories/2006/03/06/focus3.html (accessed May 2, 2011).

72. Ibid.

73. Karin Rush-Monroe, "New UCSF Robotic Pharmacy Aims to Improve Patient Safety," March 7, 2011, http://www.ucsf.edu/news/2011/03/9510/new-ucsf-robotic-pharmacy-aims-improve-patient-safety (accessed March 21, 2011).

74. Institute for Safe Medication Practices (ISMP), "Guidance on the Interdisciplinary Safe Use of Automated Dispensing Cabinets," 2008, http://www.ismp.org/tools/guidelines/ADC_Guidelines_Final.pdf asp (accessed May 2, 2011); "Follow ISMP Guidelines to Safeguard the Design and Use of Automated Dispensing Cabinets (ADCs)," February 12, 2009, https://www.ismp.org/Newsletters/acutecare/articles/20090212.asp (accessed April 22, 2011).

75. Michael D. Murray, "Automated Medication Dispensing Devices," Chapter 11 in *Making Health Care Safer: A Critical Analysis of Patient Safety Practices*, prepared for the Agency for Healthcare Research and Quality, contract no. 290-97-0013, 2001, http://archive.ahrq.gov/clinic/ptsafety/chap11.htm (accessed May 2, 2011).

76. "Cardinal Health Launches First 'Smart Pump' System to Feature New Bar Code Reader for Safer IV Medication Administration," November 24, 2007, http://www.biohealthmatics.com/News/PressReleases/2005/10/31/000000003450.aspx (accessed May 2, 2011).

77. Bryan Houlston, "Integrating RFID Technology into a Drug Administration System, Healthcare and Informatics Review Online," December 1, 2005, http://www.naccq.ac.nz/bacit/0301/2005Houliston_RFID.htm (accessed May 2, 2011).

78. Tim Vanderveen, "IVs First: A New Barcode Implementation Strategy, Patient Safety and Quality Healthcare," May–June 2006, http://www.psqh.com/mayjun06/ivs.html (accessed May 2, 2011).

79. Harris, "Report Finds a Heavy Toll from Medication Errors."

80. "How RFID Works," http://www.technovelgy.com/ct/Technology-Article.asp?ArtNum=2 (accessed May 2, 2011).

81. "RFIDs: The Pros and Cons Every Consumer Needs to Know about Radio Frequency Tags," June 4, 2005, http://www.waywiser.com/node/5294 (accessed May 2, 2011).

82. Shelley Freierman, "Most Wanted: Drilling Down/Online Pharmacies; and No Doctor's Scribble," April 11, 2005, http://query.nytimes.com/gst/abstract.html?res=F50710F83E5A0C728DDDAD0894DD404482&fta=y&archive:article_related (accessed May 2, 2011).

83. Ukens Carol, "Pharmacy Shortage Boosts Telepharmacy," June 3, 2002, http://drugtopics.modernmedicine.com/drugtopics/article/articleDetail.jsp?id=116637 (accessed May 2, 2011).

84. Ibid.

85. "Telepharmacy Robotic Medicine Delivery Unit 'TRMDU' Assessment," March 17, 2011, http://clinicaltrialsfeeds.org/clinical-trials/show/NCT01007006 (accessed March 21, 2011).

86. Pamela Lewis Dolan, "Navy Launching Telepharmacy Project: The System Will Connect More Than 100 Navy Sites, Allowing Pharmacists to Staff Several Locations Remotely," May 6, 2010, http://www.ama-assn.org/amednews/2010/05/03/bisf0506.htm (accessed March 21, 2011).

87. Steve Mitchell, "Scientists Create 'Pharmacy in a Chip'," October 19, 2003, http://www.upi.com/Science_News/2003/10/19/Scientists-create-pharmacy-in-a-chip/UPI-17331066588560/ (accessed May 2, 2011).

88. Special Report: Emerging Technologies, "Implanted Chips That Deliver Your Drugs," June 18, 2002, http://www.businessweek.com/technology/content/jun2002/tc20020618_5119.htm (accessed May 2, 2011).

89. "'Liquid Pistons' Could Drive New Advances in Camera Lenses and Drug Delivery," January 11, 2011, http://insciences.org/article.php?article_id=9775 (accessed May 3, 2011).

90. David Bois, "A Big Breakthrough in Cancer Treatment Via Nanotechnology," March 23, 2010, http://www.tonic. com/p/nanotechnology-breakthrough-cancer-treatment-rna-interference/ (accessed February 15, 2011).

91. Kenneth Chang, "Nanotechnology gets Star Turn at Speech," January 25, 2011, http://www.nytimes.com/2011/01/26/science/26light.html (accessed February 10 2011).

92. Jodi Thornton, "MRSA and Nanotechnology," November 27, 2010, http://www.ehow.com/facts_7412190_mrsa-

nano-technology.html (accessed February 21, 2011); Catherione de Lange, "Nanoparticle Bandages Could Detect and Treat Infection," July 9, 2010, http://www. newscientist.com/article/dn19158-nanoparticle-bandages-could-detect-and-treat-infection.html (accessed February 21, 2011).

93. "Nanotechnology Treatment for Burns Reduces Infection, Inflammation," September 9, 2009, http://insciences.org/article.php?article_id=6785 (accessed February 16, 2011).

# Additional Resources

"1000 Genomes Project Publishes Analysis of Complete Pilot Phase: Produces Tool for Research into Genetic Contributors to Human Disease." October 27, 2010. http://www.genome. gov/27541917 (accessed February 21, 2011).

"36 Million Americans Have Bought Medications Online without a Doctor's Prescription. Research about Dangerous Practice—and the 11 Internet Commerce Companies Partnering Together to Protect Patients—Announced as part of White House Forum." December 14, 2010. http://www.safeonlinerx.com/news/ (accessed March 22, 2011).

"About the Human Genome Research Project." August 9, 2000. http://www.healthieryou.com/complete.html (accessed May 3, 2011).

"Adult Skin Cells Converted Directly to Beating Heart Cells." January 31, 2011. http://www.sciencedaily.com/releases/2011/01/110130213901.htm (accessed January 31, 2011).

"Alliance for Safe Online Pharmacies Formed; Launches Website." May 19, 2010. http://legitscriptblog.com/2010/05/alliance-for-safe-online-pharmacies-formed-launches-website/ (accessed March 22, 2011).

Baase, Sara. *A Gift of Fire*. Upper Saddle River, NJ: Prentice Hall, 2002: 22–3.

Bois, David. "A Big Breakthrough in Cancer Treatment via Nanotechnology," March 23, 2010. http://www.tonic. com/p/nanotechnology-breakthrough-cancer-treatment-rna-interference/ (accessed February 15, 2011).

Chang, Kenneth. "Nanotechnology Gets Star Turn at Speech." January 25, 2011. http://www.nytimes.com/2011/01/26/science/26light.html (accessed February 10 2011).

"Conflicts-of-Interest in Drug Studies Sneaking Back into Medical Journals, Say Investigators." March 11, 2011. http://www.sciencedaily.com/releases/2011/03/110308172830.htm (accessed April 22, 2011).

"Cybercrime and Doing Time." December 12, 2010. http://garwarner.blogspot.com/2010/12/36-million-americans-buy-drugs-online.html (accessed March 22, 2011).

de Lange, Catherine. "Nanoparticle Bandages Could Detect and Treat Infection." July 9, 2010. http://www.newscientist. com/article/dn19158-nanoparticle-bandages-could-detect-and-treat-infection.html (accessed February 21, 2011).

Department of Health and Human Services. "PDUFA Reauthori zation Good for American Patients." 2002. http://archive. hhs.gov/news/press/2002pres/20020618.html (accessed May 3, 2011).

Dolan, Pamela Lewis. "Navy Launching Telepharmacy Project: The System Will Connect More Than 100 Navy Sites, Allowing Pharmacists to Staff Several Locations Remotely." May 6, 2010. http://www.ama-assn.org/amed-news/2010/05/03/bisf0506.htm (accessed March 21, 2011).

"Ethical Issues in Studying the Safety of Approved Drugs." July 9, 2010. http://iom.edu/Reports/2010/Ethical-Issues-in-Studying-the-Safety-of-Approved-Drugs-Letter-Report. aspx (accessed February 21, 2011).

"FDA Approves Avastin, a Targeted Therapy for First-Line Metastatic Colorectal Cancer Patients." February 26, 2004. http://www.mesotheliomacenter.com/mesothelioma-news/2004/02/26/fda-approves-avastin-a-targeted-therapy-for-first-line-metastatic-colorectal-cancer-patients-first-anti-angiogenesis-treatment-approved-for-treating-cancer/ (accessed May 3, 2011).

"FDA Approves Herceptin for Breast Cancer." September 29, 1998. http://www.pslgroup.com/dg/b1c82.htm (accessed May 3, 2011).

"FDA Approves Xolair, Biotechnology Breakthrough for Asthma." June 20, 2003. http://reports.huginonline.com/908721/119702.pdf (accessed May 3, 2011).

"FDA-Industry PDUFA V Reauthorization Meeting." January 10, 2011. http://www.fda.gov/downloads/ForIndustry/UserFees/PrescriptionDrugUserFee/UCM238732.pdf (accessed March 19, 2011).

"FDA to Make Big Change to Risk Benefit Equation Under PDUFA V." March 9, 2011. http://www.gekkowire.com/?p= 7305 (accessed March 19, 2011).

"Find the Best Drug Prices from Verified Online Pharmacies." 2011. http://www.pharmacychecker.com/ (accessed March 22, 2011).

Fleiger, Ken. "Getting SMART: Drug Review in the Computer Age." October 1995. *FDA Consumer.* http://findarticles.com/p/articles/mi_m1370/is_n8_v29/ai_17412072/ (accessed May 3, 2011).

"Follow ISMP Guidelines to Safeguard the Design and Use of Automated Dispensing Cabinets (ADCs)." February 12, 2009. https://www.ismp.org/Newsletters/acutecare/articles/20090 212.asp (accessed April 22, 2011).

"Genentech Presents Positive Preliminary Six-Month Data from Phase Ib/II Study for Lucentis in Age-Related Macular Degeneration (AMD)." August 18, 2003. http://www.gene.com/gene/news/press-releases/display.do?method=detail&id=6487 (accessed May 3, 2011).

"Genentech Receives FDA Fast-Track Designation for Avastin." June 26, 2003. http://www.gene.com/gene/news/press-releases/display.do?method=detail&id=6367 (accessed May 3, 2011).

Greenberg, Sally. "Examining the Prescription Drug User Fee Act." April 10, 2011. http://www.nclnet.org/health/106-prescription-drugs/390-examining-the-prescription-drug-user-fee-act (accessed March 18, 2911).

"Health Plans for Virtual Human." May 17, 1999. http://news.bbc.co.uk/2/hi/health/345762.stm (accessed May 3, 2011).

Hennessy, Sean, and Brian Strom. "PDUFA Reauthorization—Drug Safety's Golden Moment of Opportunity?" April 26, 2007. *The New England Journal of Medicine.* http://health-policyandreform.nejm.org/?p=11579 (accessed May 3, 2011).

"Isn't There a New Federal Law to Address Online Pharmacy Drug Safety?" June 10, 2010. http://www.safeonlinerx.com/2010/06/isnt-there-a-new-federal-law-to-address-online-pharmacy-drug-safety-.html (accessed March 22, 2011).

Leape, Lucian L., and Donald M. Berwick. "Five Years after 'To Err Is Human': What Have We Learned?" May 27, 2005. http://www.commonwealthfund.org/Content/Publications/In-the-Literature/2005/May/Five-Years-After--To-Err-Is-Human---What-Have-We-Learned.aspx (accessed May 2, 2011).

Levitt, Gabriel. "Alliance for Safe Online Pharmacies (safeonlinerx.com)—Really an "Alliance against Safe and Affordable Online Pharmacies?" June 28, 2010. http://pharmacycheckerblog.com/alliance-for-safe-online-pharmacies-safeonlinerx-com-%E2%80%93-really-an-%E2%80%9Calliance-against-safe-and-affordable-online-pharmacies%E2%80%9D (accessed March 22, 2011).

Mandal, Ananya. "Obama's Next Target: Medical Error Reduction for Patient Safety." April 12, 2011. http://www.news-medical.net/news/20110412/Obamae28099s-next-target-medical-error-reduction-for-patient-safety.aspx (accessed May 3, 2011).

Morrison, Trista. "2010 FDA Approvals Could Lead to Launch of Eight Blockbuster Biotech Drugs." February 8, 2010. http://www.cbsnews.com/8301-505123_162-33746564/2010-fda-approvals-could-lead-to-launch-of-eight-block-buster-biotech-drugs/ (accessed March 20, 2011).

Mosquera, Mary. "GAO: CMS Should Reconcile E-Prescribing, EHR Incentive Reporting." February 18, 2011. http://gov-healthit.com/news/gao-cms-should-reconcile-e-prescribing-ehr-incentive-reporting (accessed March 5, 2011).

Muzzin, Suzanne Taylor. "Sticky Synthetic Molecules Aid Fight against Prostate Cancer." August 26, 2010. http://insciences.org/article.php?article_id=9451 (accessed April 22, 2011).

"Nanotechnology Treatment for Burns Reduces Infection, Inflammation." September 9, 2009. http://insciences.org/article.php?article_id=6785 (accessed February 16, 2011).

Neergaard, Lauran. "DNA to Aid in Tailoring Prescription for Patient." *Star-Ledger,* November 3, 2003, 23.

"New Study Shows Safety of Ordering Prescription Drugs from Foreign Pharmacy Websites Verified by PharmacyChecker.com." August 13, 2010. http://pharmacychecker.com/news/internet_pharmacy_study_shows_strength_of_pharmacy-checker_verification_program%20_081310.asp (accessed March 22, 2011).

Ouellette, Jennifer. "Biomaterials Facilitate Medical Break throughs." October/November 2001. American Institute of Physics. http://www.aip.org/tip/INPHFA/vol-7/iss-5/p18.pdf (accessed May 3, 2011).

"Physicians Hospital of El Paso Set to Deploy Pyxis Safetynet Technology to Reduce Medical Errors." October 10, 2002. http://www.himss.org/asp/ContentRedirector.asp?Content Id=22358 (accessed May 3, 2011).

Polito, John R. "Senate Tobacco Bill Would Alter FDA's Mission." February 27, 2007. http://whyquit.com/pr/022 707.html (accessed May 2, 2011).

Pollack, Andrew. "Drug Testers Turn to 'Virtual Patients' as Guinea Pigs." November 10, 1998. http://www.nytimes.com/1998/11/10/health/drug-testers-turn-to-virtual-patients-as-guinea-pigs.html (accessed May 3, 2011).

Pollack, Andrew. "Merck and Partner Form Alliance to Develop Drugs Based on RNA." September 9, 2003. http://www.nytimes.com/2003/09/10/business/merck-and-partner-form-alliance-to-develop-drugs-based-on-rna.html (accessed May 3, 2011).

Pollack, Andrew. "Mixed Data Leave Doubts on Cancer Drug," September 12, 2003. http://www.nytimes.com/2003/09/11/business/mixed-data-leave-doubts-on-cancer-drug.html/ (accessed May 3, 2011).

"Preventing Death and Injury from Medical Errors Requires Dramatic, System-Wide Changes." December 1, 1999. http://www.sciencedaily.com/releases/1999/12/991201072044.htm (accessed May 3, 2011).

Raschke, Robert, Bea Gollihare, Thomas A. Wunderlich, et al. "A Computer Alert System to Prevent Injury from Adverse Drug Events." *Journal of the American Medical Association* 280, no. 15 (1998): 1317–20.

"RNA Interference Fact Sheet." March 21, 2011. http://www.nigms.nih.gov/News/Extras/RNAi/factsheet.htm (accessed April 22, 2011).

Rush-Monroe, Karin. "New UCSF Robotic Pharmacy Aims to Improve Patient Safety." March 7, 2011. http://www.ucsf.edu/news/2011/03/9510/new-ucsf-robotic-pharmacy-aims-improve-patient-safety (accessed March 21, 2011).

"Safe Online Pharmacy Coalition Lauds New Intellectual Property Plan: Plan Recognizes the Problem of Illegal Online Drug Sellers." July 7, 2010. http://www.safeonlinerx.com/2010/07/safe-online-pharmacy-coalition-lauds-new-intellectual-property-plan-plan-recognizes-the-problem-of-i.html (accessed March 22, 2011).

Sardinha, Carol. "Electronic Prescribing: The Next Revolution in Pharmacy." January–February 1998. *Journal of Managed Care Pharmacy.* http://www.amcp.org/data/jmcp/vol4/num1/spotlight.html (accessed May 3, 2011).

Schwarz, Harold, and Bret Brodowy. "Implementation and Evaluation of an Automated Dispensing System." *American Journal of Health-System Pharmacy* 52, no. 8 (April 15, 1995): 823–28. http://www.ncbi.nlm.nih.gov/pubmed/7634117 (accessed May 3, 2011).

Sink, G. "One in Three Patients Affected by Medical Mistakes, Study Says." April 7, 2011. http://www.injuryinsider.com/2011/04/07/one-in-three-patients-affected-by-medical-mistakes-study-says/ (accessed May 3, 2011).

Sullivan, Thomas. "FDA Receives Input on Prescription Drug User Fee Act Reauthorization 2012." January 11, 2011. http://www.policymed.com/2011/01/fda-receives-input-on-prescription-drug-user-fee-act-reauthorization-2012.html (accessed March 19, 2011).

"Tarceva (Erlotinib HCl) Phase II Clinical Trials Initiated in Patients with Malignant Glioma." August 8, 2003. http://www.astellas.us/docs/us/OSIP_News_2003_8_8_General_Releases.pdf (accessed May 3, 2011).

"Telepharmacy Robotic Medicine Delivery Unit 'TRMDU' Assessment." March 17, 2011. http://clinicaltrialsfeeds.org/clinical-trials/show/NCT01007006 (accessed March 21, 2011).

"Thompson Approves Demos to Expand Safety-Net Patients' Access to Prescription Drugs and Pharmacy Services, Lower Drug Prices." December 18, 2001. U.S. Department of Health and Human Services. http://archive.hhs.gov/news/press/2001pres/20011228.html (accessed May 3, 2011).

Thornton, Jodi. "MRSA and Nanotechnology." November 27, 2010. http://www.ehow.com/facts_7412190_mrsa-nanotechnology.html (accessed February 21, 2011).

"Top 25 Biotech Drugs: The Next Biosimilars Targets?" October 19, 2009. http://www.gabionline.net/layout/set/print/content/view/full/306 (accessed March 20, 2011).

Ukens, Carol. "Manuel the Robot Earns HIS Long-Term Care Keep." July 10, 2006. http://drugtopics.modernmedicine.com/drugtopics/article/articleDetail.jsp?id=353150 (accessed May 3, 2011).

Ukens, Carol. "New Bar-Code Scanner Simplifies Drug Ordering." August 7, 2006. http://www.drugtopics.com/drugtopics/author/authorDetail.jsp?id=6373 (accessed May 3, 2011).

Usdin, Steve. "Sidebar: Elastic PDUFA Deadlines." November 6, 2010. http://www.biocentury.com/biotech-pharma-news/politics/2010-11-08/fda-bio-phrma-dickering-over-longer-review-times-in-pdufa-v-a17 (accessed March 19, 2011).

Van Brunt, Jennifer. "Biotech Drug Approvals: A Year of Firsts." February 9, 2010. http://www.signalsmag.com/signalsmag.nsf/0/3DE9EAD5D34E5B8D882576C400810419?Open (accessed March 20, 2011).

Van Den Bos, Jill, Karan Rustagi, Travis Gray, Michael Halford, Eva Ziemkiewicz, and Jonathan Shreve. "The $17.1 Billion Problem: The Annual Cost of Measurable Medical Errors" [Abstract] April 2011. http://content.healthaffairs.org/content/30/4/596 (accessed May 3, 2011).

Wade, Nicholas. "A Decade Later, Genetic Map Yields Few New Cures." June 12, 2010. http://www.nytimes.com/2010/06/13/health/research/13genome.html (accessed February 21, 2011).

Webster, Lisa, and Rachelle F. Spiro. "Health Information Technology: A New World for Pharmacy." February 2010. http://pharmacytoday.org/pdf/2010/CE/CE_Feb2010.pdf (accessed February 16, 2011).

"What Is a Helix? And What Is RNA and DNA." http://www.chemistry-school.info/what_is_a_helix.htm (accessed February 20, 2012).

"White House Launches Program to Target Medical Errors; New Billion-Dollar Patient Safety Initiative Will Lead to Introduction of Visual Healthcare Quality Assurance Technology." April 28, 2011. http://www.prnewswire.com/news-releases/white-house-launches-program-to-target-medical-errors-new-billion-dollar-patient-safety-initiative-will-lead-to-introduction-of-visual-healthcare-quality-assurance-technology-120863869.html (accessed May 3, 2011).

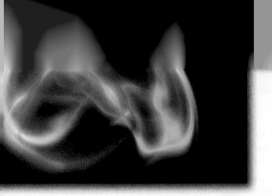

## CHAPTER 9

# Information Technology in Dentistry

## CHAPTER OUTLINE

- Review Exercises
- Notes
- Additional Resources

## LEARNING OBJECTIVES

In this chapter, the reader will learn many of the many ways that computer technology has impacted the practice of dentistry. Upon completion of this chapter, the reader will be able to:

- Describe the use of computers in education.
- Discuss the significance of the electronic patient record in integrating practice management and clinical applications.
- Discuss the impact of changing demographics on dental practice.
- Describe the use of computers in endodontics, periodontics, and cosmetic dentistry.
- Define diagnostic tools including the X-ray, digital X-ray, electronic concordance, and the new tools that use light.
- Define minimally invasive dentistry.
- List the uses of computers in dental surgery.
- Describe the trend toward growing specialization.
- Describe the emerging field of teledentistry.

## OVERVIEW

Computers have been transforming dentistry for many years. **Dental informatics** combines computer technology with dentistry to create a basis for research, education, and the solution of real-world problems in oral health care using computer applications. Studies are being done on the role of information technology on the dentist–patient relationship.[1]

From the time the patient calls the office for an appointment recorded in an electronic appointment book to the services offered and the instruments in use, even to the pain the patient senses, digital technology plays a role. The earliest application of information technology in the dentist's office, as in so many other offices, was administrative—related to bookkeeping and accounting, including submitting insurance claims and generating recall notices.

Many dental offices use computers for some aspect of their practice. Computer technology can be utilized in dentistry to help reduce medical errors; to train dentists; to facilitate communication between dentists; to perform administrative, clerical, and managerial functions in the dental office; and not least to enhance patient care.

The practice of dentistry has also been affected by demographic changes in our society over the last century. Younger people (with the significant exceptions of the poor, minorities, and immigrants) have few cavities because of preventive care. Older people are subject to periodontal disease.

## EDUCATION

Dentists can surf the Web for online information specific to their professional interests and use e-mail to communicate with each other and their patients. Computer-generated treatment plans are used to help educate patients (Figure 9.1▶). These plans can be presented on DVDs.

Although not yet common, virtual reality simulations are beginning to be used in the education of dentists and dental surgeons. Case Western Reserve University, which installed

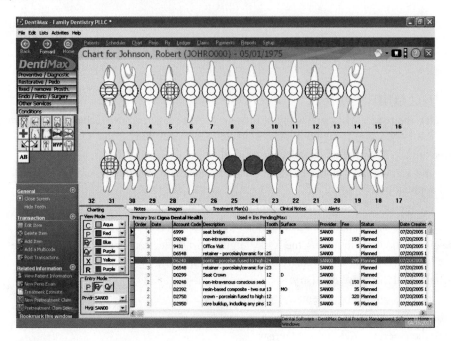

▶ **Figure 9.1**    Treatment plan.
*Source:* Courtesy of DentiMax.

virtual dentistry equipment at a cost of $2 million in 2002, is very satisfied with the part virtual reality can play in dental education. The simulators are always available, so students can learn at their own pace. According to faculty members, students learned much faster; they report that students learned drilling techniques in 2 weeks instead of one full semester. Each station includes a mannequin, drill, syringes, suction, light, cabinets, and a computer monitor—simulating a dentist's office. A camera watches the student's work and sends the student messages. The student is shown what the tooth should look like, and images and evaluations of the student's work via the monitor.[2]

**DentSim** is a program that uses virtual reality. Its purpose is to teach technical dexterity to dental students. Several small studies have been completed. One found that students "learn faster, arrive at the same level of performance, accomplish more practice procedures per hour, and request more evaluations per procedure or per hour than in our traditional laboratories." Another

study found the use of DentSim "encouraging," but also found problem areas. A later study found the experience "generally positive."[3]

## ADMINISTRATIVE APPLICATIONS

From the moment a patient calls to arrange an appointment to the electronic submission of the bill to the insurance company, computer technology may be involved. Many dental offices, like other medical offices, use computerized appointment calendars; thus, appointments can be made (and viewed) from any room in the office that has a networked computer (Figure 9.2, A–C ▶). Insurance claims can also be submitted electronically. (Figure 9.3, A–C ▶). Software also generates recall notices. (Figure 9.4, A–D ▶). Specialized software helps to create treatment plans, to explain plans to patients, and to give postoperative instructions. In offices using fully integrated practice management software, any screen is accessible from any other, simply by clicking the mouse.

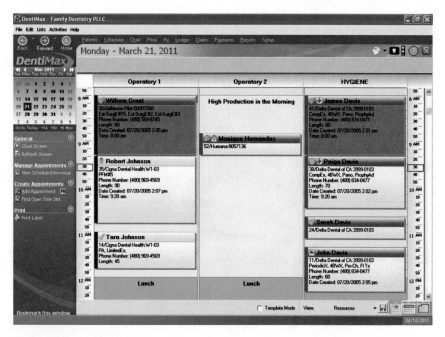

▶ **Figure 9.2**    (A) Electronic scheduling: day's view
*Source:* Courtesy of DentiMax.

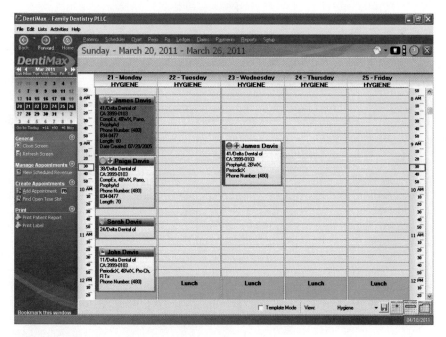

▶ **Figure 9.2**    (B) week's view
*Source:* Courtesy of DentiMax.

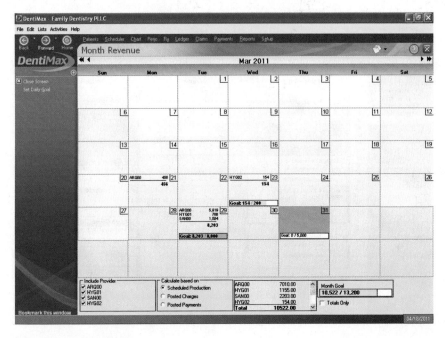

▶ **Figure 9.2** (C) month's view.
*Source*: Courtesy of DentiMax.

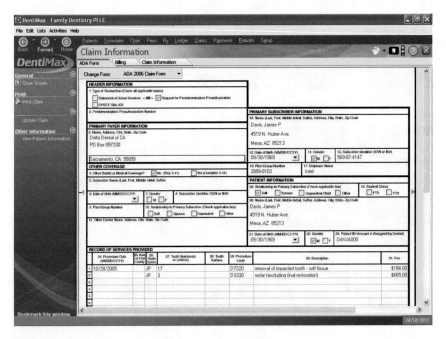

▶ **Figure 9.3** (A) Insurance claim.
*Source:* Courtesy of DentiMax.

**Dental Claim Form**   © American Dental Association, 2006

**HEADER INFORMATION**

1. Type of Transaction (Check all applicable boxes)
   ☐ State of Actual Services -OR-   ☑ Request for Predetermination/Preauthorization
   ☐ EPSDT/Title XIX

2. Predetermination / Preauthorization Number

**PRIMARY PAYER INFORMATION**

3. Name, Address, City State, Zip Code

Delta Dental of CA
PO Box 997330
Sacramento, CA. 95899

**OTHER COVERAGE**

4. Other Dental or Medical Coverage?   ☑ No (Skip 5-11)   ☐ Yes (Complete 5-11)

5. Subscriber Name (Last, First, Middle Initial, Suffix)

6. Date of Birth (MM/DD/CCYY)

7. Gender  ☐ M  ☐ F

8. Subscriber Identifier (SSN or ID#)

9. Plan/Group Number

10. Relationship to Primary Subscriber (Check Applicable box)
    ☐ Self  ☐ Spouse  ☐ Dependent Child  ☐ Other

11. Other Carrier Name, Address, City, State, Zip Code

**PRIMARY SUBSCRIBER INFORMATION**

12. Name (Last, First, Middle Initial, Suffix, Address, City, State, Zip Code

Davis, James P

4519 N. Huber Ave.

Mesa, AZ 85213

13. Date of Birth (MM/DD/CCYY)  09/30/1969

14. Gender  ☑ M  ☐ F

15. Subscriber Identifier (SSN or ID#)  569-87-4147

16. Plan/Group Number  3999-0103

17. Employer Name  Intel

**PATIENT INFORMATION**

18. Relationship to Primary Subscriber (Check applicable box)
    ☐ Self  ☐ Spouse  ☐ Dependent Child  ☐ Other

19. Student Status  ☐ FTS  ☐ PTS

20. Name (Last, First, Middle Initial, Suffix, Address, City, Zip Code

Davis, James P

4519 N. Huber Ave.

Mesa, AZ 85213

21. Date of Birth (MM/DD/CCYY)  09/30/1969

22. Gender  ☑ M  ☐ F

23. Patient ID/Account #(Assigned by Dentist)  DAVJA000

**RECORD OF SERVICE PROVIDED**

| | 24. Procedure Date (MM/DD/CCYY) | 25. Area of Oral Cavity | 26. Tooth System | 27. Tooth Numbers(s) or Letter(s) | 28. Tooth Surface | 29. Procedure Code | 30. Description | 31. Fee |
|---|---|---|---|---|---|---|---|---|
| 1 | | JP | 3 | | | D3330 | molar (excluding final restoration) | 665.00 |
| 2 | | JP | 17 | | | D7220 | removal of impacted tooth - soft tissue | 184.00 |
| 3 | | | | | | | | |
| 4 | | | | | | | | |
| 5 | | | | | | | | |
| 6 | | | | | | | | |
| 7 | | | | | | | | |
| 8 | | | | | | | | |
| 9 | | | | | | | | |
| 10 | | | | | | | | |

**MISSING TEETH INFORMATION**

34. (Place an 'X' on each missing tooth)

Permanent: 1 2 3 4 5 6 7 8 9 10 11 12 13 14 15 16 / 32 31 30 29 28 27 26 25 24 23 22 21 20 19 18 17

Primary: A B C D E F G H I J / T S R Q P O N M L K

32. Other Fee(s)

33. Total Fee  849.00

35. Remarks

**AUTHORIZATIONS**

36. I have been informed of the treatment plan and associated fees. I agree to be responsible for all charges for dental services and materials not paid by my dental benefit plan, unless prohibited by law, or the treating dentist or dental practice has a contractual agreement with my plan prohibiting all or a portion of such charges. To the extent permitted by law, I consent to your use and disclosure of my protected health information to carry out payment activities in connection with this claim.

X  Signature on file   11/22/2005
Patient/Guardian Signature   Date

37. I hereby authorize and direct payment of the dental benefits otherwise payable to me, directly to the below named dentist or dental entity.

X  Signature On File   11/22/2005
Subscriber Signature   Date

**BILLING DENTIST OR DENTAL ENTITY** (Leave blank if dentist of dental entity is not submitting claim on behalf of the patient or insured/subscriber)

48. Name, Address, City, State, Zip Code

David M Arquette DDS
4455 N. Broadway
Suite 109
Mesa, AZ 85206

49. NPI

50. License Number  9942

51. SSN or TIN  03-0545987

52. Phone Number (480) 969-3688

52A. Additional Provider ID  9942

**ANCILLARY CLAIM/TREATMENT INFORMATION**

38. Place of Treatment (Check applicable box)
    ☑ Provider's Office  ☐ Hospital  ☐ ECF  ☐ Other

39. Number of Enclosures (00 to 99)  Radiograph(s)  Oral image(s)  Model(s)

40. Is Treatment for Orthodontics?  ☑ No (Skip 41-42)  ☐ Yes (Complete 44)

41. Date appliance placed (MM/DD/CCYY)

42. Months of Treatment remaining

43. Replacement of Prosthesis?  ☑ No  ☐ Yes (Complete 44)

44. Date prior placement (MM/DD/CCYY)

45. Treatment Resulting from (Check applicable box)
    ☐ Occupational illness/injury  ☐ Auto accident  ☐ Other accident

46. Date of Accident (MM/DD/CCYY)

47. Auto Accident State

**TREATING DENTIST AND TREATMENT LOCATION INFORMATION**

53. I hereby certify that the procedures as indicated by date are in progress ( for procedures that require multiple visits) or have been completed and that the fees submitted are the actual fees I have charged and intend to collect for those procedures.

Signed (Treating Dentist)   Date

54. NPI

55. License Number  9942

56. Address, City, State, Zip Code
4455 N. Broadway
Mesa, AZ 85206

56A. Provider Specialty Code  1223G0001X

57. Phone Number (480) 969-3688

58. Treating Provider Specialty  987896

▶ **Figure 9.3**   (B) Dental claim form.

## The Electronic Dental Chart

Computers were first used by dentists in the 1960s as accounting tools. In the 1980s, computers were used for practice management. The American Dental Association (ADA) began developing guidelines for the fully integrated computerized dental office. The electronic appointment book, electronic accounting software, and electronic record keeping, in which the patient's record includes images, charting, and photos, will become more and more common. Software that computerizes some clinical procedures (charting, probing, and digital imaging) is beginning to be used. In the future, a patient record that links practice management with all clinical procedures may be developed.

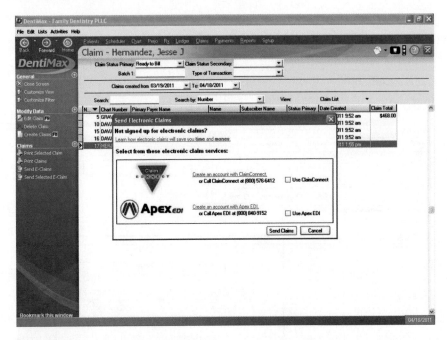

▶ **Figure 9.3** (C) Insurance claims can be sent electronically.
*Source:* Courtesy of DentiMax.

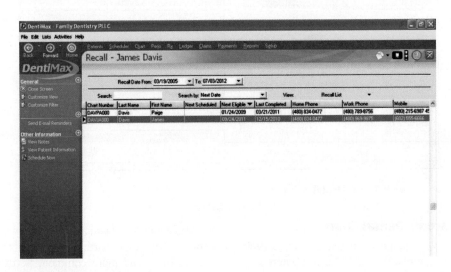

▶ **Figure 9.4** (A) Recall.
*Source:* Courtesy of DentiMax.

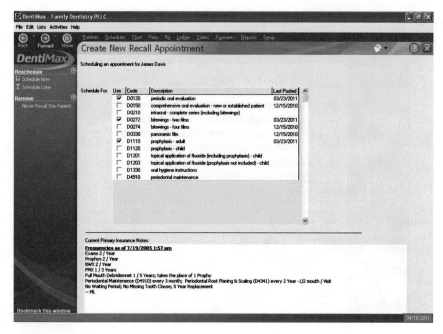

▶ **Figure 9.4** (B) Create new recall appointment screen.
*Source:* Courtesy of DentiMax.

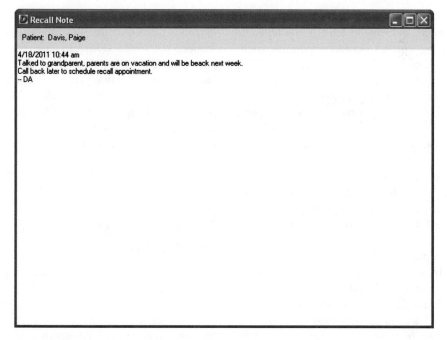

▶ **Figure 9.4** (C) Recall note.
*Source:* Courtesy of DentiMax.

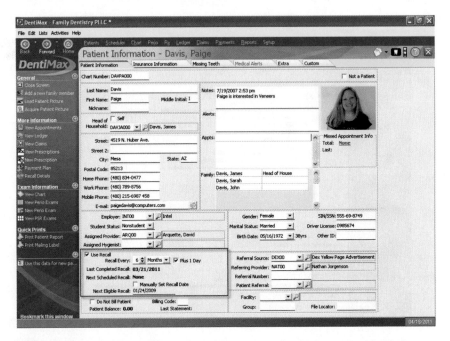

▶ **Figure 9.4**   (D) Patient information page with recall information highlighted.
*Source:* Courtesy of DentiMax.

The **electronic dental chart** is standardized, easy to search, and easy to read. It can integrate practice management tasks (administrative applications) with clinical information. It can include all of the patient's conditions and treatments, including images. The record must include codes for treatment and diagnosis, which will come from the American Dental Association (ADA). In February 2011, the ADA Standards Committee met to further develop standards. As of 2011, there were 80 standards for both information technology (IT) and products, and more are under development.[4] The electronic chart should include the following: the ability to find patients by name, patient identification numbers, health information such as allergies or conditions that would affect dental care, treatment planning, procedures performed and planned, treatments completed, medical history, and ADA codes. As additions are made, they must be dated, and an audit trail of who edited each record must be kept. Files must be password protected. The record includes graphics and text. The chart will be created on a patient's first visit and updated every visit. Not only does it contain clinical information, but transactions can also be posted. It also includes the fee schedule and the patient's insurance information (including co-payment and deductible). Because much of the chart is made up of images, it is easy for the patient to understand. The patient and dentist can develop treatment plans that take into account medical needs and finances. The chart can be electronically transmitted to specialists.

## DEMOGRAPHICS AND THE TRANSFORMATION OF DENTISTRY

In 2000, the surgeon general issued a first report on dental health. The report pointed to changes over the last hundred years. In 1900, most people lost their teeth by middle age. By the middle of the 20th century, the baby boom generation was taught to take care of their teeth. Bacteria (usually Streptococcus) were found to be the cause of tooth decay and periodontal disease in the 1950s and 1960s.

By the beginning of the 21st century, many children were drinking fluoridated water, having their teeth regularly cared for, and thus suffering less decay. This meant that they did not lose their teeth as they aged. However, according to the surgeon general, there is still an "epidemic of oral disease." Victims of this epidemic are low-income, minority, and some immigrant populations. One study traced the high number of cavities in poor children to increased lead levels in the children's blood, plus shortages in calcium and vitamin C.[5] However, dental health in general has improved over the last century. These trends—successful preventive treatments in middle-class children and an increasing aging population who have kept their teeth—have changed the conditions dentists are treating and the expectations of patients. Dentists are filling fewer teeth, but increasingly and aggressively treating the more affluent portion of the aging population. This population now seeks dental care to save their teeth. However, this may make the dentist's job more difficult because this population is both old and may be in poor health.

According to a 2010 report from the Centers for Disease Control and Prevention in 2010, "Oral Health Problems Are Preventable, Common, and Painful":

- Tooth decay affects more than one-fourth of U.S. children aged 2–5 and half of those aged 12–15. About half of all children and two-thirds of children aged 12–19 from low-income families have had decay.
- Children and adolescents of some racial and ethnic groups and those from lower-income families have more untreated decay. For example, 40% of Mexican American children aged 6–8 have untreated decay, compared with 25% of non-Hispanic whites. Twenty percent of all adolescents aged 12–19 years currently have untreated tooth decay.
- Advanced gum disease affects 4%–12% of adults. Half of the cases of severe gum disease in the United States are the result of cigarette smoking. Three times as many smokers have gum disease as people who have never smoked.
- One-fourth of U.S. adults aged 65 and older have lost all of their teeth.
- African American and Mexican American adults have twice the amount of untreated decay as non-Hispanic whites.

*Source:* Oral Health 2010 (Courtesy of the Centers for Disease Control)

Oral health problems are still more prevalent among some minority populations and among low-income families.[6]

## COMPUTERIZED INSTRUMENTS IN DENTISTRY

Computerized instruments have been entering the field of dentistry for several years. From a very expensive machine that creates crowns immediately to fiber optic digital cameras and digital X-rays, computer technology is changing some aspects of dentistry. The **fiber optic camera** is analogous to the endoscope used in surgery. It is used to view an area that is normally difficult to see. The dentist aims a fiber optic wand at the area of the mouth to be examined. The image can be viewed on a monitor by the patient and the dentist. The image can help the dentist see and diagnose problems at a very early stage. An electronic periodontal probe has been developed to replace the sharp steel probe dentists use to measure pockets between teeth and gums. It is more accurate and, one would hope, less painful than its predecessor.

Computer-controlled injections are administered by the WAND (Milestone Scientific)™. The **WAND**™ includes a microprocessor that measures tissue density; this ensures a steady flow of anesthetic. The microprocessor delivers anesthesia ahead of the needle, numbing the tissue before the needle touches it. It numbs only the injection site—not the tongue, lips, or face.

## ENDODONTICS

**Endodontics** is the dental specialty that diagnoses and treats diseases of the pulp. Endoscopes make use of fiber optics to take pictures of the root canal and show them on a screen. Both the dentist and the patient can see and discuss the images, which helps in both diagnosis and educating the patient.

The precision of ultrasonic instruments helps in performing root canal therapy. They are flexible and accurate and allow the dentist to clean out the root without harming the surrounding tissue.

If a patient needs a crown, computers can be used to create a model of the affected tooth. This computer-generated model can be electronically transmitted to another company that uses it to prepare the crown. Too expensive to be common, computer-aided design/computer-aided manufacturing (CAD/CAM) is used by a new machine to create crowns.

## PERIODONTICS

**Periodontics** is concerned with diagnosing and treating diseases of the gums and other structures supporting the teeth. Periodontal disease is caused by bacteria. Untreated, periodontal disease can lead to both tooth and bone loss. The sequence of the genome associated with the pathogen causing gum disease has been identified; this might lead to the development of effective treatments.[7] Tooth loss because of periodontal disease is related to (does not necessarily cause) heart disease. It may even be an "early warning sign of heart disease."[8] Gum disease is also linked to premature birth.[9] Periodontal disease is more prevalent in older people who have kept their natural teeth. It is also prevalent among African-Americans.[10] Periodontal disease is related to stroke and cancers, especially pancreatic cancer in men.[11] Gum disease, which affects about 50 million Americans, may be a sign of other diseases, for example, diabetes.[12]

The standard method of measuring periodontal pockets (the spaces between teeth and gums) involves probing with a steel-tipped tool, measuring the pockets, and noting the depth on a patient's chart (Figures 9.5, A and B ▶). An electronic probe with a flexible tip may be more accurate and less painful. Currently, voice-activated charting is beginning to be used.

Although not widely accepted, lasers are used by some dentists to treat periodontal disease. They

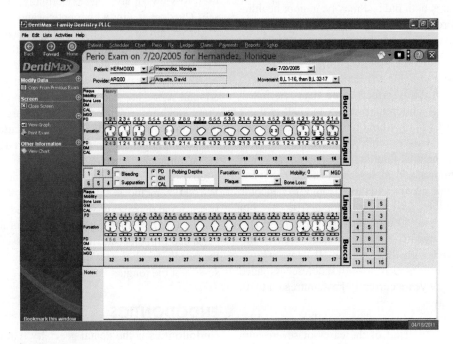

▶ **Figure 9.5** (A) Perio charting.
*Source:* Courtesy of DentiMax.

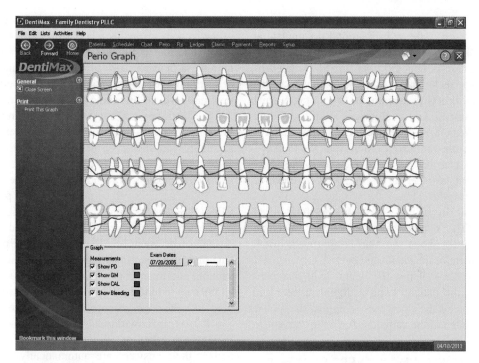

▶ **Figure 9.5** (B) Perio charting.
*Source:* Courtesy of DentiMax.

apply lasers to soft tissue and root surfaces. This can be added to traditional treatment. However, there is little or no evidence that it is effective.[13]

The change in the conditions for which people seek dental care is related to demographic changes mentioned earlier. Older adults with their own teeth are more likely to suffer from periodontal disease. Gums recede; roots are exposed and may develop cavities. The more teeth a person keeps, the more these problems develop, and the more visits to the dentist. Furthermore, affluent older adults may seek cosmetic dentistry: "smile make-overs," tooth whitening, and orthodontics.

## COSMETIC DENTISTRY

**Cosmetic dentistry** is becoming more and more widely available: 84 percent of dentists now offer cosmetic treatments.[14] Cosmetic dentistry attempts to create a more attractive smile. To do this, several procedures may be employed. Tooth bleaching may be done at home with bleaching kits or at the dentist's office using lasers. One procedure is called ZOOM. Porcelain veneers may be applied to create a whiter-looking tooth. **Bonding** involves the application of a material to the tooth that can be shaped and polished. **Dental implants** can be used to replace missing teeth; computers help plan the exact placement of the implant. Cosmetic dentists and orthodontists employ digital cameras and graphics software.

Dental implants used to take several months to complete. Many needed two surgeries. By 2007, dentists could use three-dimensional computed tomography (CT) scans. This allows dentists to "... visualize the bone ... [and] visualize how the teeth will be ...." to make a three-dimensional model of the mouth. The model allows the dentist to examine the bone at any angle. The dentist can see the exact spot for the implant. The technique also involves making the surface of the implant porous with an acid solution and an electronic charge. The implant can then be more quickly fixed to the bone. A biomaterial of titanium is used as a bonding agent, which "actively enables integration with human bone and soft tissue growth around the implant at the gumline." It is a one-visit procedure.[15]

Some orthodontics is performed via teledentistry. The technician is with the patient, and the clinician directs the technician from afar. Virtual reality three-dimensional images allow the patient to view herself or himself before and after any procedure. Some software even morphs the image—from the face before to the face after—to show the patient how her or his face will be changed by the procedure. Using the virtual reality image, the technician can move individual teeth in virtual reality. The dentist can review the procedure via the Web. When the plan is approved, a real realignment of the teeth can begin.[16]

In other systems, the dental hygienist photographs the patient using a digital camera and simply makes the changes by dragging the mouse on the image of the patient's face on the screen.

## DIAGNOSIS AND EXPERT SYSTEMS

Diagnosis is not always clear and simple; dentists need to analyze all sorts of data, such as the clinical presentation of the patient and general medical information. No individual can have all the current information at her or his fingertips. But knowing how to phrase questions and find facts for decision-making is a crucial skill. There are several collections of evidence-based articles and reviews categorized by topic that, dentists can search online. Journals, such as the *Journal of Evidence-Based Dental Practice*, give summaries of articles. Databases, such as MEDLINE, can also be helpful. When doing the search, the dentist needs to be able to frame questions that provide enough information. The question should state the problem clearly and the desired outcome. The computerized search should be of peer-reviewed, evidence-based relevant material.

The dentist then needs to apply the correct factual information to the particular situation to make a diagnosis. In dentistry, as in other fields, expert systems or **clinical decision-support systems (CDSS)** can help. Expert systems are a branch of artificial intelligence, which attempts to model computer logic on human behavior. An expert system maintains a large collection of facts relevant to the discipline (dentistry) and rules on how these facts are used in decision-making. The dentist may type in symptoms, and the expert system may respond by asking for more information; finally, diagnoses are suggested. The diagnosis is in the form of an inference: If the patient exhibits swelling, then she or he may have an infection. Expert systems are meant as an aid in diagnosis, not a replacement for the judgment of the dentist.

Today's CDSS can be tailored to each patient. CDSS "are computer programs that are designed to provide expert support for health professionals making clinical decisions . . . . To help . . . analyze patient data and make decisions regarding diagnosis, prevention, and treatment."[17] Like any expert system, CDSS may remind the practitioner of conditions and diagnoses she or he has not recently encountered.

Patient information is kept in a database. Patients are asked to fill out electronic questionnaires; their answers are automatically sent to the database. The system generates automatic alerts to remind the dentist of any health problems the patient may have. While examining the patient, all charting is done on the computer; cavities and periodontal health are electronically recorded. The CDSS automatically asks the dentist risk assessment questions; the program then classifies the patient's risk assessment. The CDSS then generates a treatment plan for the particular patient. It also informs the patient of specific risk factors, for example, smoking.

## DIAGNOSTIC TOOLS

A basic diagnostic tool is a clinical examination using a probe. This method is not completely accurate. More cavities are found by X-rays than by traditional exams.

### X-Rays

Traditional X-rays have been used for more than 100 years to diagnose cavities. X-rays are more effective than clinical examination. X-rays can be used because as the mineral content of the tooth decreases, the X-ray shows the cavity as darker.

The dentist must then interpret the X-ray correctly. This is not a foolproof method of diagnosis and may not detect cavities at an early stage when minimal intervention is necessary.

## Digital Radiography

As an aid in diagnosis, digital X-rays have some advantages. They take less time and expose the patient to 60 to 90 percent less radiation (Figures 9.6, A–C ▶). There is a cost savings on film and processing. Dentists will no longer have to store film. The image needs no developing, and the image can be viewed immediately on a monitor, by both the dentist and the patient. The dentist can also enhance the image. The patient can see the digital image more clearly than a small film, and aspects of the digital X-ray can be enhanced to show specific problem areas. Computers can be used to scan X-ray images into a patient's digital file. Like the traditional X-ray, the digital X-ray also needs interpretation. Several studies, however, have found no significant differences in diagnosis between digital and traditional imaging.

## Cone Beam Computed Tomography Scanner

**Cone beam CT (CBCT) scanners** produce accurate three-dimensional images. They use a cone-shaped beam. Digital processing produces a "virtually distortion-free 3-D image." Although the use of this technology is controversial—critics maintain that all the positive reviews are from people and groups with a financial interest in the technology[18]—some dentists are using CBCT scanners for planning dental implants, planning extractions, orthodontia, to finding periodontal defects, and, in endodontics, to measuring root canals and their configuration. CBCT imaging is also used in maxillofacial surgery, and to find bony defects in the temporomandibular joint, and to study sinuses.[19]

Those who support the use of CBCT scanners point to lower cost, more patients served in less time, and better images. They also maintain that the patient is exposed to less radiation than in conventional scans.[20] However, "A report in the *British Journal of Radiology* last year concluded

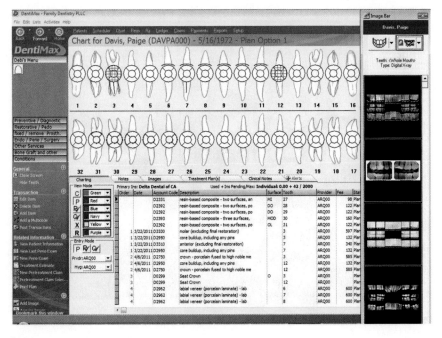

▶ **Figure 9.6**   (A) Digital image of patient's teeth.
*Source:* Courtesy of DentiMax.

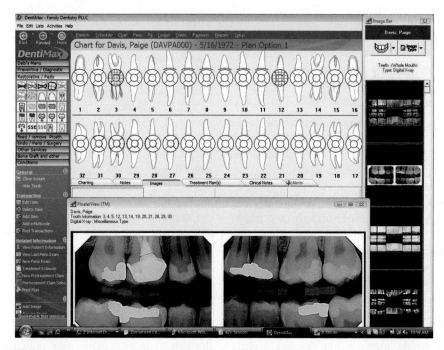

▶ **Figure 9.6** (B) Digital image of patient's teeth.
*Source:* Courtesy of DentiMax.

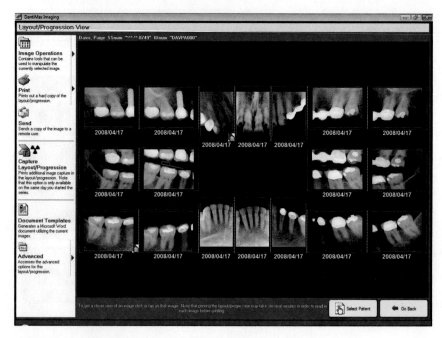

▶ **Figure 9.6** (C) Digital image of patient's teeth.
*Source:* Courtesy of DentiMax.

that cone-beam CT scans produced 'significantly higher' levels of radiation than conventional dental imaging. The standard orthodontic scan for the i-CAT produces five times as much radiation as a 2-D panoramic scan, said Dr. Ludlow, the North Carolina radiation researcher. Depending upon the model and setting, other scanners produce 4 to 67 times as much as conventional X-rays, he added."[21] More and objective studies are needed.

### Electrical Conductance

**Electrical conductance** is also currently used to diagnose cavities. An electric current is passed through a tooth, and the tooth's resistance is measured. A decayed tooth has a different resistance reading than a healthy tooth. Studies differ on the accuracy of this method, but tend to rate it high in detecting substantial cavities, but not early lesions.

### Other Methods

Traditional clinical exams and X-rays can detect cavities only after they are somewhat advanced. New methods use light to attempt to identify cavities earlier. Studies disagree on their effectiveness. New techniques have also been developed to stop demineralization, which occurs with caries; however, the success of these treatments is not yet known.

LIGHT ILLUMINATION Several methods use light to help diagnose tooth disease. These show promise in diagnosing early lesions. To find decay, a bright light is used to illuminate the tooth, revealing color differences. Decay looks darker because the light is absorbed when a cavity changes the structure of enamel.

**Fiber optic transillumination** found early lesions (affecting enamel) but was limited in diagnosing advanced caries.

**Digital imaging fiber optic transillumination (DIFOTI®)** involves using a digital camera to obtain images of teeth illuminated with laser light. The images are analyzed using computer algorithms. "They showed a direct correlation . . . between loss of fluorescence and the presence of caries . . . [and] a quantitative correlation of that loss and the amount of caries present."[22]

DIFOTI® can find cavities developing behind metal fillings that X-rays would not diagnose.

**Intraoral fiber optic cameras** allow both patient and dentist to get a close-up tour of the patient's mouth. A fiber optic device is aimed at an area of the patient's mouth, and the image appears on the screen. The image can be magnified to show problems, such as small cracks, which might otherwise remain unnoticed until the tooth breaks.

## LASERS IN DENTISTRY

**Laser** stands for **light amplification by stimulated emission of radiation**. Lasers deliver light energy. Depending on the target, the light travels at different wavelengths. Each target absorbs one wavelength and reflects other wavelengths, so each instrument is different. There are several uses of lasers in dentistry. Low-level lasers can find pits in tooth enamel that may become cavities. The Food and Drug Administration (FDA) has approved laser machines for drilling and filling cavities; lasers also reduce the bacteria in the cavity.

Minimally invasive dentistry uses lasers. When surgical lasers are used in place of drills, they burst cells by heating them. One laser works on hard tissue, another on soft tissue. Lasers can quickly harden the material used to fill the tooth, reducing the time a filling takes to complete. Lasers cannot be used where previous fillings or crowns exist.

Lasers are used by periodontists; they can reshape the gums. They can also be used to remove bacteria from periodontal pockets. However, their use is limited in root canal therapy. The FDA has approved one laser for treating root canals. Lasers can be used in some instances to help clean out the root canal and to remove bacteria. However, they can only be used in straight canals because the instruments are glass and do not bend. If the temperature is too high, the canal space can be charred, and the tooth and surrounding tissue can be damaged.

Lasers also have uses in cosmetic dentistry. Dentists can apply whitening solutions to teeth and activate the solutions using lasers. This can cause the tooth to lighten in a very short time.

## MINIMALLY INVASIVE DENTISTRY

**Minimally invasive dentistry** emphasizes prevention and the least possible intervention. Teeth are constantly affected by acids, which **demineralize** the surfaces. Early lesions beneath the enamel can be treated with calcium, phosphate, and fluoride, which help **remineralize** teeth. Preventive measures include antibacterial rinses and toothpastes, fluoride, diet, sealants, and the use of sugarless gum to increase saliva. The widespread use of fluoride has strengthened tooth enamel but not the dentin. Many cavities that appear in X-rays, are simply not found by traditional clinical examination. Cavities often appear in hard-to-see fissures in a tooth. Sealants may be used as a preventative measure. If a cavity is there, minimally invasive techniques may be used to prepare the tooth. Air abrasion can remove small amounts of a tooth; it involves aiming high-speed particles at the tooth. It can be used for the removal of cavities, for removal of defects in the enamel, and to detect cavities in fissures by opening them for inspection. It is relatively painless. It removes less of the tooth than a traditional drill.

Minimally invasive dentistry also makes use of lasers. The laser vaporizes decay by directing a stream of light at the affected area. The lasers are so precise that they affect only the decay, not the tooth. Very few patients require pain medication, and those who do are sensitive to the cold water used, not the laser. The machine is much more expensive than the conventional drill, but it allows fillings to be done so quickly that many more patients can be treated.

## SURGERY

Computers play a part in dental surgery, from the delivery of anesthesia to the planning and creation of dental implants. Computerized monitoring devices can keep track of a patient's vital signs. For patients requiring implants, software can create a three-dimensional view of the patient: This allows the dentist to see the exact relationship of the planned implant to the patient's bone. The surgery can be done as a simulation; dental CT scans allow the surgeon to rotate the implant on the screen so that by the time the patient is operated on, the surgery is planned down to the last detail. The software can measure bone density from the image and predict whether or not bone grafts will be needed. Procedures take less time and are easier for both patient and dentist.

The latest surgical alternative does not use scalpels. It is radiosurgery. According to the Academy of General Dentistry, "radiosurgery is a technique that uses radio waves to produce a pressureless, bloodless incision instead of knives." It is used for the following procedures: cosmetic surgery (to heat bleaching agents), gum surgery, root canal therapy, the removal of a muscle that grows between the two front teeth, and biopsies. There is no bleeding, and healing is faster.[23]

## THE GROWTH OF SPECIALIZATION

In the last quarter of the 20th century, only 10 percent of dentists were specialists. By 2004, 22 percent of dentists were specialists.[24] This is expected to rise to about 30 percent. This is due in part to the decrease in the number of dentists trained, whereas the number of specialists trained remains constant, so that specialists form a greater proportion. It is also because of changing demographics. As life expectancy increases and dental health improves, more affluent patients who feel they need to be attractive will seek cosmetic dentistry. With the aging population, some dentists will specialize in geriatrics. New technologies that allow dental problems to be diagnosed and treated earlier will result in dentists who specialize in diagnostics. Group practices may increase. In 2000, 108 million people in the United States lacked dental insurance. This number remained the same in 2010. Twenty-five million children in the United States go without dental insurance. Many dental plans fail to adequately cover some procedures such as dental implants.[25] However, there is the possibility of the inclusion of dental services under health maintenance organizations (HMOs), which will expect preventive care and economical service. Patients may educate themselves via the Internet and expect more from their dentists.

## TELEDENTISTRY

**Teledentistry** programs have been developed to help dentists access specialists, improving patient care. One system uses the Internet and requires a computer and digital camera.

The general dentist can e-mail a patient's chart, including images, to the specialist who can suggest both diagnosis and treatment. This saves the patient time and travel and gives her or him access to expert advice.

# IN THE NEWS

According to "Radiation Worries for Children in Dentists' Chairs" by Walt Bogdanich and Jo Craven McGinty published on November 22, 2010, in *The New York Times*, dentists are using equipment that emits higher levels of radiation than necessary; and they are using it with children, who are more likely to be affected by radiation.

Although children are more susceptible to the harmful effects of radiation than adults, many dentists' offices still use old-fashioned X-ray film, which emits more radiation than necessary. Some dentists are also using a new technology called a cone-beam CT scanner. The cone-beam CT scanner exposes the patient to more radiation than an X-ray. Although the manufacturers of the device say that it is safe, there is no independent confirmation of this claim. The manufacturers sponsor conferences and have even financed an issue of the *Journal of the American Dental Association* that dealt with the cone beam scan. Although one of the

articles in the journal stated that the cone beam scan was equivalent to an airport scan, independent researchers contend that it emits hundreds of times more radiation.

According to Keith Horner, a professor of oral radiology at the University of Manchester in Britain, who is coordinating a study of cone beam scanners for the European Commission, "All these different cone-beam CT scanners came out to a world that was unprepared. . . . They are just pushed out there by manufacturers with the message that a 3-D image is always going to be better than a 2-D image, and that isn't the case."

Digital cameras can also be used to create a three-dimensional image. They use no radiation but are not as fast as a cone beam scanner. Cone beam scanners are not regulated in most states, and when they are, they do not measure the radiation absorbed by patients.

# Chapter Summary

Computers are used in all aspects of dentistry, from educating dentists and patients to helping in surgery.

- The electronic patient record may standardize the dental chart and integrate the practice by including all of a patient's information, including financial, insurance, and clinical information.

- Changing demographics and improved dental health for most children have combined to change the tasks performed by dentists.

- Computer technology is making the tools used by periodontists, endodontists, and surgeons more precise.

- Traditional diagnostic tools are being supplemented by methods based on digital technology and fiber optics.
- Minimally invasive dentistry emphasizes prevention and the least possible intervention.
- Computers play a role in dental surgery, from delivering anesthesia to monitoring a patient's vital signs.
- Lasers are used in many branches of dentistry.
- More and more dentists are specializing in a particular field.
- Teledentistry can deliver expert consults, especially during surgery, at a distance.
- Some experts are concerned about the exposure of children to excess radiation.

# Key Terms

bonding

clinical decision-support systems (CDSS)

cone beam CT (CBCT) scanners

cosmetic dentistry

demineralize

dental implants

dental informatics

DentSim

digital imaging fiber optic transillumination (DIFOTI)

electrical conductance

electronic dental chart

endodontics

fiber optic camera

fiber optic transillumination

intraoral fiber optic cameras

laser (light amplification by stimulated emission of radiation)

minimally invasive dentistry

periodontics

remineralize

teledentistry

WAND

# Review Exercises

## Multiple Choice

1. The _____ is analogous to the endoscope used in surgery.
   a. digital X-ray
   b. laser
   c. fiber optic camera
   d. None of the above

2. _____ is the dental specialty that diagnoses and treats diseases of the pulp.
   a. Periodontics
   b. Endodontics
   c. Cosmetic dentistry
   d. Digital dentistry

3. _____ is the dental specialty that diagnoses and treats diseases of the gums.
   a. Periodontics
   b. Endodontics
   c. Cosmetic dentistry
   d. Digital dentistry

4. _____ is the dental specialty concerned with smile makeovers.
   a. Periodontics
   b. Endodontics
   c. Cosmetic dentistry
   d. Digital dentistry

5. _____ emphasizes prevention and the least possible intervention.
   a. Periodontics
   b. Endodontics
   c. Cosmetic dentistry
   d. Minimally invasive dentistry

6. _____ can find cavities developing behind metal fillings.
   a. Traditional examination
   b. DIFOTI
   c. Traditional X-rays
   d. Digital X-rays

7. _____ found early lesions (affecting enamel) but was/were limited in diagnosing advanced caries.
   a. X-rays
   b. Magnetic resonance imaging
   c. CT scans
   d. Fiber-optic transillumination

8. _____ can remove small amounts of a tooth; it involves high-speed particles aimed at the tooth.
   a. DIFOTI
   b. Light illumination
   c. Air abrasion
   d. None of the above

9. _____ deliver(s) light energy. Depending on the target, the light travels at different wavelengths.
   a. Lasers
   b. X-rays
   c. Air abrasion
   d. All of the above

10. One study traced the high number of cavities in poor children to _____ .
    a. increased lead levels in the children's blood
    b. shortages in calcium
    c. shortages in vitamin C
    d. All of the above

## True/False

1. Some orthodontics is performed via teledentistry. The technician is with the patient, and the clinician directs the technician from afar. _____
2. Dental health in general has improved over the last century. _____
3. Teeth are constantly affected by acids, which demineralize the surfaces. _____

4. The percentage of dentists who are specialists is not expected to rise. _____
5. The change in the conditions for which people seek dental care is related to demographic changes. _____
6. The laser vaporizes decay by directing a stream of light at the affected area. _____
7. The earliest application of information technology in the dentist's office was administrative—related to bookkeeping and accounting. _____
8. Lasers can always be used to help clean out a root canal and to remove bacteria. _____
9. Lasers are used in cosmetic dentistry. _____
10. Traditional clinical exams and X-rays can detect cavities only after they are somewhat advanced. _____

## Critical Thinking

1. What are the primary functions of computer technology in the dentist's office? In your answer, refer to clinical, administrative, and special-purpose applications.
2. How do you envision dentistry 10 years from now?
3. How would you address the need for proper dental care for children who are disadvantaged?
4. What methods would you incorporate to educate people about good oral health care?
5. How would you close the gap between the poor, health care-deficient populace and the affluent, who can afford proper, regular dental care?
6. With an aging population, dentistry will have to reflect the demand for cosmetic surgery. Do you think that insurance should cover this? Why or why not?

# Notes

1. M. Kirshner, "The Role of Information Technology and Informatics Research in the Dentist-Patient Relationship," December 2003, http://adr.sagepub.com/content/17/1/77.full.pdf (accessed May 4, 2011).
2. "Virtual Toothache Helps Student Dentists," July 24, 2008, http://www.sciencedaily.com/releases/2008/07/080721114604.htm (accessed May 4, 2011).
3. A. Welk, C. Splieth, M. Rosin, B. Kordass, and G. Meyer, "DentSim - A Future Teaching Option for Dentists," [Abstract] *International Journal of Computerized Dentistry* 7, no. 2 (April 2004): 123–30, http://www.ncbi.nlm.nih.gov/pubmed/15516090 (accessed May 4, 2011); J. S. Rees, S. M. Jenkins, T. James, et al., "An Initial Evaluation of Virtual Reality Simulation

in Teaching Pre-clinical Operative Dentistry in a UK Setting," [Abstract] *European Journal of Prosthodontics and Restorative Dentistry* 15, no. 2 (June 2007): 89–92, http://www.ncbi.nlm.nih.gov/pubmed/17645072 (accessed May 4, 2011); J. A. Buchanan, "Experience with Virtual Reality-Based Technology in Teaching Restorative Dental Procedures," [Abstract] *Journal of Dental Education* 68, no. 12 (December 2004): 1258–65, http://www.ncbi.nlm.nih.gov/pubmed/15576814 (accessed May 4, 2011).

4. "Upcoming Standards Meetings to Eye Electronic Health Records, Imaging and Dental Products," January 3, 2011, http://www.ada.org/news/5187.aspx (accessed May 4, 2011).

5. S. Carpenter, "Lead and Bad Diet Give a Kick in the Teeth—Poor Children Are Most Susceptible to Lead Toxicity," June 26, 1999, http://www.highbeam.com/doc/1G1-55165309.html (accessed May 4, 2011).

6. "Oral Health: Preventing Cavities, Gum Disease, Tooth Loss, and Oral Cancers: At a Glance 2010," February 19, 2010, http://www.cdc.gov/chronicdisease/resources/publications/aag/doh.htm (accessed May, 4, 2011).

7. "TIGR Scientists Complete the First Genome Sequence of an Oral Pathogen Associated with Severe Adult Periodontal Disease," June 12, 2001, http://www.JCVI.org (accessed May 4, 2011); Christoph Schaudinn, Amita Gorur, Duane Keller, Parish P. Sedghizadeh, and J. William Costerton, "Periodontitis, an Archetypical Biofilm Disease," August 1, 2009, http://jada.ada.org/content/140/8/978.abstract (accessed May 4, 2011).

8. Jennifer Garvin, "Study Links Tooth Loss, Heart Disease," 2009, http://dentalimplants-usa.com/conditions/heart1.html (accessed May 4, 2011); "Tooth Loss Could Be Sign of Heart Disease," May 4, 2011, http://www.dailymail.co.uk/health/article-190811/Tooth-loss-sign-heart-disease.html (accessed May 4, 2011).

9. Nicholas Bakalar, "Gum Disease Is Linked to Rates of Early Birth," October 11, 2005, http://query.nytimes.com/gst/fullpage.html?res=9501EEDD163FF932A25753C1A9639C8B63 (accessed May 4, 2011).

10. "What Is Periodontitis?" May 4, 2011, http://www.news-medical.net/health/What-is-Periodontitis.aspx (accessed May 4, 2011).

11. "Link Found between Periodontal Disease and Pancreatic Cancer," January 16, 2007, http://www.hsph.harvard.edu/news/press-releases/2007-releases/press01162007b.html (accessed May 4, 2011).

12. Jay Adlersberg, "Gum Disease and Diabetes," March 29, 2010, http://abclocal.go.com/wabc/story?section=news/health&id=7356664 (accessed May 4, 2011).

13. Charles M. Cobb, "Lasers in Periodontics: A Review of the Literature," [Abstract] April 2006, http://www.ncbi.nlm.nih.gov/pubmed/16584335 (accessed May 4, 2011).

14. Chapel Lane, "The Facts and Fiction about Cosmetic Dentistry," April 10, 2010, http://articles.everyquery.com/articles-the-facts-and-fiction-about-cosmetic-dentistry-24034.html (accessed May 4, 2011).

15. "3D Dental Implants: Prosthodontists Devise Technique to Insert Dental Implants in a Single Surgery," October 1, 2007, http://www.sciencedaily.com/videos/2007/1011-3d_dental_implants.htm (accessed March 2, 2011).

16. Alton Bishop, Randol Womack, and Mitra Derakhshan, "An Esthetic and Removable Orthodontic Treatment Option for Patients: Invisalign," *Dental Assistant*, September–October 2002, http://www.invisaligncec.jp/research/pdfs/WomackReprint.pdf (accessed May 4, 2011).

17. Eneida Mendonca, "Clinical Decision Support Systems: Perspectives in Dentistry," *Journal of Dental Education* 68, no. 6 (2004): 589–97, http://www.jdentaled.org/cgi/content/full/68/6/589 (accessed May 4, 2011).

18. Walt Bogdanich and Jo Craven Mcginty, "Radiation Worries for Children in Dentists' Chairs," November 22, 2010, http://www.nytimes.com/2010/11/23/us/23scan.html (accessed March 23, 2011).

19. "From the Dental Advisor: Cone Beam CT Scanners," February 16, 2010, http://www.dentistryiq.com/index/display/article-display.articles.dentistryiq.clinical.2010.02.From-THE-DENTAL-ADVISOR_-Cone-beam-CT-scanners.html (accessed March 23, 2011).

20. Ibid.

21. Bogdanich and Mcginty, "Radiation Worries for Children in Dentists' Chairs."

22. Kevin E. Smith, "Caries Detection: At Best an Inexact Science: Part II," *Global Dental Newsjournal*, 2000, http://www.global-dental.com/clinical.html (accessed May 4, 2011).

23. Academy of General Dentistry, "Blade-Free Radiosurgery Offers New Cosmetic Surgery," 2006, http://www.smile-science.net/dental_information/blade_free_radio_surgery_offers.htm (accessed May 4, 2011).

24. Eric Solomon, "The Future of Dentistry," November 2004, http://www.globusdental.com/thefutureofdentistry (accessed May 4, 2011).

25. Jessica Gorman, "The New Cavity Fighters," *Science News*, August 19, 2000, http://findarticles.com/p/articles/mi_m1200/is_8_158/ai_65301573/ (accessed May 4, 2011); Sharon Bell, "The Bad Side of Dental Tourism," 2011, http://www.streetdirectory.com/travel_guide/110409/dental_surgery/tha_bad_side_of_dental_tourism.html (accessed May 4, 2011).

# Additional Resources

"3D Dental Implants: Prosthodontists Devise Technique to Insert Dental Implants in a Single Surgery." October 1, 2007. http://www.sciencedaily.com/videos/2007/1011-3d_dental_implants.htm (accessed March 2, 2011).

Alipour-Rocca, L., V. Kudryk, and T. Morris. "A Teledentistry Consultation System and Continuing Dental Education via Internet." *Journal of Medical Internet Research* 1 (1999). http://www.ncbi.nlm.nih.gov/pmc/articles/PMC1761814/ (accessed May 4, 2011).

American Association of Cosmetic Dentists. "Seniors Benefit from Cosmetic Dentistry." June 3, 2002. http://www.aacdaccreditation.net/index.php?module=cms&page=91&CTGTZO=-420&CTGTZL=-480 (accessed May 4, 2011).

Angier, Natalie. "Dentistry, Far Beyond Drilling and Filling." August 5, 2003. http://www.nytimes.com/2003/08/05/science/dentistry-far-beyond-drilling-and-filling.html (accessed May 4, 2011).

Bell, Sharon. "The Bad Side of Dental Tourism." 2011. http://www.streetdirectory.com/travel_guide/110409/dental_surgery/tha_bad_side_of_dental_tourism.html (accessed May 4, 2011).

Bogdanich, Walt, and Jo Craven Mcginty. "Radiation Worries for Children in Dentists' Chairs." November 22, 2010. http://www.nytimes.com/2010/11/23/us/23scan.html (accessed March 23, 2011).

Clark, Glenn T. "Teledentistry: Genesis, Actualization, and Caveats." *Journal of the California Dental Association* (2000). http://www.cda.org/library/cda_member/pubs/journal/jour0200/intro.html (accessed May 4, 2011).

Delrose, Daniel C., and Richard W. Steinberg. "The Clinical Significance of the Digital Patient Record." *Journal of the American Dental Association* 131 (June 2000): 57s–60s.

Diagnosis and Management of Dental Caries. "Summary." Evidence Report/Technology Assessment: Number 36. AHRQ Publication No. 01-E055. February 2001. http://archive.ahrq.gov/clinic/epcsums/dentsumm.htm (accessed May 4, 2011).

Douglas, Chester W., and Cherilyn Sheets. "Patients' Expectations of Oral Health in the 21st Century." *Journal of the American Dental Association* 131 (June 2000): 3s–7s.

Dove, S. Brent. "Radiographic Diagnosis of Dental Caries." August 29, 2003. http://www.jdentaled.org/cgi/reprint/65/10/985.pdf (accessed May 4, 2011).

Drisco, Connie H. "Trends in Surgical and Nonsurgical Periodontal Treatment." *Journal of the American Dental Association* 131 (June 2000): 31s–38s.

Forrest, J. L., and S. A. Miller. "Evidence-Based Decision Making in Action: Part 1—Finding the Best Clinical Evidence." [Abstract] *Journal of Contemporary Dental Practice* 3, no. 3 (2002). http://www.ncbi.nlm.nih.gov/pubmed/12239574 (accessed May 4, 2011).

"From the Dental Advisor: Cone Beam CT Scanners." February 16, 2010. http://www.dentistryiq.com/index/display/article-display.articles.dentistryiq.clinical.2010.02.From-THE-DENTAL-ADVISOR_-Cone-beam-CT-scanners.html (accessed March 23, 2011).

Garvin, Jennifer. "Study Links Tooth Loss, Heart Disease." 2009. http://dentalimplants-usa.com/conditions/heart1.html (accessed May 4, 2011).

Glickman, Gerald N., and Kenneth Koch. "21st-Century Endodontics." June 2000. http://jada.ada.org/content/131/suppl_1/39S.abstract (accessed May 4, 2011).

Kurtzweil, Paula. "Dental More Gentle with Painless 'Drillings' and Matching Fillings." *FDA Consumer*, May–June, 1999. http://findarticles.com/p/articles/mi_m1370/is_3_33/ai_54612389/ (accessed May 4, 2011).

Lane, Chapel. "The Facts and Fiction about Cosmetic Dentistry." April 10, 2010. http://articles.everyquery.com/articles-the-facts-and-fiction-about-cosmetic-dentistry-24034.html (accessed May 4, 2011).

"Oral Health: Preventing Cavities, Gum Disease, Tooth Loss, and Oral Cancers: At a Glance 2010." February 19, 2010. http://www.cdc.gov/chronicdisease/resources/publications/aag/doh.htm (accessed May, 4, 2011).

Parks, E. T., and G. F. Williamson. "Digital Radiography: An Overview." *Journal of Contemporary Dental Practice* 3, no. 4 (2002): 23–39. http://www.thailanddentist.com/digital xray/kodak/rvg5000/digital%20radiography.pdf (accessed May 4, 2011).

Scanlon, Jessie. "Say Ahhh (and Watch the Monitor)." September 4, 2003. http://www.nytimes.com/2003/09/04/technology/say-ahhh-and-watch-the-monitor.html (accessed May 4, 2011).

Schneiderman, A., M. Elbaum, T. Shultz, S. Keem, M. Greenebaum, and J. Driller. "Assessment of Dental Caries with Digital Imaging Fiber-Optic Transillumination (DIFOTI): In Vitro Study." [Abstract] 1997. http://www.ncbi.nlm.nih.gov/pubmed/9118181 (accessed May 4, 2011).

Stabholz, A., R. Zeltser, M. Sela, et al. "The Use of Lasers in Dentistry: Principles of Operation and Clinical Applications." December 2003. http://www.ncbi.nlm.nih.gov/pubmed/14733160 (accessed May 4, 2011).

Stookey, George, and Carlos Gonzalez-Cabezas. "Emerging Methods of Caries Diagnosis." October 2001. http://www.ncbi.nlm.nih.gov/pubmed/11699969 (accessed May 4, 2011).

"Virtual Toothache Helps Student Dentists." July 24, 2008. http://www.sciencedaily.com/releases/2008/07/080721114604.htm (accessed May 4, 2011).

White, Joel M., and W. Stephen Eakle. "Rationale and Treatment Approach in Minimally Invasive Dentistry." June 2000. http://jada.ada.org/content/131/suppl_1/13S.full (accessed May 4, 2011).

# Related Web Sites

The National Oral Health Surveillance System (http://www.cdc.gov/nohss) links data from various state-based systems, including state oral health surveys and the Behavioral Risk Factor Surveillance System.

The State Dental Program Synopses (http://apps.nccd.cdc.gov/synopses/index.asp) present state population demographics and information about the activities and funding levels of state dental programs.

Centers for Disease Control and Prevention also manages the Data Resource Center (http://drc.hhs.gov), a joint project with the National Institute of Dental and Craniofacial Research, which assembles oral health data and other information needed to support research, policy development, and program evaluation.

PEARSON
**myhealthprofessionskit**™

Go to www.myhealthprofessionskit.com to access the Companion Web site created for this textbook. Simply select "Basic Health Science" from the choice of disciplines. Find this book and register to access self-assessment quizzes, flashcards, and more.

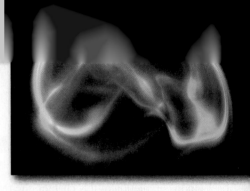

# Informational Resources: Computer-Assisted Instruction, Expert Systems, Health Information Online

- Review Exercises
- Notes
- Additional Resources
- Related Web Sites

## LEARNING OBJECTIVES

Upon completion of this chapter, the reader will be able to:

- List the many informational resources that computer technology and the Internet have made available and their use in the health care fields.
- Describe the use of computer-assisted instruction (CAI) in health care education.
- Discuss the Visible Human Project; many simulation programs use data from this project.
- Describe simulation programs, such as ADAM, that make use of text and graphics.
- Describe simulation programs that make use of virtual reality (VR) to teach surgical procedures, dentistry, and other skills.
- Define patient simulators.
- Be aware of the existence of distance learning programs in health care education.
- Discuss the role of expert systems, such as INTERNIST, MYCIN, and POEMS, in health care.
- Describe the resources on the Internet, including medical literature databases, physicians' use of e-mail, general information and misinformation, and support groups, and be able to discuss both the positive and negative consequences of using the Internet as a resource for health information.
- Describe health-related uses of smartphones and tablet computers.
- Discuss the availability of self-help software.
- Discuss the uses of computers in psychiatry.

## OVERVIEW

Computers and the Internet have made increasing amounts of information available to more people than in the past and have changed the way we teach and learn in many fields. Health care is no exception. Software exists to teach both providers and consumers of health care. The Internet makes vast stores of information available to patients and health care providers and can provide support for people with various illnesses. Self-help programs present information for consumers of health care. Databases, such as MEDLINE, and expert systems, such as MYCIN and INTERNIST, make the latest medical research easily available to health care professionals. The existence of these new informational resources has made it possible for health care professionals to learn in a variety of environments, via distance learning. These same developments have made it necessary for health care providers to be computer literate to take advantage of new and expanding sources of information.

## EDUCATION

### The Visible Human Project

The **Visible Human Project** is a computerized library of human anatomy at the National Library of Medicine (Figure 10.1, A and B ▶). It began in 1986 and is an ongoing project. It has created "complete, anatomically detailed, three-dimensional representations of the male and female human body." The images are accessible over the Internet. Hundreds of people have used these images on computer screens where they can be rotated and flipped and taken apart and put back together. Structures can be enlarged

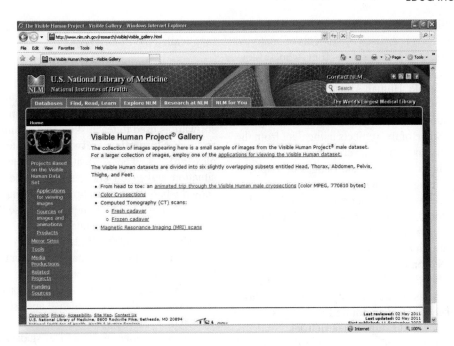

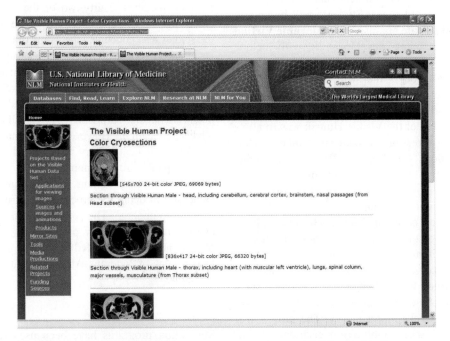

▶ **Figure 10.1** (A) The Visible Human Project gallery and (B) the Visible Human Project: Color Cryosections.
*Source:* (A) National Library of Medicine, http://www.nlm.nih.gov/research/visible/visible_gallery.html; accessed March 29, 2011; (B) National Library of Medicine, http://www.nlm.nih.gov/research/visible/photos. html; accessed March 29, 2011.

and highlighted. The images, also available on CD-ROM, have been used by students of anatomy, researchers, surgeons, and dentists who discovered a new face muscle. There is some speculation that the Visible Human's virtual cadavers may replace actual cadavers in medical education. The Visible Human is available for both teaching and research. Some of the projects using data from the Visible Human include several three-dimensional views of the human body and images of magnetic resonance imaging (MRI) and computed tomography (CT) scans. ADAM, a program that is used to teach anatomy, uses data from the Visible Human. The data provided by the Visible Human are the source for a virtual colonoscopy.

The National Library of Medicine is moving the project "From Data to Knowledge." Some current aspects of the Visible Human will allow users to see *and feel* anatomic flythroughs on the Web and to see surrounding structures. Students can use a wand to create three-dimensional structures from two-dimensional structures or from segmented slices. Students will be able to build and palpate organs. An **Explorable Virtual Human** is being developed. It will include authoring tools that engineers can use to build anatomical models that will allow students to experience how real anatomical structures feel, appear, and sound.

One goal of the Visible Human was to allow the use of three-dimensional anatomical models in education. The **Vesalius Project** (Columbia University) is creating these models (called maximal models) of anatomical regions and structures to be used in teaching anatomy.[1]

A project called the **Virtual Human Embryo** is digitizing some of the 7,000 human embryos lost in miscarriages that have been kept by the National Museum of Health and Medicine of the Armed Forces Institute of Pathology since the 1880s. An embryo develops in 23 stages over the first 8 weeks of pregnancy. The project will include at least one embryo from each stage. It will be sectioned and sliced. Each slice will be placed under a microscope, and digital images will be created. Users will be able to access the images on DVDs and CDs and manipulate and study them.

Images are now available in a mobile application (app) called the Embryo App.[2]

## Computer-Assisted Instruction

Computer-assisted instruction (CAI) is used at all stages of the educational process. Drill-and-practice software is used to teach skills that require memorization. **Simulation software** simulates a complex process. The student is presented with a situation and given choices. The student is then shown what effect that choice would have on the situation. Early simulation programs used text and graphics to describe a situation. Later, animation and sound were added. Today, some programs use virtual reality (VR) so that the student actually feels as if he or she were there.

What is the effect of CAI on education for health care professionals? A quantitative analysis was performed of 47 studies of the use of CAI in the health science professions in 1992. The studies all compared student performance in CAI with traditional teaching methods. Thirty-two of the studies concluded that CAI is superior. However, the analysis of the studies also concluded that some of the 47 studies jumped to conclusions that were unsupported by the data they collected. The statistical analysis concludes that CAI does have a "moderate-sized effect." A later review of literature on CAI found that computers are having "surprisingly . . . a small impact on medical education." However, it was found to be a helpful supplement in some areas of study.

Hospitals are beginning to use "electronic informed consent programs." The programs explain aloud and in detail the procedures that the patient is going to undergo. The patient can ask questions and receive answers. The patient is also informed of risks and benefits. **iMedConsent** is used at the Department of Veterans Affairs and at 190 U.S. hospitals.[3]

## Simulation Software

Simulation programs have been used for many years in nursing education. As early as 1963, computer-based nursing courses were developed using **PLATO (Programmed Logic for Automatic Teaching Operations)**. The student sat before her or his "television screen and . . . electronic keyset similar to . . . a standard typewriter" and was presented with hypothetical patients to evaluate, problems to solve, and questions to answer. The program used both text and graphics. It was judged to be successful in allowing students to progress at their own pace and in their own style of learning. At that time, most schools did not have the computers necessary to use these programs. Now computers are used throughout the educational system, and simulation programs are a taken-for-granted part of health care education. Programs such as **ILIAD** have been used for years and provide hypothetical cases for the student to evaluate. The student's diagnostic abilities are then compared to the computer's. **ADAM** teaches anatomy and physiology. It uses two- and three-dimensional images (some of them created from the Visible Human data) and has versions available for both patients and professionals. It is interactive, allowing the user to click away over 100 layers of the body and see more than 4,000 structures! Using multiple windows, the user can compare different views of one anatomical structure. A program called eXpert Trainer helps students learn the skills needed for minimally invasive surgery (MIS) (see Chapter 7).

## Virtual Reality Simulations

During the 1990s, several trends emerged to make VR surgical simulators possible. First, the Visible Human makes three-dimensional models possible. Second, "the rapid adoption of . . . minimally invasive procedures enabled surgeons to perform operations from outside the body and observe their actions on a video monitor." VR simulations can show exactly what the surgeon would see on the monitor. Third, haptic force-feedback systems allow the user to actually feel and manipulate objects in VR.[4]

The newest simulations use VR techniques, requiring the power of supercomputers. Simulations using VR can make medical education safer and more effective. They are particularly useful in teaching procedures, such as colonoscopies, which are guided by *haptic* clues (sense of feel) and where a mistake can seriously harm a patient (Figure 10.2 ▶).

Now, before a medical resident operates on a live patient, surgery can be simulated. Students can manipulate surgical instruments while watching a computer monitor. Motors in the instruments provide resistance so that the student learns how much pressure is required for a particular task (Figure 10.3 ▶).

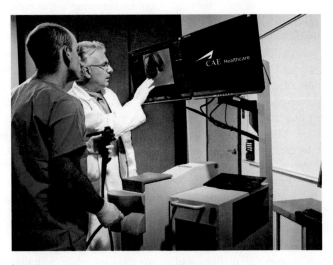

▶ **Figure 10.2** Simulation of a colonoscopy.
*Source:* CAE Endoscopy VR simulator. Reproduced by permission of CAE Healthcare. Copyright © 2011 CAE Healthcare. All rights reserved.

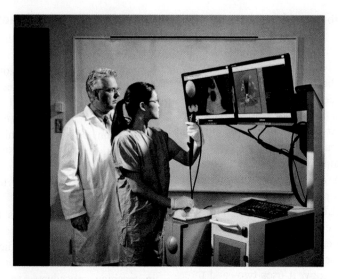

▶ **Figure 10.3** Simulation of a bronchoscopy.
*Source:* CAE Endoscopy VR simulator. Reproduced by permission of CAE Healthcare. Copyright © 2011 CAE Healthcare. All rights reserved.

Using a device developed by Dr. Thomas Krummel, of the Penn State College of Medicine, the student can "feel the operation in their hands as they see it on a computer screen". Dr. Krummel has developed another device using a mannequin and computer imaging, which allows medical students to practice inserting a bronchoscope into a child's trachea. Dr. Krummel has also designed a program to teach surgical skills to new students at Pennsylvania State. The school uses a four-step program, which first teaches skills and then uses a three-dimensional anatomical program. The third step is to perform the tasks learned while monitored by a computer. The last step involves performing the operation on a simulator that mimics the human body and its responses.

VR simulations are also being used to train surgeons to perform minimally invasive operations.[5] Because the surgeon operates in a restricted field that she or he cannot directly see, MIS requires extensive training. One MIS trainer (called **KISMET**) uses "a rough imitation of the . . . abdomen . . . [so] the trainee [can] manipulate the instruments in the usual way . . . . KISMET does all the necessary calculations and generates the virtual endoscopic view."[6] KISMET also allows the student to feel and see how soft tissue reacts to grasping and cutting in real time.

Simulations using VR are currently being developed to teach the administration of an epidural anesthetic, which requires the insertion of a catheter in the epidural space of the spinal column; the only guide is one's sense of feel. A mistake could leave a patient paralyzed. The epidural simulator allows the student to perform the procedure while feeling the resistance of the tissue, but without endangering a live patient. Students can learn to administer an intravenous (IV) injection from a simulation program instead of practicing on a rubber arm. "The student is able to sense the tactile response of needle and catheter insertion—from the 'pop' as the needle enters the skin through entry into the vein lumen." Simulations are also being used to help teach surgeons to operate on the prostate. As MIS becomes more common, VR simulators that mimic the sights, sounds, and feel of these procedures are being further developed. The Food and Drug Administration (FDA) approved the use of VR simulations to insert a catheter into the carotid artery.[7]

In dentistry, VR simulations make use of mannequins to allow students to practice filling cavities while watching both the mannequin and a monitor. The student feels the tooth via the instruments, learning to distinguish between a healthy and a diseased tooth. The student's work is immediately evaluated. The procedure can be repeated numerous times.

In 2002, researchers created the virtual stomach, a computer simulation. The stomach can be used to study how medications and nutrients decompose and are dispersed. Using the virtual stomach has already led to new knowledge: Tablets break down at the bottom of the stomach, and the density of the tablets is important to the speed with which they break down.

PATIENT SIMULATORS Human patient simulators (HPS) are programmable mannequins on which students can practice medical procedures (Figure 10.4, A–I▶). The simulator has liquids flowing through its blood vessels, inhales oxygen and exhales carbon dioxide, produces heart and lung sounds, and has eyes that open and close, pupils that dilate, and a tongue that can swell to simulate an allergic reaction. The student can perform an electrocardiogram, take the pulse, and measure blood pressure and temperature. Medications can be administered intravenously; the mannequin reads the barcode and reacts as it has been programmed to react. Students can practice intubations. They can learn needle decompression of pneumothorax; chest tubes may be inserted. Different kinds of patients can be simulated, including a healthy adult, a woman experiencing problems with pregnancy, and a middle-aged man suffering from hypertension. There are patient simulators built for specific medical training programs, such as nursing education or emergency care. **BabySim** teaches the skills needed to work with infants. Another mannequin, called **PediaSim**, is a virtual child. It can be programmed also, for instance, to have an allergic reaction to peanuts.

**iStan**, according to its manufacturer, METI, is "the first real breakthrough in medical mannequin technology in 30 years." It is completely wireless. It was designed around a human-like skeleton. Its arms, neck, spine, and hips move. Its skin looks and feels human. It can sweat, breathe, drool, cry, and bleed. Its eyes are "fully reactive." Patient sounds are clearer than in previous simulators. Procedures such as defibrillation, chest tube catheterization, and needle decompression can be performed on iStan. iStan comes with new patient monitoring software identical to a real patient monitor that is wireless and can run on a touch screen or tablet computer.[8]

In 2008, the American Board of Internal Medicine let cardiologists renew their board certification by performing procedures on Simantha. **Simantha** is a life-size patient simulator for cardiologists. The simulation includes monitors that mimic displays in angiographic suites and multimedia characters.[9]

These mannequins can be used in classrooms or in simulated emergency situations. A crowded corner of an emergency room can be simulated, with noise, time limits, and physical constraints for the student. This brings the simulation even

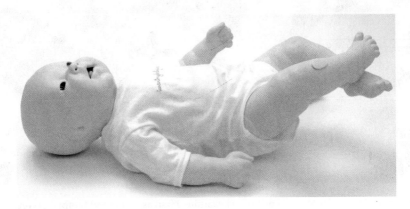

▶ **Figure 10.4** (A) BabySim.
*Source:* Courtesy of METI.

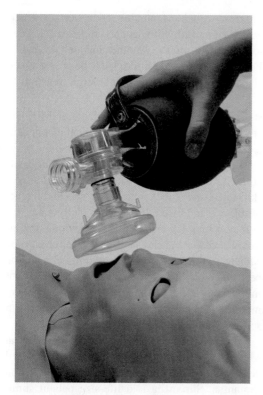

▶ **Figure 10.4**   (B) PediaSim.
*Source:* Courtesy of METI.

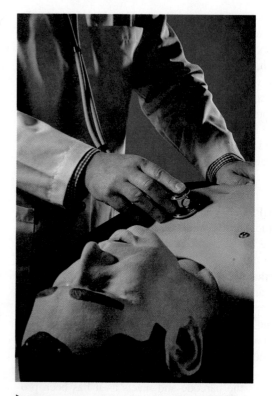

▶ **Figure 10.4**   (C) A doctor examines iStan.
*Source:* Courtesy of METI.

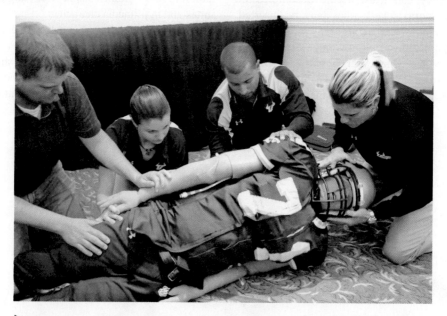

▶ **Figure 10.4**   (D) Medical personnel examine iStan as an injured football player.
*Source:* Courtesy of METI.

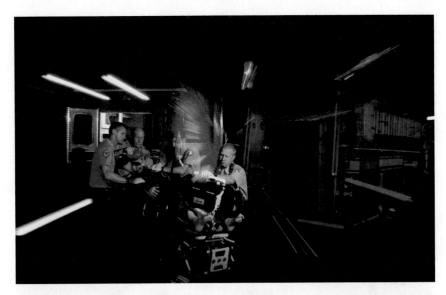

▶ **Figure 10.4**  (E) Emergency medical services (EMS) personnel treat METIman in a virtual emergency.
*Source:* Courtesy of METI.

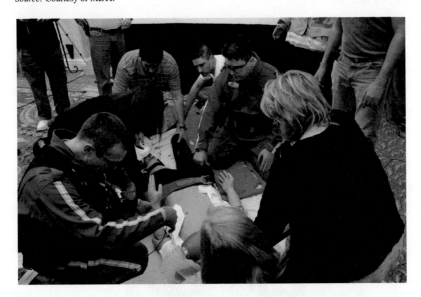

▶ **Figure 10.4**  (F) Medical personnel treat Airman METIman.
*Source:* Courtesy of METI.

closer to reality. **METI LiVE** lets the user create hospitals or disasters using several patient simulators. Patient simulators can be transferred virtually "from ER, to OR or ICU and create a real hospital environment or any health care environment with multiple patients in various stages of treatment, multiple points of care and multiple care givers."[10]

There are many patient simulators that focus on a particular type of patient and specific skills. The first childbirth simulator (not a VR simulator) was created in 1949; now there are several. There

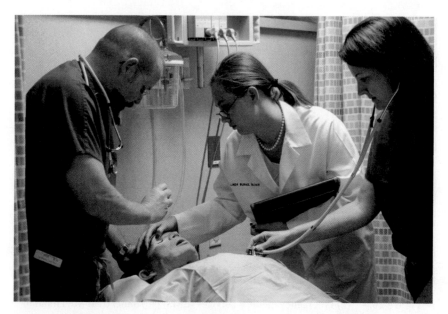

▶ **Figure 10.4** (G) Nurses examine METIman.
*Source:* Courtesy of METI.

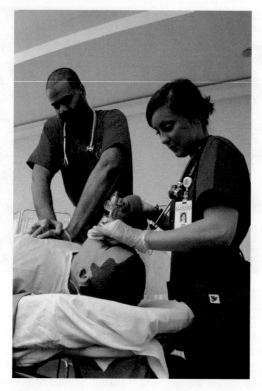

▶ **Figure 10.4** (H) Nursing students practice on METIman.
*Source:* Courtesy of METI.

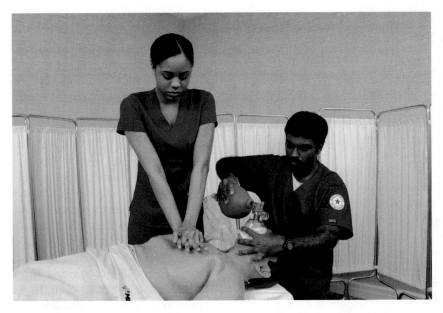

▶ **Figure 10.4** (I) Nursing students practice on METIman.
*Source:* Permission granted, Courtesy of METI.

are simulators for teaching laparoscopic and endoscopic procedures in interaction with models. PelvicExamSIM teaches medical students how to do pelvic exams. There are simulations of "heart attack, drug overdose, vehicular accidents, effects from weapons of mass destruction, [and] bio-terrorism."[11] SimMom is an interactive birthing simulator made by Laerdal, which also makes an infant CPR simulator.[12]

## Distance Learning

The expansion of information and telecommunications technology has made it possible to learn in a variety of settings—not just the traditional classroom. Distance learning refers to learning in an environment where student and instructor are not physically face-to-face. It may mean anything from simply picking up assignments on the Internet and e-mailing a paper to a professor, to a complete videoconference system where teacher and students see and hear each other via cameras, monitors, and microphones. Distance learning for health care professionals usually falls somewhere

in between. A course may use Internet resources, videotapes, and CD-ROMs, along with traditional textbooks and other printed material. Both health science institutions and the government have made educational resources available over the Internet. Through the Learning Center for Interactive Technology, the National Library of Medicine's Cognitive Science Branch provides links to databases, information, and tutorials for health care professionals, making it possible for them to continue learning wherever there is a computer with a link to the Internet. It also is attempting to expand the opportunities for distance learning for health care professionals and to link existing distance learning sites. Some traditional colleges and universities have degree programs at the graduate and undergraduate level in health sciences that do not require the student to be on campus, but do require self-discipline and access to a computer and the Internet. Public health workers may also learn via distance learning. The **Virtual Hospital** provides online courses for credit for health care professionals.

## DECISION SUPPORT: EXPERT SYSTEMS

An expert system (or computerized decision-support system) is an attempt to make a computer an expert in one narrow field. Both facts and rules about how the facts are used to make decisions in the field are entered in the computer. Expert systems are a branch of artificial intelligence, which examines how computers behave like human beings, that is, in "intelligent" ways. Expert systems have been used in medicine since the 1950s. They are meant to be decision-support systems, which help, but do not replace, medical personnel. They are especially useful when there is a limited, well-defined area of knowledge needed for a decision, which will be based on objective data. The doctor enters symptoms, test results, and medical history. The computer either asks for more information or suggests a diagnosis, and perhaps treatment. Some systems give the diagnosis in the form of a probability.

The computer can suggest conditions that the doctor has not thought of since medical school or has simply not considered. However, it is up to the health care professional to confirm the suggestion by tests. Although these systems are very helpful, they have their drawbacks. Each system is an expert in only one limited area. Expert systems may also spend time eliminating conditions that human experts would not even need to consider. However, with the amount of information available today, a computer's ability to organize is crucial.

Studies of diagnostic software have had mixed results. One study of emergency room patients with chest pain found a 97 percent accuracy rate for computers diagnosing heart attacks compared with a rate of 78 percent for doctors. A study of four programs found them to give correct diagnoses 50 to 75 percent of the time. In 1989, a trial using 31 undiagnosed cases compared the diagnosis of an expert system in the area of internal medicine, called QMR, to the best guess of the attending physician and found the following: The accuracy of the physician was 80 percent ompared with 85 percent for the expert system and 60 percent for the house staff.

One early medical expert system was developed at Stanford University in 1970. Called **MYCIN**, it aids in the diagnosis and treatment of bacterial infections. The doctor types in data about the patient's symptoms; the computer asks for more information until it has enough to suggest a diagnosis. The computer then asks about any drug sensitivities the patient might have, so that treatment may be suggested. MYCIN's diagnostic accuracy equals or surpasses that of human specialists. **INTERNIST** is another expert system developed at the University of Pittsburgh. It contains information about 500 diseases and their 2,900 associated symptoms. A newer expert system developed in England is called **Postoperative Expert Medical System (POEMS)**, which focuses on patients who become sick while recovering from surgery. The **Databank for Cardiovascular Disease** at Duke University is a highly specialized expert system that combines computer monitoring with extensive collections of information on cardiac patients.

Starting in 2009, doctors in New York State emergency departments can use a computer application containing "concise guidelines for starting prompt drug treatment that can reduce the risk of becoming infected" with human immunodeficiency virus (HIV). The guidelines include all relevant information and are constantly updated. This approach to HIV is called postexposure prophylactic treatment: It works to keep the infection localized by stopping the virus from multiplying. "The immune system can prevent it from entering the bloodstream." Clinical trials conclude that immediate drug treatment reduces the risk of infection by 80 percent.[13]

An interesting decision support system could in the near future come in the form of IBM's Watson. Watson could act as a computerized physician's assistant, a tool to digest and summarize information. Watson could look at all data including patient history, labs, articles, genomic data, and clinical data. It could digest and summarize a patient's records and see, for example, how specific treatments worked on similar patients.[14]

In October 1998, a review of decision-support systems was published in the *Journal of the American Medical Association* (*JAMA*).

The review looks at studies of the use of some of the systems during the past quarter century. The quality of expert systems varies. However, in certain areas, specifically drug use and preventive medicine, "these systems have been shown to improve physician performance and, less frequently, improve patient outcomes." Later studies have also had mixed results. They have found that decision-support systems prevent medication errors ("incorrect decisions"), but their effect on adverse drug events ("harm to patients") is not so clear. Outcomes were improved on the "use of deep vein thrombosis (DVT) prophylaxis." Results with diabetes were mixed. Diagnostic decision-support systems do remind doctors to consider more options and diagnoses.[15]

# HEALTH INFORMATION ON THE INTERNET

Both doctors and consumers who have access to it use the Internet as a source of health care information. Care should be used when searching for health information; the consumer is required to give personal information. This information is being mined for several purposes, including profiling the person most in need of a product or service. Several groups of health care professionals have created a suggested code of conduct for health-related Web sites: (1) that they disclose any information that consumers would find useful, including financial ties; (2) that they distinguish scientific information from advertising; (3) that they attempt to assure the high quality of information; and (4) that they disclose privacy risks and take steps to ensure privacy. Any health care professional giving advice or other information over the Web should abide by professional standards. The site needs to make it clear to consumers how they can get in touch with the site manager and should encourage feedback. Due to the concern over the reliability (or unreliability) of health information, a professor at the University of Minnesota created a site to rate newspaper and magazine health articles.[16]

Some sites, including medical literature databases, are specifically meant for health care professionals. Sixty percent of doctors surveyed said they found Internet information helpful. Many sites are directed to consumers. There are at least 10,000 health-related sites on the Web (excluding support groups). According to the Federal Trade Commission, "consumer online searches for health information are increasing dramatically."[17] Tens of millions of people log on to the Internet looking for information about medication and disease, suggested cures, and support groups. The Internet (with all of its misinformation) has some reliable sites, for example, Mayo's Symptom Checker,[18] providing good information.

It should be noted that access to health-related information on the Internet is not equally distributed throughout society, but is restricted to those with access to computers with an Internet connection and the knowledge to make use of them. The digital divide refers to the gap between information haves and have-nots. Whites and Asian-Americans, those with higher incomes, and those with higher education are more likely to have computer and Internet access than low-income people, less educated people, and African-Americans and Hispanics. People in rural areas have less access to the Internet than people in urban areas. A February 2002 report from the federal government maintained that the digital divide was disappearing quickly. The Bush Administration then lowered funding to government programs that supported community computing centers. However, a 2003 study by sociologist, Dr. Steven Martin at the University of Maryland, concluded that, "Computer ownership and Internet use may actually be spreading less quickly among poorer households than among richer households." Between 1998 and 2001, Internet use grew from 14 to 25 percent among families with annual incomes of less than $15,000; it grew from 59 to 79 percent among families with incomes greater than $75,000. The odds that a poor family would use the Internet grew by a factor of 2.1, whereas the odds for an affluent family grew by 2.6 percent. Dr. Martin predicts that it will be another 20 years before 90 percent of the poorest quarter of the population owns computers.[19]

By 2003, 61.8 percent of U.S. households owned computers, and of those, 87.6 percent were linked to the Internet. The percentage of households with broadband connections grew from 9.1 to 19.9 percent from 2001 to 2003. People with broadband connections are more likely to use the Internet than those with dial-up connections.[20] Although the digital divide is shrinking, it still persisted in 2006, according to a federal report. Race and ethnicity, family income, and education all influence Internet use among students. At school, among white students, 67 percent use the Internet; this compares to 58 percent of Asian-American, 47 percent of African-American and Native-American, and 44 percent of Hispanic students. At home, 54 percent of white students, 27 percent of African-American students, and 26 percent of Hispanic students use the Internet. The higher the family income, the more likely a student is to use the Internet (at home or in school). The more education a parent has, the higher is the Internet use. Lower use in some ethnic groups is tied to poverty.[21] However, many states have library networks that give people free online access to information.

In a Pew survey reported in *The New York Times* in March 2006, among adults age 18 and older, "74 percent of whites go online, 61 percent of African-Americans do and 80 percent of English-speaking Hispanic adults report using the Internet." This compares to the results of a similar study completed in 1998: 42 percent of white adults, 40 percent of Hispanic adults, and 23 percent of African-American adults reported using the Internet. Among adults, as well as among children, higher household income and education are correlated positively with Internet use. Age also correlates negatively with Internet use.[22]

In 2011, the digital divide still exists. According to a survey done by the Pew Internet Project at the end of 2009, 74 percent of all Americans age 18 and older use the Internet (79 percent of English-speaking adults). According to the study's director, "The gap hasn't tremendously shrunk. The disparity still exists even as more people are online." Sixty percent of American adults have a broadband connection, and 55 percent connect to the Internet wirelessly. However, Internet use is not spread equally through our society. The biggest differences are by age, income, and education. A later Pew report (2011) added health to the list of variables affecting Internet use. Ninety-three percent of adults between the ages of 18 and 29 use the Internet, whereas only 38 percent of those age 65 and over use the Internet. Sixty percent of people with household incomes of less than $30,000 per year use the Internet, whereas 94 percent of those with incomes of $75,000 and over do. Thirty-nine percent of people with less than a high school education use the Internet, whereas 94 percent of college graduates and those with advanced degrees use it.[23]

A Pew survey conducted in 2010 found that many Americans with disabilities lack access to the Internet: 81 percent of healthy adults use the Internet, compared with 62 percent of Americans with disabilities; 2 percent report that they have a disability that prevents them or makes it harder for them to use the Internet. Once online, however, those with an illness or disability are more likely to look up health-related information and use social media.[24]

## Medical Literature Databases

The capacity of computers to store and organize huge collections of data, to make the data accessible, and to transmit the data over telecommunications lines forms the basis of online medical literature databases. The National Library of Medicine provides a collection of computerized databases called **MEDLARS (Medical Literature Analysis and Retrieval System).** The 40 databases contain 18 million references. They are available free via the Internet and can be searched for bibliographical lists or for information.

**MEDLINE** is a comprehensive online database of current medical research including publications from 1946 to the present containing 18 million articles from 5,561 journals. Between 2005 and 2011, 2,000 to 4,000 references were added each Tuesday, Wednesday, Thursday, Friday, and Saturday. In 2010, almost 700,000 citations were added.[25] It has been used in hospitals for years. MEDLINE can be used for academic research or to help a doctor identify a patient's problem. Because

MEDLINE is updated almost daily, it gives access to the most up-to-date information to health care personnel. Although the information in MEDLINE is meant for professionals, some of its users are patients. **SDILINE (Selective Dissemination of Information Online)** contains only the latest month's additions to MEDLINE. Other MEDLARS databases include AIDSLINE, AIDSTRIALS, and CANCERLIT. DIRLINE is a guide to online information. MEDLARS also contains a database of "Images in the History of Medicine." It includes posters (Figure 10.5, A and B▶).

**CINAHL (Cumulative Index to Nursing and Allied Health Literature)** is a group of four databases specifically geared to the needs of nurses and other professionals in 17 allied health fields. This includes the fields of dental hygiene, occupational therapy, and radiology. CINAHL includes an index of 3,000 journals with 2.3 million records from 1982 to the present; bibliographic citations of books, pamphlets, software, and standards of practice; abstracts or full text of articles where they are available; journals; and descriptions of Web sites.

In 1998, the National Library of Medicine introduced MedlinePlus, which is meant for the general public (Figure 10.6▶). It contains information on more than 800 diseases and conditions. The information is selected using strict guidelines to guarantee accuracy and objectivity.

Databases of drug information are also online. **Medi-Span** is a collection of data on drug/drug and drug/food interactions. **Clinical Pharmacology** is a database for health care professionals, with the latest information on drugs. It also contains information for doctors to distribute to their patients. **New Medicines in Development** provides information on drugs that have been recently approved and those awaiting approval. **ClinicalTrials.gov** was launched in February 2000; it lists 105,168 clinical trials in 174 countries. It is searchable by disease and location—for

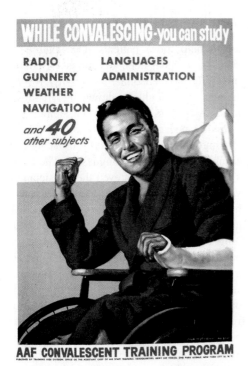

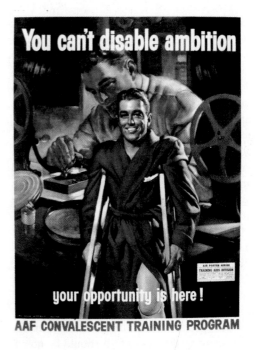

▶ **Figure 10.5** (A and B) Army and Air Force posters from the 1940s.
*Source:* Courtesy of the National Library of Medicine.

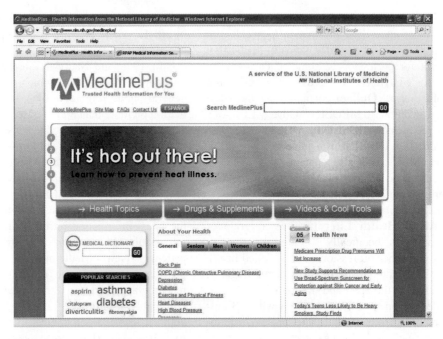

▶ **Figure 10.6** MedlinePlus is a database maintained for consumers.
*Source:* Courtesy of the National Institutes of Health.

example, cancer AND Los Angeles. In 2011, its pages were viewed 50 million times per month, with 65,000 daily visitors. "ClinicalTrials.gov offers up-to-date information for locating . . . clinical trials for a wide range of diseases and conditions. A clinical trial . . . is a research study in human volunteers to answer . . . health questions. Interventional trials determine whether experimental treatments or new ways of using known therapies are safe and effective under controlled environments. Observational trials address health issues in large groups of people or populations in natural settings."[26]

**CenterWatch** maintains a Web site that is a source of information on clinical trials for both patients and medical professionals. It includes a database of trials that are looking for volunteers, as well as information on completed trials and educational resources. It allows you to search for specific clinical trials and sign up for e-mails about specific trials.[27] It should be noted, however, that the purpose of drug trials is to test the effectiveness and safety of the medication,

not to help those patients participating in the trial. There have been questions raised regarding ethics and adequate safeguards for human subjects who might be drawn into participating in clinical trials by desperation stemming from illness or poverty. Only one-half of the people who participate in clinical drug trials are actually administered the drug being tested. The other half is given a placebo. Not even the physician knows which patient is receiving which substance. For those interested in the records of drugs that are already on the market, the U.S. FDA's Center for Drug Evaluation and Research maintains a site that provides information on the safety records of drugs and on drug companies and advertisement campaigns. Of course, you should judge information from the FDA as you would information from any other site, bearing in mind that much of the FDA's drug evaluation budget comes from the drug companies it oversees.

Although the existence of these resources is widely known, the effect of their use is not. A review of the literature on the use and effectiveness of electronic information retrieval systems was published in *JAMA* in October 1998. The study found that use is limited: Although "physicians have 2 unanswered questions for every 3 patients," they use a computer to search for information only "0.3 to 9 times per physician per month."[28] Further, "most searches retrieve only one fourth to one half of the relevant articles," and how the information retrieved is actually used is not known. A later study (2009) found a "high frequency of failure to attend to the CDS alerts and recommendations," and that clinical decision-support (CDS) systems are of limited use and effectiveness, but stated that when CDS systems are properly designed to fit into the work flow of those who will use them, they may have a positive impact on health care.[29]

## E-Mail

A majority of health care consumers who go online to search for advice would prefer information from their own doctors online. Many patients want to establish an e-mail connection with their own physicians. Not only is the information likely to be reliable, but some found an e-mail consultation less intimidating than a face-to-face meeting, enabling them to ask questions that they would not otherwise ask. Yet, few doctors make it available. Doctors express concerns with the time it would take to read and respond to e-mail, problems of liability, and issues of confidentiality and privacy. However, one 3-year study of a pediatric practice, which offered free e-mail as an option, found it was an effective way for doctors and patients and their families to communicate. In 33 months, a total of 1,239 e-mails were received from parents (81 percent) and health care providers (19 percent) alike. Some requested general information (69 percent); others had specific questions (22 percent). Most (87 percent) were answered immediately with suggested treatment and the recommendation to see a doctor. "On average, reading and responding to each e-mail took slightly less than 4 minutes."[30]

Other practices do not deal with e-mail in the same way. In a study of unsolicited e-mail, a fictitious patient sent e-mail to 58 dermatology Web sites around the world. Although the message asked for help with a problem that required attention immediately, only one-half of the sites responded. However, of those that responded, more than 90 percent recommended that the patient see a doctor, and 59 percent diagnosed the condition correctly. A questionnaire was sent to the sites that had responded: 28 percent said that they usually do not answer any patient e-mail. Only 24 percent said they answer e-mail communications individually.

In April 2002, a survey was conducted asking doctors and patients for their attitudes toward e-mail. It found that 90 percent of patients would like to exchange e-mail with their physicians, whereas only 15 percent of doctors do exchange e-mail with their patients. Doctors cite concerns with liability (a paper trail), privacy, time, the possibilities of misunderstanding, and the slowness of e-mail compared with conversation. The small percentage of doctors who provide e-mail state that patients are calmer when they know there is an open line to their physicians and therefore do not need to communicate as much. Some doctors who provide e-mail for their patients maintain that "no malpractice lawsuits . . . had been filed in which e-mail played a role."[31]

By 2013, the American Recovery and Reinvestment Act (ARRA) of 2009 calls for including secure e-mail between doctors and patients as part of the electronic health record (EHR). Although use of electronic health records and practice management software has increased over the past several years, the increase in the use of e-mail to communicate with patients is "modest . . . [with] little adherence to recognized guidelines." This remained true at least through 2006, before the ARRA was passed, according to a study published in the *Journal of Medical Internet Research*.[32]

The American Medical Association published guidelines for the use of e-mail between patient and physician. They include establishing a turnaround time; keeping copies of e-mails; discussing privacy with the patient and telling the patient who will read the e-mail; restricting e-mail to appropriate topics such as scheduling and prescription refills, not HIV status or mental health; requiring patients to put the subject of the e-mail on the subject line and their name and patient identification number in the e-mail; sending an automatic acknowledgement of receipt of the e-mail and having patients do the same; being able to save and retrieve e-mails; keeping a mailing list of patients but using blind copies to send group e-mails; avoiding libel; including the physicians name, contact information, and reminders of privacy concerns in each e-mail; and requiring that patients keep e-mails short.[33]

In a recent study, 4,203 physicians were surveyed about their use of e-mail. Only 16 percent used e-mail for patient communications, whereas only 2.9 percent used it frequently. A mere 6.7 percent followed at least half of the e-mail guidelines. Barely 1.6 percent followed all of the e-mail guidelines. Older doctors and those of Asian descent were less likely to use e-mail. Doctors in large (50+) practices and those who practiced in cities were more likely to use e-mail. E-mail was used more by surgeons and family physicians than by other doctors. The study found that doctors use e-mail to communicate with everybody but patients. Another study found that younger, female, university-based doctors were more likely to use e-mail than community-based physicians.[34] A 2007 study of e-mail between doctors and patients in seven countries in Europe had similar findings: 1.8 percent of the populations had requested prescriptions via e-mail; 3.2 percent had scheduled an appointment; and 2.5 percent had asked a question. In both the United States and European countries, patients wanted to be able to use e-mail to communicate with their doctors.[35]

In California, the Kaiser Permanente health system began using e-mail in 2004. By 2008, 35,423 patients and 3,092 doctors were using it. In one study, 630,807 e-mails (from March 2006 to December 2008) were analyzed and compared to the data of the year before. Patients initiated 85 percent of e-mail communication. Among patients with diabetes and/or hypertension who used e-mail, 2.4 to 6.5 percent "saw improvements . . . in blood sugar control and screening, cholesterol screening and control as well as screening for retinopathy and . . . kidney disease . . . . [M]ore patients with diabetes or hypertension alone

achieved blood pressure levels under 140/90." The more a patient e-mailed the doctor, the more the patient improved.[36]

## Self-Help on the Web

Tens of millions of adults search the Web for health-related information. Some people visiting health-related Web sites may just be doing academic research or seeking to learn. However, many are looking for a diagnosis, treatment, and cure. The numbers of sites either providing advice or linking to sites that provide advice are too numerous to list. Many sites include disclaimers stating in general that, although they attempt to include only accurate information, they are not responsible for the validity of the information presented. The disclaimer may further advise that a medical professional be consulted before any treatment is either started or discontinued. There are sites devoted to almost any disease, condition, treatment, and drug. You can find self-help for depression, stress, addiction, and almost any personal problem you can name. You do not even need to name your problem. One site shows you a human body and invites you to click where it hurts. You are then presented with a list of possible body parts and their possible diseases. If you continue to click, you will be linked to sites that can provide you with information and advice, from "how to treat your own . . . " to where to go for professional help.

Information is not the only online health-related resource. A possibly dangerous development is the availability of both prescription and nonprescription drugs on the Web. The sale of drugs over the Internet is virtually unregulated. A person can log on in one state, find a pharmacy in another state, and "consult" (over telecommunications lines) with a doctor, who will then write a prescription, which will be filled through the mail. The prescriptions are signed by physicians whose "examination" of the "patient" may consist of a review of a short questionnaire. This is illegal in some states. Under federal law "dispensing prescription drugs without a valid physician order is a violation of the FDCA [Federal Food, Drug, and Cosmetics Act]."[37] Nonprescription drugs are also available.

In 2010, Google launched its **Body Browser**. From an Internet window, the user can look into the human body, rotate it, and zoom in or out. The user can peel back layers and look at bones, muscles, or blood vessels. You can focus on one organ or the whole body.[38]

## Support Groups on the Web

The Web provides online support. There are support groups for hospitalized children, for people with cancer and other diseases, and for patients' families and caregivers. Newsgroups, e-mail discussion groups, and live chat groups are available that link people with health- or disease-related interests. **Starbright World** is a network linking 30,000 seriously ill children in 100 hospitals and many homes in North America. Children in the network can play games, chat, and send and receive e-mail. They can also get medical information. Children and teenagers suffering with asthma use Starbright World to discuss their experiences with others in similar situations.[39]

Support groups exist for virtually every illness. When Dr. Ken Mott, a public health physician, was diagnosed with cancer, he had to travel to receive the treatment he needed. Illness can be isolating. Being in a strange city can compound the isolation. But Dr. Mott, like many other patients, found support and community on the World Wide Web. "Physical disability and pain . . . physical and emotional isolation occur . . . [and] the . . . side effects of treatment . . . leave victims susceptible to depression and withdrawal. But on the Internet and through e-mail I find dimensions of communication for emotional and psychological support that you may not have imagined."[40] It is especially helpful for people with rare diseases. Takayasu arteritis occurs in between 1.2 and 2.6 people per million scattered over the world, making it virtually impossible to form face-to-face support groups. Yet, now the Internet is being used to build a community and disseminate information and give support.

For people isolated by illness or disability, special social networks may be their only social connections. Although these people are less likely to have Internet access, when they do access the

Internet, it may become their whole social world—a lifeline, according to a woman with multiple sclerosis. Some of the bigger patient networks include PatientsLikeMe, Health Central, Inspire, CureTogether, and Alliance Health Network. Diabetic Connect has 140,000 members. Other networks are started by patients and are much smaller. Nin was started by a person with lupus in 2008. Currently, it has 2,300 members. People use these networks to share experiences with others who know how they feel. Friends and doctors, unless they are living with disabilities, don't understand. The networks are used to share experiences, to get tips on coping with the disease, "to get a real-life perspective," and just "to interact with people without worrying about the stigma of the disease." The networks are clear that they are not a substitute for medical advice. However, a recent Pew study found that "just 2% of adults living with chronic disease report being harmed by following medical advice found on the Internet." According to some research, "emotions can be contagious." If the people on your network are negative about the disease, you can become negative; on the other hand, you can catch a positive attitude too.[41]

## Judging the Reliability of Health Information on the Internet

Anyone can offer information on the Web, with possibly dangerous results. A compliance officer at the FDA related one instance, "A physician was browsing the Web when he came across a site that contained a fraudulent drug offering . . . the person who maintains the site claimed he had a cure for a very serious disease, and advised those with the disease to stop taking their prescription medication. Instead they were told to buy the product he was selling, at a cost of several hundred dollars." Web sites can be run by anyone. More and more sites providing medical information are being operated by unidentified sources, vendors, and manufacturers; many sites are produced by patients. Judging the reliability of a Web site can be difficult. The U.S. Department of Health and Human Services has established a site called http://healthfinder.gov to help guide people toward reliable sources of information.

The American Medical Association advises users to judge Web sites as critically as they would judge printed information. The major concern of people using the Web for medical information is privacy. Even though most sites have stated privacy policies, a study found that most do not adhere to them. Users have no way of knowing this. The actual content of the site should be judged on the following criteria: Is there information on the author, and is the author reliable? Are the sources of information clear and reliable? Are the sources of funding revealed? Are there any conflicts of interest, for example, does the author or site receive money from any source interested in steering the user toward a particular treatment? Is the information up-to-date? Conflicts of interest bearing on money received from a drug or device company are the most important information to reveal. This does not necessarily make the information invalid. However, you should be very careful using that information and should find backup from another source.

Even reliable sites can provide partial information to doctors as well as to patients. According to one physician, the Web is as attractive to physicians as it is to patients. But even the best sites are incomplete at best. A MEDLINE search produces abstracts of articles, not the articles themselves. The abstract states the conclusion of a study, for example, that a heart drug was found to be effective, but that is not enough information. The abstract leaves out the necessary details: Who were the participants and how were they selected? What other medications were they taking? How was the data analyzed? Who designed and financed the study?

Reliable sites do exist. The Virtual Hospital was a comprehensive and authoritative site, maintained by the University of Iowa. The information it collected continues to be available on the Internet at http://www.uihealthcare.com/vh/. It provides information for patients and health care providers. Its information is provided by health care professionals. Material is presented in a multimedia format and is organized both by type of information (e.g., textbook) and by problem. A health care provider can read a chapter on upper respiratory conditions and view a video clip of the condition.[42] The Virtual Hospital provides information for

patients on disease prevention, including immunizations, diet, and cancer screening. Reliable information is also available through **Medscape**, which provides a collection of medical journals online.

## HEALTH-RELATED SMARTPHONE AND TABLET COMPUTER APPS

Some of the newest informational resources are smartphone and tablet computer apps (Figure 10.7▶). There are too many to mention here. Several apps have to do with fitness; they help you keep track of diet and exercise. Others help you keep track of the food, calories, and sugar you have consumed. Some allow you to calculate your body mass index, base metabolic rate, and blood alcohol level, and how many calories you are burning when you exercise. There are other apps that give you information on medications, inform you of whether or not your lab results are normal, and let you see what your symptoms could indicate. One allows you to give yourself an eye exam. Another examines drugs and their side effects. IHeartRate shows you your heart rate at any time. Fast Food calorie counter counts the calories in 9,000 fast foods available at 73 fast food establishments. Water Your Body shows you how much water you should drink per day and lets you keep track of how much you do drink. Health Remedy provides information on common illnesses. The Ovulation Calendar may help a woman become pregnant, after which

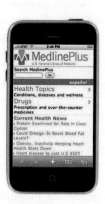

▶ **Figure 10.7**   MedlinePlus is available on mobile phones.
*Source:* Courtesy of the National Library of Medicine.

Ipregnant lets her calculate the due date. After the baby is born, Trixie Tracker keeps track of his or her sleeping and feeding. You can use KidsCheckup to see what your child's symptoms indicate—whether to go to the doctor or the emergency room; it also shows you where the hospital is. Brush Timer makes sure you are brushing your teeth long enough.[43]

Several smartphone apps deal with more serious health issues. One uses videos to show you what to do in various emergency situations, such as choking or having a cardiac episode. One app puts information on who to call in an emergency with phone numbers on your phone. It also lists your allergies. A Pocket First Aid Guide gives life-saving first aid information. Another can keep a history of your blood pressure. A similar app lets the user keep track of blood sugar.[44]

The T2 Mood Tracker, which was developed by the National Center for Telehealth and Technology (T2), was released by the Department of Defense. It allows soldiers and veterans to use their smartphones to "self-monitor their mental health and keep track of their moods and behaviors after a deployment." It is an electronic version of older pen and paper self-monitoring tools. It can be used alone or in conjunction with therapy. It keeps a record of emotional experience. It automatically generates graphs. Notes can be added on medications, stressors, and other events. Because the data belong to the user, the Health Insurance Portability and Accountability Act is not relevant.[45]

## SELF-HELP SOFTWARE

For those without an Internet connection, self-help software on CD-ROM provides information, suggests diagnosis and treatment, and may even act as a therapist for people with mild-to-moderate emotional problems, including stress, eating disorders, sexual dysfunction, and depression. Before attempting any self-treatment or taking any medication (even over-the-counter nonprescription medications) and before taking advice on the Internet, you should always check with your physician.

Family health guides on CD-ROM provide more information than a book and are easier to search.

The information you need is on your screen at the click of a mouse. The *Mayo Clinic Family Health Book on CD-ROM* is a comprehensive source of information on health, illness, and medications. From text, graphics, and video, the user can quickly learn, for example, how to stop a bleeding cut. The *Doctor's Book of Home Remedies* is a source of 300 healing tips for 138 illnesses. It includes helpful information on conditions from high cholesterol to headaches, dandruff, and snoring.

*Medical House Call* allows the user to enter his or her symptoms and responds with possible diagnoses, as well as advice on calling the doctor. Some programs allow the user to enter complete medical histories for each family member. Other guides focus on medications, fitness, or a specific condition.

## COMPUTERS AND PSYCHIATRY

Computers play a part in psychiatry from diagnosis to treatment. **CIDI (Composite International Diagnostic Interview)** is an interview that screens for depression and anxiety. Computers have been used as a tool to screen teenagers for a variety of conditions including suicidal tendencies. A program developed at the Columbia University College of Physicians and Surgeons prompts the interviewer to ask 3,000 questions and follow-ups. Anyone flagged by the computer is seen by a psychologist who then makes the diagnosis. Many psychological diagnostic tests, such as **CIDI-Auto** are self-administered. One company advertises self-administered tests that they claim will help diagnose addiction, thought errors, and even criminal tendencies. They do warn, however, that these diagnoses are meant as suggestions only; they are not conclusive.

The first uses of computers in psychotherapy were in testing; later studies found the online tests comparable to traditional testing. Computers can be better at information gathering than clinicians. Some studies found that some people are more open with a computer-administered interview. More people were willing to participate in a computer-administered interview. A series of studies in 2004 found that computers and the Internet were helpful aids to therapy. "Technological applications . . . include self-help Internet sites, computer-administered therapy, [and] virtual reality therapy" to name a few.[46] The **Web-based Depression and Anxiety Test (WB-DAT)** was found to be effective in diagnosing anxiety disorders and depression. "In computer-guided therapy, the computer itself both determines and provides the feedback to the patient." In a test in which the data concerning 193 subjects was taken from two studies of gamblers and one of major depressives, the WB-DAT did well in identifying people suffering from major depressive disorder, social phobias, obsessive-compulsive disorder (OCD), and posttraumatic stress disorder.[47] Several programs that are effective include Fear Fighter for phobias and panic, BTSteps for OCD, and Overcoming Depression for depression.

Two programs have been found helpful for drinking—Behavioral Self-Control Program for Windows and Drinker's Checkup. Beating the Blues uses cognitive-behavioral therapy for depression and anxiety. Seven out of 10 people who used it would recommend it to friends.[48] Although all patients using computer-aided therapies were in telephone contact with live therapists, computers apparently do a good job at some sorts of therapies. There is computer-aided self-help for phobia/panic, nonsuicidal depression, and OCD. Some patients with OCD and depression were given a self-help book with a telephone number to call a computer-operated interactive voice system. Self-help exposure programs on the Internet or on a personal computer aided people with panic disorder. Clients can carry palmtops that remind them of techniques to be used in everyday life; this is used as an aid in treating people with generalized anxiety disorder and social phobia. The Web can bring therapy to patients whose conditions may make them unlikely to seek treatment (including those with agoraphobia or OCD).

Later studies tended to confirm the 2004 studies. Online screening programs for anxiety and mood disorders have been "generally equivalent" to assessment by a therapist.[49] Some self-help programs on computers have been shown to be

effective; on the Internet, users can get feedback, making the programs more helpful. Internet-based treatment was found to be as effective as face-to-face treatment in a number of randomized clinical trials. The use of VR in treating certain phobias has also been tested in randomized clinical trials and found to be effective. VR is being used to treat soldiers returning from Iraq with posttraumatic stress disorder.[50] Internet therapy (**interapy**) for those suffering from posttraumatic stress disorder was found to be very effective through self-reports. Interapy was also found to be effective in treating depression. The Internet-based treatment was cognitive-behavioral therapy in all cases studied. Because interapy is relatively new, the evidence is limited concerning its effectiveness.[51] Anxiety disorders have been treated for many years with controlled exposure to whatever provokes the anxiety. Investigations are being performed to see whether the exposure can be done using VR technology.

In 2010, advances in computer technology and artificial intelligence allowed the creation complex virtual situations. These advances allow people to be exposed to situations that in real life they find threatening and frightening. They find the virtual situations threatening, but know that they are safe. Researchers are using these virtual environments to see how people with certain conditions react to certain virtual situations (e.g., how heavy drinkers feel when a virtual bartender offers them a drink; how gamblers react to virtual slot machines; how people with social anxiety give a speech to a virtual room full of virtual people). Because the therapist is in the situation at the moment, she or he can give immediate advice. Some experiments have shown that the advice does have an effect on actual behavior in the real world. Researchers are also attempting to use virtual people to improve the ability of autistic children to think and talk while surrounded by others. Use of virtual worlds in therapy is called **cybertherapy**, and it is a growing field. It is not meant to replace human therapy, but to be used as a tool along with it.[52]

In some situations, cybertherapists are being used. **Angelina** is a virtual human, programmed to "nod sympathetically" and be "socially sensitive." Talking with a student with a social anxiety disorder, Angelina's "eyes and expression, guided by video cameras and microphones stay in sync with the student's, as an empathetic therapist's would." While not looking quite human, Angelina is mobile and human enough to conduct a conversation that is somewhat natural. A recent study at the University of Southern California found that people tell her more of their fears than they tell live therapists. Angelina does not diagnose, but she asks if you want to see a therapist and can give you a list of therapists.[53]

At the University of Quebec in Outaouais, people who suffer from social anxiety were put in two groups. One group was given talk therapy 1 hour per week for 14 weeks, and the other was given talk therapy with cybertherapy. Both groups improved, and research is continuing, to see if a combination of real and virtual therapy speeds recovery.[54]

The U.S. Army is developing SimCoach, based on Angelina. **SimCoach** will conduct interviews with veterans and their families to see what problems they are experiencing. The veterans will be able to use SimCoach anonymously and receive a list of therapists if needed.[55]

Researchers at Stanford University had people inhabit **avatars** (virtual bodies). Each avatar interacted with a researcher. The researchers then made subtle changes to some of the avatars. Some were made taller, some shorter. No one noticed the changes. They found that the "taller" avatars were more aggressive with their partners than those made shorter. When the headsets were taken off, the behavior remained. Researchers concluded that people identify strongly with their avatars and that "what we learn in one body is shared with other bodies we inhabit, whether virtual or physical." Experiments are being done that put young people into virtual old peoples' bodies to increase appreciation of the older person's point of view.[56]

Computer programs have been used for several years in the treatment of drug addiction. In 2003, a study found that people who had both traditional drug counseling and used a computer program designed to change their behavior "failed fewer drug tests and stayed 'clean' longer" than those who did not have access to the computer-based education. In 2008, a study was published in the

*American Journal of Psychiatry* on people who used **Computer-based Training in Cognitive Behavioral Therapy (CBT4CBT)**, a computer program designed to treat addiction. In the study, 77 people who had used drugs or alcohol during the preceding month were randomly assigned to two groups. One group had traditional drug counseling; the other had counseling plus the use of the program. After 8 weeks, "53 percent of the weekly urine specimens submitted by the treatment-as-usual group tested positive for drugs compared with 34 percent of the specimens submitted by those who also used the CBT4CBT program." Follow-up studies showed that the group who used the computer program continued to improve, while the other group did not. According to the researchers, the participants "love the program." The program includes several modules, each focusing on a different skill such as avoiding risky situations, preventing HIV, and how to handle cravings. They include film clips, graphics, games, and assignments. The program is a user friendly and inexpensive way to provide extra support for patients.[57]

## CONCLUSION

Information technology, specifically the explosive growth of the Internet, has made more information available to more people than ever before. However, the quality of the information varies. Moreover, access is not equally distributed across society. Both health care professionals and consumers use these informational resources. The effects of the use of expert systems and extensive medical literature databases available to health care professionals have not been extensively studied. They apparently do enhance physician performance in some areas. However, there is much room for improvement in these programs. The many health-related apps available for tablet computers and smartphones are used by both consumers and health care professionals. There is accurate general information available for health care consumers. However, extreme caution must be exercised in using the Internet or self-help software as a source of health care information. The use of computers in psychiatry has increased in recent years.

# IN THE NEWS

According to "Prescription for Fear," by Virginia Heffernan published on February 4, 2011, in *The New York Times*, if you search for health information on the Internet, you should be careful to use objective sources, not Web pages covered with ads.

Many health-related Web sites, including WebMD, have relationships with pharmaceutical companies that influence the information found on the site. However, there are sites that are nonprofit and objective. One of these is the Mayo Clinic

Web site. If you are looking for objective information, stay away from sites that are filled with ads and drug peddling.

In 2010, WebMD began as an ad-supported site with $504 million. However, as mentioned earlier, the Mayo Clinic is nonprofit. WebMD's site for headaches begins with recommendations of medications, whereas the Mayo Clinic site makes no mention of medications until the eighth page and mentions other headache treatments.

# Chapter Summary

Chapter 10 introduces the reader to the vast informational resources made available by computer technology and the Internet.

- Computer-assisted instruction has been used in the education of health care professionals since the 1960s.

  - Drill-and-practice software teaches facts that require memorization.

  - Simulations teach students to evaluate situations and solve problems, as well as teaching skills. Some simulation programs use data from the Visible Human, an ongoing project that contains thousands of images of one male and one female cadaver.

  - Currently, simulation programs are making use of virtual reality techniques, so that the student actually feels as if he or she is performing a procedure. Simulations using virtual reality are used to teach many skills including surgical procedures, administration of epidural anesthesia, and dentistry.

  - Patient simulators provide realistic programmable mannequins on which students can practice procedures.

- Computers and telecommunications have made distance learning possible.

- Expert systems such as INTERNIST, MYCIN, and POEMS are used as decision-support systems to help in diagnosis.

- The Internet makes a huge amount of information (and misinformation) available to both health care providers and patients. The effects of its use have not yet been evaluated.

  - Medical literature databases such as MEDLINE provide access to the latest research.

  - The Internet provides opportunities for lifelong, distance learning for health care professionals.

  - Health-related information on the Web can be accurate (such as that provided by the Virtual Hospital) or of dubious value. The user must use caution and common sense. The Internet also has online support groups for people with illnesses and for their families.

- Self-help software is available on CD-ROM and, if used with caution, may provide useful information.

- The many health-related apps available for tablet computers and smartphones are used by both consumers and health care professionals.
- Some computer programs appear to help those with various conditions, such as OCD, panic disorders, and posttraumatic stress disorder. Computer programs are increasingly being used in psychiatry.

- Information should be carefully and critically scrutinized. Always look at the credentials of authors and who is paying for the research. Look for any ties between researchers and the devices and medications they are investigating. Be aware of conflicts of interest.

# Key Terms

ADAM

Angelina

avatars

BabySim

Body Browser

CenterWatch

CIDI (Composite International Diagnostic Interview)

CIDI-Auto

CINAHL (Cumulative Index to Nursing and Allied Health Literature)

Clinical Pharmacology

ClinicalTrials.gov

Computer-based Training in Cognitive Behavioral Therapy (CBT4CBT)

cybertherapist

cybertherapy

Databank for Cardiovascular Disease

Explorable Virtual Human

human patient simulators

ILIAD

iMedConsent

interapy

INTERNIST

iStan

KISMET

Medi-Span

MEDLARS (Medical Literature Analysis and Retrieval System)

MEDLINE

Medscape

METI LiVE

MYCIN

New Medicines in Development

PediaSim

PLATO (Programmed Logic for Automatic Teaching Operations)

Postoperative Expert Medical System (POEMS)

SDILINE (Selective Dissemination of Information Online)

Simantha

SimCoach

simulation software

Starbright World

Vesalius Project

Virtual Hospital

Virtual Human Embryo

Visible Human Project

Web-based Depression and Anxiety Test (WB-DAT)

# Review Exercises

## Multiple Choice

1. The most comprehensive medical literature database is _____ .
   a. SDILINE
   b. AIDSLINE
   c. MEDLINE
   d. None of the above

2. _____ is a programmable mannequin of a child on which students can practice procedures.
   a. Childsim
   b. PediaSim
   c. The Small Virtual Patient
   d. None of the above

3. _____ is an expert system that helps in diagnosis.
   a. MYCIN
   b. INTERNIST
   c. None of the above
   d. A and B are both expert systems

4. \_\_\_\_\_ is a computerized library of human anatomy.
   a. The Visible Human
   b. The Virtual Hospital
   c. The Databank of Cardiovascular Disease
   d. None of the above

5. The best place to look for *authoritative* general health care information online for consumers would be \_\_\_\_\_ .
   a. MedlinePlus
   b. CenterWatch
   c. Any search will find authoritative information
   d. There is no reliable information on the Internet

6. Which of the following is likely to be a source of reliable health care information on the Internet?
   a. A site maintained by a drug company
   b. A site maintained by a patient
   c. A site maintained by a university
   d. None of the above is likely to provide reliable information

7. \_\_\_\_\_ is a database of the most recent additions to MEDLINE.
   a. MEDLARS
   b. AIDSLINE
   c. NEWLINE
   d. SDILINE

8. Which of the following is currently being taught with the aid of simulations using virtual reality?
   a. Minimally invasive surgical techniques
   b. The administration of epidural anesthesia
   c. Some aspects of dentistry
   d. All of the above

9. \_\_\_\_\_ is a program that teaches anatomy by allowing the student to use a mouse to click away layers of the body.
   a. ILIAD
   b. ADAM
   c. KISMET
   d. None of the above

10. It is not difficult to find support groups on the Web. Starbright World \_\_\_\_\_ .
    a. attempts to link seriously ill children in hospitals in the United States
    b. is a network of AIDS patients
    c. is a network of people with cancer
    d. is a network of families of people with cancer

## True/False

1. Expert systems will eventually replace doctors. \_\_\_\_\_

2. All the information on the Internet is reliable and accurate. \_\_\_\_\_

3. MEDLARS is a collection of medical literature databases. \_\_\_\_\_

4. The Visible Human provides anatomically detailed, three-dimensional representations of the male and female human body. \_\_\_\_\_

5. The Virtual Hospital was a service of the University of Iowa that provided up-to-date, accurate health-related information on the Web. \_\_\_\_\_

6. In order to post health-related information on the Internet, a person needs to pass a rigorous exam. \_\_\_\_\_

7. Information on current clinical drug trials is available on the Internet. \_\_\_\_\_

8. Some studies have contended that there are programs that are helpful in treating mild clinical depression. \_\_\_\_\_

9. ADAM is a program that teaches anatomy. \_\_\_\_\_

10. Simulation programs were used in health care education as far back as 1949. \_\_\_\_\_

## Critical Thinking

1. Discuss the advantages and disadvantages of using virtual reality simulations in health care education.

2. It is possible to become a physician assistant in a distance learning program without being physically present on a campus or setting foot

in a classroom. How do you think this might affect education?

3. Given the many uses of information technology in health care today, anyone entering a health care field must be computer literate and computer competent. Discuss this statement.

4. The Internet provides unparalleled informational resources for both consumers and providers of health care. This may be helpful. However, it may be quite dangerous. Comment on the positive and negative aspects of the availability of health-related information on the Internet.

5. One of the characteristics of the Internet is anonymity—you can hide your identity, and so can anyone else. Discuss the possible effects of this on Internet support groups.

# Notes

1. Celina Imielinska and Pat Molholt, "Incorporating 3D Virtual Anatomy into the Medical Curriculum," *Communications of the ACM* 48, no. 2 (2005): 49–54.

2. Florence Haseltine, John Cork, Ray Gasser, Elizabeth Lockett, Ying Sun, and Emily Wilson, "The Mobile Embryo Application," No date, http://nmhm.washingtondc.museum/news/EmbryoAppPoster.pdf (accessed May 5, 2011); "Medical Museum, NIH Partners Debut 'Embryo App' Featuring Images from World-Renowned Carnegie Collection of Embryology," April 28, 2011, http://nmhm.washingtondc.museum/news/embryo_app_2011.html (accessed May 5, 2011).

3. "Hospitals Turn to Digital Informed Consent Tools To Educate Patients," November 12, 2010, http://www.ihealthbeat.org/articles/2010/11/12/hospitals-turn-to-digital-informed-consent-tools-to-educate-patients.aspx (accessed November 15, 2010).

4. Mark Scerbo, "Medical Reality Simulators: Have We Missed an Opportunity?" 2005, http://www.hfes.org/web/BulletinPdf/bulletin0505.pdf (accessed May 5, 2011).

5. Anthony G. Gallagher, E. Matt Ritter, Howard Champion, Gerald Higgins, Marvin P. Fried, Gerald Moses, C. Daniel Smith, and Richard Satava, "Virtual Reality Simulation in the Operating Room," http://www.ncbi.nlm.nih.gov/pmc/articles/PMC1356924/ (accessed May 5, 2011).

6. "The 'Karlsruhe Endoscopic Surgery Trainer': A 'Virtual Reality' Based Training System for Minimally Invasive Surgery," http://www-kismet.iai.fzk.de/KISMET/docs/UKMITAT.html (accessed May 5, 2011).

7. "Virtual Reality Simulation Technology Improves Carotid Angiography Skills," Medical Studies/Trials, May 3, 2006, http://www.news-medical.net/news/2006/05/03/17717.aspx (accessed May 5, 2011).

8. Joshua Schwimmer, "The iStan Medical Mannequin: It Sweats, Bleeds, and Breathes," April 19, 2008, http://www.healthline.com/health-blogs/tech-medicine (accessed March 24, 2011); "Company FAQs: METI Learning," 2010, http://meti.com/index.html (accessed March 25, 2011); "iStan–Most Advanced Wireless Human Patient Simulator from METI," 2010, http://www.meti.com/products_ps_istan.htm (accessed March 25, 2011).

9. Joshua Schwimmer, "Interventional Cardiologists Tested on Virtual Patient Simulators," March 31, 2008, http://www.healthline.com/health-blogs/tech-medicine/interventional-cardiologists-tested-virtual-patient-simulators (accessed March 24, 2011).

10. "Company FAQs: METI Learning."

11. AIMS Industry Council, "What Is Medical Simulation?" 2011, http://www.medsim.org/whatissimulation.php (accessed May 5, 2011); "Company FAQs: METI Learning."

12. "Improving Patient Safety," 2011, http://www.laerdal.com/us/ (accessed July 19, 2011).

13. Roni Caryn Rabin, "Tools to Offer Fast Help for HIV Exposure," September 8, 2009, http://www.nytimes.com/2009/09/08/health/08hiv.html (accessed February 16, 2011).

14. Levi Sumagaysay, "After Man vs. Machine on 'Jeopardy,' What's Next for IBM's Watson?" February 17, 2011, http://blogs.siliconvalley.com/gmsv/2011/02/after-man-vs-machine-on-jeopardy-whats-next-for-ibms-watson.html (accessed February 17, 2011); Frank D. Roylance, "'Watson in the Examining Room?' University of Maryland and IBM Working on a Computerized Physicians' Assistant," February 17, 2011, http://articles.baltimore-sun.com/2011-02-17/health/bs.md-watson-medicine-20110217_1_watson-medical-privacy-patient (accessed February 17, 2011); "IBM's Watson Could Usher New Era in Medicine," February 17, 2011, http://www.pcworld.com/article/219904/ibms_watson_could_usher_new_era_in_medicine.html (accessed February 17, 2011).

15. E. S. Berner, *Clinical Decision Support Systems: State of the Art.* AHRQ Publication No. 09-0069-EF. Rockville, MD: Agency for Healthcare Research and Quality, June 2009.

16. "Web Site to Rate Content of Health Care News," *Star-Ledger,* April 17, 2006.

17. "2001 Report to Congress on Telemedicine," February 2001, ftp://ftp.hrsa.gov/telehealth/report2001.pdf (accessed May 5, 2011).

18. Virginia Heffernan, "A Prescription for Fear," February 4, 2011, http://www.nytimes.com/2011/02/06/magazine/06 FOB-Medium-t.html (accessed February 10, 2011).

19. Lisa Guernsey, "A Dissent on the Digital Divide," September 18, 2003, http://www.nytimes.com/2003/09/18/technology/a-dissent-on-the-digital-divide.html (accessed May 5, 2011).

20. U.S. Department of Commerce, "A Nation Online: Entering the Broadband Age," September, 2004, http://www.ntia.doc.gov/reports/anol/NationOnlineBroadband04.htm (accessed May 5, 2011).

21. Ben Feller, "Digital Divide Still Separates Students," September 5, 2006, http://www.msnbc.msn.com/id/14685703/ns/technology_and_science-tech_and_gadgets/t/digital-divide-still-separates-students/ (accessed May 5, 2011).

22. Michel Marriott, "Digital Divide Closing as Blacks Turn to Internet," March 31, 2006, http://www.nytimes.com/2006/03/31/us/31divide.html (accessed May 5, 2011).

23. Pew Internet and American Life Project, " Report: Internet, Broadband, and Cell Phone Statistics," 2011, http://www.pewinternet.org/Reports/2010/Internet-broad band-and-cell-phone-statistics.aspx (accessed March 25, 2011); Kelly Heyboar, "Digital Divide: The Internet's Haves and Have-Nots," January 15, 2010, http://blog.nj.com/njv_kelly_heyboer/2010/01/digital_divide_the_internets_h.html (accessed March 25, 2011).

24. Susannah Fox, " Americans Living with Disability and Their Technology Profile," January 21, 2011, http://www.pewinternet.org/Reports/2011/Disability.aspx (accessed March 25, 2011); Susannah Fox and Kristen Purcell, "Chronic Disease and the Internet," March 24, 2010, http://pewresearch.org/pubs/1537/chronic-disease-internet-use (accessed March 25, 2011).

25. U.S. National Library of Medicine National Institutes of Health, "Fact Sheet MEDLINE®," January 26, 2011, http://www.nlm.nih.gov/pubs/factsheets/medline.html (accessed March 29, 2011).

26. "Frequently Asked Questions about Clinical Trials," 2011, http://health.ucsd.edu/clinicaltrials/Pages/faq.aspx (accessed May 5, 2011).

27. "About CenterWatch," No date, http://centerwatch.com/about-centerwatch/index.htm (accessed March 29, 2011).

28. Robert Trowbridge, and Scott Weingarten, "Clinical Decision Support Systems," Chapter 53 in *Making Health Care Safer: A Critical Analysis of Patient Safety Practices*, prepared for the Agency for Healthcare Research and Quality, contract no. 290-97-0013, 2001, http://www.ahrq.gov/clinic/ptsafety (accessed May 5, 2011).

29. Berner, "Clinical Decision Support Systems: State of the Art."

30. Stephen Borowitz and Jeffrey Wyatt, "The Origin, Content, and Workload of E-mail Consultations," *JAMA* 280, no. 15 (1998): 1321–24.

31. Katie Hafner, "'Dear Doctor' Meets 'Return to Sender,'" June 6, 2002, http://www.nytimes.com/2002/06/06/technology/dear-doctor-meets-return-to-sender.html (accessed May 5, 2011).

32. Robert Brooks and Nir Menachemi, "Physicians Use of Email with Patients: Factors Influencing Electronic Communication and Adherence to Best Practices," March 7, 2006, http://www.jmir.org/2006/1/e2/ (accessed March 26, 2011).

33. "Guidelines for Physician-Patient Electronic Communications," 2011, http://www.ama-assn.org/ama/pub/about–ama/our-people/member-groups-sections/young-physicians-section/advocacy-resources/guidelines-physician-patient-electronic-communications.page (retrieved March 27, 2011).

34. Brooks and Menachemi, "Physicians Use of Email with Patients: Factors Influencing Electronic Communication and Adherence to Best Practices."

35. Silvana Santana, Berthold Lausen, Maria Bujnowski-Fedek, Catherine Chronaki, Per Egil Kummervold, Janne Rasmussen, and Tove Sorensen, "Online Communications between Doctors and Patients in Europe: Status and Perspectives," [Abstract] 2010, http://www.jmir.org/2010/2/e20/ (accessed March 28, 2011).

36. Amanda Gardner, " Patients Who E-Mail with Doctors See Health Improvements," July 12, 2010, http://www.usatoday.com/news/health/2010-07-11-doctor-email_N.htm (accessed March 24, 2011).

37. "A Pharmaceutical Candy Store: Internet Offers Unregulated Access to Dangerous Drugs," 2009, http://www.addiction-treatment-centers.com/addiction-articles/a-pharmaceutical-candy-store-internet-offers-unregulated-access-to-dangerous-drugs (accessed May 5, 2011); Constance H. Fung, Hawkin E. Woo, and Steven M. Asch, "Controversies and Legal Issues of Prescribing and Dispensing Medications Using the Internet," February 2004, http://www.mayoclinicproceedings.com/content/79/2/188.full.pdf (accessed May 5, 2011).

38. Terrence O'Brien, "Google Body Browser Brings Search to 3-D Human Models," December 19, 2010, http://www.switched.com/2010/12/19/google-body-browser-offers-3-d-view-of-human-body-sans-skin?icid=sphere_blog-smith_inpage_engadget (accessed March 23, 2011); Sindya N. Bhandoo, "New from Google: The Body Browser," December 23, 2010, http://well.blogs.nytimes.com/2010/12/23/new-from-google-the-body-browser/ (accessed February 15, 2011).

39. Pat Bass, "Asthma," January 27, 2010, http://www.asthma.about.com (accessed March 25, 2011).

40. Ken Mott, "Cancer and the Internet," *Newsweek,* August 19, 1996, 19.

41. Claire Cain Miller, "Social Networks a Lifeline for the Chronically Ill," March 24, 2010, http://www.nytimes.com/2010/03/25/technology/25disable.html (accessed March 26, 2011).

42. "The Virtual Hospital," 2009, http://www.uihealthcare.com/vh/ (accessed March 29, 2011).

43. "iFit: 50 Coolest Fitness and Health Apps for the iPhone," 2007, http://www.nursingdegree.net/blog/28/ifit-50-coolest-fitness-and-health-apps-for-the-iphone/ (accessed November 11, 2010).

44. R. Elizabeth and C. Kitchen, "iPhone Apps that Could Save Your Life," August 30, 2010, http://www.healthguideinfo.com/health-testing-technology/p85038/ (accessed February 16, 2011).

45. Phil Hornshaw, "Fresh iPhone Apps for Nov. 11: For Veterans, T2 Mood Tracker, CNET Reviews," November 11, 1010, http://www.appolicious.com/articles/3912-fresh-iphone-apps-for-nov-11-forveterans-t2-mood-tracker-cnet-reviews (accessed February 28, 2011).

46. Michelle G. Newman, "Technology in Psychotherapy: An Introduction," *JCLP* 60, no. 20 (2004), http://web.cs.wpi.edu/~hofri/Readings/CTh-3.pdf (accessed May 5, 2011).

47. "Welcome to the Web-Based Depression and Anxiety Test," March 30, 2011, http://telljp.wb-dat.net/ (accessed March 30, 2011); Peter Farvolden, Carolina McBride, R. Michael Bagby, and Paula Ravitz, "A Web-Based Screening Instrument for Depression and Anxiety Disorders in Primary Care," August 5, 2003, http://www.ncbi.nlm.nih.gov/pubmed/14517114 (accessed March 30, 3011)

48. "Beating the Blues," 2011, http://www.beatingtheblues.co.uk/ (accessed March 29, 2011).

49. Paul M. G. Emmelkamp, "Technological Innovations in Clinical Assessment and Psychotherapy," 2005, http://www.ncbi.nlm.nih.gov/pubmed/16244509 (accessed May 5, 2011).

50. Carlos Bergfeld, "A Dose of Virtual Reality," July 26, 2006, http://www.businessweek.com/print/technology/content/jul2006/tc20060725_012342.htm (accessed May 5, 2011).

51. "Interapy (Internet-Based Therapy)," June 15, 2010, http://www2.som.uq.edu.au/som/Research/PTSD/treatments/Lists/Treatments/View_Treatment_v2.aspx?List=b54278cc%2D10ab%2D4c68%2Db0ea%2Dd71bb87c15af&ID=10 (accessed April 8, 2011).

52. Benedict Carey, "In Cybertherapy, Avatars Assist with Healing," November 22, 2010, http://www.nytimes.com/2010/11/23/science/23avatar.html (accessed February 2, 2011); Sergiu Vidican, "The Power of Cybertherapy," November 23, 2010, http://www.metrolic.com/the-power-of-cybertherapy-148529/ (accessed March 25, 2011).

53. Carey, "In Cybertherapy, Avatars Assist with Healing"; Vidican, "The Power of Cybertherapy."

54. Vidican, "The Power of Cybertherapy."

55. Carey, "In Cybertherapy, Avatars Assist with Healing."

56. Ibid.

57. "Modern Trends in Drug and Alcohol Addiction Treatment," 2003, http://www.drug-addiction.com/modern_drug_treatments.htm (accessed February 21, 2011); Rebecca A. Clay, " New Hope for Substance Abuse Treatment: Delivering Cognitive Behavioral Therapy Via Computer Enhances Outcomes, Research Suggests," March 2009, http://www.apa.org/monitor/2009/03/substance.aspx (accessed March 25, 2011).

# Additional Resources

"About CenterWatch." No date. http://centerwatch.com/about-centerwatch/index.htm (accessed March 29, 2011).

"About ClinicalTrials.gov." April 2, 2008. http://clinicaltrials.gov/ (accessed March 29, 2011).

ADAM. 2011. http://www.adam.com (accessed May 5, 2011).

Aschoff, Susan. "A Diehard Patient." April 30, 2002. http://www.sptimes.com/2002/04/30/Floridian/A_diehard_patient.shtml (accessed May 5, 2011).

Association of Schools of Public Health Distance Programs. 2010. http://www.asph.org (accessed May 5, 2011).

Bass, Pat. "Asthma." January 27, 2010. Asthma.about.com (accessed March 25, 2011).

Beamish, Rita. "Computers Now Helping to Screen for Troubled Teen-Agers." *The New York Times,* December 17, 1998, G9.

"Beating the Blues." 2011. http://www.beatingtheblues.co.uk/ (accessed March 29, 2011).

Berner, ES. *Clinical Decision Support Systems: State of the Art.* AHRQ Publication No. 09-0069-EF. Rockville, MD: Agency for Healthcare Research and Quality, June 2009.

Bhandoo, Sindya N. "New from Google: The Body Browser." December 23, 2010. http://well.blogs.nytimes.com/2010/12/23/new-from-google-the-body-browser/ (accessed February 15, 2011).

Bitzer, Maryann D., and Martha C. Boudreaux. "Using a Computer to Teach Nursing." In *Computers in Nursing,* ed. Rita D. Zielstorff, 171–85. Rockville, MD: Aspen, 1982.

Brooks, Robert, and Nir Menachemi. "Physicians Use of Email with Patients: Factors Influencing Electronic Communication and Adherence to Best Practices." March 7, 2006. http://www.jmir.org/2006/1/e2/ (accessed March 26, 2011).

Carey, Benedict. "In Cybertherapy, Avatars Assist with Healing." November 22, 2010. http://www.nytimes.com/2010/11/23/science/23avatar.html (accessed February 2, 2011).

Classen, D. C. "Clinical Decision Support Systems to Improve Clinical Practice and Quality of Care." *JAMA* 280, no. 15 (1998): 1360–1.

Clay, Rebecca A. "New Hope for Substance Abuse Treatment: Delivering Cognitive Behavioral Therapy Via Computer Enhances Outcomes, Research Suggests." March 2009. http://www.apa.org/monitor/2009/03/substance.aspx (accessed March 25, 2011).

"Company FAQs: METI Learning." 2010. http://meti.com/index.html (accessed March 25, 2011).

Eisenberg, Anne. "The Virtual Stomach (No, It's Not a Diet Aid)." October 31, 2002. http://www.nytimes.com/2002/10/31/technology/circuits/31next.html (accessed May 5, 2011).

Elizabeth, R., and C. Kitchen. "iPhone Apps That Could Save Your Life." August 30, 2010. http://www.healthguideinfo.com/health-testing-technology/p85038/ (accessed February 16, 2011).

Eng, Thomas R., A. Maxfield, K. Patrick, et al. "Access to Health Information and Support: A Public Highway or a Private Road?" *JAMA* 280, no. 15 (1998): 1371–5.

Epstein, Randi Hutter. "Sifting through the Online Medical Jumble." January 28, 2003. http://www.nytimes.com/2003/01/28/health/sifting-through-the-online-medical-jumble.html (accessed May 5, 2011).

"Evaluating Medical Information on the Web." November 17, 2003. http://www.ornl.gov/sci/techresources/Human_Genome/posters/chromosome/evaluate.shtml (accessed May 5, 2011).

"Fact Sheet. The Visible Human Project." May 4, 2010. http://www.nlm.nih.gov/research/visible/visible_human.html (accessed May 5, 2011).

Farvolden, Peter, Carolina McBride, R. Michael Bagby, and Paula Ravitz. "A Web-Based Screening Instrument for Depression and Anxiety Disorders in Primary Care." August 5, 2003. http://www.ncbi.nlm.nih.gov/pubmed/14517114 (accessed March 30, 3011).

Ferguson, Tom. "Digital Doctoring—Opportunities and Challenges in Electronic Patient–Physician Communication." *JAMA* 280, no. 15 (1998): 1361–2.

Fisk, Sandra. "Doc in a Box a Home Health Software Guide." *Better Homes and Gardens,* August 1995, 44–52.

Fox, Susannah. "Americans Living with Disability and Their Technology Profile." January 21, 2011. http://www.pew internet.org/Reports/2011/Disability.aspx (accessed March 25, 2011).

Fox, Susannah, and Kristen Purcell. "Chronic Disease and the Internet." March 24, 2010. http://pewresearch.org/pubs/1537/chronic-disease-internet-use (accessed March 25, 2011).

Gardner, Amanda. "Patients Who E-Mail with Doctors See Health Improvements." July 12, 2010. http://www.usatoday.com/news/health/2010-07-11-doctor-email_N.htm (accessed March 24, 2011).

"Guidelines for Physician–Patient Electronic Communications." 2011. http://www.ama-assn.org/ama/pub/about-ama/our-peo ple/member-groups-sections/young-physicians-section/advocacy-resources/guidelines-physician-patient-electronic-communications.page (retrieved March 27, 2011).

Heffernan, Virginia. "A Prescription for Fear." February 4, 2011. http://www.nytimes.com/2011/02/06/magazine/06FOB-Medium-t.html (accessed February 10, 2011).

Hersh, William, and David Hickam. "How Well Do Physicians Use Electronic Information Retrieval Systems? A Framework for Investigation and Systematic Review." *JAMA* 280, no. 15 (1998): 1347–52.

Heyboar, Kelly. "Digital Divide: The Internet's Haves and Have-Nots." January 15, 2010. http://blog.nj.com/njv_kelly_heyboer/2010/01/digital_divide_the_internets_h.html (accessed March 25, 2011).

Hornshaw, Phil. "Fresh iPhone Apps for Nov. 11: For Veterans, T2 Mood Tracker, CNET Reviews." November 11, 1010. http://www.appolicious.com/articles/3912-fresh-iphone-apps-for-nov-11-forveterans-t2-mood-tracker-cnet-reviews (accessed February 28, 2011).

"Hospitals Turn to Digital Informed Consent Tools to Educate Patients." November 12, 2010. http://www.ihealthbeat.org/articles/2010/11/12/hospitals-turn-to-digital-informed-consent-tools-to-educate-patients.aspx (accessed November 15, 2010).

"How to Evaluate Health Information on the Internet: Questions and Answers." No date. http://ods.od.nih.gov/Health_Infor mation/How_To_Evaluate_Health_Information_on_the_Inter net_Questions_and_Answers.aspx (accessed May 5, 2011).

"IBM's Watson Could Usher New Era in Medicine." February 17, 2011. http://www.pcworld.com/article/219904/ibms_watson_could_usher_new_era_in_medicine.html (accessed February 17, 2011).

"iFit: 50 Coolest Fitness and Health Apps for the iPhone." 2007. http://www.nursingdegree.net/blog/28/ifit-50-coolest-fit ness-and-health-apps-for-the-iphone/ (accessed November 11, 2010).

"Interapy (Internet-Based Therapy)." June 15, 2010. http://www2.som.uq.edu.au/som/Research/PTSD/treatments/Lists/Treatments/View_Treatment_v2.aspx?List=b5427

8cc%2D10ab%2D4c68%2Db0ea%2Dd71bb87c15af& ID=10 (accessed April 8, 2011).

"iStan—Most Advanced Wireless Human Patient Simulator from METI." 2010. http://www.meti.com/products_ps_istan.htm (accessed March 25, 2011).

"KISMET Medical Applications." July 10, 2001. http://iregt1.iai.fzk.de/KISMET/kis_apps_med.html (accessed May 5, 2011).

Kolata, Gina. "Web Research Transforms Visit to the Doctor." March 6, 2000. http://www.nytimes.com/library/tech/00/03/biztech/articles/06inte.html (accessed May 5, 2011).

Le, Tao. "Medical Education and the Internet: This Changes Everything." *JAMA* 285, no. 6 (2001): 809.

Lindberg, Donald A. B. "The National Library of Medicine's Web Site for Physicians and Patients." *JAMA* 285, no. 6 (2001): 806.

Maddox, Peggy Jo. "Ethics and the Brave New World of E-Health." November 21, 2002. http://www.nursingworld.org/MainMenuCategories/ANAMarketplace/ANAPeriodicals/OJIN/Columns/Ethics/Ethicsandehealth.aspx (accessed May 5, 2011).

Miller, Claire Cain. "Social Networks a Lifeline for the Chronically Ill." March 24, 2010. http://www.nytimes.com/2010/03/25/technology/25disable.html (accessed March 26, 2011).

"Modern Trends in Drug and Alcohol Addiction Treatment." 2003. http://www.drug-addiction.com/modern_drug_treatments.htm (accessed February 21, 2011).

National Library of Medicine. "The Visible Human Project." May 4, 2010. http://www.nlm.nih.gov/research/visible/visible_human.html (accessed May 5, 2011).

O'Brien, Terrence. "Google Body Browser Brings Search to 3-D Human Models." December 19, 2010. http://www.switched.com/2010/12/19/google-body-browser-offers-3-d-view-of-human-body-sans-skin?icid=sphere_blogsmith_inpage_engadget (accessed March 23, 2011).

O'Connor, Anahad. "Images of Preserved Embryos to Become a Learning Tool." March 25, 2003. http://www.nytimes.com/2003/03/25/science/images-of-preserved-embryos-to-become-a-learning-tool.html (accessed May 5, 2011).

Patsos, Mary. "The Internet and Medicine: Building a Community for Patients with Rare Diseases." *JAMA* 285, no. 6 (2001): 805.

Pew Internet and American Life Project. "Report: Internet, Broadband, and Cell Phone Statistics." 2011. http://www.pewinternet.org/Reports/2010/Internet-broadband-and-cell-phone-statistics.aspx (accessed March 25, 2011).

Prutkin, Jordan. "Cybermedical Skills for the Internet Age." *JAMA* 285, no. 6 (2001): 808.

Rabin, Roni Caryn. "Tools to Offer Fast Help for HIV Exposure." September 8, 2009. http://www.nytimes.com/2009/09/08/health/08hiv.html (accessed February 16, 2011).

Rajendran, Pam R. "The Internet: Ushering in a New Era of Medicine." *JAMA* 285, no. 6 (2001): 804–5.

Roylance, Frank D. "'Watson in the Examining Room?' University of Maryland and IBM Working on a Computerized Physicians' Assistant." February 17, 2011. http://articles.baltimoresun.com/2011-02-17/health/bs.md-watson-medicine-20110217_1_watson-medical-privacy-patient (accessed February 17, 2011).

Rubin, Rita. "Prescribing On Line . . . Industry's Rapid Growth, Change Defy Regulation." *USA Today,* October 2, 1998, 1, 2.

Santana, Silvana, Berthold Lausen, Maria Bujnowski-Fedek, Catherine Chronaki, Per Egil Kummervold, Janne Rasmussen, and Tove Sorensen. "Online Communications between Doctors and Patients in Europe: Status and Perspectives." [Abstract] 2010. http://www.jmir.org/2010/2/e20/ (accessed March 28, 2011).

Schwimmer, Joshua. "Interventional Cardiologists Tested on Virtual Patient Simulators." March 31, 2008. http://www.healthline.com/health-blogs/tech-medicine/interventional-cardiologists-tested-virtual-patient-simulators (accessed March 24, 2011).

Schwimmer, Joshua. "The iStan Medical Mannequin: It Sweats, Bleeds, and Breathes." April 19, 2008. http://www.healthline.com/health-blogs/tech-medicine (accessed March 24, 2011).

Speilberg, Alissa. "On Call and Online, Sociohistorical, Legal and Ethical Implications of E-mail for the Patient–Physician Relationship." *JAMA* 280, no. 15 (1998): 1353–9.

"Starbright World." 2010. http://www.starbright.org (accessed May 5, 2011).

Sumagaysay, Levi. "After Man vs. Machine on 'Jeopardy,' What's Next for IBM's Watson?" February 17, 2011. http://blogs.siliconvalley.com/gmsv/2011/02/after-man-vs-machine-on-jeopardy-whats-next-for-ibms-watson.html (accessed February 17, 2011).

Terry, Nicolas. "Access vs Quality Assurance: The e-Health Conundrum." February 14, 2001. http://jama.ama-assn.org/content/285/6/807.full (accessed May 5, 2011).

"The Virtual Hospital." 2009. http://www.uihealthcare.com/vh/ (accessed March 29, 2011).

"The Visible Human Project: From Data to Knowledge." May 3, 2011. http://www.nlm.nih.gov/research/visible/data2knowledge.html (accessed May 5, 2011).

U.S. National Library of Medicine National Institutes of Health. "Fact Sheet MEDLINE®." January 26, 2011. http://

www.nlm.nih.gov/pubs/factsheets/medline.html (accessed March 29, 2011).

Vidican, Sergiu. "The Power of Cybertherapy." November 23, 2010. http://www.metrolic.com/the-power-of-cybertherapy-148529/ (accessed March 25, 2011).

"Welcome to the Web-Based Depression and Anxiety Test." March 30, 2011. http://telljp.wb-dat.net/ (accessed March 30, 2011).

Winker, Margaret A., Annette Flanagin, Bonnie Chi-Lum, et al. "Guidelines for Medical and Health Information on the Internet." [Abstract] August 7, 2001. http://jama.ama-assn.

org/content/283/12/1600.abstract?cited-by=yes&legid=jama;283/12/1600 (accessed May 5, 2011).

"World Health Organization (WHO) Composite International Diagnostic Interview (CIDI)." 2004. http://www.hcp.med.harvard.edu/wmhcidi/ (accessed May 5, 2011).

Zuger, Abigail. "HEALTH: Hospital, Clinic, Practice: 3 Views of Doctors and the Web; Reams of Information, Some of It Even Useful." October 25, 2000. http://www.nytimes.com/2000/10/25/business/health-hospital-clinic-practice-3-views-doctors-web-reams-information-some-it.html (accessed May 5, 2011).

# Related Web Sites

The Federal Trade Commission (FTC) looks into complaints about false health claims on the Internet. Their Web page can help consumers evaluate claims. The FTC's "Operation Cure. All" page can be found at http://www.ftc.gov/opa/2001/06/cureall.shtm.

The Food and Drug Administration (FDA) regulates drugs and medical devices. "Buying Medicines and Medical Products Online" can be found at http://www.fda.gov/Drugs/Resources ForYou/Consumers/BuyingUsingMedicineSafely/Buying MedicinesOvertheInternet/ucm202675.htm.

The Harvard School of Public Health provides consumers with "Health Insight" at http://www.health-insight-harvard.org/.

*The Journal of the American Medical Association* is available at http://jama.ama-assn.org.

The National Cancer Institute is located at http://cancer.gov.

The National Library of Medicine provides access to MEDLINE and MedlinePlus at http://www.nlm.nih.gov.

**PEARSON**
**myhealthprofessionskit**

Go to www.myhealthprofessionskit.com to access the Companion Web site created for this textbook. Simply select "Basic Health Science" from the

choice of disciplines. Find this book and register to access self-assessment quizzes, flashcards, and more.

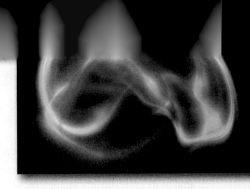

# Information Technology in Rehabilitative Therapies: Computerized Medical Devices, Assistive Technology, and Prosthetic Devices

## CHAPTER OUTLINE

- Additional Resources
- Related Web Sites

## LEARNING OBJECTIVES

Upon completion of this chapter, the reader will be able to:

- Describe the contribution made to the design of medical devices by information technology and be able to discuss the advantages of computerized medical monitoring systems over their predecessors.
- Describe the use of computerized devices in delivering medications.
- Discuss the Americans with Disabilities Act of 1990 and be able to discuss the impact digital technology has had on assistive devices for people with physical challenges.
  - List assistive devices for those with impaired vision, speech, hearing, and mobility.
  - Discuss speech recognition devices, speech synthesizers, and screen readers.
- Describe the contributions computer technology has made to the development of prosthetics.
  - Discuss the contribution of computer technology to the improvement of myoelectric limbs.
  - Discuss the contributions computer technology has made to improving sight for the blind and hearing for the deaf.
- Define functional electrical stimulation.
  - List its uses in implanted devices such as pacemakers.
  - Discuss its use in simulating physical workouts for paralyzed muscles and restoring movement to paralyzed limbs.
- Discuss the risks posed by implants.
- Discuss the uses of computers in rehabilitative therapies.

## OVERVIEW

Digital technology, particularly the microprocessor, has had an enormous impact on the creation, design, and manufacture of medical devices, adaptive devices, and prosthetics. Computers have improved the design of some devices with health care applications and made possible a whole range of new ones. In hospitals and medical offices, **computerized medical instruments** with embedded microprocessors are more accurate than their predecessors. In the work place and the home, the impact of information technology on people who are physically challenged is tremendous. Assistive, or adaptive, technology allows some people with disabilities to work and/or live independently.

**Prosthetic devices** (replacement limbs and organs) that contain motors and respond to electrical signals existed prior to computers. However, prosthetic devices designed and manufactured with the help of computers and containing microprocessors are more sensitive, lighter, and more flexible and can work almost as well as natural limbs. **Computerized functional electrical stimulation (CFES or FES)** is a technology that involves delivering low-level electrical stimulation to muscles. Used for many years in pacemakers, CFES is now being used to strengthen muscles paralyzed by spinal cord injury or stroke. CFES is being used experimentally to restore the ability to stand and walk to paraplegics.

## COMPUTERIZED MEDICAL INSTRUMENTS AND DEVICES

Computerized medical instruments are "electronic devices equipped with microprocessors [which] provide direct patient services such as monitoring . . . [and] administering medication or treatment."[1] Computerized drug delivery systems are used to give medications. Insulin pumps include a battery-operated pump and a computer chip. The pump is not automatic. However, the chip allows the user to control the amount of insulin administered. Insulin is administered via a plastic tube inserted under the skin; the tube is changed every 2 or 3 days. The pump is worn externally and continually delivers insulin according to the user's program. In March 2001, the Food and Drug Administration (FDA) approved a new device for glucose testing. It is worn like a watch and takes fluid through the skin using electric currents; electrodes measure the glucose. The measurements are taken every 20 minutes, and an alarm goes off if the levels are too low. Tests showed that this method was not as accurate as the finger prick and is not meant to replace it, but to reveal trends. Electronic intravenous (IV) units not only are programmable, but also can detect incorrect flow and sound an alarm. Some units can be programmed to administer several drugs through several channels. IV anesthesia can be administered via a mechanical syringe infusion pump, controlled by complex and sophisticated software.

Computerized monitoring systems that collect data directly from patients via sensors have been used for many years. These devices can provide continuous oversight of a patient's condition and can be programmed to sound an alarm under certain conditions to notify human personnel of a change. Computerized **physiological monitoring systems** that analyze blood, **arrhythmia monitors** that monitor heart rates, **pulmonary monitors** that measure blood flow through the heart and respiratory rate, **fetal monitors** that measure the heart rate of the fetus, and **neonatal monitors** that monitor infant heart and breathing rates are devices that are standard and accepted.

Computerized instruments are both more accurate and more reliable than their predecessors. For example, an infusion pump can be set at the desired rate and that rate will be maintained. Its predecessor, whose flow had to be estimated, could have its rate changed by the patient's movements. Computerized cardiac monitors are able,

unlike their predecessors, to distinguish between cardiac arrest and a wire coming loose.

Monitoring devices may or may not be linked to a network. Stand-alone devices include IV pumps, electrocardiograms (ECG) (Figure 11.1▶) and cardiac monitors, defibrillators, temperature pulse respiration (TPR), and blood pressure monitors. When devices are networked, patients can be monitored from a central location within the hospital, such as a nurses' station, or even from a physician's home. Networked devices can interact with each other; for example, a cardiac monitor can communicate with a medication delivery device. Networked equipment is most common in emergency rooms, operating rooms, and critical and intensive care units. Because a network

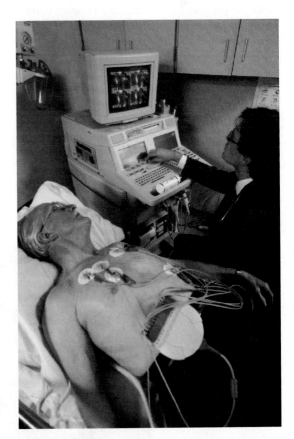

▶ **Figure 11.1** An electrocardiogram (ECG) records the electrical activity of a heart.
*Source:* Brand X Pictures/Jupiter Images.

makes patient's information immediately available anywhere in the hospital and allows a specialist to consult with the emergency room online, it can reduce response time in emergencies.

In 2011, researchers at Massachusetts General Hospital developed a portable device costing $200 that can be linked to a smartphone. It can analyze tissue and predict whether a tumor is malignant and apt to spread. The results take 1 hour. The findings are displayed on a smartphone. Although the technology has not yet undergone clinical testing, in an early test, its predictions were quite accurate. "By looking at a combination of four biomarkers in . . . [samples of biopsies of abnormal stomach tissue], the researchers correctly predicted whether 48 of the patients had benign or malignant" tumors. The accuracy of predictions was 96 percent for the first 50 people; current methods achieve 84 percent accuracy. The test was used on a second group of 20 people with 100 percent accuracy.[2]

Different kinds of devices for detecting cancer are in various stages of development. Researchers in Israel are developing breath nanosensors. These sensors can identify patients with cancer, as well as distinguish among patients with "lung, breast, bowel and prostate cancers." In California, researchers have created a small laser scanner for finding breast cancer, that, by measuring

"hemoglobin, fat and water content, tumor, oxygen consumption and tissue density . . . provides detailed metabolic information" of the breast. It uses no radiation and can also be used to show the effectiveness of various treatments. It provides the information fast and can be analyzed immediately, which could lead to more effective treatments.[3]

## Computerized Devices in Optometry/ Ophthalmology

An ophthalmologist is a doctor who treats eye diseases. An optometrist examines the eye and prescribes glasses. Computerized devices help make eye care, from preliminary vision testing to surgery, more precise. Computerized instruments are used to measure refractive error and the shape of the cornea (Figure 11.2 ►). The **Optomap Panoramic200** examines the retina without dilation using low-powered red and green lasers. The image of 90 percent of the retina can be reviewed right away and is larger than that produced by conventional examination. It can help in the early detection of retinal tears, macular degeneration, and diabetic retinopathy. Tools called **biomicroscopes** are used for diagnosis of cataracts.[4] **Tonometers** check the health of the optic nerve by measuring pressure from fluid in the eye.[5] **Corneal topography** uses a computer to create

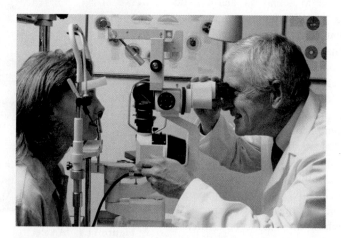

► **Figure 11.2**   A computerized eye exam.
*Source:* Courtesy of Thinkstock.

an accurate three-dimensional map of the cornea so that the health care professional can see the shape and power of the cornea. The **Heidelberg retinal tomograph (HRT)** uses lasers to scan the retina, resulting in a three-dimensional description. This technique can detect glaucoma before any loss of vision.[6] **GDx Access** uses an infrared laser to measure the thickness of the retinal nerve fiber. It is used for the early detection of glaucoma.[7] Computers help to make cataract surgery more precise. In such surgery, the eye's lens is replaced by an intraocular lens (IOL). The most precise measurements are needed to determine which IOL to implant. **Optical biometry** refers to the IOL calculations. Traditionally, ultrasound was used for the measurement; it required anesthesia. The IOLmaster takes precise measures in a shorter time and requires no anesthesia. The **Tracey visual function analyzer** measures how well you can see by measuring how your eye focuses light. It can examine both eyes in 1 minute without touching the eye. It "measures 64 points on the retina by projecting a thin beam of light . . . through the pupil in less than 50 milliseconds." Software analyzes the results and finds any abnormalities. These data help in surgical or laser vision correction. Computers are also used to custom design contact lenses.[8]

Several types of glasses may improve the vision of people with tunnel vision, which can be the result of retinitis pigmentosa or glaucoma. One device "combines a camera, computer and transparent computer display on a pair of glasses." People using these glasses would be able to see through the transparent part of the lens, but would also see a tiny version of a wider (peripheral) field superimposed on the lens. Prism glasses, which also expand the field of vision, did well in two clinical trials.[9]

The FDA has approved the testing of retinal implants, and some are in various stages of trials. In a healthy eye, the retina changes light into electrical signals. The retinal implant contains thousands of light detectors; it also changes light into electric signals. Currently, scientists around the world are studying computer chips that will replace the retina. One major disagreement is where the chip should be implanted:

under the retina close to light-detecting cells or near the retinal layer that sends nerve impulses to the brain. The way light is sent to the implant also differs—through a camera or via infrared signals that come from a device mounted on lens frames. The chip will (if successful) treat retinitis pigmentosa and macular degeneration. Some early implants improved vision enough for the participants to see light and shapes. A chip developed in Germany is in clinical trials. Two successful implants in previously blind people were performed in 2005.[10] Clinical trials on the German subretinal implants started in 2005 and lasted for 5 years. In 2010, Retinal Implant, AG of Germany announced that its first clinical trial "improved the eyesight of 11 patients to the point they were able to recognize objects . . . [and] read at a basic level at normal reading distance and in regular light conditions." Now clinical trials are beginning on 50 people. In the new version, the power supply is behind the ear, under the skin, and connected to the eyeball. The device "is a three-by-three millimeter microelectric chip (0.1 millimeter thick), containing about 1500 light-sensitive photodiodes, amplifiers and electrodes." Implanted under the retina, it "stimulat[es] inner retina nerve cells" to generate vision. The tiny chip converts light into electricity by stimulating retinal nerves, and the electricity is sent to the brain via the optical nerve. The brain receives an image made up of $38 \times 40$ pixels, "points of light that are . . . brighter or dimmer according to the light that falls on the chip."[11]

Another approach to the retinal implant is the epiretinal implant placed under the conjunctiva, which "directly stimulates the ganglia using signals sent from a camera and power sent from an external transmitter, both mounted on a pair of glasses." This approach is being tested in Europe and has been successful. For the first time in three decades, a 73-year-old man was able to see. However, this approach requires that a camera be mounted on glasses; and to see around him or her, the patient must move his or her head, not just the eyeball.[12]

In California, a different method of combating macular degeneration has been approved for

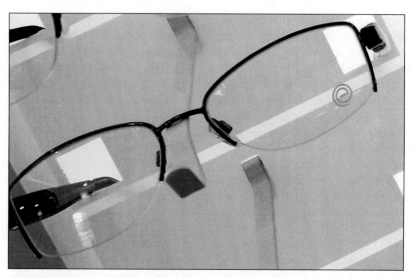

▶ **Figure 11.3** emPower electronic glasses charging.
*Source:* Kevin E. Schmidt/ZUMA Press/Newscom.

sale in the United States (2010). Vision Care Technologies has developed a tiny telescope. It has been implanted into one of a patient's eyes. It is an out-patient procedure. "The IMT [implantable miniature telescope] renders enlarged central vision over a wide area of the retina to improve central vision, while the nonoperated eye provides peripheral vision for mobility and orientation." Even though it has been approved, the company is studying patient outcomes.[13]

New electronic glasses called emPower are being sold in the United States (Figure 11.3▶). The frames contain batteries, and the lenses contain liquid crystals. The liquid crystals (like the thickness of the lenses in traditional glasses) affect the way the light is refracted. To turn emPower into reading glasses, the user touches the frame, and the batteries "send along a current that changes the orientation of the molecules in the crystals." To turn off the reading function, the user touches the frame again. The glasses do have to be charged. They cost between $1,000 and $2,000.[14]

In 2010, researchers in Finland created a pair of "**smart glasses**." They are attached to a small computer. The computer can "recognize" both people and objects, by looking them up in a database. The information is displayed "on the inside of the glasses . . . but appear[s] to hover near the object." The researchers hope to develop a way for the glasses to connect to the Internet wirelessly, focus on an object, use artificial intelligence, and display what the user would want to know about the object or person. Theoretically, these glasses could "introduce" people on the street to you, with information found on the Internet.[15]

In ophthalmic surgical training programs, virtual reality simulations are beginning to be used. The **EYESI surgical simulator** is a virtual reality simulator that allows doctors to learn new surgical skills and techniques "in preparation for surgery on the human eye." In 2006, the program was being evaluated by New York University to test its effectiveness.[16]

## ASSISTIVE DEVICES

The **Americans with Disabilities Act of 1990** (ADA) prohibits discrimination against people with disabilities and requires that businesses with more than 15 employees provide "reasonable accommodation" to allow the disabled to perform their jobs. On July 26, 2010 (the 20th anniversary of the ADA), President Obama signed an executive order designed "to establish the Federal Government as a model employer of individuals with disabilities," by increasing recruitment and training of people living with disabilities.[17] In addition, there are changes in the Department of Justice's regulations implementing the ADA. These will affect parts of the ADA, including, for example, accessibility of recreational facilities and public facilities, sale of tickets for accessible seating, and allowing wheelchairs and scooters in all pedestrian areas.[18]

Under the ADA, employers are required to provide not only entrance ramps for people in wheelchairs, but also hardware and software that make computers usable by people with disabilities. Many assistive devices have been developed. **Adaptive technology** makes it possible for people with disabilities to exercise control over their home and work environments. Some assistive devices allow people with physical challenges to work with computers and other office equipment. Others simply improve the quality of life. For example, at Boston University, scientists are developing a system based on computer-generated noise that helps elderly people keep their balance. It sends random vibrations to the feet, which automatically adjust their balance.

Wheelchairs are being developed that not only help move people around, but also climb stairs and allow them to reach a high shelf. The iBOT wheelchair stands up on its back wheels if the user needs to climb stairs and raises the seat to allow reaching. An even smarter wheelchair is being developed. It includes sensors and a computer, and the user can simply tell it where to go or use a touch panel. The wheelchair finds its way, using laser radar to find objects in its way; a computer calculates a new path if necessary.

A tongue-driven wheelchair has been shown in a clinical trial to enable people with high-level spinal cord injuries to issue commands. The same tongue device can also be used to issue computer commands. "Trial participants were able to easily remember and correctly issue tongue commands to play computer games and drive a powered wheelchair around an obstacle course with very little prior training." The user gives commands via a rice-grain-size magnet attached to the tongue. Sensors on wireless headphones detect the tongue movement. The signals output by the sensors are transmitted to a computer on the wheelchair. "The signals were processed to determine the relative motion of the magnet with respect to the array of sensors." That information then moved a cursor or the wheelchair. The tongue was used because it is directly connected to the brain by a nerve. Each subject trained the computer to understand his or her specific tongue movements. He or she then used the tongue magnet to move a cursor to play computer games and then to drive the wheelchair. They were told to move forward and backward, to do U-turns, to change direction, and to do all this as fast as possible while avoiding accidents. The wheelchair operates in discrete mode, where the stop command is issued automatically after a command, and continuous mode, in which the wheelchair is in continuous motion. In the trial, only six commands were used. However, the Tongue Drive system can use many more.[19]

Sensors can be embedded in fabrics and clothing. The sensors detect motion and send signals to a computer that displays the activity. Smart clothing can help to monitor chronically ill patients, such as those with heart conditions.[20] In Europe, a smart fabric has been developed that can help prevent repetitive stress injuries by sensing muscular overload. Measuring the electrical activity of a muscle is very difficult. However, the sensors embedded in the fabric of the clothing can sense muscle contraction. The same researchers are working on a belt worn by a pregnant mother that would monitor a fetus's heartbeat during pregnancy and shirts for athletes that would sense muscle fatigue.[21]

Computer technology can help those with impaired vision, hearing, speech, and mobility. People with low or no vision can use speech recognition systems as input and speech synthesizers for output. Brain input systems are being developed for people who lack the muscle control to use alternative input devices.

Hearing impairment is not a barrier to computer use. However, computers do expand the means of communication that hearing-impaired people can access. Computers can be used as text telephones and can send and receive e-mail. Special modems can communicate with both **text telephones** and computers. Computer-aided transcription makes use of a typist entering verbal communications at a meeting. The communications are then displayed as text on a monitor.

**Assistive technology** encompasses many areas. People with low vision can use a large type display on a monitor. Braille keyboards allow the blind to type. Blind users can use keyboard alternatives to mouse clicks as commands (for example, [ALT]-F-O, instead of clicking on the open icon). In 2003, a Braille telephone organizer was developed. It combines the functions of the cell phone, note taker, and wireless Internet connector. It can receive information and either read it to the user or allow the user to read it in Braille. Text can be entered using its Braille keyboards.

**Speech recognition** is useful for people who do not have the use of their hands and for the vision impaired. It promises that you can give computer commands or dictate text. Speech recognition hardware includes a microphone and a chip inside the computer that converts the spoken word to digital data that the computer can process. The digitized word is compared to a database of words in the computer's memory; if a match is found, the word is recognized. Speech recognition systems enable the user to give voice commands to their computers instead of clicking with a mouse, and to write, edit, and format text documents by dictating instead of typing. Great progress has been made in recent years, until speech recognition is almost perfect. Speech recognition systems that may not be able to distinguish between some English words and phrases—for example, "hyphenate" sounds exactly like "-8" (hyphen eight) and "the right or left" sounds like "the writer left"—can now be corrected by voice. The newest systems have error rates close to zero.

Using **page scanners**, speech synthesizers, and screen reader software, printed text can be digitized and input and then read aloud by the computer. A scanner converts printed text into a form the computer can accept as input; that is, it digitizes it. Speech synthesis refers to the ability

of a computer to talk; voice output devices turn digital data into speech-like sounds, allowing the computer to talk or read *to* a vision-impaired user or speak *for* a speech-impaired user. Speech synthesis requires both hardware and software. The **speech synthesizer** is really a computer in itself with a processor, memory, and an output device. The software is loaded into the synthesizer's memory. The microprocessor generates speech output and translates binary code to speech. A speaker and amplifier are also necessary. **Screen reader software** tells the speech synthesizer what to say, for example, to read the text description of an icon.

Ray Kurzweil (2006) invented a portable speech-synthesizing device that uses a digital camera and a handheld organizer called the Kurzweil–National Federation of the Blind Reader. The device takes a picture of the written text, scans it, and reads it. You do not have to be near a computer to use it. It also contains a memory that can save pages.[22]

People with impaired vision are not the only users of speech recognition software. People who have lost the use of their hands also find it useful; instead of typing, they can talk to the computer. Other input devices include the **head mouse**, which moves the cursor according to the user's head motions. **Puff straws** allow people to control the mouse with their mouths.[23] Some computers allow input through eye movement. Some eye input systems do not require the user to stare at letter after letter, but allow the eye to move down a column of letters and stop on one. The chosen letter floats on the screen, and the software predicts the next most likely letters. For example, if the user selected a "q", "u" would be the next most likely letter. After the "u", the next letter would be an "a," "e," "i," or "o." Users of this system can type at 25 words per minute, compared with 15 words per minute using an onscreen keyboard.[24]

Perhaps, most amazing are programs that attempt to translate electrical impulses from the brain into a mouse click. A quadriplegic can, after a period of training, click a mouse by contracting facial muscles or simply thinking. In 2003, a system that enabled a user to give a command by furrowing his or her brow on which a sensor was taped was demonstrated. Robotic arms and computer mice could be controlled using the sensor. Paralyzed stroke patients could speak on the telephone.

## Augmentative Communication Devices

An **augmentative communication device** is any device that helps a person communicate. Medicare began covering these devices in 2002. Those who lack the ability to speak or whose speech is impaired can have a computer speak for them. The device should allow the user to communicate basic needs, carry on conversations, work with a computer, and complete assignments for work or school. It should work with environmental controls at home, but travel with the user. It should enable the user to communicate with anyone, and say anything. It should be easy to use. There are devices that allow the user to type a message on a traditional keyboard and the computer speaks aloud. Some keyboards can be easily operated by one finger. Other devices, as you recall, allow the user to select letters by gazing at an area on the screen, which displays the characters. For people whose speech is impaired, there are devices that enhance speech—making the unintelligible comprehensible—and allow normal communication. Many of these devices are user friendly, that is, easy for people with no computer background to use. Some are specifically designed for children—allowing the user to move an electric pointer to select a picture symbol. Some devices for children have the words organized by part of speech, the English word appearing above the symbol. These devices include synthesized voices. More sophisticated devices included spelling, word prediction, and preprogrammed messages. Portable devices allow the user to communicate anywhere. A device, which the user wears on a belt, allows a user to communicate by pressing buttons to play pre-recorded messages and carry on simple conversations.

## Electronic Aids to Daily Living

**Electronic aids to daily living (EADL)** (formerly called **environmental control systems [ECS]**) help physically challenged people control their environments. Speech recognition technology can be used in the home to control appliances. Butler-in-a-Box has been made by Mastervoice since 1986. It not only understands and obeys voice commands, but also responds in a human voice. Using this system, one can control home appliances with voice commands. It also acts as a speaker phone that will dial or answer calls on command. Other EADLs allow the installation of a single switch to control the operation of several appliances (including other controllers). A device even exists that holds the book the user is reading and turns the pages.

EADLs can transmit signals to electrical devices. They can be used to control any electrical appliance in the home. This would include lights, telephones, computers, appliances, air conditioners, infrared devices, security systems, sprinklers, doors, curtains, and electric beds.[25] Voice, joysticks, or switches may control the system. This may enable physically challenged people to live independently at home. Several studies have found "increased levels of independence," an increase in feelings of security, help in adjusting to the disability, increased feelings of competence, and decreased frustration among people who use EADLs. In 2005, one study of people with cervical spinal cord injuries "found that users had greater independence and function in performing daily tasks than those who did not use EADLs."[26]

Another use of environmental controls is to help in language development in children. Many environmental controls include infrared capability. One possibility is using an action toy that moves back and forth to teach the concepts of backwards and forwards or fast/slow. In toys that require children to take turns, phrases such as "My turn" and "Your turn" could be taught.[27] Research is also being done into the possibility of using augmentative communication devices for patients who are only voiceless for a short time, because of illness or surgery.

## PROSTHETIC DEVICES

Prostheses are attempts to replace natural body parts or organs with artificial devices. **Myoelectric limbs**—artificial limbs containing motors and responding to the electrical signals transmitted by the residual limb to electrodes mounted in the socket—predate computers. However, computer-related research has improved myoelectric limbs and had an immense impact on prosthetics in general. Developments related to computers include the tiny circuitry used by the sensors that receive the electrical signals and the motors that move the limb, the use of computers in the design and manufacture of limbs, and the improvement of the sensors used in prostheses.

Today, microprocessors can be embedded in a prosthetic limb and make the limb more useful and flexible. Sensors are attached to muscles in the residual limb. The patient must be able to control these muscles. Contracting the muscles generates electrical impulses. A microprocessor processes and amplifies the electrical impulses, sending them as control signals to the prosthesis. The microprocessor controls the tiny motor that moves the artificial limb. Combined with natural-looking prostheses, the results can be a life like limb (Figure 11.4▶).

Computer-aided design and manufacturing (CAD/CAM) systems also improve prostheses by making the fit better. The artificial limb must be fitted to the natural limb. CAD/CAM systems have been developed to design both the socket and limb. With CAD/CAM, thousands of measurements can be taken and a three-dimensional model created on the computer screen to create a perfect custom fit for each patient. CAD/CAM is also used in dentistry to help create individually fitted prostheses.

Computers have made other advances possible. A knee socket has been developed that includes a computer chip that allows patients to walk naturally. Energy-storing feet contain plastic springs or carbon fibers, which are designed to help move the prosthesis. A lower leg prosthesis is called the **C-Leg** or computerized leg. It includes a prosthetic knee and shin system controlled by a microprocessor. It is made of lightweight carbon fiber and gets its power from a rechargeable battery. With a traditional prosthesis, the user has to think about each step. But the C-Leg analyzes gait 50 times per second; it anticipates movement and thus thinks for the patient. It is supposed to adjust to uneven ground by itself, but results from studies are mixed. It requires less energy for walking at speeds slower or faster than usual, but not at the walker's usual speed; the user does not have to think about changing walking speed. In small studies, patient satisfaction was found to be high. Most study participants chose to keep the C-Leg as opposed to a conventional prosthesis. However, in water, the C-Leg has been known to short out in at least one instance.[28] By 2011, more than 30,000 people were using the C-Leg. It can now be set by the user for a particular activity such as bicycle riding.[29]

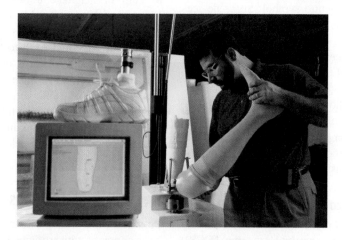

▶ **Figure 11.4** Computers help design and manufacture life like limbs.
*Source:* Brand X Pictures/Jupiter Images.

**eLegs exoskeleton** is a bionic device that helps paraplegics walk. It is wearable and artificially intelligent. It weighs 45 pounds. It can fit people who weigh less than 220 pounds and are between 5 foot 2 inches and 6 foot 4 inches tall. eLegs is attached to the person by Velcro, clips, and shoulder straps. It is worn over clothes and shoes and, after some practice, takes 1 or 2 minutes to put on or take off. It allows a more natural human gait than other devices and allows the person wearing it to walk at over 2 MPH. It is powered by batteries and "employs a gesture-based human-machine interface which—utilizing sensors— observes the gestures the user makes . . . and then acts accordingly. A real-time computer draws on sensors and input devices to orchestrate every aspect of a single stride."[30]

People with computerized prosthetic limbs not only walk but can play sports, run, climb mountains, and—using a prosthetic hand developed at Rutgers University in 1998 with fingers that can be controlled separately—even play the piano! Prosthetic limbs now enable a person to experience touch and temperature. "Patients can . . . have nerves from their hands and finger tips transferred to muscles in their biceps. This gives them the sensation of touch."[31] Other avenues of research for developing a sense of touch are being followed on using cyber-nerves. "'Cyber-nerves' are created from a revolutionary material called Pedot that conducts electricity like a wire and which can encourage the growth of new cells." It may be ready for human trials in a few years.[32] The Pentagon and Johns Hopkins have developed a mind-controlled prosthetic limb, the **Modular Prosthetic Limb (MPL)**, which is currently being tested in human beings. It has fingers that move independently. It weighs about 9 pounds (the weight of a human arm). "[T]he MPL will offer the first hard-wired neural control of bionic body parts, whether lost to injury or neurodegenerative disease." The Defense Advanced Research Projects Agency is working with several universities on this project. Because the neural implant degenerates in 2 years, many surgeries are required. Research is being done to attempt to solve this problem.[33]

At Johns Hopkins in Baltimore, researchers are attempting to "rerout[e] an amputee's remaining nerves in a lost limb to his or her chest" in patients who retain some nerve capacity. According to Dr. Michael McLoughlin, the head to the project, when you think about moving a limb, the chest muscles contract, moving the artificial limb. This research is in its very early stages.[34]

In 2005, the FDA approved a pilot clinical study of the **BrainGate Neural Interface System** for amyotrophic lateral sclerosis (ALS, or Lou Gehrig's disease). The system involves implanting a chip in the brain that converts brain cell impulses to computer signals.[35] In 2006, in the pilot clinical trial, "A man with paralysis of all four limbs could directly control objects around him . . . using only his thoughts." The device, called BrainGate, is surgically implanted. It includes a sensor that records brainwaves and interprets them. It can read brain impulses using implanted wires and translate them into commands.[36] "BrainGate uses a tiny (4×4 mm, about the size of a baby aspirin) silicon electrode array to read neural signals directly within brain tissue." A quadriplegic woman without the power of speech had received a BrainGate implant. She was still able to control a computer cursor accurately even after having the implant for 1,000 days. BrainGate allowed her to use only her thoughts to control the cursor. Others have used BrainGate to control artificial limbs. According to the author of a paper appearing in the *Journal of Neural Engineering*, "Our objective with the neural interface is to reach the level of performance of a person without a disability using a mouse."[37]

In Israel, researchers are working on a sniff-activated sensor. It "translates changes in nasal air pressure into electrical signals that are passed to a computer." By sniffing in a particular way, a person can "select letters or numbers to compose text, . . . or control a mouse." The device can also be used to control a wheelchair. It has been used successfully with two quadriplegics. Its cost at $385 is far lower than other devices such as eye-tracking devices that cost up to $20,000.[38]

Work is beginning in Italy using nanotechnology to attempt to repair spinal cord injuries. These injuries involve the permanent destruction of nerves. In order to regrow new neural tissue, researchers created neural prosthetics of nano-materials filled with drugs that can regenerate growth, which were injected into cavities or cysts in rats' spinal cords. They found that "the cyst [was] replaced by newly formed tissue . . . that provided the appropriate environment for . . . regeneration."[39]

There are several groups of researchers (2010) developing touch-sensitive artificial skin. One type would be based on sensors that can detect the slightest pressure—even the weight of a fly weighing 20 mg. This is achieved through "a large array of pixel pressure sensors on a flexible and stretchable substrate." The project is based on organic electronics. The skin could be used on robots to improve their ability to pick up breakable objects and to help surgeons with the tools of minimally invasive surgery. The researchers hope to develop the skin's sensitivity to the point where it could tell the difference between a smooth surface and an irregular surface. Another project is developing e-skin to increase the sensitivity of touch. E-skin uses nanowire transistors. Its crystalline semiconductor would be able to sense the touch needed for a keyboard. Although it would use less electricity and be more chemically stable than skin based on pixel pressure sensors, it may be less durable.[40]

**Osseointegration** is a technology that allows the integration of living bone with titanium implants. The bone actually grows around the implant, which is thus integrated into the body. It has been used in dentistry, and in cranial and maxillofacial reconstruction, since 1952. In 1990, its use was expanded to other prostheses. It has many benefits over traditional prostheses, including more control and less pain. Among the disadvantages are the necessity for two surgeries, long rehabilitation, and risk of infection that can lead to reamputation.[41]

Work is being done (2011) in nanotechnology to develop smart implants. They would be able to release antibiotics and anti-inflammatory drugs from the surface of the implant. The implant would be coated by a polymer created from nanotubes. Nanostructured materials can also "sense and promote new bone growth."[42] The field of

nanobiology can help improve the communication between human tissue and artificial implants. One of the implants they are working on is an artificial retina, which will be able to see in color.[43]

Computer technology is also helping people who are hearing impaired. A digital hearing aid (essentially a tiny computer), which can be programmed to meet individual needs and adjust to background noise, became available in 1996. Although it cannot help the profoundly deaf, many people found it better at picking up faint sounds than older models. Digital technology has also made possible the development of the cochlear implant (cleared by the FDA in 1996), a device that has been shown to be of some benefit to hearing-impaired people with intact auditory nerves (Figure 11.5▶).

The implant device consists of an internal element surgically implanted behind the ear and a small computer that can be carried. The computer, which is a speech processor, digitizes sound. It is attached to the implant by a cord. The computer sends the digitized code to the implant and then to the inner ear where it is interpreted as sound. Although called an implant, because of its size, most of it is not actually implanted. The size is needed to accommodate the power needs of translating analog to digital signals. The National Institutes of Health National Institute on Deafness and Other Communication Disorders continues to conduct research on improving the implants. According to the manufacturer, the newest implants give "an average of 46%" in hearing improvement and use a 36 percent smaller sound processor than previous implants. They also use rechargeable batteries.[44] In 2003, a researcher from the Massachusetts Institute of Technology (MIT) began working on a low-power analog device that would be fully implanted. In 2010, MIT finished creating what is essentially a "bionic ear"—small, implantable, and running on rechargeable batteries that should last 30 years.[45]

One of the problems of hearing aids is that they may amplify sound but do not indicate where the sound is coming from. A system was developed in 2006 that includes microphones in eyeglasses; when the sound is heard, it is analyzed by a computer.

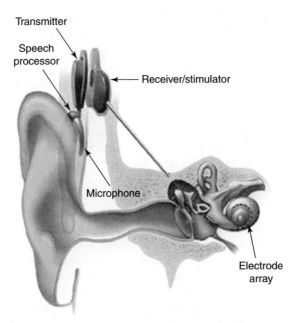

Transmitter

Speech processor

Receiver/stimulator

Microphone

Electrode array

**Ear with cochlear implant**

▶ **Figure 11.5**   Ear with a cochlear implant.
*Source:* Courtesy of NIH Medical Art.

Pads in the frames of the glasses will vibrate, telling the user where the sound originated.[46]

Hearing aids include "digital processing and directional microphones." Sound is more natural. Speech is clearer. Background noise is minimized. They are worn behind the ear; only a small tube enters the ear. If you wear hearing aids in each ear, the wireless e2e (ear-to-ear) system coordinates the hearing aids for better sound. Hybrid implants "combine a traditional hearing aid with a modified electrode similar to . . . a cochlear implant." They provide the best sound.[47] Currently a program is in clinical trials that supplements devices that enhance hearing with computerized auditory training.[48]

The **Acceleglove** uses sensors that detect hand and finger movement and sends signals to the computer. The computer associates the hand movements with a particular word. It then translates the sign language into text and speech.[49] The newest Acceleglove takes the arm into account,

so that more gestures can be recognized. The Acceleglove recognizes the gestures of American Sign Language with over 90 percent accuracy.[50]

## COMPUTERIZED FUNCTIONAL ELECTRICAL STIMULATION TECHNOLOGY

Myoelectrically controlled prostheses, you recall, use the electrical impulses transmitted by muscles to stimulate movement in artificial limbs. CFES (or FES) directly applies low-level electrical stimulation to muscles that cannot receive these signals from the brain. CFES technology was originally developed by NASA. FES has been used for many years in pacemakers and other implanted devices. It is now used to strengthen paralyzed muscles with exercise. It can be used to simulate a full cardiovascular workout for people who are paralyzed, reducing the secondary effects of paralysis. FES even makes it possible to restore movement to some limbs paralyzed by stroke and spinal injury. By stimulating the correct muscles, people who are paralyzed can walk. The amount of electricity is controlled by a microprocessor, which uses feedback from the body to adjust itself.

A normal arm or leg moves because a specific muscle contracts in response to an electrical signal from the brain. A spinal cord injury can prevent these signals from traveling between the brain and any muscle below the injury. Although the muscles still have the ability to move, they do not receive the necessary signals. FES stimulates the muscles directly, sending the electrical signals using electrodes on the skin's surface. On April 1, 2003, Medicare began covering the Parastep system, one system using FES (called functional neuromuscular stimulation) that allows paraplegics to walk. In 2003, in a 17-year follow-up study of two patients using FES, it was found that "[a]lthough the FES system was devised as a temporary means of achieving functional activation . . . it was found to be effective and relatively safe for more than 17 years."[51] In 2002, the National Institutes of Health gave a $3.1 million grant to the University of Delaware's Center for Biomedical Engineering to develop a system using FES and robots that will assist paralyzed stroke patients. The robot will help move the patient's legs to teach him or her to walk. They hope to develop an FES device that is small and wearable.

FES is used in many implanted medical devices, some of which we have come to take for granted. Computers delivering electrical stimulation to the heart are permanently embedded in the human body as pacemakers. A more advanced pacemaker, based on two-way communications technology developed by NASA, allows the doctor to regulate the pacemaker from outside the patient's body, even via the Internet. More complicated than a pacemaker, an implantable cardioverter defibrillator monitors heart rate and gives a jolt of electricity when needed. According to the U.S. FDA, in a clinical study, it restored normal heart rate in 91 percent of the patients. Devices are being tested and approved constantly. In 2006, the FDA planned to have outside experts

monitor devices (such as defibrillators) once they were on the market.[52] In September 1997, the FDA approved an implanted neural prosthesis that restores some hand movement to quadriplegics. The device includes a tiny battery and microprocessor "implanted in the chest and connected to electrodes wired under the skin to eight thumb and finger muscles of the dominant hand. Jerking an externally mounted device on the opposite shoulder signals the implant to move the thumb and fingers." After a period of training, the device enabled quadriplegics to feed themselves and hold a pen. An implantable defibrillator can monitor the heart, and, when it detects an arrhythmia, it converts it to a normal heart rhythm. In March 1998, the FDA approved a breathing pacemaker. It controls breathing by sending electrical impulses to the phrenic nerve.

In July 1997, the FDA approved an implanted device that reduces seizures in people with epilepsy by delivering electrical signals to the brain. Implanted pacemakers (Activa) for the brain are also used to help control the tremors of Parkinson's disease. This device has wires that connect to the electrodes in the brain. Pacemakers for the brain are being tested for the treatment of bipolar disorder and depression. As of 2010, a brain implant (which is not actually implanted in the brain) is being improved in an attempt to make brain pacemakers "more precise." The process involves connecting a chip "to tiny electrodes that provide precisely controlled stimulation to diseased areas." Current devices become less useful "because of overstimulation of the brain." The new device, ReNaChip (Rehabilitation Nano Chip), can analyze the brain's activity and deliver stimulation only when it is needed."[53] In 2011, it was found that FES helped to improve paralyzed people's ability to grasp.[54] Electronic stimulation is also being used to prevent chronic pain. Electronic devices are implanted and send low levels of electrical energy to nerves. This does not allow the pain signals to reach the brain.[55]

In 2006, an implantable device using FES—a **neuroprosthesis**—was developed. It is still being used in 2011. It uses "low levels of electricity in order to activate nerves and muscles in order to restore movement." The electrodes are implanted. They are powered by a switch outside the body. When it is turned on, the patient can move limbs that had been paralyzed.[56]

In 2004 and 2005, the FDA approved two devices (**Neuromove** and **Biomove 3000**) for stroke patients. Both devices help to stimulate the muscles to avoid atrophy and increase both the range of motion and blood circulation. The devices help to communicate with paralyzed muscles through electrical stimulation of the brain. The devices work as follows: "When you think about moving a muscle and the device detects the . . . signal in the muscle, the Biomove then sends a stimulation signal to that muscle to cause it to contract providing positive reinforcement by active biofeedback. In most cases, repetitive use causes the brain to assign new brain cells to control that muscle."[57]

**Neuromodulation** is a field that helps treat disorders of the central nervous system including chronic pain. It "involves implanting an electrode within the nervous system, such as on or below the surface (cortex) of the brain, the spinal cord or the peripheral nerve. A pacemaker-like device called a neurostimulator is implanted in the upper chest and connected under the skin to the electrode. The device is programmed to deliver an electrical current to stimulate targeted nerve cells and nerve fibers in the brain, spinal cord and peripheral nerve."[58] Neuromodulation is used to treat such diverse conditions as Parkinson's disease, obsessive-compulsive disorder, pain, chronic nausea, urinary control, and benign prostate disease. Percutaneous neuromodulation therapy was recently approved by the FDA. It is used to treat back pain in an office procedure. It treats back pain by inserting electrodes (three times thinner than a human hair) into the tissue near the part of the spine causing the pain. The stimulation by the electrodes helps "calm...the nerves," alleviating the pain.[59]

## RISKS POSED BY IMPLANTS

Many of the developments we have mentioned in this chapter involve surgically implanting chips or mechanical devices in human beings. These include heart pacemakers, neural implants, drug delivery systems, and some devices under development. Although millions of people are walking around with implants, we should remember that implants pose some risks, including rejection of the implant and infection at the site. Some implants can cause blood clots and require the user to take anticlotting medications. Research is currently being done to lower the risks of implants. Some scientists are focusing on creating more user-friendly materials that the human body will accept. Research was completed at Rensselaer Polytechnic Institute in New York. Using a technique called **microdialysis**, the project looked at the body's response to an implant at the cellular level. A tiny probe took a sample of fluid at the point where the implant and body meet. The analysis of this fluid can show early signs of rejection or infection.

## COMPUTERS IN REHABILITATIVE THERAPIES

A computerized program called **HELEN (HELp Neuropsychology)** contains diagnostic analyses that keep track of specific tests and tasks performed by the stroke patient. The tasks and methods of solving them are kept in a database. HELEN also contains a rehabilitative module. Tasks are provided for the patient. The methods used to solve the task become information for the neuropsychologist. Interactive procedures allow the patient to try different solutions to the problem. "The system contains tasks that relate to perception, memory and attention, including writing, reading, and counting." Deficits can be pinpointed, and problems that engage the intact portion of the brain can be presented. The patient can control the pace of rehabilitation. HELEN hopes to supplement the program with virtual reality to make it more interesting for the patients. Some of the tasks are used with the Internet, for example, the patient is asked: How many pictures do you see? How many black and white? Patients are also asked to put sentences in order.[60]

**MotionMonitor** is a "computer-based system [which] gives physical therapists real-time, objective measures of the motion of each joint in the patient's body." It involves the placing of electrodes on the patient; they are read by magnetic trackers. This information becomes an animation that both the physical therapist and patient can see in real time.[61] It results in objective measures of how a limb is moving for the therapist. It is also used to educate patients to avoid harmful movements.

In Israel researchers are using software to identify brain injuries, "calculate the probability of recovery and recommend . . . ways to treat the patient." Using virtual reality, patients use a mouse or joystick while viewing themselves on a screen. When the patient makes a small mouse movement, this creates "large virtual movements of the patient's arm, hand, or shoulder on the screen." The patient views the virtual motion. "The virtual experience . . . induces a therapeutic effect on the brain that reduces pain and increases function." The patient sees his or her arm moving without feeling pain, and this leads to "the brain under[going] a corrective learning process."[62]

Currently (2011) researchers are developing devices that could be used in stroke rehabilitation to regain hand and arm movement. The devices are attempting to give people a sense of touch. The devices include one that vibrates but does not give the patient the sense of holding something; a device that is driven by a motor to squeeze, which does give the user the sense of holding something; and a "'shape memory alloy' device which has thermal properties and creates a sensation like picking up a cup of tea."[63] In Ireland, computer games are being developed specifically to help people recover some of the deficits caused by stroke. The games help keep people engaged in the rehabilitative process.[64]

FES has been used for many years in several forms of rehabilitation. Electrical stimulation can help to simulate a workout for muscles that are not being used because of injury. This may prevent the atrophy of the muscles. It can be used for strengthening the muscles and helping in voluntary activity. A physical therapist must place the electrodes correctly and adjust the amount of electricity.

Virtual reality is being used experimentally to help people with amputations control phantom pain. The system gives the illusion that the amputated limb is still there. Using a headset, the patient sees himself or herself with two arms or legs. They are able to use the physical limb to control the virtual limb. Five patients have tried the system. "Four out of the five patients report[ed] improvement in their phantom limb pain."[65]

Many people lose their eyesight because of a neurological condition or disease. Magnetic resonance imaging (MRI) and computed tomography (CT) scans can be used to diagnose these conditions. Some stroke victims lose their vision following a stroke. New therapies have emerged. "The approach is predicated on a revolution sweeping the field of neurobiology: the discovery that the adult brain isn't fixed . . ., but rather has the ability to 'rewire' itself." **Vision replacement therapy** (VRT) retrains the brain. Using dots on a computer screen, the aim is to stimulate peripheral vision. This therapy can be effective years after the stroke occurred. The therapy may be used to treat other conditions such as obsessive-compulsive disorder.[66]

**PARO** is a therapeutic robot developed in Japan. It looks and feels like a little furry seal. Through the use of sensors, it can see light and feel being touched or slapped or held. It can remember what action produced stroking or slapping and change its behavior accordingly. It knows a few words. It is used with patients with dementia to reduce stress and to promote interaction among patients, caregivers, and others.[67] It can be used where real animals cannot be used. It moves its head and legs and has the voice of a baby seal.

There are several new portable devices that can be used for pain control at home. One is an ultrasound device that uses sound waves and massage. A second uses electromagnetic waves. A third reduces muscle pain "by using an electrical current . . . and massage."[68]

## CONCLUSION

Information technology has made possible major improvements in medical devices. This chapter could not be an exhaustive survey because new devices are being developed and approved every year. Computerized monitors can continuously collect data from patients, notifying hospital personnel of a change. Adaptive technology will continue to improve the quality of life of people with disabilities. Assistive devices make it possible for people who are physically challenged to work and live independently. Computerized prostheses have been developed that work almost as well as natural limbs. FES is used in implanted devices, such as pacemakers, and to restore movement to paralyzed limbs. Computer programs are now being used in the rehabilitation of stroke patients.

# IN THE NEWS

According to "The Boss Is Robotic, and Rolling Up Behind You," by John Markoff published on September 4, 2010, in *The New York Times*, doctors can use robots as assistants on site while the doctor is at another site.

Many hospitals and assisted-living facilities are using robots in place of doctors and other caregivers.

Some robots use artificial intelligence. A doctor can, through a robot, talk to a patient, see the cardiac monitor, and judge the patient's condition.

Robots are also being used for the elderly. Eventually they may be used to visit the elderly in place of relatives. They may also be used by the elderly to visit friends, museums, and relatives.

# Chapter Summary

Chapter 11 introduces the reader to the uses of digital technology in medical instruments, adaptive and assistive devices, and prostheses, and to the use of FES technology.

- Computerized medical instruments with embedded microprocessors are used to monitor patients and administer medication.
  - Computerized drug delivery systems are programmable and can detect incorrect flow.
  - Computerized monitoring devices include physiological monitoring systems, arrhythmia monitors, pulmonary monitors, fetal monitors, and neonatal monitoring systems. They continuously monitor a patient's condition and can be programmed to sound an alarm and notify personnel of a dangerous change.

- Some monitors are part of a network; this makes it possible to check the patient's condition from a central location and can decrease response time in emergencies.
- Information technology has had a tremendous impact on people with disabilities.
- The Americans with Disabilities Act of 1990 requires employers to provide "reasonable accommodation" for people with disabilities on the job. Digital technology has made this possible.
- Speech recognition technology allows people without sight or without the use of their hands to interact with computers. Other special input devices include head mice and puff straws.

- Page scanners, speech synthesizers, and screen readers enable the computer to speak to you if you cannot see the screen and for you if you cannot speak.
- Speech recognition can also be used to control appliances in the home, allowing disabled people to live independently.
- Prostheses are artificial replacement limbs and organs.
  - Myoelectric limbs contain a microchip and motor and respond to contractions of the muscle of the natural limb. They work almost as well as natural limbs.
  - CAD/CAM is used in the design and manufacture of prosthetic limbs.
  - Computer technology has contributed to the development of a prosthetic hand whose fingers can be separately controlled and prostheses that can sense hot and cold.

- Computer technology is also contributing to developments that help restore hearing and sight and movement to paralyzed limbs.
- Computer technology with neural interfaces is allowing stroke victims and people with spinal cord injuries to control their bodily movements and to some degree their environments.
- Computerized functional electrical stimulation delivers low-level electrical stimulation to muscles.
  - It is used in implanted devices such as pacemakers and to stimulate paralyzed muscles, even enabling the paralyzed to walk.
- Implants pose the risk of infection and rejection.
- Computer programs that recognize that the brain is not a fixed entity are now being used in the rehabilitation of stroke patients, even years after the stroke occurred.

# Key Terms

Acceleglove

adaptive technology

Americans with Disabilities Act of 1990

arrhythmia monitors

assistive technology

augmentative communication device

biomicroscopes

Biomove 3000

BrainGate Neural Interface System

C-Leg

computerized functional electrical stimulation (CFES or FES)

computerized medical instrument

corneal topography

electronic aids to daily living (EADL)

eLegs exoskeleton

environmental control systems

EYESI surgical simulator

fetal monitors

GDx Access

head mouse

Heidelberg retinal tomograph (HRT)

HELEN (HELp Neuropsychology)

microdialysis

Modular Prosthetic Limb (MPL)

MotionMonitor

myoelectric limbs

neonatal monitors

neuromodulation

Neuromove

neuroprosthesis

optical biometry

Optomap Panoramic200

osseointegration

page scanners

PARO

physiological monitoring systems

prosthetic devices

puff straws

pulmonary monitors

screen reader software

smart glasses

speech recognition

speech synthesizer

text telephones

tonometers

Tracey visual function analyzer

vision replacement therapy

# Review Exercises

## Multiple Choice

1. _____ help(s) physically challenged people control their environments.
   a. Nanogate
   b. Thinkgate
   c. Electronic aids to daily living (EADLs)
   d. None of the above

2. Networked devices _____ .
   a. can reduce response time in emergencies
   b. are most often found in emergency rooms, critical care units, and intensive care units
   c. cannot display findings in a central location
   d. All of the above

3. Puff straws, head mice, and speech recognition software could be characterized as _____ .
   a. prosthetic devices
   b. assistive devices
   c. adaptive devices
   d. B or C

4. The computer in these glasses can "recognize" both people and objects, by looking them up in a database. These glasses are known as _____ .
   a. spy glasses
   b. smart glasses
   c. crystal glasses
   d. All of the above

5. _____ is an alternate input device that a blind person could use.
   a. Braille keyboard
   b. speech recognition software
   c. A or B
   d. screen reader

6. The system that involves implanting a chip in the brain that will convert brain cell impulses to computer signals is called _____ .
   a. Verichip
   b. Brainchip
   c. Thinkgate
   d. BrainGate

7. CFES delivers low-level electrical stimulation and is used _____ .
   a. in pacemakers
   b. to simulate workouts for paralyzed muscles
   c. to restore movement to paralyzed muscles
   d. All of the above

8. The _____ restores some measure of hearing to deaf people with intact auditory nerves.
   a. artificial ear
   b. cochlear implant
   c. hearing pacemaker
   d. prosthetic ear

9. Prosthetic limbs, which contain motors and respond to signals transmitted by the muscles in the residual limb, are called _____ .
   a. energy-storing limbs
   b. myoelectric limbs
   c. computerized limbs
   d. motorized limbs

10. Discrimination against people with disabilities is prohibited by the _____ .
    a. Civil Rights Act
    b. Fourteenth Amendment to the U.S. Constitution
    c. Americans with Disabilities Act
    d. None of the above

## True/False

1. It is possible to control a mouse pointer with brain waves. _____
2. The Acceleglove uses sensors that detect hand and finger movement and sends signals to the computer. _____
3. Hardware and software exist that will allow you to control your home environment by giving voice commands. _____
4. Myoelectric limbs are made possible by computers. _____
5. A computerized program called HELEN (HELp Neuropsychology) contains diagnostic analyses that keep track of specific tests and tasks performed by the stroke patient. _____

6. Electronic stimulation is being used to prevent chronic pain. _____

7. Implanted pacemakers for the brain are used to help control the tremors of Parkinson's disease. _____

8. Networked devices can interact with each other. _____

9. Computerized cardiac monitors cannot distinguish between cardiac arrest and a wire coming loose. _____

10. The C-Leg analyzes gait 50 times per second; it anticipates movement and thus thinks for the patient. _____

## Critical Thinking

1. Evaluate your work space at home, school, or work. How would you design an adaptive environment for people who are mobility impaired?

2. How would you design an adaptive environment for people with speech impairments?

3. How would you design an adaptive environment for people who are blind?

4. The quality of life can be greatly enhanced with the extraordinary CFES technology and advances in prosthetic devices. However, the present cost to the patient can be prohibitive. How would you make this technology available to anyone who needs it?

5. How will the health care professions be affected by all the computerized and technical advances concerning disabilities?

# Notes

1. Lawrence Krieg, "Introduction to Computerized Medical Instrumentation," August 31, 2009, http://courses.wccnet.edu/computer/ mod/mod-m.htm (accessed May 6, 2011).

2. Carolyn Y. Johnson, "Device Linked to Smartphone Helps Diagnose Cancer: Early Trials Show Promising Results, Researchers Say," February 24, 2011, *The Boston Globe*, http://articles.boston.com/2011-02-24/business/29343388_1_ovarian-cancer-cancer-care-smartphone (accessed February 26, 2011).

3. Alan Naditz, "Medical Connectivity: New Frontiers: Telehealth Innovations of 2010," *Telemedicine and e-Health* 16, no. 10 (December 2010): 986–92.

4. "Technology: Optomap Panoramic200," May 7, 2010, http://www.joneseyecenters.com/index.cfm/technology/optomap (accessed April 4, 2011).

5. "Tonometer," No date, http://www.optivision2020.com/tonometer.html (accessed April 4, 2011).

6. "Technology: Heidelberg Retina Tomograph," May 7, 2010, http://www.joneseyecenters.com/index.cfm/technology/heidelbergretina (accessed April 4, 2011).

7. "GDx Access," 2011, http://www.omnieyeatlanta.com/index.cfm/technology/gdx (accessed April 4, 2011).

8. "Technology: Tracey Visual Function Analyzer," May 7, 2010, http://www.joneseyecenters.com/index.cfm/technology/tracey (accessed April 4, 2011).

9. "Computer Display on Glasses Helps to Overcome Tunnel Vision," September 11, 2006, http://www.eri.harvard.edu/faculty/peli/gang/mtbeurope.info.pdf (accessed May 6, 2011); "Senior Scientist Dr. Eli Peli of Schepens Eye Research Institute Wins 2010 Edwin H. Land Medal," August 18, 2010, http://coalgeology.com/senior-scientist-dr-eli-peli-of-schepens-eye-research-institute-wins-2010-edwin-h-land-medal/5804/ (accessed April 5, 2011).

10. Dan Roberts, "Microchip Implantation," February 10, 2007, http://www.mdsupport.org/library/chip.html (accessed May 6, 2011).

11. Larry Greenemeier, "Vision Quest: Retinal Implants Deliver the Promise of Sight to Damaged Eyes," June 15, 2010, https://www.scientificamerican.com/article.cfm?id=retinal-implant-vision (accessed March 30, 2011); Elizabeth Armstrong Moore, "Trials of Human Retinal Implants Quite Successful," 2010, http://news.cnet.com/8301-27083_3-10469657-247.html (accessed March 30, 2011); "Retinal Implant Brightens Future for the Blind," November 3, 2010, http://news.discovery.com/tech/retinal-implant-brightens-future-for-blind.html (accessed March 30, 2011); Neal Kurtzman, "Retinal Implants," March 25, 2010, http://medicine-opera.com/2010/03/retinal-implants/ (accessed March 30, 2011).

12. Greenemeier, "Vision Quest: Retinal Implants Deliver the Promise of Sight to Damaged Eyes"; Moore, "Trials of Human Retinal Implants Quite Successful"; "Retinal Implant Brightens Future for the Blind"; Kurtzman, "Retinal Implants."

13. Naditz, "Medical Connectivity: New Frontiers: Telehealth Innovations of 2010."

14. Anne Eisenberg, "Have You Charged Your Eyeglasses Today?" February 12, 2011, http://www.nytimes.

com/2011/02/13/business/13novel.html (accessed March 30, 2011).

15. Michelle Bryner, "'Smart' Eyeglasses Fill You In on What You're Looking At," December 23, 2010, http://www.livescience.com/10920-smart-eyeglasses-fill-youre.html (accessed April 5, 2011).

16. "Virtual Reality Gaining Acceptance in Ophthalmic Surgical Training Programs," August 1, 2006, http://www.orbis.org/Default.aspx?cid=5778&lang=1html (accessed May 6, 2011).

17. "Executive Order–Increasing Federal Employment of Individuals with Disabilities," July 26, 2010, http://www.whitehouse.gov/the-press-office/executive-order-increasing-federal-employment-individuals-with-disabilities (accessed May 6, 2011).

18. Tracy Russo, "President Obama Announces Revised ADA Regulations," July 26, 2010, http://blogs.usdoj.gov/blog/archives/913 (accessed May 6, 2011).

19. "Clinical Trial Shows Quadriplegics Can Operated Powered Wheelchair with Tongue Drive System," July 6, 2009, http://www.hoise.com/vmw/09/articles/vmw/LV-VM-08-09-4.html (accessed March 30,2011); "Tongue-Drive Wheelchair Electrical and Computer Engineers Design Wheelchair Controlled by a Magnet on the User's Tongue," November 8, 2008,http://www.sciencedaily.com/videos/2008/1112-tonguedrive_wheelchair.htm (accessed November 15, 2010); Val Willingham, "Wheelchair Mobility at the Tip of the Tongue," January 25, 2010, http://articles.cnn.com/2010-01-25/health/hm.wheelchair.tongue_1_tongue-drive-system-spinal-cord-maysam-ghovanloo?_s=PM:HEALTH (accessed March 30,2011); "EYESI Simulator," No date, http://www.vrmagic.com/simulators/eyesi-surgical/ (accessed April 4, 2011).

20. "Smart Pants: Computer Engineers Develop Clothes That Sense and Interpret Movements," April 1, 2006, http://www.aip.org/dbis/HFES/stories/15151.html (accessed May 6, 2011).

21. ICT Results, "Smart Fabrics Make Clever (Medical) Clothing," October 2008, http://www.sciencedaily.com/releases/2009/10/081021190640.htm (accessed April 5, 2011).

22. J. D. Biersdorfer, "A Scanner-Reader to Take Along Anywhere," July 13, 2006, http://www.nytimes.com/2006/07/13/technology/13blind.html (accessed May 6, 2011).

23. "The Dasher Project," August 2, 2006, http://www.inference.phy.cam.ac.uk/dasher/ (accessed August 2, 2006).

24. Ibid.

25. "VoiceIR Environmental Control System: Voice Controller," 2007, http://www.broadenedhorizons.com/voiceir.htm (accessed April 5, 2011).

26. C. Oddo 2011. "Electronic Aids to Daily Living." In: J. H. Stone, M. Blouin, eds. *International Encyclopedia of Rehabilitation*, 2011, http://cirrie.buffalo.edu/encyclopedia/en/article/279 (accessed May 6, 2011).

27. Annalee Anderson, "Language Learning Using Infrared Toys," 2003 ConferenceProceedings, www.csun.edu/cod/conf/2003/proceedings/68.htm (accessed May 6, 2011).

28. Steven Rainwater, "Heroic Cyborg to Receive Medal," February 2006, http://robots.net/article/1826.html (accessed May 6, 2011).

29. "How the C-Leg® Works," 2011, http://www.sierraortho.com/content/c-leg-microprocessor-knee-otto-bock (accessed April 5, 2011).

30. "Introducing eLEGS, Exoskeleton by Berkeley Bionics Enables Paraplegics to Walk," October 7, 2010. http://berkeleybionics.com/2010/introducing-elegs/# (accessed April 1, 2011).

31. Carol Pearson, "Bionic Arm Can Move, Feel: Nerves from Amputated Limb Are Attached to the Remaining Muscle," April 15, 2011, http://www.voanews.com/english/news/usa/Bionic-Arm-Can-Move-Feel-119921104.html (accessed April 23, 2011).

32. Wayne Renardson, "Artificial Nerves Strands of Pedot and Sense of Touch in Prosthetics," August 30, 2010, wayne at renardson.org (accessed April 23, 2011).

33. Drew Halley, "Mind-Controlled Artificial Arm Begins the First Human Testing," August 3, 2010, http://singularityhub.com/2010/08/03/mind-controlled-artificial-arm-begins-the-first-human-testing/ (accessed April 23, 2011).

34. Allen Naditz. "Medical Connectivity: New Frontiers: Telehealth Innovations of 2010."

35. Catherine Calacanis, "FDA Approves Research to Study Brain Chip for ALS," August 3, 2005, http://www.medicalinformaticsinsider.com/2005/08/25/fda-approves-research-to-study/ (accessed May 6, 2011).

36. Leigh Hochberg, Mijail D. Serruya, Gerhard M. Friehs, et al., "Neuronal Ensemble Control of Prosthetic Devices by a Human with Tetraplegia," *Nature* 442 (2006): 164–71, http://www.nature.com/nature/journal/v442/n7099/abs/nature04970.html (accessed May 6, 2011); Aaron Saenz, "Braingate Frees Trapped Minds," May 20, 2009, http://singularityhub.com/2009/05/20/braingate-frees-trapped-minds/ (accessed February 21, 2011).

37. "BrainGate Neural Interface Reaches 1,000-Day Milestone," March 24, 2011,http://news.brown.edu/press-releases/2011/03/braingate (accessed April 23, 2011); Paul Harris, "BrainGate Gives Paralysed the Power of Mind Control: A Tiny Chip Implant Is Enabling Paralysed and Injured People to Move Objects by the Power of Their Thoughts–and, in Time, Researchers Hope It Could Help Them Walk Again," *The Observer*, Sunday April 17, 2011.

38. Naditz, "Medical Connectivity: New Frontiers: Telehealth Innovations of 2010."

39. "Nanostructured Scaffolds Offer a Promising Route to Repairing Spinal Cord Injuries." February 2, 2011. http://www.nanowerk.com/spotlight/spotid=19962.php (accessed April 2, 2011).

40. Naditz, "Medical Connectivity: New Frontiers: Telehealth Innovations of 2010."

41. Miki Fairley, "Osseointegration: In the Wave of the Future?" September 2006, http://www.oandp.com/edge/issues/articles/2006-09_03.asp (accessed May 6, 2011).

42. Michael Berger, "Nanotechnology Research Lays the Foundation for Smart Implants," January 25, 2011, http://www.nanowerk.com/spotlight/spotid=19835.php (accessed February 16, 2011).

43. "Towards an Artificial Retina for Color Vision," January 26, 2011, http://www.nanowerk.com/spotlight/spotid=19863.php (accessed March 31, 2011).

44. "Cochlear Implants," March 2011, http://www.nidcd.nih.gov/health/hearing/coch.asp (accessed April 5, 2011); "Nucleus 5 Upgrade Program," 2010, http://products.cochlearamericas.com/support/cochlear-implants/upgrade-program (accessed April 5, 2011).

45. "The Future of Cochlear Implants," April 15, 2010, http://graysdeafblog.wordpress.com/tag/fully-implanted-cochlear-implants/ (accessed April 5, 2011).

46. David Copithorne, "Varibel Hearing-Aid Glasses Integrate Eight Directional Microphones," April 17, 2006, http://hearingmojo.com/varibel-hearing-aid-glasses-integrate-eight-directional-microphones (accessed April 23, 2011).

47. "New Help for Hearing Loss," January 10, 2008, http://www.parade.com/articles/editions/2006/edition_05-14-2006/Hearing_Loss (accessed May 6, 2011).

48. "Supplementing Hearing Aids with Com-puterized Auditory Training (LACE)," February 15, 2011, http://clinicaltrials.gov/ct2/show/NCT00727337 (accessed April 5, 2011).

49. "Breaking Sound Barriers," March 1, 2006, http://www.sciencedaily.com/videos/2006/0310-breaking_sound_barriers.htm (accessed May 6, 2011).

50. Mike Hanlon, "The AcceleGlove–Capturing Hand Gestures in Virtual Reality," http://www.gizmag.com/go/2134/ (accessed April 6, 2011); Peter Puya Abolfathi, "Interpreting Sign Language Is Just the Beginning for the AcceleGlove Open Source Dataglove," July 23, 2009, http://www.gizmag.com/acceleglove-open-source-dataglove/12252/ (accessed April 6, 2011).

51. S. Agarwal, R. Kobetic, S. Nandurkar, and E. B. Marsolais, "Functional Electrical Stimulation for Walking in Paraplegia: 17-Year Follow-up of 2 Cases," [Abstract] Spring 2003, http://www.ncbi.nlm.nih.gov/pubmed/12830975 (accessed May 6, 2011).

52. Barry Meier, "FDA Plans to Intensify Oversight of Heart Devices," April 7, 2006, http://www.nytimes.com/2006/04/07/business/07device.html (accessed May 6, 2011).

53. Naditz, "Medical Connectivity: New Frontiers: Telehealth Innovations of 2010."

54. "Benefits of Electrical Stimulation Therapy Found with People Paralyzed by Spinal Cord Injury," February 18, 2011, http://www.sciencedaily.com/releases/2011/02/110217125113.htm (accessed April 23, 2011).

55. Thomas M. Wascher, "Rechargeable Spinal Cord Stimulators for Chronic Pain," http://www.spine-health.com/treatment/pain-management/rechargeable-spinal-cord-stimulators-chronic-pain-research-article (accessed May 6, 2011).

56. Cynthia Bowers, "New Device Gives Hope to Paralyzed," July 17, 2006, http://www.cbsnews.com/stories/2006/07/17/earlyshow/health/main1808040.shtml (accessed May 6, 2011); "Challenges in Neuroprosthesis Use," 2010, http://www.scireproject.com/rehabilitation-evidence/upper-limb/neuroprostheses/challenges-in-neuroprosthesis-use (accessed April 23, 2011).

57. "Some Biomove 3000 and Biomove 5000 Questions," April 22, 2010, http://www.biomoveusa.com/FAQ-Biomove.htm (accessed May 6, 2011); "Zynex Medical's NeuroMove™ System Citedin New Clinical Study of Stroke RecoveryTherapies," *Business Wire,* October 26, 2005, http://www.businesswire.com/news/home/20051026005179/en/Zynex-Medicals-NeuroMove-TM-System-Cited-Clinical (accessed May 6, 2011); "Biomove 3000 System," January 27, 2005, http://www.accessdata.fda.gov/cdrh_docs/pdf4/K042650.pdf (accessed May 6, 2011).

58. "The Neurostimulator: Pacemaker for the Brain," September 2006, http://www.froedtert.com/HealthResources/ReadingRoom/FroedtertToday/September2006Issue/PacemakerfortheBrain.htm (accessed May 6, 2011).

59. "Medtronic Neuromodulation Business Overview, FY 2010 Revenue," November 19, 2010, http://www.medtronic.com/ (accessed April 6, 2011); Mary Claire Walsh, "Percutaneous Neuromodulation Therapy (PNT)," January 12, 2010, http://www.spineuniverse.com/treatments/pain-management/percutaneous-neuromodulation-therapy-pnt (accessed April 6, 2011).

60. Cecilia Sik Lànyi, Julianna Szabò, Attila Pàll, and Ilona Pataky, "Computer Controlled Cognitive Diagnostics and Rehabilitation Method for Stroke Patients," *ERCIM News* No. 61, April 2005, http://www.ercim.eu/publication/Ercim_News/enw61/lanyi.html (accessed May 6, 2011).

61. "Sports Injury Prevention & Performance: 3D Imaging System Helps Athletes Recover from Injuries." December 1, 2006, http://www.sciencedaily.com/videos/2006/1203-sports_injury_prevention_amp_performance.htm (accessed May 6, 2011); "The MotionMonitor," 2011, http://www.innsport.com/ (accessed April 23, 2011).

62. Roland Piquepaille, "Virtual Reality Used for Stroke Rehabilitation." March 17, 2008, http://www.zdnet.com/blog/emergingtech/virtual-reality-used-for-stroke-rehabilitation/866 (accessed April 7, 2011).

63. University of Southampton, "Scientists Develop New Technology for Stroke Rehabilitation," April 6, 2011, http://www.sciencedaily.com/releases/2011/04/110405102204.htm (accessed April 7, 2011).

64. "Computer Games Help Stroke Patients," April 10, 2010, http://www.science.ie/science-news/computer-games-stroke-patients.html (accessed April 7, 2011).

65. "Virtual Reality Lets Amputees 'Control' Missing Limbs," November 15, 2006, http://www.sciencedaily.com/releases/2006/11/061115093227.htm (accessed May 6, 2011).

66. Sharon Begley, "*Wall Street Journal* Feature: NovaVision™ VRT™ Research & Improvements for Stroke Vision Loss Patient," February 1, 2005, http://www.self-healing.org/vision-therapy-for-stroke/ (accessed May 6, 2011).

67. "Paro Therapeutic Robot," 2010, http://www.parorobots.com/ (accessed November 12, 2010).

68. Lashan Clarke, "Portable Home Medical Devices for Pain Control," December 31, 2010, http://www.healthguideinfo.com/health-testing-technology/p101529/ (accessed February 15, 2011).

# Additional Resources

"$3.1 Million NIH Grant Funds Research to Help Stroke Patients." October 17, 2002. http://www.udel.edu/PR/UDaily/01-02/NIHgrant101702.html (accessed May 6, 2011).

Abolfathi, Peter Puya. "Interpreting Sign Language Is Just the Beginning for the AcceleGlove Open Source Dataglove." July 23, 2009. http://www.gizmag.com/acceleglove-open-source-dataglove/12252/ (accessed April 6, 2011).

"Benefits of Electrical Stimulation Therapy Found with People Paralyzed by Spinal Cord Injury." February 18, 2011. http://www.sciencedaily.com/releases/2011/02/110217125113.htm (accessed April 23, 2011).

Berger, Michael. "Nanotechnology Research Lays the Foundation for Smart Implants." January 25, 2011. http://www.nanowerk.com/spotlight/spotid=19835.php (accessed February 16, 2011).

Bhattacharjee, Yudhijit. "Smart Wheelchairs Will Ease Many Paths." May 10, 2001. http://www.nytimes.com/2001/05/10/technology/10NEXT.html?ex=1198904400&en=49d403d1d3597ed8&ei=5070 (accessed May 6, 2011).

Bhattacharjee, Yudhijit. "So That's Who's Talking: A Hearing Aid Points to the Sound." September 27, 2001. http://query.nytimes.com/gst/fullpage.html?res=9D03E1D6133AF934A1575AC0A9679C8B63 (accessed May 6, 2011).

"BrainGate Neural Interface Reaches 1,000-Day Milestone." March 24, 2011. http://news.brown.edu/pressreleases/2011/03/braingate (accessed April 23, 2011).

Bryner, Michelle. "'Smart' Eyeglasses Fill You In on What You're Looking At." December 23, 2010. http://www.livescience.com/10920-smart-eyeglasses-fill-youre.html (accessed April 5, 2011).

Bryner, Michelle. "Brainpower: Human Minds May Soon Control Prosthetic Limbs." February 23, 2011. http://www.technewsdaily.com/2114-brainpower-human-minds-may-soon-control-prosthetic-limbs.html (accessed April 3, 2011).

Carroll, Linda. "Doctors Look Ahead to 'Pacemakers for the Brain.'" February 18, 2003. http://www.raven1.net/mcf/news/pacemakers-for-brain.htm (accessed May 6, 2011).

"Challenges in Neuroprosthesis Use." 2010. http://www.scire-project.com/rehabilitation-evidence/upper-limb/neuroprostheses/challenges-in-neuroprosthesis-use (accessed April 23, 2011).

Clarke, Lashan. "Portable Home Medical Devices for Pain Control." December 31, 2010. http://www.healthguideinfo.com/health-testing-technology/p101529/ (accessed February 15, 2011).

"Clinical Trial Shows Quadriplegics Can Operated Powered Wheelchair with Tongue Drive System." July 6, 2009. http://www.hoise.com/vmw/09/articles/vmw/LV-VM-08-09-4.html (accessed March 30, 2011).

"Cochlear Implants." March 2011. http://www.nidcd.nih.gov/health/hearing/coch.asp (accessed April 5, 2011).

"Computer Games Help Stroke Patients." April 10, 2010. http://www.science.ie/science-news/computer-games-stroke-patients.html (accessed April 7, 2011).

Copithorne, David. "Varibel Hearing-Aid Glasses Integrate Eight Directional Microphones." April 17, 2006. http://hearingmojo.com/varibel-hearing-aid-glasses-integrate-eight-directional-microphones (accessed April 23, 2011).

"Early Infection and Rejection Detection: Microdialysis Technique May Help Implants Stay Put Longer." July 28, 2003. http://news.rpi.edu/update.do?artcenterkey=154 (accessed May 5, 2011).

Eisenberg, Anne. "Analog over Digital? For a Better Ear Implant, Yes." May 29, 2003. http://www.nytimes.com/2003/05/29/technology/what-s-next-analog-over-digital-for-a-better-ear-implant-yes.html (accessed May 6, 2011).

Eisenberg, Anne. "Beyond Voice Recognition, to a Computer That Reads Lips." September 11, 2003. http://www.nytimes.com/2003/09/11/technology/what-s-next-beyond-voice-recognition-to-a-computer-that-reads-lips.html (accessed May 6, 2011).

Eisenberg, Anne. "A Chip That Mimics a Retina but Strains for Light." August 9, 2001. http://www.nytimes.com/2001/08/09/technology/what-s-next-a-chip-that-mimics-a-retina-but-strains-for-light.html (accessed May 6, 2011)

Eisenberg, Anne. "A Gaze That Dictates, with Intuitive Software as the Scribe." September 12, 2002. http://www.nytimes.com/2002/09/12/technology/what-s-next-a-gaze-that-dictates-with-intuitive-software-as-the-scribe.html (accessed May 6, 2011).

Eisenberg, Anne. "Have You Charged Your Eyeglasses Today?" February 12, 2011. http://www.nytimes.com/2011/02/13/business/13novel.html (accessed March 30, 2011).

Eisenberg, Anne. "The Kind of Noise That Keeps a Body on Balance." November 14, 2002. http://www.nytimes.com/2002/11/14/technology/what-s-next-the-kind-of-noise-that-keeps-a-body-on-balance.html (accessed May 6, 2011).

Eisenberg, Anne. "What's Next: A Chip That Mimics Neurons, Firing Up the Memory." June 2, 2002. http://www.nytimes.com/2002/06/20/technology/what-s-next-a-chip-that-mimics-neurons-firing-up-the-memory.html (accessed May 6, 2011).

Eisenberg, Anne. "What's Next: Glasses So Smart They Know What You're Looking At." June 28, 2001. http://www.nytimes.com/2001/06/28/technology/what-s-next-glasses-so-smart-they-know-just-what-you-re-looking-at.html (accessed May 6, 2011).

Eisenberg, Anne. "When the Athlete's Heart Falters, a Monitor Dials for Help." January 9, 2003. http://www.nytimes.com/2003/01/09/technology/what-s-next-when-the-athlete-s-heart-falters-a-monitor-dials-for-help.html (accessed May 6, 2011).

"EYESI Simulator." No date. http://www.vrmagic.com/simulators/eyesi-surgical/ (accessed April 4, 2011).

"FDA Approves NESS Device for Moving Paralyzed Legs." November 2006. http://www.ishitech.co.il/1106ar5.htm (accessed April 6, 2011).

Felton, Bruce. "Technologies That Enable the Disabled." September 14, 1997. http://www.nytimes.com/1997/09/14/business/earning-it-technologies-that-enable-the-disabled.html (accessed May 6, 2011).

"The Future of Cochlear Implants." April 15, 2010. http://graysdeafblog.wordpress.com/tag/fully-implanted-cochlear-implants/ (accessed April 5, 2011).

Gallagher, David. "For the Errant Heart, a Chip That Packs a Wallop." August 16, 2001. http://www.nytimes.com/2001/08/16/technology/circuits/16HOWW.html (accessed May 6, 2011).

Garibaldi, Matthew. "Myoelectric Prostheses Offer Advantages." Winter 2006. http://www.ucsfhealth.org/newsletters/orthopaedic_surgery_news/winter_2006/myoelectric/ (accessed May 6, 2011).

"GDx Access." 2011. http://www.omnieyeatlanta.com/index.cfm/technology/gdx (accessed April 4, 2011).

Glassman, Mark. "A Braille Phone Organizer Connects the Dots and the User." April 17, 2003. http://www.nytimes.com/2003/04/17/technology/watch-accessibility-braille-phone-organizer-connects-dots-user.html (accessed May 6, 2011).

Greenemeier, Larry. "Vision Quest: Retinal Implants Deliver the Promise of Sight to Damaged Eyes." June 15, 2010. https://www.scientificamerican.com/article.cfm?id=retinal-implant-vision (accessed March 30, 2011).

Halley, Drew. "Mind-Controlled Artificial Arm Begins the First Human Testing." August 3, 2010. http://singularityhub.com/2010/08/03/mind-controlled-artificial-arm-begins-the-first-human-testing/ (accessed April 23, 2011).

Hanlon, Mike. "The AcceleGlove—Capturing Hand Gestures in Virtual Reality." http://www.gizmag.com/go/2134/ (accessed April 6, 2011).

Harris, Paul. "BrainGate Gives Paralysed the Power of Mind Control: A Tiny Chip Implant Is Enabling Paralysed and Injured People to Move Objects by the Power of Their Thoughts—and, in Time, Researchers Hope It Could Help Them Walk Again." *The Observer*, Sunday April 17, 2011.

Happ, Mary Beth, Tricia Roesch, and Sarah Kagan. "Patient Communication Following Head and Neck Cancer Surgery: A Pilot Study Using Electronic Speech-Generating Devices." November 2005. http://lib.bioinfo.pl/paper:16270113 (accessed May 6, 2011).

"How the C-Leg® Works." 2011. http://www.sierraortho.com/content/c-leg-microprocessor-knee-otto-bock (accessed April 5, 2011).

ICT Results. "Smart Fabrics Make Clever (Medical) Clothing." October 2008. http://www.sciencedaily.com/releases/2009/10/081021190640.htm (accessed April 5, 2011).

"Introducing eLEGS, Exoskeleton by Berkeley Bionics Enables Paraplegics to Walk." October 7, 2010. http://berkeleybionics.com/2010/introducing-elegs/# (accessed April 1, 2011).

Johnson, Carolyn Y. "Device Linked to Smartphone Helps Diagnose Cancer: Early Trials Show Promising Results, Researchers Say." February 24, 2011. *The Boston Globe.* http://articles.boston.com/2011-02-24/business/29343388_1_ovarian-cancer-cancer-care-smartphone (accessed February 26, 2011).

Junker, Andrew H. "A Revolutionary Approach to Computer Access: Coherent Detected Periodic Brainwave Computer Control." 2003. http://www.csun.edu/cod/conf/2003/proceedings/235.htm (accessed May 6, 2011).

Klonoff, David C. "Diabetes and Telemedicine: Is the Technology Sound, Effective, Cost-effective, and Practical?" 2003. http://care.diabetesjournals.org/cgi/content/full/26/5/1626 (accessed May 6, 2011).

Krcmar, Stephen. "The Stuff of Dreams." April 2006. http://www.rehabpub.com/features/42006/7.asp (accessed May 6, 2011).

Kurtzman, Neal. "Retinal Implants." March 25, 2010. http://medicine-opera.com/2010/03/retinal-implants/ (accessed March 30, 2011).

Marriott, Michel. "Wired by a Kindred Spirit, the Disabled Gain Control." April 24, 2003. http://www.nytimes.com/2003/04/24/technology/wired-by-a-kindred-spirit-the-disabled-gain-control.html (accessed May 6, 2011).

Mathur, Ruchi, and William C. Shiel. "Insulin Pump for Diabetes Mellitus." November 14, 2007. http://www.medicinenet.com/insulin_pump_for_diabetes_mellitus/article.htm (accessed May 6, 2011).

"Medicare to Pay for FES Walking System." 2002. http://sci.rutgers.edu/forum/archive/index.php/t-47354.html (accessed May 6, 2011).

"Medtronic Neuromodulation Business Overview, FY 2010 Revenue." November 19, 2010. http://www.medtronic.com/ (accessed April 6, 2011).

Moore, Elizabeth Armstrong. "Trials of Human Retinal Implants Quite Successful." 2010. http://news.cnet.com/8301-27083_3-10469657-247.html (accessed March 30, 2011).

"MotionMonitor." 2011. http://www.innsport.com/ (accessed April 23, 2011).

Naditz, Allen. "Medical Connectivity: New Frontiers: Telehealth Innovations of 2010." *Telemedicine and e-Health* 16, no. 10 (December 2010): 986–92.

"Nanostructured Scaffolds Offer a Promising Route to Repairing Spinal Cord Injuries." February 2, 2011. http://www.nanowerk.com/spotlight/spotid=19962.php (accessed April 2, 2011).

"New Device Approval: GlucoWatch Automatic Glucose Biographer—P990026." June 29, 2009. http://www.fda.gov/MedicalDevices/ProductsandMedicalProcedures/DeviceApprovalsandClearances/Recently-Approved Devices/ucm089158.htm (accessed May 6, 2011).

"New Device Approvals: Medtronic Model 7250 Jewel AF Implantable Cardioverter Defibrillator System—P980050/S1." June 29, 2009. http://www.fda.gov/Medical Devices/ProductsandMedicalProcedures/Device ApprovalsandClearances/Recently-ApprovedDevices/ucm089056.htm (accessed May 6, 2011).

"Nucleus© 5 Upgrade Program." 2010. http://products.cochlearamericas.com/support/cochlear-implants/upgrade-program (accessed April 5, 2011).

Nussbaum, Debra. "Bringing the Visual World of the Web to the Blind." *The New York Times,* March 26, 1998, G8.

Oddo, C. "Electronic Aids to Daily Living." In: J. H. Stone, M. Blouin, eds. *International Encyclopedia of Rehabilitation.* 2011. http://cirrie.buffalo.edu/encyclopedia/en/article/279 (accessed May 6, 2011).

"Otto Bock C-leg®: A Review of Its Effectiveness for Special Care Services." WCB Evidence Based Group, Dr. Craig W. Martin, Senior Medical Advisor. November 27, 2003. http://www.worksafebc.com/health_care_providers/Assets/PDF/Otto_Bock_Cleg.pdf (accessed May 6, 2011).

"Pacemaker for the Brain May Offer Hope for Parkinson's Disease." 2011. http://mentalhealth.about.com/library/sci/0102/blparkins0102.htm (accessed May 6, 2011).

"A Pacemaker for Your Brain." June 28, 2010. http://www.physorg.com/news196958657.html (accessed May 6, 2011).

"Paro Therapeutic Robot." 2010. http://www.parorobots.com/ (accessed November 12, 2010).

Pearson, Carol. "Bionic Arm Can Move, Feel: Nerves from Amputated Limb Are Attached to the Remaining Muscle." April 15, 2011. http://www.voanews.com/english/news/usa/Bionic-Arm-Can-Move-Feel-119921104.html (accessed April 23, 2011).

Piquepaille, Roland. "Virtual Reality Used for Stroke Rehabilitation." March 17, 2008. http://www.zdnet.com/blog/emergingtech/virtual-reality-used-for-stroke-rehabilitation/866 (accessed April 7, 2011).

Rachkesperger, Tracy. "Growing Up with AAC." 2006. http://www.asha.org/public/speech/disorders/GrowingUpAAC.htm (accessed May 6, 2011).

"Retinal Implant Brightens Future for Blind." November 3, 2010. http://news.discovery.com/tech/retinal-implant-birghtens-future-for-blind.html (accessed March 30, 2011).

Saenz, Aaron. "Braingate Frees Trapped Minds." May 20, 2009. http://singularityhub.com/2009/05/20/braingate-frees-trapped-minds/ (accessed February 21, 2011).

Saenz, Aaron. "Braingate 2: Your Mind Just Went Wireless." June 17, 2009. http://singularityhub.com/2009/06/17/braingate2-your-mind-just-went-wireless/ (accessed February 21, 2011).

"Senior Scientist Dr. Eli Peli of Schepens Eye Research Institute Wins 2010 Edwin H. Land Medal." August 18, 2010. http://coalgeology.com/senior-scientist-dr-eli-peli-of-schepens-eye-research-institute-wins-2010-edwin-h-land-medal/5804/ (accessed April 5, 2011).

Skillings, Jonathan. "Prosthetics Go High Tech." August 3, 2005. http://www.news.com/Prosthetics-go-high-tech/2008-1082_3-5816267.html (accessed May 6, 2011).

"Supplementing Hearing Aids with Computerized Auditory Training (LACE)." February 15, 2011. http://clinicaltrials.gov/ct2/show/NCT00727337 (accessed April 5, 2011).

Taub, Eric. "Typing with Two Hands, No Fingers." May 1, 2003. http://www.nytimes.com/2003/05/01/technology/news-watch-keyboards-typing-with-two-hands-no-fingers.html (accessed May 6, 2011).

"Technology: Heidelberg Retina Tomograph." May 7, 2010. http://www.joneseyecenters.com/index.cfm/technology/heidelbergretina (accessed April 4, 2011).

"Technology: Optomap Panoramic200." May 7, 2010. http://www.joneseyecenters.com/index.cfm/technology/optomap (accessed April 4, 2011).

"Technology: Tracey Visual Function Analyzer." May 7, 2010. http://www.joneseyecenters.com/index.cfm/technology/tracey (accessed April 4, 2011).

"Tongue-Drive Wheelchair Electrical and Computer Engineers Design Wheelchair Controlled by a Magnet on the User's Tongue." November 8, 2008. http://www.sciencedaily.com/videos/2008/1112-tonguedrive_wheelchair.htm (accessed November 15, 2010).

"Tonometer." No date. http://www.optivision2020.com/tonometer.html (accessed April 4, 2011).

"Towards an Artificial Retina for Color Vision." January 26, 2011. http://www.nanowerk.com/spotlight/spotid=19863.php (accessed March 31, 2011).

Tran, N., and T. J. Webster. "Nanotechnology for Bone Materials." [Abstract] 2009. http://www.ncbi.nlm.nih.gov/pubmed/20049801 (accessed April 5, 2011).

University of Southampton. "Scientists Develop New Technology for Stroke Rehabilitation." April 6, 2011. http://www.sciencedaily.com/releases/2011/04/110405102204.htm (accessed April 7, 2011).

"VoiceIR Environmental Control System: Voice Controller." 2007. http://www.broadenedhorizons.com/voiceir.htm (accessed April 5, 2011).

Walsh, Mary Claire. "Percutaneous Neuromodulation Therapy (PNT)." January 12, 2010. http://www.spineuniverse.com/treatments/pain-management/percutaneous-neuromodulation-therapy-pnt (accessed April 6, 2011).

Weingarten, Marc. "For an Irregular Lens, an Optical Blueprint." September 12, 2002. http://www.cs.berkeley.edu/~barsky/NYTimes.article/For.6.htm (accessed May 7, 2011).

Wiener, Jon. "USC Ophthalmologists Announce Launch of Permanent Retinal Implant Study." April 30, 2002. http://www.eurekalert.org/pub_releases/2002-04/uosc-uoa_1043002.php (accessed May 7, 2011).

Willingham, Val. "Wheelchair Mobility at the Tip of the Tongue." January 25, 2010. http://articles.cnn.com/2010-01-25/health/hm.wheelchair.tongue_1_tongue-drive-system-spinal-cord-maysam-ghovanloo?_s=PM:HEALTH (accessed March 30, 2011).

# Related Web Sites

ALS Association. http://www.alsinfo.org

National Institutes of Health. http://www.nih.gov

Telemedicine Insider. http://www.telemedicineinsider.com

U.S. Department of Veterans Affairs. http://www.va.gov

U.S. Food and Drug Administration. http://www.fda.gov

PEARSON
**myhealthprofessionskit**

Go to www.myhealthprofessionskit.com to access the Companion Web site created for this textbook. Simply select "Basic Health Science" from the choice of disciplines. Find this book and register to access self-assessment quizzes, flashcards, and more.

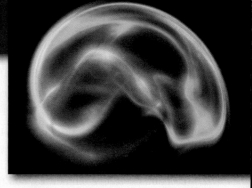

CHAPTER **12**

# Security and Privacy in an Electronic Age

## CHAPTER OUTLINE

- Learning Objectives
- Security and Privacy—An Overview
- Threats to Information Technology
  - *Computer Technology and Crime*
  - *Security*
- Privacy
  - *Databases*
    - Government Databases
    - Private Databases
    - Databases and the Internet
- Privacy, Security, and Health Care
  - *Health Insurance Portability and Accountability Act of 1996 (HIPAA) and HITECH*
    - Privacy of Medical Records under HIPAA, HITECH, and the USA Patriot Act
    - Telemedicine and Privacy
    - E-Mail and Privacy
    - Privacy and Genetic Information
    - Privacy and Electronic Health Records
- Security Breaches
- In the News
- Chapter Summary
- Key Terms
- Review Exercises
- Notes
- Additional Resources
- Related Web Sites

## LEARNING OBJECTIVES

Upon completion of this chapter, the reader will be able to:

- Define security and privacy.
- Discuss threats to information technology, including crimes, viruses, and the unauthorized use of data.
- Discuss security measures including laws, voluntary codes of conduct, restriction of access to computer systems, biometrics, and the protection of information on networks.
- Describe the impact of information technology on privacy, including the existence of large computerized databases of information kept by both government and private organizations, some of which are on networks linked to the Internet.
- Describe the relationship of privacy and security to health care and appreciate the importance of the privacy of electronic medical records.
- Discuss the Health Insurance Portability and Accountability Act of 1996 (HIPAA), the Health Information Technology for Economic and Clinical Health Act of 2009 (HITECH), and the USA Patriot Act (2001), specifically their effects on privacy protections.
- Discuss the enforcement of HIPAA, as amended by HITECH.

## SECURITY AND PRIVACY— AN OVERVIEW

Information technology (IT) and the expansion of the Internet have changed the way we live. Almost all of our institutions—schools, businesses, hospitals, and government agencies—depend on computers. By 2014, hospitals are supposed to have installed computerized hospital information systems; eventually, all health care institutions will be linked electronically. Computers enable the collection, storage, and processing of enormous amounts of information quickly and efficiently. At the same time, any harm to computer systems is more threatening to the normal conduct of business. Safeguarding computer systems becomes critical. Guaranteeing the accuracy and **security** and protecting the **privacy** of electronic records, including medical records, are crucial. Our initial discussion of security and privacy, although general, also applies to medical issues of security and privacy. It is an ongoing challenge. Old unused records should be removed and destroyed to avoid disclosure. In April 2011, Texas Comptroller Susan Combs announced that a publicly accessible state computer server had contained the personal information for 3.5 million people for at least a year. The information included names, addresses, Social Security numbers, some dates of birth, and driver's license numbers.[1]

In April 2011, a college in the United Kingdom e-mailed a list intended for staff to a class of students. The list contained the names, medical histories, and medical conditions of 300 students. The students listed had physical, mental, or learning disabilities. One student with a brain tumor was named; another named student had anorexia. Detailed descriptions were included. The students who received the e-mails were asked to delete them.[2] In December 2010, a computer at St. Louis University in Missouri was hacked, leading to unauthorized access to personal information including Social Security numbers of 12,000 employees. The computer also contained health information ("names, dates of birth, dates of service, testing assessments, diagnoses and treatments") of 800 students who had been counseled by the Student Health Service.[3] In February 2011, several of Health Net's (a California health insurer) servers containing personal information and demographic data for 1.9 million patients nationally "went missing." The data included names, Social Security numbers, and "sensitive health information." The same company lost data on 1.5 million people in 2009.[4] Data on computers are not secure.

Privacy has many aspects. Among them is the ability to control personal information and the right to keep it from misuse. Computer technology makes this much more difficult. Security measures attempt to protect computer systems, including information, from harm and abuse; the threats may stem from many sources including natural disaster, human error, or crime including the spreading of **viruses**. Protection may take the form of anything from professional and business codes of conduct, to laws, to restricting access to the computer.

This chapter deals with threats to information technology, stressing dangers to the privacy of information in electronic databases, as well as measures to protect the security of computer systems. Massive government and private databases on the Internet pose dangers to personal privacy. This chapter also deals with computers and trends in health care delivery, including the growth of health maintenance organizations and medical insurance companies, the relationship of telemedicine to issues of privacy and security, the use of electronic health records and e-mail. The electronic sharing of health records can help save lives by assuring continuity of care. However, the lack of security in computer systems in health care organizations and on networks in general endangers doctor–patient confidentiality and the privacy of medical information. Even under the Health Insurance Portability and Accountability Act of 1996 (HIPAA), medical records are accessible not only to your physicians, but also to insurance companies, laboratories, pharmacies, and hospital clerical staffs. Under the Health Information Technology for Economic and Clinical Health Act of 2009 (HITECH), part of the American Recovery and Reinvestment Act of 2009, the privacy protections of HIPAA are strengthened and expanded significantly to, for example, businesses that work with your health care provider. Included in this chapter is a discussion of attempts to make electronic health records secure, including federal legislation protecting the privacy of medical records—HIPAA and HITECH.

## THREATS TO INFORMATION TECHNOLOGY

Threats to information technology include hazards to hardware, software, networks, and data including information stored in electronic databases. **Data accuracy** and security are what is most relevant to the use of computerized health records. However, computer hardware, software, and data can be damaged by anything from simple carelessness to power surges, crime, and computer viruses Computer systems, like any other property, can be hurt or destroyed by disasters such as floods and fires.

### Computer Technology and Crime

Computer technology has led to new forms of crime. Crimes involving computers can be crimes using computers or crimes against computer systems. Many times they are both—using computers to harm computer systems. Computer crime includes committing fraud and scams over the Internet, unauthorized copying of software protected by copyright (called **software piracy**), and **theft of services** such as cable TV. Software piracy costs the software industry billions of dollars a year. According to the Business Software Alliance, over 30 percent of software is pirated.[5] **Theft of information**, including breaking into a medical database and gaining access to medical records, is also considered a crime.

One common computer crime is **fraud**—such as using a computer program to illegally transfer money from one bank account to another or printing payroll checks to oneself. Fraudulent purchases over the Internet are common. Purchases over the Internet are increasing. A favorite target of Internet thieves is software. Because software is delivered instantly—electronically—it is received before credit card numbers are checked.

Viruses can also damage hardware, software, and data. A virus is a program that attaches itself

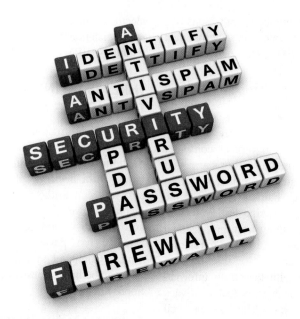

▶ **Figure 12.1**   Antivirus software can help protect your
computer.
*Source:* almagami/Shutterstock.com

to another program and replicates itself. A virus
may do damage to your hardware or destroy your
data, or it may simply flash an annoying message.
Most states and the federal government make it
a crime to intentionally spread a computer virus.
Federal law makes it a felony to do $1,000 or
more worth of damage to any computer involved
in interstate commerce; this includes any personal
computer connected to the Internet. The penalties for damaging computer systems have been
severely increased by the USA Patriot Act and
the Homeland Security Act. Spreading viruses
is a kind of high-tech vandalism. Virus detection
software can find and get rid of many but not all
viruses (Figure 12.1▶).

One of the most valuable resources of any
organization is data or information. An accurate
list of a business's customers with their purchases
and credit records, or of a doctor's patients with
their confidential medical histories, is a vital asset
that cannot be replaced. It is crucial that this information be correct and secure. However, this is

not always the case. Data may be incorrect simply because of carelessness in data entry; that is,
information in a database is erroneous because
of faulty entry or an inaccurate source. However,
data may be correct and still vulnerable to misuse.
Some information, including medical records, is
highly personal and subject to abuse. Protecting
the privacy of records kept on electronic databases and on networks is extremely difficult, if not
impossible.

**Identity theft** involves someone using your
private information to assume your identity.
Identity theft rose between 2000 and 2003; however, it has now stabilized: "Identity fraud victims
as a percent of the United States adult population . . . declined slightly from 4.7% to 4.0%
between 2003 and 2006." According to Javelin
Strategy and Research, which issues a report on
identity fraud every year, identity fraud continued to rise each year until, in 2010, the number
of victims decreased 28 percent. Identity fraud
reached an 8-year low. The decreases in fraud

could be due to stricter standards and checks by lenders and increased security and law enforcement.[6] However, the average amount that fraud victims had to pay increased from $387.00 to $681.00. They trace the increased dollar amount per victim to new account fraud. In new account fraud, someone opens an account without your knowledge. New account fraud cost $27 billion in 2010. The only type of identity fraud that rose was theft by someone known to the victim (a relative or roommate); this grew by 7 percent. This report also finds that data breaches are down from 221 million to 26 million records. However, according to the Identity Theft Resource Center, data breaches ("event[s] that potentially put a person's name, Social Security number, drivers license number, medical record or financial record (credit or debit card) potentially at risk, either in electronic or paper form . . .") increased 33 percent from 2009 to 2010. In 2010, there were 662 data breaches putting 16,167,542 records at risk. Twenty percent of these were paper breaches.[7] Whichever number you choose to believe—and the discrepancy could be due to differences in definition or counting or sampling error—data breaches are a big problem. There were 250,854 complaints of identity theft that reached the Federal Trade Commission in 2010; this constituted 19 percent of the complaints received, the "top . . . consumer complaint . . . for the 11th year in a row."[8]

Although identity theft predates computers, the existence of computer networks, the centralization of information in databases, and the posting of public information on the Internet could make information much easier to steal. An identity thief needs only a few pieces of information (such as Social Security number and mother's maiden name) to steal your identity. Under this false identity—your identity—the thief can apply for credit cards, take out loans, buy houses, and even commit crimes. Identity theft is extremely difficult to prosecute. It is also not easy for the victim to correct all the negative information that the thief has created. False negative information may keep appearing in response to every routine computer check. Currently, some cities are putting all public

records including property and court records on the Internet, making identity theft even easier to commit. Think of the information (including your signature) on the ticket you were issued last month.

Because it is such a serious problem costing so much money, many states have introduced and passed legislation regarding identity theft. In 2009, 37 states and the District of Columbia had legislation introduced on identity theft. Twenty-three of them passed the legislation. In 2010, 30 states and the District of Columbia introduced such legislation and 15 states passed it. In 2011, 34 states introduced such legislation.[9] On the federal level, two senators have introduced a bill on identity theft. The bill would create a "national framework" defining personal information as "any information that can be used to steal from a consumer, commit identity theft, or be used for other criminal activities." If information is breached, the victim must be notified. The law covers any concern that collects information such as businesses, governments, and schools. All breaches must be disclosed. It introduces no new penalties. The bill has been introduced before, but has a chance to pass this year.[10]

Biometric methods are used in identification systems to safeguard your identity. Some biometric methods use "keystroke dynamics, a form of behavioral biometrics, to recognize valid users" and prevent unauthorized access to computers.[11] Worldwide, people are concerned over bank card fraud and identity theft, according to a Unisys biannual global study in 2009. The study also found increasing acceptance of biometric methods of protecting data, especially in the United Kingdom, where "95% . . . who said they would . . . provide biometric data . . . would be willing to provide fingerprint data; 90% . . . would provide an eye scan; and 82% would agree to a facial scan." Although the United Kingdom had the highest acceptance rates of these methods, other countries also had high acceptance rates.[12]

As of 2011, some threats to computer systems include the following. **Spyware** is software that can be installed without the user's knowledge to track their actions on a computer. **Adware** may display unwanted pop-up advertisements on your monitor; the advertisements may be related to the sites you search on the Web or even the content of your e-mail. A **fraudulent dialer** can connect the user with numbers without the user's knowledge; the dialer may connect the user's computer to an expensive 900 number. The user will be totally unaware until he or she receives the telephone bill. The additional money is collected by the person who gave out the fraudulent number. A dialer is usually installed with free software. Because a dialer needs a phone, broadband connections are usually not affected. **Keylogging** can be used by anyone to track anyone else's keystrokes, e-mail addresses typed, and Web sites visited. **Malware** (short for malicious software) is software designed to harm your computer. It can change or destroy data. **Phishing** involves sending fraudulent messages via e-mail or instant message that purport to be from a legitimate source such as a social network or information technology (IT) administrator. The user is directed to a fake Web site and asked to enter information. A **Trojan horse** appears to be a normal program such as computer game but "conceals malicious functions." An **e-mail bomb** or **denial-of-service attack** sends so much e-mail to one address that the server stops working. A **botnet** is comprised of a collection of automatic software robots. Botnets can remove software or send spam. Social media (such as Facebook) is now a major way of spreading harmful computer programs. Also, mobile devices may become targets.[13] Antivirus software can help protect your computer.

## Security

Security measures attempt to protect computer systems and the privacy of computerized data. They can include anything from laws and **codes of conduct**, to training employees, to audit trails, to restricting access to computers, to **encryption**—scrambling of data so that it does not make sense. There are federal laws that attempt to protect computer systems and aspects of privacy (Figures 12.2 and 12.3▶).

There are also codes of conduct within some businesses and organizations that attempt to safeguard information. Protecting privacy on the

Internet is a much more difficult problem. An early attempt at self-regulation occurred in December 1997. To forestall government regulation, several computer companies and look-up services reached an agreement on a code of conduct to limit public access to personal data on the Internet. The code would allow people to have their names removed from databases, but it includes no way of informing people what is online about them or giving them a way to correct it. A person would have to contact all 14 companies and ask to have his or her name removed from each database. The agreement also would ask marketers to "voluntarily limit the collection of personal data." Encryption would be used to protect private information. Social Security numbers, mother's maiden name, birth date, credit and financial records, and medical records would no longer be available to the general public; private investigators and law enforcement agencies would have access to this information.

Many organizations restrict access to their computers. This can be done by requiring authorized users to have **personal identification numbers (PINs)** or use **passwords**. Locking computer rooms and requiring employees to carry ID cards and keys are also used to restrict access. **Biometric methods**, including **fingerprints**, **hand prints**, **retina scans** or **iris scans**, **lip prints**, **facial thermography**, **body odor sensors**, **voice recognition**, and **DNA** also help make sure only authorized people have

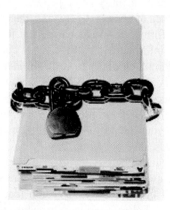

▶ **Figure 12.2**  Summary of the HIPAA Privacy Rule.
*Source*: Courtesy of the Department of Health and Human Services (HHS.gov).

## Partial List of Federal Legislation on Computers and Privacy

- **1970— The Fair Credit Reporting Act** regulates credit agencies. It allows you to see your credit reports to check the accuracy of information and challenge inaccuracies. Amended several times, the Fair and Accurate Credit Transaction Act of 2003 preempts some state privacy protections, but mandates that you can have a free credit report each year.[14]

- **1974— Privacy Act** prohibits disclosure of government records to anyone except the individual concerned, except for law enforcement purposes. It also prohibits the use of information except for the purpose for which it was gathered. It deals with the use and disclosure of Social Security numbers.[15]

- **1978—Right to Financial Privacy Act** (RFPA) establishes procedures for the federal government to follow when looking at bank records. RFPA was amended due to the USA Patriot Act of 2001 to permit the disclosure of financial information to any intelligence or counterintelligence agency in any investigation related to international terrorism (October, 2001).[16]

- **1984 (amended in 1994)—Computer Fraud and Abuse Act** prohibits unauthorized access to federal computers.[17]

- **1984—Cable Communications Policy Act** protects the personal information of customers of cable service providers.[18]

- **1986—Electronic Communications Privacy Act** prohibits government agencies from intercepting electronic communications without a search warrant. It also prohibits individuals from intercepting e-mail. However, there are numerous exceptions, and the courts have interpreted this to allow employers to access employees' e-mail. This law does not apply to communications within an organization.[19]

- **1988— Video Privacy Protection Act** prohibits video rental stores from revealing what tapes you rent.[20]

- **1988 (amended in 1990)—Computer Matching and Privacy Protection Act** limits the use of computer matching.[21]

- **1994—Computer Abuse Amendments Act** makes it a crime to "gain unauthorized access to a computer system [used in interstate commerce] with the intent to obtain anything of value, to defraud the system, or to cause more than $1000 worth of damage." This applies to any computer linked to the Internet. It specifically prohibits the transmission of viruses. (Note: Section 1030 was amended on October 26, 2001, by the USA Patriot antiterrorism legislation.)[22]

- **1996—National Information Infrastructure Protection Act** establishes penalties for interstate theft of information and for threats against networks and computer system trespassing.[23]

- **1996—Health Insurance Portability and Accountability Act (HIPAA)** puts a national floor under privacy protections for medical information.

- **1997—Driver Privacy Protection Act** limits disclosure of personal information in Motor Vehicles records.[24]

- **1999—The Financial Modernization Act** governs collection and disclosure of customers' personal financial information by financial institutions.[25]

▶ **Figure 12.3**  Federal laws intended to protect computer systems and privacy of individuals.

- **2000—Children's Online Privacy Protection Act** requires Web sites targeting children aged 13 or under to get parental consent to gather information on the children.[26]

- **2001—The USA Patriot Act** gives law enforcement agencies greater power to monitor electronic and other communications, with fewer checks.[27]

- **2002—The Homeland Security Act** expands and centralizes the data gathering allowed under the Patriot Act.[28]

- **2003—Fair and Accurate Credit Transactions Act (FACTA)** added new sections to the federal Fair Credit Reporting Act intended to help consumers fight identity theft. Accuracy, privacy, limits on information sharing, and new consumer rights to disclosure are included in FACTA.[29]

- **2004—Social Security Protection Act**: to amend the Social Security Act and the Internal Revenue Code of 1986 to provide additional safeguards for Social Security and Supplemental Security Income beneficiaries with representative payees, to enhance program protections, and for other purposes.[30]

- **2004—Video Voyeurism Act** would prohibit video voyeurism in the maritime and territorial jurisdiction of the United States.[31]

- **2005— Combat Methamphetamine Epidemic Act**: A new part of the USA Patriot Act that requires anyone who buys cough medicine containing pseudoephedrine to present photo ID.[32]

- **2005—Online Privacy Protection Act** requires the Federal Trade Commission to prescribe regulations to protect the privacy of personal information collected from and about individuals who are not covered by the Children's Online Privacy Protection Act of 1998 on the Internet, to provide greater individual control over the collection and use of that information, and for other purposes.[33]

- **2009—Health Information Technology for Economic and Clinical Health Act** (HITECH Act) made significant changes to the privacy and security rules of the Health Insurance Portability and Accountability Act of 1996 (HIPAA), extending their reach and imposing breach notification requirements on HIPAA-covered entities and their business associates.

▶ **Figure 12.3**  *(Continued)*

access to computer systems. Biometric technology can use facial structure to identify individuals. **Biometric keyboards** can identify a person by behavior, for example, by fingerprint, voice, and gait. None of these methods is foolproof. Even biometric methods, which for a time were seen as more reliable, are far from perfect. PINs and passwords can be forgotten or shared, and ID cards and keys can be lost or stolen. Biometric methods also pose a threat to privacy, because anyone who can gain access to the database of physical characteristics gains access to other, possibly private information about you. Some biometric measures are inherently different than other security measures. In more traditional methods, such as fingerprinting, you are aware that your identity is being checked. However,

iris and retina scans, facial thermographs, **facial structure scans**, and body odor sensors allow your identity to be checked without your knowledge, cooperation, or consent. This can be seen as an invasion of privacy. Now there is the possibility of implanted radio frequency identification (RFID) tags as a security measure.

Since September 11, 2001, the federal government has attempted to increase airport security using various measures to screen passengers and baggage. Many U.S. airports are using a whole body imaging technique using backscatter X-ray machines. It has been referred to as a virtual strip search because "The level of detail uncovered [is] akin to . . . disrobing in public: the images seen by the screeners reveal the outlines of nipples and genitalia."[34] Privacy groups have sued to stop the procedure as "unlawful, invasive, and ineffective." Others have questions about the possible long-term cancer risk from this exposure to "penetrating radiation [which] causes genetic mutations, which set all living cells on the path to cancer."[35]

Protecting information that is kept on a network is much more difficult because no one knows who can access a network. Even top-secret defense systems have been broken into. One way of protecting data is through encryption. Only authorized persons can see the decrypted data. Electronic blocks (called **firewalls**) can be used to limit access to networks. None of these measures guarantees security; therefore, a protection plan that includes backing up data is always necessary. This guarantees that you have an accurate copy of the data you need, but does nothing to protect data from misuse.

However, on April 12, 2011, assistant director of the Federal Bureau of Investigation's (FBI) Cyber Division, Gordon Snow, told the Senate Judiciary Crime and Terrorism Subcommittee, that criminals can "penetrate any system that is accessible from the Internet." This means, he continued, that "government networks and the nation's critical infrastructure could be degraded, disrupted, or destroyed." Even when a crime is detected, it is very difficult to know where it originated or who did it.[36]

# PRIVACY

Computer technology has transformed the way we assemble, store, and protect data—including highly confidential material. It has also changed the way we work at jobs. Almost every white-collar worker has a microcomputer on his or her desk. The personal computer has replaced the typewriter. E-mail is replacing the memo and telephone call. This makes both our words and our work more subject to scrutiny and less private. People think of e-mail as private; it is not. According to Barry Lawrence of the Society of Human Resource Management, "e-mail [is] like a postcard. Anyone can read it along the way." Employees are fired for using e-mail for private communications or to send messages critical of their bosses. The **Electronic Communications Privacy Act of 1986** has been interpreted to allow employers access to employees'

e-mail. Not only are your words subject to scrutiny; so is your work. When you are working on your office PC, every keystroke may be monitored and counted by your employer. The Act "as amended, protects wire, oral, and electronic communications while those communications are being made, are in transit, and when they are stored on computers. The Act applies to email, telephone conversations, and data stored electronically." However, some of the act's privacy protections were changed by "the Communications Assistance to Law Enforcement Act (CALEA), the USA PATRIOT Act in 2001, the USA PATRIOT reauthorization acts in 2006, and the FISA Amendments Act of 2008."[37]

As an employee, you have a very restricted right to privacy. In 1977, the Federal Privacy Protection Commission, under pressure from business groups, did not ask Congress to make it a crime for employers to gather information "unrelated to job performance" about employees. As a consumer, when you make a purchase with a credit card, your name, address, and credit card number, along with your purchases, are recorded. The information becomes part of your credit history, and a profile of your buying habits can be put together and sold to direct marketers. Records that used to be kept in physically separate places—your credit history in one store's credit file; your health records in your doctor's office; or a city's records of births, marriages, and vehicle ownership in a county courthouse—are now organized in databases, stored on computers, linked to networks, and available to anyone with a computer and a connection to the Internet.

Smart cards are currently being used as driver's licenses. These cards can contain information about the driver and links to government and private databases. However, in May 2005, as part of the military spending bill, President Bush signed the **Real ID Act of 2005** into law. Prior to this, the states were cooperating with the federal government to establish acceptable federal standards. However, the Real ID Act "directly imposes prescriptive federal driver's license standards" by the federal government on the states.[38] This law requires every American to have an electronic identification card. By 2008, states were supposed to start providing ID cards that meet the standards set up by the Real ID Act. "You'll need a federally approved ID card to travel on an airplane, open a bank account, collect Social Security payments . . ." And practically speaking, your driver's license likely will have to be reissued to meet federal standards. To be issued a card, you will need to appear (in person) at a state motor vehicle agency with photo identity, "document your birth date and address, and show that your Social Security number is what you had claimed it to be." This information must be verified, digitized, and stored by the Department of Motor Vehicles (DMV). Your prior licenses and immigration status must also be verified.

For the states to be able to check the information an applicant provides, databases containing this information must be put online and standardized so that each state can access the information. The cards will contain (in machine-readable form) at least the following information: name, date of birth, sex, ID number, a digital photo, and address. The Department of Homeland Security may unilaterally add other items like a fingerprint or an iris scan.[39] The Department of Homeland Security, the states, and Departments of Motor Vehicles (DMV) are working to set up guidelines; they have not as yet determined what technology or technologies to use: RFID, barcode, or magnetic stripe. The cards must contain features that make them secure against tampering or copying. Data must be encrypted. Cardholders will be able to block transmission of the information and "ha[ve] to be informed about how the agency issuing the card intended to use it, what information [i]s being collected . . . , the basic risks of the technology . . . , and which precautions [a]re available."[40] State DMVs must share all of the information in their databases with all other state DMVs' databases. This creates a huge database. Police can demand ID from anyone. The law also sets up a "requirement for background checks on employees." However, by 2011, according to some sources, the Real ID Act had "been put in limbo after 25 states adopted legislation opposing it."[41] Even if this is true, it is not legal. Federal law cannot legally be nullified by a state.

A new threat to personal privacy may come from implanted RFID tags according to privacy advocates. The tags are radio transmitters that give off a unique signal, which can be read by a receiver. The person with the tag implanted does not need to know it is being read. Tags have been used in pets and products. The U.S. Food and Drug Administration (FDA) has approved the tags for medical use.[42] In 2006, two employees of an Ohio company had RFID tags embedded in their arms. The company said "it was testing the technology as a way of controlling access to a room."[43]

However, these chips are very easily counterfeited—"you could have a chip implanted, and then your front door would unlock when your shoulder got close to the reader. Let us imagine that you did this; then, I could sit next to you on the subway, and read your chip's ID. This takes less than a second. At this point I can let myself in to your house, by replaying that ID. So now you have to change your ID; but as far as I know, you cannot do this without surgery."[44]

Computer technology and the Internet allow for the inexpensive and easy gathering and distribution of personal information—from the most mundane to the most intimate details of our lives—which may be collected without our consent or knowledge. Laws have been proposed to create some minimal privacy rights on the Internet; for example, sites now have to get parental consent before collecting information from children. The computer may gather information about you without your knowledge as you browse the Net. Cookies are small files that a Web site may put on your hard drive when you visit. Cookies can be programmed to track your movements, collecting information that helps advertisers target you. This information may be sold and shared; the fact is that you do not control your information once it is in cyberspace.

## Databases

An electronic **database** is an organized collection of data that is easy to access, manipulate, search, and sort. Gathering facts is not new. A decennial census is mandated by the U.S. Constitution, so that representation in Congress can be determined. Records of birth, marriage, death, divorce, property ownership, taxes, driving, and bankruptcy are all on file. The local library even keeps records of the books you check out until they are returned. These records have always been kept. However, they used to be kept in the local courthouse or DMV—every file physically and logically separate from every other file. To access the records, you had to travel to where the file was kept. Today, with the use of computerized databases on networked computers, this is not the case. Through the use of Social Security numbers as identifiers, the information in one database can be linked to information in other databases, and a complete and detailed portrait of any individual can be painted.

GOVERNMENT DATABASES Large databases of information are kept by the federal and local governments as well as by private businesses. Agencies of the federal government maintain more than 2,000 databases. The FBI's National Crime Information Center includes millions of records. The Internal Revenue Service (IRS) keeps a database on the sources and amounts of income we earn and the taxes we pay. The Social Security Administration has records that are used to determine your eligibility for benefits. The Department of Defense has a database that includes your draft status. The National Directory of New Hires is a database that the federal government was required to start on October 1, 1997, by the 1996 welfare law. Every time a person is hired, his or her name must be reported along with address, Social Security number, and wages. Wage reports are required every 3 months. The data collected by the Census Bureau are now computerized, although by law, they cannot be used against a respondent.

Agencies of the government may use computer matching to link data in several databases. For example, the IRS uses computer matching to match tax records with vehicle registration and other records kept by state governments and with private records of large transactions kept by banks. The IRS looks for expensive purchases, such as cars and boats, and for large cash transactions. The National Directory of New Hires will be matched against the Department of Health and Human Services' (HHS) list of everyone owing or owed child support, and the lists will be checked against each other. The purpose of the National Directory of New Hires is to provide a national database of "employment and unemployment

insurance information that will enable state Child Support Enforcement . . . agencies to be more effective in locating noncustodial parents, establishing child support orders and enforcing child support orders." States and other federal agencies provide the information.[45]

Some federal agencies (including the IRS, Social Security Administration, and Secret Service) use computer profiling—a technique that puts together a portrait of a person "likely" to commit a crime. Computer profiling was being used by the Computer Assisted Passenger Screening Program, which used dozens of criteria, most of them secret, to screen for air travelers likely to be terrorists. However, in 2010, the Department of Homeland Security instituted the Secure Flight program, which gathers more biographic information from passengers and matches them against terrorist watch lists.[46] Although data gathered by the government are subject to some regulation, data gathered by private companies are not. Government and private companies do cooperate in the gathering of data. Currently, certain jurisdictions are putting all their records online. This means your signature is available on a traffic ticket, and the details of your divorce can be read like a novel.

Since September 11, 2001, Congress, concerned with security, passed two bills that affect privacy: the USA Patriot Act (2001) and the **Homeland Security Act** (2002). The **USA Patriot Act** gives law enforcement agencies greater power to monitor electronic and other communications, with fewer checks. It allows increased sharing of information between the states, the FBI, and the Central Intelligence Agency (CIA). The law expands the authority of the government to allow roving wiretaps, which intercept communications, wherever the person is. Both e-mail and voicemail may be seized under a search warrant.[47] The government may track Web surfing and request information from Internet Service Providers (ISPs) about their subscribers. The law establishes a DNA database that will include anyone convicted of a violent crime. Some of these provisions were originally scheduled to sunset or expire in 2005. However, on March 9, 2006, President Bush signed an extension of the USA Patriot Act. The 16 provisions will not expire.

The Homeland Security Act expands and centralizes the data gathering allowed under the Patriot Act. A new federal Department of Homeland Security is established to analyze data collected by other agencies. The law includes expanded provision for the government to monitor electronic communications and authority for the government to mine databases of personal information, at the same time that it limits Congressional oversight. Any government body at any level can now request information from your ISP without a warrant or probable cause, as long as there is a "good faith" belief that national security is involved. Your local library is required to turn over any record to the FBI, if asked. The act limits an individual's access to information under the Freedom of Information Act. If a business states that its activities are related to security, that information will be kept secret.[48] The law gives government committees more freedom to meet in secret. It limits liability for companies producing antiterrorism products including vaccinations, at the same time that the government would gain wider power to declare national health emergencies and quarantines and order forced vaccinations.

In February 2011, a limited extension of the USA Patriot Act was passed by both the House and Senate. The extensions included provisions "permitting surveillance of individuals and groups not connected to identified terrorist groups, . . . granting access to any tangible items of individuals under surveillance, and . . . authorizing the FBI's use of roving wiretaps." Discussions are taking place in the Senate Judiciary Committee on extending the provisions until 2013, but with increased oversight.[49]

Since September 11, "new mechanisms . . . for data sharing and mining" have been developed.[50] Many private businesses have been pressed to give customer information to the federal government. One instance of this, which was revealed in 2006, involved large telecommunications companies giving the telephone records of millions of Americans to the National Security Administration without warrants.[51]

In an action that defies classification, "the text of a secret agreement that the Department of Homeland Security executed with the Centers for Disease Control to share airline data" has been revealed. This violates an agreement that the United States reached with the European Union that the latter would share data despite "the lack of privacy laws in the United States. . . . DHS agreed that the passenger data would not be used for any purpose other than the prevention of serious crime." However, the Department of Homeland Security has broken the agreement.[52]

PRIVATE DATABASES Private organizations keep computerized databases of employees and potential customers. Hospitals keep records of patients. You may not be aware that data are being gathered or that the data gathered may be entered in a database. The information in the databases may be available to the general public over the Internet. Unaware of the existence of the information, you have no opportunity to check its accuracy. When you buy something using a credit card at the supermarket, fill out a warranty card, subscribe to a magazine, fill out a survey questionnaire, or rent a movie, data are collected about your purchasing habits. When you make a telephone call, a record is kept of the telephone number, time, and length of the call. All of this information is collected for commercial purposes; businesses can buy your profile and analyze it, looking for likely customers. However, you do not control what happens to information about you or who will become aware of the brand of soap you use in the shower.

The **MIB Group, Inc.** (formerly the **Medical Information Bureau**) is of particular interest. It is comprised of 470 insurance companies. Its database contains health information on about 15 million Americans and Canadians. Although the information in the database is not supposed to be the sole reason to determine coverage,[53] according to the Annualmedicalreport.com, the information (whether true or not) in this huge database is used by medical insurers to help determine insurance rates and whether to grant or deny someone medical coverage and even to drop coverage. According to *Business Week*, "two-thirds of all insurance companies are using consumers' medical histories and personal information to deny coverage, charge higher premiums, and exclude certain medical conditions from policies."[54] However, the MIB Group, Inc. denies this, stating that "MIB Members . . . are strictly forbidden from using MIB information about you as the basis for determining your eligibility for insurance. MIB Members only use MIB's information as an 'alert' or 'red flag,' which prompts them to obtain additional information through traditional underwriting tools and methods."[55] The medical histories in this database are not protected by doctor–patient privilege and are specifically exempt from HIPAA.[56] Although some members of the MIB Group are covered by HIPAA regulations, the MIB itself operates under the Fair Credit Reporting Act as amended by the **Fair and Accurate Credit Transaction Act of 2003 (FACTA)**, which added some protections against identity theft to the earlier law. Consumers have the right to one copy of their MIB file per year and to attempt to correct any inaccurate information.[57] The privacy department of the MIB, according to an April 2011 e-mail to the author, states that "We do adhere to both of these privacy protections."[58]

Credit bureaus receive information from businesses and banks. From this, they compile a credit history and credit report. Your credit report is used as a basis for granting or denying you a credit card, mortgage, or student loan. It may also be requested by a potential employer and may be used to deny you a job. Although the use and content of credit reports are regulated by the **Fair Credit Reporting Act of 1970**, it is extremely difficult to remove inaccurate negative information. FACTA limits information sharing and adds new consumer protection rights, especially against identity theft. (For a full discussion of FACTA, see "Fact Sheet 6a: Facts on FACTA, the Fair and Accurate Credit Transactions Act," February 2011, http://www.privacyrights.org/fs/fs6a-facta.htm.)

Some private companies (data warehouses) exist for the sole purpose of collecting and selling personal information. They sell information to credit bureaus and to employers for background checks. Since September 11, the demand for background checks on prospective (or even current) employees has increased. One company experienced a 33 percent increase in the demand for background checks.

The linking of information is making these background checks more thorough. Electronic databases are now being linked into larger and more comprehensive super databases. For example, in November 2001, one company linked together criminal records from all U.S. jurisdictions (a database of 20 million convictions). Before that, each jurisdiction had to be searched separately.

DATABASES AND THE INTERNET When files were first computerized, they were kept in separate computer systems; security could be as easy as locking the door to the computer room and requiring each authorized user to have valid identification. Today, computerized files are kept on networks, many of which are linked to the Internet. The information includes highly personal data such as Social Security numbers, dates of birth, mothers' maiden names, and unlisted phone numbers. Companies such as Lexis-Nexis and Equifax sell credit and financial information and medical records to banks, insurance companies, and direct marketers. You are not aware of the information that is available about you, where it is stored, or its accuracy. The impact of this is serious. Anyone with access to your Social Security number can gain access to information about you and even assume your identity. Recently (April 2011), it was revealed that iPhones and iPads keep location data logs.[59] According to a recent study, the logs are put "in a secret file, then transfer[red] . . . to the user's computer." One of the researchers stated that it is now "possible for almost anybody—a jealous spouse, a private detective—with access to your phone or computer to get detailed information about where you've been."[60]

## PRIVACY, SECURITY, AND HEALTH CARE

The privacy of medical records is something people are very concerned about. Several trends combine to threaten the security and privacy of health care information. First, health care information has traditionally been protected by state law. Now, however, this information routinely crosses state lines, which means it needs federal protection. It is very difficult to protect information on computer networks, especially the Internet. The privacy protections of the Health Information Portability and Accountability Act began going into effect on April 14, 2003. HIPAA provides the first federal protection for the privacy of medical records, which was extended by HITECH in 2009.

## Health Insurance Portability and Accountability Act of 1996 (HIPAA) and HITECH

Given the facts of current medical practice—the use of the electronic medical record stored on networks, telemedicine, and information that routinely crosses state lines—federal protection has become a necessity.

In 1996, Congress passed the **Health Insurance Portability and Accountability Act (HIPAA)**. Guidelines to protect electronic medical records were developed by the Department of Health and Human Services (HHS). By encouraging the use of the electronic medical record and facilitating the sharing of medical records among health care providers, it can assure continuity of care and thus save lives. If you are in an accident far from home, the availability of your medical history can prevent medical catastrophes such as allergic reactions to medications. However, the more easily your records are available, the less secure they are. Medical information can be used against you. According to a report by the U.S. Congress cited in the *Telemedicine Newsletter*, it is crucial to safeguard the privacy of health information because, "Inaccuracies in the information or its improper disclosure, can deny an individual access to . . . basic necessities of life, and can threaten an individual's personal and financial well-being."

HIPAA and HITECH "encourage electronic transactions, but . . . also require new safeguards to protect the security and confidentiality" of health information.[61] The new safeguards do not override stronger state protections.

For the first time, all patients have the right to see their medical records and *request* changes; patients will have some knowledge of the use of their medical records and must be notified in writing of their providers' privacy policy. HIPAA gives patients more control over their medical information. Under the rule, medical records must be supplied within 30 days of the patient's request, and the patients are allowed to review and copy their own records as they wish. Prior to HIPAA, many states did not give patients the legal right to see their records. Additionally, the patient can request amendments be made to their records if their appeal is justifiable.

HIPAA regulations began going into effect on April 14, 2001; health plans, clearinghouses, and providers who use electronic billing and funds transfer had until April 14, 2003, to comply. Other entities had until April 2006 to comply. In 2006, the enforcement portion of the law went into effect; that is, health care institutions can be fined for disobeying the law. The regulations cover "all medical records and other individually identifiable health information used or disclosed by a covered entity in any form, whether electronically, on paper, or orally." Higher standards apply to psychotherapy notes, which are not considered part of a medical record under this law and "are never intended to be shared with anyone else." The law applies to both public and private providers and institutions. Providers must give patients a written explanation of how their health information may be used; patients may see, copy, and *request* changes in their medical records. Providers need to make a good faith effort to get a patient's consent before using his or her information. Health information may no longer be used by employers or banks to make decisions regarding employment or loans. Except for the sharing of information for the purpose of treatment, payment, or business operations, "disclosures . . . will be limited to the minimum necessary."[62] In practice, this may mean that any health care business can see personal health information with little regard for treatment.

Health care providers and institutions may design their own procedures to meet the new standards; however, they must be written and must include the following information: who has access to patient information, how this information will be used, and the conditions under which it may be shared. Health care providers are responsible for seeing that those with whom they do business also protect patient privacy. Employees must be trained to respect patient privacy and follow privacy procedures, and one person must be chosen to ensure that the privacy procedures are followed. Under specific conditions, health information may be shared without the patient's consent (e.g., for public health needs, research, and some law enforcement activities, and when the interests of national defense and security are involved). Under HIPAA, violations of the law can be punished by both civil and criminal penalties.[63]

Some of the original privacy protections have been weakened, for example, the requirement of a patient's written consent for disclosure of health information.[64] Because of this, some privacy advocates stress the weaknesses of the privacy protection. However, with all its weaknesses, HIPAA provides the first national minimum privacy protections for health information.[65]

HIPAA requires health care facilities (protected entities) to conduct a risk analysis to "evaluate risks . . . and to implement policies and procedures to address those risks."[66] Risk management requires the entity to put into place security measures. The use of virus protection software, specifically **Spybot Search and Destroy**, would be advisable. One of the security measures that health care organizations can use is Single Sign On— Password Management. Single Sign On makes use of smart cards and biometrics. It makes it possible for multiple users to share a workstation without compromising security. It keeps track of users.

Before 2008, the law enforcement agency responsible for HIPAA (the HHS Office of Civil Rights) tended to simply respond to complaints. It only completed a few compliance reviews. In addition, the HHS Office of Civil Rights had chosen not to prosecute high-profile cases, including "the theft of millions of veterans' records . . . , [a] California health plan that left personal information about patients on a public Web site for years, and a Florida hospice that sold . . . personal patient information to other hospices."[67]

Between 2003 and 2006, there were 19,420 grievances, most of them alleging privacy violations or difficulty in getting records. There were

two criminal prosecutions. "One man was sentenced to 16 months . . . in prison for stealing credit card information from a cancer patient; a woman was convicted of selling an FBI agent's medical records." The government responded to 73 percent of the complaints by saying there was no violation or allowing the violating entity to fix the problem. The HHS preferred to work for voluntary compliance and settle complaints through "corrective action plans." This has been criticized by privacy advocates who state that "the administration's decision not to enforce the law more aggressively has not safeguarded . . . medical records." According to a health care privacy expert at Columbia University, "The law was put in place to give people some confidence when they talk to their doctor or file a claim with their insurance company, that information isn't going to be used against them. [Because] they have done almost nothing to enforce the law . . . we're dangerously close to having a law that is essentially meaningless." HIPAA compliance was falling in 2005. Five hundred cases were open.[68]

By June 30, 2008, 37,200 complaints had reached the Office for Civil Rights (OCR). Eighty percent were resolved; 6,648 were investigated, and corrective action was taken. In July 2008, for the first time, a covered entity was required to pay a fine. After receiving 31 complaints about one company, the Office for Civil Rights and Centers for Medicare and Medicaid Services (CMS) investigated and required the company to pay $100,000. There has also been an increase in criminal prosecutions by the Department of Justice.[69]

HITECH, passed in 2009 as part of the stimulus, further defines compliance with HIPAA's privacy and security requirements. It also expands HIPAA standards that help electronic exchange of health information. It establishes incentives for adopting EHRs. It increases penalties for noncompliance and requires encryption.[70] HITECH is also intended to implement a "national health technology infrastructure," which could lead to the extension of telemedicine.[71]

On August 3, 2009, HHS took enforcement of HIPAA's Security Rule out of the hands of the CMS and put the Office for Civil Rights in charge.

"This change reflects the growing seriousness of HHS and others about enforcing federal privacy and security mandates for health information." HITECH requires HIPAA to implement new breach regulations, encourages the use of electronic health records (EHRs), increases civil and criminal penalties for violations of the Privacy Rule, prohibits sales of health information without the consent of the patient, and tightens other HIPAA restrictions on disclosures of health information. Perhaps the most important thing that HITECH does is extend HIPAA privacy protections to businesses that work with HIPAA-covered entities. If a covered entity does not follow HIPAA's privacy rule, "it is almost entirely exclude[d] from receiving monetary incentives for introducing EHRs."[72] HITECH defines a breach as "unauthorized acquisition, access, use or disclosure of protected health information which compromises the security or privacy of such information."[73]

In 2009, criminal prosecutions under HIPAA increased. Two hospital employees in Florida were indicted for theft of patient records to use in a fraud scheme that included credit card fraud. In Arkansas, three healthcare workers pleaded guilty to violating HIPAA's privacy rule. Civil prosecutions are also increasing. CVS Pharmacy paid a $2.25 million settlement and had to change the way it disposed of patient information.[74] In February 2011, the first civil money penalty for HIPAA violations was imposed. Cignet Health of Prince Georges County in Maryland had to pay $4.3 million for violating 41 patients' rights by not allowing them their medical records and for failing to either cooperate with the investigation or produce the records for the Office for Civil Rights. The amount of the penalty is partly due to the violations and partly to the increased penalties under HITECH.[75]

HITECH requires that breaches of the security of health information be reported to each individual affected. If the breach involves fewer than 500 people, it can be reported to HHS yearly. However, breaches involving 500 people or more must be reported to HHS and are published on the HHS Web site. February 22, 2010 was the compliance deadline. One recent page of breach notifications on the HHS's Web site listed well over 100 entities, each with breaches affecting 500 or more people. Some affected 40,000, 60,000, or 130,000 individuals' personal health information. The breaches involved theft of laptops, unauthorized access to servers, improper disposal of paper records and e-mails, and the simple loss of records.[76]

PRIVACY OF MEDICAL RECORDS UNDER HIPAA, HITECH, AND THE USA PATRIOT ACT Under these laws, there are many circumstances that allow police access to your medical records without a warrant. HIPAA allows the release of private medical information in some situations including the assertion that you are a suspect or witness to a crime or a missing person. Your information may also be released if national security or intelligence is involved or for the protection of VIPs including the president and foreign dignitaries. The government may also access your medical records under the USA Patriot Act "for an investigation to protect against international terrorism or clandestine intelligence activities" (Section 215). The HITECH section of the American Reinvestment and Recovery Act includes some strong privacy protections for medical records. It prohibits the unauthorized sale of medical records but provides exceptions for research, public health, and treatment. "The Act also limits marketing, requires covered entities and business associates to keep an audit trail of personnel having access to the information, mandates policies setting standards for technology systems to restrict sensitive information, use data encryption and directs breach notifications. The new law prescribes monetary penalties for violations and requires monitoring of contracts and reporting on compliance."[77]

TELEMEDICINE AND PRIVACY Telemedicine refers to any kind of health care administered over telecommunications lines. This would include the use of e-mail by physicians to communicate with patients and colleagues, distance exams and consultations, teleradiology, and telepsychiatry, among other specialties. Health care information, comprised of medical records, live videos, psychiatric consultations, and radiologic images, has traditionally been protected by state regulations. But now, this information routinely crosses state lines. Therefore, HIPAA protection is of special importance to this information. HIPAA requires that e-mail be secured either by using encryption or by controlling access. HIPAA specifically discusses privacy issues of telemedicine, including the presence of nonmedical personnel (e.g., camera people and other technicians) and the fact that the more stringent privacy protection (federal or state) has precedence.[78]

E-MAIL AND PRIVACY For some doctors and their patients, e-mail is not yet a common form of communication. It can be used as a practical, easy, inexpensive way of confirming or changing appointments, asking and answering questions, and maintaining communication over long distances. Some physicians also see it as a way to rebuild the traditional personal doctor–patient relationship that existed prior to managed care. Some doctors see e-mail as an intimate form of communication. However, e-mail has not been private. It is not like a telephone conversation; a permanent record of e-mail communications exists. Although e-mail is private in transit, it is not protected while stored. As mentioned, courts have ruled that employers have the legal right to read employees' e-mail, and today, many doctors are employees of health maintenance organizations. E-mail may be read on any of the computer systems it passes through on its way between doctor and patient. Because of the threats to the privacy of medical information, many doctors are now refusing to use e-mail. The requirements of HIPAA that e-mail be encrypted may help with these issues.

PRIVACY AND GENETIC INFORMATION Information-based medicine depends on genetic information. As research focuses on genetics and an individual's genetic predisposition to develop certain diseases, privacy issues arise. Although this research could eventually lead to treatments and cures tailored to each person, it also raises darker possibilities. Employers and insurance companies could use it against employees and consumers.[79] Polls have

consistently shown that Americans fear that genetic information would be used against them; one poll found that "63 percent of workers would not take genetic tests if employers could get access to the results." Some individuals become so desperate about negative genetic information that they resort to stealing pages of their medical records.[80] There have been some instances where employers did genetic tests on workers without their knowledge. The government sued, and a $2.2 million settlement was reached.[81] In 2005, IBM stated it would not "use genetic information in hiring or in determining eligibility for its health care benefits."

**GINA, the Genetic Information Nondiscrimination Act**, became law on May 21, 2008. Its basic purpose is to protect people from discrimination by health insurers and employers based on genetic information. In a proposed 2009 rule clarifying GINA, genetic information was defined as health information. Health plans were prohibited from using it in "eligibility determinations, premium computations, applications of any pre-existing condition exclusions." The latest updates on GINA, effective in 2011, clarify who the law covers in regard to employment: applicants, trainees, apprentices, and current and former employees. The definition of genetic information is very broad. The law may be violated with no intent to violate it. Genetic information includes genetic tests of the person and family members. It also includes family medical history as well as an individual's request for genetic counseling. An employer may not gather genetic information or even inadvertently come into possession of it. He or she may not do an Internet search on an individual that will result in the acquisition of genetic information, listen to conversations to hear genetic information, or make a request for health information in a way that is likely to elicit genetic information.[82]

PRIVACY AND ELECTRONIC HEALTH RECORDS Your medical records include information about your total physical and mental make-up. They may discuss your relationships with family members, sexual behavior, and drug- or alcohol-related problems. One particularly sensitive piece of information is one's human immunodeficiency virus (HIV) status. On a personal level, knowing that anyone has access to intimate details of your life may be humiliating.

Computerizing medical records and making them easily available over networks is, of course, essential to good medical care and can save lives. However, access to networked medical records is not limited to medical personnel. The issues of privacy and the easy availability of records kept on networked databases have special impact on health care and medical ethics. Most people assume the confidentiality of the doctor–patient relationship. This confidentiality is challenged by several trends. The movement to computerize medical records and possibly put them on the Internet, the expanding use of telemedicine, the increasing use of e-mail by health care workers, the increased use of health maintenance organizations, and reliance on third parties to pay for medical care all raise serious questions of patient confidentiality and medical ethics. Under HIPAA and HITECH, however, health care providers and their business associates have put some privacy protections in place.

A National Research Council report issued in March 1997 found that although electronic medical records were becoming more and more common, they were not secure, and little was being done to protect them. The report stated that certain precautions can be taken to limit access to medical records. However, 6 years later, medical records were still not secure. In March 2003, less than 1 month before HIPAA required privacy protection of medical records, Texas reported that the computer network shared by 16 state agencies and 225 private and public organizations lacked protection for medical records. Some proposed protections include requiring the use of passwords by authorized users, biometrics, using electronic blocks (called firewalls) to limit the access to networks, and keeping track of who actually sees a record through audit trails. The most obvious precaution is to train personnel not to leave patient information displayed on a computer screen. Under current law, encryption is required.

Many people now receive health care through health maintenance organizations. Under managed care, people are seen by several health care providers, and records are shared. For example, a patient seen by a general practitioner can be referred to a gastroenterologist for magnetic resonance imaging (MRI) and blood work. The patient's records are seen by primary care physicians, hospital and laboratory personnel, radiologists, pharmacists, consultants, and office staffs. Patients' records are also available to state health organizations and researchers. This electronic paper trail is then monitored by the health insurance provider and may be seen by an employer seeking to cut medical insurance costs. "Most patients would be surprised at the number of organizations that receive information about their health record," according to Dr. Paul D. Clayton of Columbia Presbyterian Medical Center in New York and Chair of the National Research Council Panel. Dr. Clayton is only referring to authorized users. Incidents have occurred in which unauthorized users (**hackers**) have gained access to hospital computer systems and changed patient information. The possibility of theft of patient information also exists.

The problems of protecting private medical information may multiply if all medical and health records are digitized and put online under a national system proposed by the Health Information Technology Decade. Of course, having a national database of health records could improve health care by making all your medical information (including allergies, medications, and most recent test results) available in any hospital, doctor's office, and emergency room. The challenge of making medical information secure is daunting. However, if data were not secure (and as yet, it seems no data are secure), marketers could tailor advertising to people with a particular disease, lenders could disqualify people on the basis of an estimate of how long they would live, and employers could deny employment or promotions. Complaints to the Federal Trade Commission in 2010 resulted in a preliminary report stating "that major drug, health, and information-technology companies might be compromising consumer privacy with tools used to gather information and market their products and services online." One of the things the Federal Trade Commission recommended was an opt-out feature for consumers that would allow them "to request that their online searching and browsing activities not be mined."[83] Even with the extended protection of HITECH, hundreds of breaches affecting millions of people still occur.

## SECURITY BREACHES

Instituting security measures (passwords, encryption, biometrics, audit trails, and so on) is of course crucial. Still, it should be recognized that breaches of security are common.

As of March 17, 2011, OCR had posted on its Web site 249 breaches. The breaches affected 8,289,236 individuals. The dates of these breaches ranged from September 22, 2009, to January 12, 2011. Most of the breaches were by covered entities, but some involved business associates. They included both electronic and paper records. Breaches are traced to unauthorized access, theft, loss of information, and hacking. Breaches of security are common; to see a more complete list, go to http://www.hhs.gov/ocr/privacy/hipaa/administrative/breachnotificationrule/postedbreaches.html.

# IN THE NEWS

According to "New Jersey Nearly Sold Secret Data," by Richard Pérez-Peña published on March 9, 2011, in *The New York Times*, New Jersey inadvertently almost sold hard drives containing personal and sensitive information.

The hard drives contained information on abused children. They also contained information on employees. They included names and addresses, birthdays, and Social Security numbers. Some of the drives had been used by high-ranking officials of the state. Several different branches of government used them. Some drives had been erased—but were easily restored. Others had not been erased.

Because of the leaks of sensitive information, the New Jersey State Treasury Department is no longer selling computers.

# Chapter Summary

Chapter 12 introduces the reader to the issue of security for computer systems and the importance of the privacy of the information on those systems—specifically medical records. Although guaranteeing the privacy of medical records was always important, keeping these records on databases on networks raises new problems.

- Threats to information technology may stem from many sources, including crime, viruses, human error, and natural disaster.
- Security measures that attempt to protect computer systems including information may include laws, codes of conduct, encryption, and restricting access. Restricting access may

be done by assigning PINs or passwords, by requiring ID cards and keys, or through biometric methods. Firewalls (electronic blocks to access) may be used to protect information on networks.

- Computer technology changes the nature of the way we work and makes work more subject to scrutiny.
- The Internet makes gathering personal information easy and inexpensive.
- The existence of networked databases of personal information, especially if they are connected to the Internet, endangers privacy by making that information accessible to anyone.

- HIPAA provides the first national standards for the privacy and security of health information. Until 2009, enforcement was lax.

- HITECH strengthens and extends HIPAA's privacy and security protections.
- Breaches of security continue to occur.

# Key Terms

adware

biometric keyboards

biometric methods

body odor sensors

botnet

cloud computing

codes of conduct

data accuracy

database

denial-of-service attack

DNA

Electronic Communications Privacy Act of 1986

e-mail bomb

encryption

facial structure scans

facial thermography

Fair and Accurate Credit Transaction Act of 2003 (FACTA)

Fair Credit Reporting Act of 1970

fingerprints

firewalls

fraud

fraudulent dialer

GINA (Genetic Information Nondiscrimination Act)

hackers

hand prints

Health Information Technology for Economic and Clinical Health Act of 2009 (HITECH),

Health Insurance Portability and Accountability Act (HIPAA)

Homeland Security Act

identity theft

iris scans

keylogging

lip prints

malware

Medical Information Bureau

MIB Group, Inc.

passwords

personal identification numbers (PINs)

phishing

privacy

Real ID Act of 2005

retina scans

security

software piracy

Spybot Search and Destroy software

spyware

theft of information

theft of services

Trojan horse

USA Patriot Act

viruses

voice recognition

# Review Exercises

## Multiple Choice

1. Threats to information technology include threats to _____ .
   a. hardware
   b. software
   c. data
   d. All of the above

2. The unauthorized copying of software protected by copyright is called _____ .
   a. theft of services
   b. software piracy
   c. A and B
   d. None of the above

3. Breaking into a medical database and gaining access to medical records is an example of a crime called _____ .
   a. theft of services
   b. theft of information
   c. software piracy
   d. network piracy

4. Which of the following is a way of attempting to protect computer systems and data from unauthorized use?
   a. Encryption
   b. Codes of conduct
   c. Restricting access through the use of PINs
   d. All of the above

5. Biometric security methods include _____ .
   a. use of passwords
   b. locking the computer room
   c. iris scans, lip prints, and body odor sensors
   d. carrying ID cards

6. Using a computer to create a description of someone who, you believe, is "likely" to commit a crime is called _____ .
   a. computer matching
   b. computer profiling
   c. computer graphics
   d. None of the above

7. Privacy means _____ .
   a. the ability to control personal information and keep it from misuse
   b. the attempt to protect a computer hardware from criminals
   c. the attempt to protect computer hardware from natural disaster
   d. None of the above

8. Threats to information technology may stem from _____ .
   a. crime
   b. human error
   c. natural disaster
   d. All of the above

9. A program that attaches itself to another program, replicates itself, and may do damage to your computer is called a _____ .
   a. network
   b. database
   c. virus
   d. None of the above

10. The first federal protection for the privacy of medical information is provided by the _____ .
    a. Homeland Security Act
    b. Health Insurance Portability and Accountability Act
    c. USA Patriot Act
    d. All of the above

11. The _____ gives law enforcement agencies greater power to monitor electronic and other communications, with fewer checks.
    a. Health Insurance Portability and Accountability Act
    b. Privacy Act
    c. USA Patriot Act
    d. All of the above

12. _____ are small files that a Web site may put on your hard drive when you visit. They can be programmed to track your movements, collecting information that helps advertisers target you.
    a. Cookies
    b. Tracers
    c. A and B
    d. None of the above

13. _____ limits disclosure of personal information in Department of Motor Vehicle records.
    a. Driver Privacy Protection Act
    b. Motor Vehicle Act
    c. Federal Privacy Act
    d. None of the Above

14. The _____ has a database that contains health histories of 15 million people.
    a. Immigration and Naturalization Service (INS)
    b. MIB Group, Inc.
    c. National Crime Information Center (NCIC)
    d. None of the above

15. _____ became law on May 21, 2008; its basic purpose is to protect people from discrimination by health insurers and employers based on genetic information.
    a. HIPAA (Health Information Portability and Accountability Act)
    b. GINA (Genetic Information Nondiscrimination Act)
    c. ARRA (American Recovery and Reinvestment Act)
    d. None of the above

## True/False

1. Most computer frauds are committed by employees of the organization being defrauded. _____

2. E-mail is a private communication. _____

3. According to the Electronic Privacy Information Center, most Web sites have privacy policies. _____

4. Computer matching links the information in one database to the information in other databases. _____

5. The MIB Group, Inc., contains medical information on millions of people, and it claims to guard the privacy of these records. _____

6. Traditionally, health care information has been protected by state law. _____

7. Computerizing medical records and making them available over networks helps facilitate sharing of medical records among health care providers and, therefore, can help assure continuity of care. _____

8. Medical records on the Internet are guaranteed to be secure. _____

9. Hackers have never gained access to hospital computer systems. _____

10. It is a crime for employers to gather genetic information about their employees. _____

11. Under HIPAA, medical records get some federal privacy protection. _____

12. Under some circumstances, government agencies have access to your medical information without a warrant. _____

13. The HITECH section of the American Reinvestment and Recovery Act includes some strong privacy protections for medical records. _____

14. Your rights under HIPAA are affected by the USA Patriot Act. _____

15. Under HIPAA, you have the right to examine your medical records. _____

## Critical Thinking

1. Assume that the information you provide when you register as a college student is kept in a networked database. This includes personal details such as your name, Social Security number, birth date, address, financial and marital status, and prior educational records. How would you safeguard the privacy of this information?

2. Numerous medical organizations are keeping records online. Some are linking their hospital networks to the Internet. How would you propose protecting the confidentiality of the doctor–patient relationship in this situation?

3. Computer profiling is being used to identify people "likely" to commit a crime. Although these people may not be automatically arrested, they may be stopped and questioned for no reason other than their profile "fits." In a democracy, people are supposed to be arrested only after a crime is committed, and even then, they are presumed innocent. Does computer profiling violate these tenets of democracy?

4. Where would you draw the line on how much private information (e.g., name, Social Security number, mother's maiden name, unlisted phone number and address, financial and medical information) should be available on the Internet? What are the pros and cons of government regulation?

5. Discuss why privacy and security are especially important issues in the new millennium.

6. How do HIPAA, HITECH, and the USA Patriot Act affect the privacy of medical information? Does the possible loss of privacy guarantee greater national security?

# Notes

1. Kelley Shannon, "Breach in Texas Comptroller's Office Exposes 3.5 Million Social Security Numbers, Birth Dates," April 11, 2011, http://www.dallasnews. com/news/state/headlines/20110411-bre ach-in-texas-comptrollers-office-expo ses-3.5-million-social-security-numbers-birth-dates.ece (accessed April 13, 2011).

2. "UK: Godalming College Email Gaffe Exposes Students Medical Details," April 7, 2011, http://www.databreaches. net/?p=17555 (accessed April 13, 2011).

3. "Hacking Incident at St. Louis University Affects over 12,000 Employees and 800 Students Receiving Counseling Services," March 16, 2011, http://www.databrea ches.net (accessed April 13, 2011).

4. Maureen McKinney, "Health Net Data Breach Affects 1.9 Million," March 15, 2011, http://www.healthcarein fosecurity.com/articles.php?art_id=3428 (accessed April 24, 2011); Karen Boruff, "Health Net data Breach Affects 1.9M Enrollees," March 16, 2011, http://www.examiner.

com/health-insurance-in-sacramento/health-net-data-breach-affects-1-9m-enrollees (accessed May 18, 2011).

5. George Beekman, *Computer Confluence: Exploring Tomorrow's Technology,* 5th ed. (Upper Saddle River, NJ: Prentice Hall, 2003).

6. John Leyden, "Credit Crunch Pushes US ID Fraud to 8 Year Low," February 9, 2011, http://www.theregister.co.uk/2011/02/09/id_fraud_slump/ (accessed April 14, 2011).

7. Matt Liebowitz, "ID Theft, Data Breaches Jumped 33 Percent in 2010," January 5, 2011, http://www.msnbc.msn.com/id/40 929975/ns/technology_and_science- security/ (accessed April 14, 2011); Jeremy Logsdon, "Identity Fraud Down 28% in 2010; Consumer Costs Up!" February 9, 2011, http://www.technologylawsource.com/2011/02/articles/privacy-1/identity-fraud-down-28-in-2010-consumer-costs-up/#axzz1JVF5ip6v (accessed April 14, 2011).

8. Blake Ellis, "No. 1 Consumer Complaint: Identity Theft," March 8, 2011, http://money.cnn.com/2011/03/08/pf/consumer_complaints/index.htm (accessed April 14, 2011).

9. "2009 Identity Theft Legislation," August 27, 2010, http://www.ncsl.org/? tabid=12538 (accessed April 14, 2011); "2010 Identity Theft Legislation," March 9, 2011, http://www.ncsl.org/?tabid=12538 (accessed April 14, 2011); "2011 Identity Theft Legislation," March 9, 2011, http://www.ncsl.org/?tabid=12538 (accessed April 14, 2011).

10. Gautham Nagesh, "Senators Try Again on Identity Theft Bill," July 14, 2010, http://thehill.com/blogs/hillicon-valley/technology/108763-senators-try-again-on-identity-theft-bill (accessed April 14, 2011).

11. "AuthenWare Selected to Protect Utahrealestate.com Website," January 19, 2011, http://www.findbiometrics.com/industry-news/i/8548/ (accessed April 14, 2011).

12. "Unisys Research Shows Growing Global Acceptance of Biometrics among Consumers for Protecting Identities and Personal Information: Bank Card Fraud and ID Theft Remain Top Fears Worldwide Despite Overall Decline in Security Concerns," November 10, 2009, http://www.unisys.com/unisys/news/detail.jsp?print=true&id=1120000 970000610143 (accessed April 14, 2011).

13. "About Spyware," 2011, http://www.spywareterminator.com/support/what-is-spyware.aspx (accessed April 14, 2011); Dimitr Alperovitch, "8 IT Security Threats for 2011," December 28, 2010, http://www.healthcareinfosecurity.com/podcasts.php?podcastID=908 (accessed April 14, 2011).

14. "Fair Credit Reporting Act and the Privacy of Your Credit Report," October 7, 2005, http://epic.org/privacy/fcra/ (accessed May 11, 2011).

15. "The Privacy Act?" http://www.hhs.gov/foia/privacy/index.html (accessed May 11, 2011).

16. "The Right to Financial Privacy Act," 2003, http://epic.org/privacy/rfpa/ (accessed May 11, 2011).

17. "Computer Fraud and Abuse Act," 2003, http://legal.web.aol.com/resources/legislation/comfraud.html (accessed May 11, 2011).

18. University of Miami, Miller School of Medicine: Privacy/Data Protection Project, "Cable Communications Protection Act of 1984," May 11, 2005, http://privacy.med.miami.edu/glossary/xd_ccpa.htm (accessed May 20, 2011).

19. "Federal Statutes Relevant in the Information Sharing Environment (ISE)," April 7, 2010, http://it.ojp.gov/default.aspx?area=privacy&page=1285 (accessed May 11, 2011).

20. "The Video Privacy Protection Act (VPPA)," May 11, 2005, http://privacy.med.miami.edu/glossary/xd_vppa.htm (accessed May 11, 2011).

21. "Overview of the Privacy Act of 1974, 2010 Edition," http://www.justice.gov/opcl/1974privacyact.pdf (accessed May 11, 2011).

22. "The Computer Fraud and Abuse Act (as Amended 1994 and 1996)," http://www.panix.com/~eck/computer-fraud-act.html (accessed May 11, 2011).

23. "National Information Infrastructure Protection Act of 1996," http://epic.org/security/1996_computer_law.html (accessed May 11, 2011).

24. "Driver Privacy Protection Act (DPPA)," http://www.accessreports.com/statutes/DPPA1.htm (accessed May 11, 2011).

25. "The Gramm–Leach–Bliley Act," No date, http://epic.org/privacy/glba/ (accessed May 11, 2011).

26. "How to Comply with the Children's Online Privacy Protection Rule," 2007, http://www.ftc.gov/oia/ftccoppareport.pdf http://www.ftc.gov/oia/ftccoppareport.pdf (accessed May 11, 2011).

27. "The USA Patriot Act," 2011, http://epic.org/privacy/terrorism/usapatriot/ (accessed May 11, 2011).

28. "A Bill: To Establish a Department of Homeland Security, and for Other Purposes," 2002, http://www.steptoe.com/assets/attachments/702.pdf (accessed May 11, 2011).

29. "Fact Sheet 6a: Facts on FACTA, the Fair and Accurate Credit Transactions Act," February 2011, http://www.privacyrights.org/fs/fs6a-facta.htm (accessed May 20, 2011).

30. 108th U.S. Congress (2003–2004), "H.R. 743 [108th]: Social Security Protection Act of 2004," http://www.govtrack.us/congress/bill.xpd?bill=h108-743 (accessed May 11, 2011).

31. 109th U.S. Congress (2005–2006), "H.R. 84 [109th]: Online Privacy Protection Act of 2005," http://www.govtrack.us/congress/bill.xpd?bill=h109-84 (accessed May 11, 2011).

32. "Combat Methamphetamine Epidemic Act 2005 (Title VII of Public Law 109-177)," http://www.deadiversion.usdoj.gov/meth/index.html (accessed May 11, 2011).

33. "Cegavske Targets 'Video Voyeurism,'" February 17, 2005, http://www.reviewjournal.com/lvrj_home/2005/Feb-17-Thu-2005/news/25883310.html (accessed May 11, 2011)

34. "Spotlight on Surveillance," 2005, http://epic.org/privacy/surveillance/spotlight/ (accessed May 9, 2011).

35. "Whole Body Imaging Technology and Body Scanners ('Backscatter' X-Ray and Millimeter Wave Screening)," January 2010, http://epic.org/privacy/airtravel/backscatter/ (accessed April 15, 2011); "Cancer Danger in Airport 'Backscatter' X-Ray Machines," January 5, 2010, http://healthfreedoms.org/2010/01/05/cancer-danger-in-airport-backscatter-x-ray-machines/ (accessed April 15, 2011).

36. Molly Bernhart Walker, "FBI: No Internet-Connected System Is Impervious to Cybercrime," April 14, 2011,

http://www.fiercegovernmentit.com/story/fbi-no-internet-connected-system-impervious-cybercrime/2011-04-14 (accessed April 14, 2011).

37. "Federal Statures Relevant in the Information Sharing Environment (ISE)," April 7, 2010, http://it.ojp.gov/default.aspx?area=privacy&page=1285 (accessed April 15, 2011).

38. "Real ID Act of 2005 Driver's License Title Summary," 2011, http://www.ncsl.org/standcomm/sctran/realidsummary05.htm (accessed May 9, 2011).

39. Declan McCullagh, "FAQ: How Real ID Will Affect You," May 6, 2005, http://www.news.com/FAQ-How-Real-ID-will-affect-you/2100-1028_3-5697111.html (accessed May 9, 2011).

40. Anush Yegyazarian, "Tech.gov: Real ID's Real Problems," October 11, 2006, http://www.pcworld.com/article/127419/techgov_real_ids_real_problems.html (May 10, 2011).

41. Matt Gouras, "Tea Party Vision for Mont. Raising concerns," February 24, 2011, http://www.msnbc.msn.com/id/41768730/ns/politics-more_politics/t/tea-party-vision-montana-raising-concerns/#.T0-XBdQ7XNU (accessed February 26, 2011); "National ID Cards and REAL ID Act," 2011, http://epic.org/privacy/id_cards/ (accessed May 12, 2011).

42. Barnaby J. Feder and Tom Zeller Jr., "Identity Chip under Skin Approved for Use in Health Care," October 14, 2004, http://query.nytimes.com/gst/fullpage.html?res=9D07EED71F3BF937A25753C1A9629C8B63 (accessed May 10, 2011).

43. Richard Waters, "US Group Implants Electronic Tags in Workers," February 12, 2006, http://www.ft.com/cms/s/2/Tec414700-9bf4-11da-8baa-0000779e2340.html (accessed May 10, 2011).

44. "Demo: Cloning a Verichip," July 2006, http://cq.cx/verichip.pl (accessed May 10, 2011).

45. "National Directory of New Hires," March 28, 2011, http://www.acf.hhs.gov/programs/cse/newhire/ndnh/ndnh.htm (accessed April 24, 2011).

46. Jay Boehmer, "Secure Flight Now Checking Watchlists for All Passengers on U.S. Carriers," June 25, 2010, http://www.businesstravelnews.com/article.aspx?id=13679&ida=Airlines&a=btn (accessed April 24, 2011).

47. Ronald Plesser, James J. Halpert, and Milo Cividanes, "Summary and Analysis of Key Sections of USA PATRIOT ACT of 2001," http://www.cdt.org/security/011031summary.shtml (accessed May 10, 2011).

48. Lauren Weinstein, "Taking Liberties with Our Freedom," *Wired News*, December 2, 2002, http://www.wired.com/politics/law/news/2002/12/56600 (accessed May 10, 2011).

49. "Senate, House Pass Limited Patriot Act Extensions," February 16, 2011, http://epic.org/privacy/terrorism/usa-patriot/ (accessed April 16, 2011).

50. Jacqueline Klosek, *The War on Privacy*. Westport, CT: Praeger, 2007.

51. Ibid.

52. "Statement of Barry Steinhardt, Director of the ACLU Technology and Liberty Program, on RFID Tags Before the Commerce, Trade and Consumer Protection Subcommittee of the House Committee on Energy and Commerce," July 14, 2004, http://www.aclu.org/technology-and-liberty/statement-barry-steinhardt-director-aclu-technology-and-liberty-program-rfid- (accessed May 10, 2011).

53. "Legal Guide: Health-Care Law Patients' Rights," 2011, http://public.findlaw.com/abaflg/flg-17-1a-2.html (accessed April 16, 2011).

54. "Know Your Health," 2011, https://www.annualmedicalreport.com/ (accessed April 16, 2011).

55. "Denied Insurance because of a Medical Coding Error," August 17, 2009, https://www.annualmedicalreport.com/tag/mib-codes/ (accessed April 16, 2011); "AnnualMedicalReport.com Portrays MIB Inaccurately While Promoting Its Service," 2011, http://www.mib.com/html/inaccurate_portrayal_of_mib.html (accessed April 16, 2011).

56. Sunshine Red, "Medical Records: About the Medical Information Bureau," June 22, 2007, http://www.associatedcontent.com/article/286156/medical_records_about_the_medical_information.html (accessed May 10, 2011).

57. "Fact Sheet 6a: Facts on FACTA, the Fair and Accurate Credit Transactions Act," February 2011, http://www.privacyrights.org/fs/fs6a-facta.htm (accessed April 15, 2011); "Consumer Protection," 2011, http://www.mib.com/html/consumer_protection.html (accessed April 15, 2011); "Some Hitech Relief in Sight," No date, http://whychat.5u.com/medfico.html (accessed April 15, 2011).

58. E-mail to Barbara Weill, dated April 19, 2011, from Sue of the Privacy Department of the MIB.

59. Chris Conley, "Sony Learns the Hard Way That Protecting User Privacy Is Not a Game," April 28, 2011, http://www.aclu.org/blog/technology-and-liberty/sony-learns-hard-way-protecting-user-privacy-not-game (accessed May 14, 2011).

60. Mark Hefflinger, "Report: iPhone Keeps Secret Log Tracking User's Location," April 20, 2011, http://www.dmwmedia.com/news/2011/04/20/report-iphone-keeps-secret-log-tracking-user039s-location (accessed May 14, 2011).

61. "Protecting the Privacy of Patients' Health Information," HHS Fact Sheet, July 6, 2001, http://aspe.hhs.gov/admnsimp/final/pvcfact2.htm (accessed May 10, 2011).

62. Ibid.

63. Ibid.

64. Office for Civil Rights—HIPAA, "Medical Privacy—National Standards to Protect the Privacy of Personal Health Information, August 14, 2002, http://www.hhs.gov/ocr/privacy/hipaa/understanding/summary/privacy.html (accessed May 10, 2011).

65. HHS Fact Sheet, "Protecting the Privacy of Patients' Health Information," May 9, 2009, http://aspe.hhs.gov/admnsimp/final/pvcfact2.htm (accessed May 10, 2011).

66. "HIPAA Security Series," June 6, 2005, http://library.ahima.org/xpedio/groups/public/documents/government/bok1_027878.pdf (accessed May 11, 2011).

67. Rob Stein, "Medical Privacy Law Nets No Fines: Lax Enforcement Puts Patients' Files at Risk, Critics

Say," Monday June 5, 2006; AO1, http://www.washingtonpost.com/wp-dyn/content/article/2006/06/04/AR2006060400672.html (accessed May 11, 2011).

68. Ibid.

69. Selma Chavis, "A HIPAA Crackdown?" September 15, 2008, http://www.radiologytoday.net/archive/rt_102008p24.shtml (accessed April 15, 2011).

70. "Summary of the HIPAA Privacy Rule," No date, http://www.edocscan.com/hipaa-privacy-rule-summary (accessed April 16, 2011); "Encryption HITECH Act Security Requirements," No date, http://www.edocscan.com/encryption-hitech-act-security-requirements (accessed April 16, 2011).

71. "Analysis of the HITECH Act's Incentives to Facilitate Adoption of Health Information Technology," March 8, 2009, http://www.hcfa.com/analysis-of-the-hitech-act%E2%80%99s-incentives-to-facilitate-adoption-of-health-information-technology/ (accessed April 16, 2011).

72. Cynthia Marcotte Stamer, "Reassignment of HIPAA Security Rule Enforcement Signals Growing Seriousness about Enforcing HIPAA," August 4, 2009, http://slphealthcareupdate.wordpress.com/2009/08/04/reassignment-of-hipaa-security-rule-enforcement-signals-growing-seriousness-about-enforcing-hipaa/ (accessed April 15, 2011); "Summary of the HIPAA Privacy Rule," No date, http://www.edocscan.com/hipaa-privacy-rule-summary (accessed April 16, 2011).

73. Richard W. Merrill Jr., "Summary of HITECH Act of 2009," July 14, 2009, http://www.jdsupra.com/post/documentViewer.aspx?fid=8464b692-4b4e-44e0-995a-c319dc71598e (accessed April 15, 2011).

74. Cynthia Marcotte Stamer, "Two Recent Criminal Prosecutions for HIPAA Privacy Rule Violations Signal Rising Criminal Enforcement Risks," September 8, 2009, http://slphealthcareupdate.wordpress.com/2009/09/08/two-recent-criminal-prosecutions-for-hipaa-privacy-rule-violations-signal-rising-criminal-enforcement-risks/ (accessed April 15, 2011).

75. "HHS Imposes a $4.3 Million Civil Money Penalty for Violations of the HIPAA Privacy Rule." February 22, 2011. http://www.hhs.gov/news/press/2011pres/02/20110222a.html (accessed February 23, 2011).

76. "Health Information Privacy," No date, http://www.hhs.gov/ocr/privacy/ (accessed April 15, 2011); Erin Brisbay McMahon, "Coming Soon: Final HITECH Regulations Will Amend HIPAA Privacy, Security and Breach Notification Requirements," March 22, 2011, http://www.valeocommunications.com/2011/03/22/coming-soon-final-hitech-regulations-will-amend-hipaa-privacy-security-and-breach-notification-requirements/ (accessed April 15, 2011); "Health Information Privacy HITECH Breach Notification Interim Final Rule," No date, http://www.hhs.gov/ocr/privacy/hipaa/understanding/coveredentities/breachnotificationifr.html (accessed April 15, 2011); "HIPAA, HITECH Act Summary," 2009, http://whatishipaa.org/hitech-act.php (accessed April 15, 2011).

77. "Medical Record Privacy," 2011, http://epic.org/privacy/medical/ (accessed May 1, 2011).

78. HIPAA Privacy Update, "Issue: Privacy and Telemedicine," 2000, http://www.connected-health.org/policy/federal-and-state/external-resources/hipaa's-privacy-rule-summarized-what-does-it-mean-for-telemedicine.aspx (accessed May 11, 2011).

79. "Medicine and the New Genetics," 2006, http://www.ornl.gov/sci/techresources/Human_Genome/publicat/primer2001/6.shtml (accessed May 11, 2011).

80. Robert Klitzman, "The Quest for Privacy Can Make Us Thieves," May 9, 2006, http://www.nytimes.com/2006/05/09/health/09essa.html (accessed May 11, 2011).

81. Steve Lohr, "I.B.M. to Put Genetic Data of Workers Off Limits," October 10, 2005, http://query.nytimes.com/gst/fullpage.html?res=990DEFD71F30F933A25753C1A9639C8B63 (accessed May 11, 2011).

82. "Health Information Privacy: Genetic Information," No date, http://www.hhs.gov/ocr/privacy/hipaa/understanding/special/genetic/index.html (accessed April 16, 2011); C. R. Wright, "The Latest on Gina," February 2011, http://www.laborlawyers.com/showarticle.aspx?The-Latest-On-GINA&Ref=list&Type=1119&Cat=3389&Show=13634 (accessed April 16, 2011).

83. "Is Your Medical Information Safe Online?" December 2, 2010, http://news.consumerreports.org/health/2010/12/online-privacy-medical-records-is-your-medical-information-safe-online.html (accessed May 11, 2011).

# Additional Resources

109th U.S. Congress (2005–2006). "H.R. 82 [109th]: Social Security On-line Privacy Protection Act." http://www.govtrack.us/congress/bill.xpd?bill=h109-82 (accessed May 11, 2011).

2009 Identity Theft Legislation. August 27, 2010. http://www.ncsl.org/?tabid=12538 (accessed April 14, 2011).

2010 Identity Theft Legislation. March 9, 2011. http://www.ncsl.org/?tabid=12538 (accessed April 14, 2011).

2011 Identity Theft Legislation. March 9, 2011. http://www.ncsl.org/?tabid=12538 (accessed April 14, 2011).

"ABA Family Legal Guide: Health-Care Law Patients' Rights." 2011. http://public.findlaw.com/abaflg/flg-17-1a-2.html (accessed April 16, 2011).

"About Spyware." 2011. http://www.spywareterminator.com/support/what-is-spyware.aspx (accessed April 14, 2011).

Alperovitch, Dimitri. "8 IT Security Threats for 2011." December 28, 2010. http://www.healthcareinfosecurity.com/podcasts.php?podcastID=908 (accessed April 14, 2011).

"Analysis of the HITECH Act's Incentives to Facilitate Adoption of Health Information Technology." March 8, 2009. http://www.hcfa.com/analysis-of-the-hitech-act%E2%80%99s-incentives-to-facilitate-adoption-of-health-information-technology/ (accessed April 16, 2011).

"AnnualMedicalReport.com Portrays MIB Inaccurately While Promoting Its Service." 2011. http://www.mib.com/html/inaccurate_portrayal_of_mib.html (accessed April 16, 2011).

"Answers to Frequently Asked Questions about Government Access to Personal Medical Information (Under the USA Patriot Act and the HIPAA Regulations)." American Civil Liberties Union. May 30, 2003. http://www.aclu.org/privacy/medical/15222res20030530.html (accessed May 11, 2011).

Austen, Ian. "A Scanner Skips the ID Card and Zooms In on the Eyes." May 15, 2003. http://www.nytimes.com/2003/05/15/technology/how-it-works-a-scanner-skips-the-id-card-and-zeroes-in-on-the-iris.html (accessed May 11, 2011).

"AuthenWare Selected to Protect Utahrealestate.com Website." January 19, 2011. http://www.findbiometrics.com/industry-news/i/8548/ (accessed April 14, 2011).

Baase, Sara. *A Gift of Fire: Social, Legal, and Ethical Issues in Computing*. Upper Saddle River, NJ: Prentice Hall, 1996.

Bernstein, Nina. "Personal Files via Computer Offer Money and Pose Threat." *The New York Times,* June 12, 1997, A1, B14.

Boehmer, Jay. "Secure Flight Now Checking Watchlists for All Passengers on U.S. Carriers." June 25, 2010. http://www.businesstravelnews.com/article.aspx?id=13679&ida=Airlines&a=btn (accessed April 24, 2011).

Burton, Brenda K., and Erik Kangas. "HIPAA Email Security Management in Email Communications, Secure Email White Paper." 2006. http://www.interman.us/extranet/pdf/HIPAA-Email.pdf (accessed May 11, 2011).

"Cancer Danger in Airport 'Backscatter' X-Ray Machines." January 5, 2010. http://healthfreedoms.org/2010/01/05/cancer-danger-in-airport-backscatter-x-ray-machines/ (accessed April 15, 2011).

Chaddock, Gail Russell. "Security Act to Pervade Daily Lives." *Christian Science Monitor.* November 21, 2002. http://www.csmonitor.com/2002/1121/p01s03-usju.html (accessed May 11, 2011).

Chavis, Selma. "A HIPAA Crackdown?" September 15, 2008. http://www.radiologytoday.net/archive/rt_102008p24.shtml (accessed April 15, 2011).

Clymer, Adam. "Conferees in Congress Bar Using a Pentagon Project on Americans." February 12, 2003. http://www.nytimes.com/2003/02/12/us/threats-responses-electronic-surveillance-congress-agrees-bar-pentagon-terror.html (accessed May 11, 2011).

"Consumer Protection." 2011. http://www.mib.com/html/consumer_protection.html (accessed April 15, 2011).

Cronin, Anne. "Census Bureau Tells Something about Everything." *The New York Times,* December 1, 1997, D10.

"Denied Insurance Because of a Medical Coding Error." August 17, 2009. https://www.annualmedicalreport.com/tag/mib-codes/ (accessed April 16, 2011).

Donovan, Larry. "Privacy Law Update." 2001. http://library.findlaw.com/2001/Feb/1/129062.html (accessed May 11, 2011).

Electronic Frontier Foundation. "PATRIOT Act—Analysis by EFF: Analysis of the Provisions of the USA PATRIOT Act That Relate to Online Activities (Oct 31, 2001)." http://www.tgorski.com/terrorism/PATRIOT_Act_Analysis_By_EFF.htm (accessed May 11, 2011).

Electronic Privacy Information Center. "Latest News." May 11, 2011. http://www.epic.org (accessed May 11, 2011).

Electronic Privacy Information Center. "Medical Privacy." 2011. http://www.epic.org/privacy/medical (accessed May 11, 2011).

Ellis, Blake. "No. 1 Consumer Complaint: Identity Theft." March 8, 2011. http://money.cnn.com/2011/03/08/pf/consumer_complaints/index.htm (accessed April 14, 2011).

"Encryption HITECH Act Security Requirements." No date. http://www.edocscan.com/encryption-hitech-act-security-requirements (accessed April 16, 2011).

"Face Recognition." January 19, 2006. http://epic.org/privacy/facerecognition/ (accessed May 11, 2011).

"Fact Sheet 6a: Facts on FACTA, the Fair and Accurate Credit Transactions Act." February 2011. http://www.privacyrights.org/fs/fs6a-facta.htm (accessed April 15, 2011).

"Federal Statures Relevant in the Information Sharing Environment (ISE)." April 7, 2010. http://it.ojp.gov/default.aspx?area=privacy&page=1285 (accessed April 15, 2011).

"The Federal Trade Commission's Settlement with ChoicePoint." March 18, 2008. http://www.ftc.gov/bcp/cases/choicepoint/ (accessed April 14, 2011).

Fein, Esther B. "For Many Physicians, E-Mail Is the High-Tech House Call." *New York Times,* November 20, 1997, A1, B8.

Fitzgerald, Thomas J. "A Trail of Cookies? Cover Your Tracks." March 27, 2003. http://www.nytimes.com/2003/03/27/technology/basics-a-trail-of-cookies-cover-your-tracks.html (accessed May 11, 2011).

Gautham Nagesh. "Senators Try Again on Identity Theft Bill." July 14, 2010. http://thehill.com/blogs/hillicon-valley/technology/108763-senators-try-again-on-identity-theft-bill (accessed April 14, 2011).

Gouras, Matt. "Tea Party Vision for Mont. Raising concerns." February 24, 2011. http://www.msnbc.msn.com/id/417687 30/ns/politics-more_politics/t/tea-party-vision-montana-raising-concerns/#.T0-XBdQ7XNU (accessed February 26, 2011).

Guernsey, Lisa. "What Did You Do before the War." November 22, 2001. http://www.nytimes.com/2001/11/22/technology/what-did-you-do-before-the-war.html (accessed May 12, 2011).

"Hacking Incident at St. Louis University Affects over 12,000 Employees and 800 Students Receiving Counseling Services." March 16, 2011. http://www.databreaches.net (accessed April 13, 2011).

Hafner, Katie. "'Dear Doctor' Meets 'Return to Sender.'" June 6, 2002. http://www.nytimes.com/2002/06/06/technology/dear-doctor-meets-return-to-sender.html (accessed May 12, 2011).

"Health Information Privacy." No date. http://www.hhs.gov/ocr/privacy/ (accessed April 15, 2011).

"Health Information Privacy: Genetic Information." No date. http://www.hhs.gov/ocr/privacy/hipaa/understanding/special/genetic/index.html (accessed April 16, 2011).

"Health Information Privacy HITECH Breach Notification Interim Final Rule." No date. http://www.hhs.gov/ocr/privacy/hipaa/understanding/coveredentities/breachnotificationifr.html (accessed April 15, 2011).

"HHS Imposes a $4.3 Million Civil Money Penalty for Violations of the HIPAA Privacy Rule." February 22, 2011. http://www.hhs.gov/news/press/2011pres/02/20110222a.html (accessed February 23, 2011).

"HIPAA, HITECH Act Summary." 2009. http://whatishipaa.org/hitech-act.php (accessed April 15, 2011).

Holtzman, David. "Homeland Security and You." January 21, 2003. http://news.cnet.com/Homeland-Security-and-you/2010-1071_3-981262.html (accessed May 12, 2011).

"Know Your Health." 2011. https://www.annualmedicalreport.com/ (accessed April 16, 2011).

Leary, Warren E. "Panel Cites Lack of Security on Medical Records." *The New York Times,* March 6, 1997, A1, B11.

Lee, Jennifer. "Dirty Laundry, Online for All to See." September 5, 2002. http://www.nytimes.com/2002/09/05/technology/dirty-laundry-online-for-all-to-see.html (accessed May 12, 2011).

Lee, Jennifer. "Identity Theft Complaints Double in '02, Continuing Rise." January 23, 2003. http://www.nytimes.com/2003/01/23/us/identity-theft-complaints-double-in-02-continuing-rise.html (accessed May 12, 2011).

Lewis, Peter H. "Forget Big Brother." *The New York Times,* March 19, 1998, G1, G6.

Leyden, John. "Credit Crunch Pushes US ID Fraud to 8 Year Low." February 9, 2011. http://www.theregister.co.uk/2011/02/09/id_fraud_slump/ (accessed April 14, 2011).

Lichtblau, Eric. "Republicans Want Terror Law Made Permanent." April 9, 2003. http://www.nytimes.com/2003/04/09/us/nation-war-liberty-security-republicans-want-terrorism-law-made-permanent.html (accessed May 12, 2011).

Liebowitz, Matt. "ID Theft, Data Breaches Jumped 33 Percent in 2010." January 5, 2011. http://www.msnbc.msn.com/id/40929975/ns/technology_and_science-security/ (accessed April 14, 2011).

Logsdon, Jeremy. "Identity Fraud Down 28% in 2010; Consumer Costs Up!" February 9, 2011. http://www.technologylawsource.com/2011/02/articles/privacy-1/identity-fraud-down-28-in-2010-consumer-costs-up/#axzz1JVF5ip6v (accessed April 14, 2011).

Markoff, John. "Guidelines Don't End Debate on Internet Privacy." *The New York Times,* December 18, 1997.

McCullagh, Declan. "Bush Signs Homeland Security Bill." November 25, 2002. http://news.cnet.com/2100-1023_3-975305.html (accessed May 12, 2011).

McKinney, Maureen. "Health Net Data Breach Affects 1.9 Million." March 15, 2011. http://www.healthcareinfosecurity.com/articles.php?art_id=3428 (accessed April 24, 2011).

McMahon, Erin Brisbay. "Coming Soon: Final HITECH Regulations Will Amend HIPAA Privacy, Security and Breach Notification Requirements." March 22, 2011. http://www.valeocommunications.com/2011/03/22/coming-soon-final-hitech-regulations-will-amend-hipaa-privacy-security-and-breach-notification-requirements/ (accessed April 15, 2011).

Merrill, Richard W. Jr. "Summary of HITECH Act of 2009." July 14, 2009. http://www.jdsupra.com/post/document Viewer.aspx?fid=8464b692-4b4e-44e0-995a-c319dc 71598e (accessed April 15, 2011).

Murphy, Dean E. "Librarians Use Shredder to Show Opposition to New F.B.I. Powers." April 7, 2003. http://www.nytimes.com/2003/04/07/national/07LIBR.html (accessed May 12, 2011).

"National Directory of New Hires." March 28, 2011. http://www.acf.hhs.gov/programs/cse/newhire/ndnh/ndnh.htm (accessed April 24, 2011).

"National ID Cards and REAL ID Act." 2011. http://epic.org/privacy/id_cards/ (accessed May 12, 2011).

Newman, Andy. "Those Dimples May Be Digits." May 3, 2001. http://www.nytimes.com/2001/05/03/technology/those-dimples-may-be-digits.html (accessed May 12, 2011).

"Over 10 Million Individuals Now Affected by Large Data Breaches, as Reported on OCR Web Site." 2009. http://www.hipaa.com/2011/04/over-10-million-individuals-now-affected-by-large-data-breaches-as-report-ed-on-ocr-web-site/ (accessed April 16, 2011).

Parsons, June, Dan Oja, and Stephanie Low. *Computers, Technology, and Society*. Cambridge, MA: ITP, 1997.

Pear, Robert. "Bush Acts to Drop Core Privacy Rule on Medical Data." March 22, 2002. http://www.nytimes.com/2002/03/22/us/bush-acts-to-drop-core-privacy-rule-on-medical-data.html (accessed May 12. 2011).

Pear, Robert. "Health System Warily Prepares for Privacy Rules." April 6, 2003. http://www.nytimes.com/2003/04/06/us/health-system-warily-prepares-for-new-privacy-rules.html (accessed May 12, 2011).

Pear, Robert. "Vast Worker Database to Track Deadbeat Parents." *The New York Times,* September 22, 1997.

"Research and Markets: 2011 Identity Fraud Survey Report: Identity Fraud Decreases but Remaining Frauds Cost Consumers More Time and Money." February 14, 2011. http://www.pymnts.com/research-and-markets-2011-identity-fraud-survey-report-identity-fraud-decreases-but-remaining-frauds-cost-consumers-more-time--money-201102140 06411/ (accessed April 14, 2011).

Reuters. "Senate Rebuffs Domestic Spy Plan." *Wired News.* January 23, 2003. http://www.wired.com/politics/law/news/2003/01/57386 (accessed May 12. 2011).

Safire, William. "You Are a Suspect." November 14, 2002. http://www.nytimes.com/2002/11/14/opinion/you-are-a-suspect.html (accessed May 12, 2011).

Schwaneberg, Robert. "Questions Leave 'Smart Card' in Limbo for Now." *Star-Ledger,* June 30, 1998, 11, 14.

Schwaneberg, Robert. "Smart Cards Take a Step in Legislature." *Star-Ledger,* June 23, 1998, 11, 15.

Schwartz, John. "Threats and Responses: Surveillance; Planned Databank on Citizens Spurs Opposition in Congress." January 16, 2003. http://www.nytimes.com/2003/01/16/us/threats-responses-surveillance-planned-databank-citizens-spurs-opposition.html (accessed May 12, 2011).

Seelye, Katharine Q. "A Plan for Database Privacy, but Public Has to Ask for It." *The New York Times,* December 18, 1997, A1, A24.

"Senate, House Pass Limited Patriot Act Extensions." February 16, 2011. http://epic.org/privacy/terrorism/usapatriot/ (accessed April 16, 2011).

Shannon, Kelley. "Breach in Texas Comptroller's Office Exposes 3.5 Million Social Security Numbers, Birth Dates." April 11, 2011. http://www.dallasnews.com/news/state/headlines/20110411-breach-in-texas-comptrollers-office-exposes-3.5-million-social-security-numbers-birth-dates.ece (accessed April 13, 2011).

Shelley, Gary, and Thomas Cashman. *Discovering Computers a Link to the Future*. Cambridge, MA: ITP, 1997.

"Some HITECH Relief in Sight." No date. http://whychat.5u.com/medfico.html (accessed April 15, 2011).

Stamer, Cynthia Marcotte. "Reassignment of HIPAA Security Rule Enforcement Signals Growing Seriousness about Enforcing HIPAA." August 4, 2009. http://slphealthcareupdate.wordpress.com/2009/08/04/reassignment-of-hipaa-security-rule-enforcement-signals-growing-seriousness-about-enforcing-hipaa/ (accessed April 15, 2011).

Stamer, Cynthia Marcotte. "Two Recent Criminal Prosecutions for HIPAA Privacy Rule Violations Signal Rising Criminal Enforcement Risks." September 8, 2009. http://slphealthcareupdate.wordpress.com/2009/09/08/two-recent-criminal-prosecutions-for-hipaa-privacy-rule-violations-signal-rising-criminal-enforcement-risks/ (accessed April 15, 2011).

"Summary of the HIPAA Privacy Rule." No date. http://www.edocscan.com/hipaa-privacy-rule-summary (accessed April 16, 2011).

"Surfer Beware: Personal Privacy and the Internet." Report of the Electronic Privacy Information Center, Washington, D., June 1997. http://epic.org/reports/surfer-beware.html (accessed May 12, 2011).

"UK: Godalming College Email Gaffe Exposes Students' Medical Details." April 7, 2011. http://www.databreaches.net/?p=17555 (accessed April 13, 2011).

"Unisys Research Shows Growing Global Acceptance of Biometrics among Consumers for Protecting Identities and Personal Information: Bank Card Fraud and ID Theft Remain Top Fears Worldwide Despite Overall Decline in Security Concerns." November 10, 2009. http://www.unisys.com/unisys/news/detail.jsp?print=true&id=1120000 970000610143 (accessed April 14, 2011).

Walker, Molly Bernhart. "FBI: No Internet-Connected System Is Impervious to Cybercrime." April 14, 2011. http://www.fiercegovernmentit.com/story/fbi-no-internet-connected-system-impervious-cybercrime/2011-04-14 (accessed April 14, 2011).

Wayner, Peter. "Code Breaker Cracks Smart Cards' Digital Safe." *The New York Times,* June 22, 1998, D1–2.

"While Identity Theft Is Down, Friendly Fraud Is Up." April 4, 2011. http://blog.nj.com/north_american_precis_syndicate/2011/04/while_identity_theft_is_down_friendly_fraud_is_up.html (accessed April 14, 2011).

"Whole Body Imaging Technology and Body Scanners ('Backscatter' X-Ray and Millimeter Wave Screening)." January 2010. http://epic.org/privacy/airtravel/backscatter/ (accessed April 15, 2011).

Wright, C. R. "The Latest on Gina." February 2011. http://www.laborlawyers.com/showarticle.aspx?The-Latest-On-GINA&Ref=list&Type=1119&Cat=3389&Show=13634 (accessed April 16, 2011).

Zuzek, Ashley. "Changes to Patriot Act Limit Medicinal Purchases." April 18, 2006. http://thedartmouth.com/2006/04/18/news/changes/ (accessed May 12, 2011).

# Related Web Sites

Biometrics Identity Management Agency. http://www.biometrics.dod.mil/

Department of Health and Human Services. http://www.hhs.gov

Department of Labor. http://www.dol.gov

Electronic Frontier Foundation. http://www.eff.org

Electronic Privacy Information Center (http://www.epic.org) is a research organization concerned with privacy issues.

It keeps a Privacy Archive with "an extensive collection of documents, reports, news items, policy analysis and laws relating to privacy issues."

Federal Trade Commission. http://www.ftc.gov

MIB Group. http://www.mib.com

Patient Privacy Rights. http://www.patientprivacyrights.org

Privacy Rights Clearinghouse. http://www.privacyrights.org

---

PEARSON
**myhealthprofessionskit**™

Go to www.myhealthprofessionskit.com to access the Companion Web site created for this textbook. Simply select "Basic Health Science" from the choice of disciplines. Find this book and register to access self-assessment quizzes, flashcards, and more.

# Glossary

**1000 Genomes Project**—"to provide a comprehensive public resource that supports researchers aiming to study . . . genetic variation that might cause human disease. [It seeks to] integrat[e] data on all types of variation that might cause human disease."

**Acceleglove**—uses sensors that detect hand and finger movement and sends signals to the computer, which associates the hand movements with a particular word and then translates the sign language into text and speech

**accounts receivable (A/R)**—include any invoice or any payment from the patient or insurance carriers to the medical practice

**acquired immune deficiency syndrome (AIDS)**—AIDS attacks the immune system, leading to susceptibility to opportunistic infection

**ADAM**—simulation software that teaches anatomy and physiology, using two- and three-dimensional images (some of them created from the Visible Human data); versions available for both patients and professionals; interactive, allowing the user to click away over 100 layers of the body and see more than 4,000 structures

**adaptive technology**—(also called assistive technology) makes it possible for people with disabilities to exercise control over their home and work environments

**adjustment**—a positive or negative change to a patient account

**administrative applications**—use of information technology for tasks such as office management, finance and accounting, and materials management

**adware**—may display unwanted pop-up advertisements on your monitor; it may be related to the sites you search on the Web or even the content of your e-mail

**American Recovery and Reinvestment Act (ARRA) of 2009**—signed into law on February 17, 2009, by President Barack Obama; includes financial incentives for adopting electronic health records

**Americans with Disabilities Act (ADA) of 1990**—federal law that prohibits discrimination against people with disabilities and requires that businesses with more than 15 employees provide "reasonable accommodation" to allow the disabled to perform their jobs

**Angelina**—a virtual human, a cybertherapist, programmed to "nod sympathetically" and be "socially sensitive"

**antibiotic resistance**—the condition where certain bacteria no longer respond to antibiotics

**antisense technology**—one experimental technology used to develop drugs to shut off disease-causing genes

**application software**—programs that perform specific tasks for the user, also called productivity software; include word processing, spreadsheet, database management, graphics, and communications programs

**Aquarius**—the only undersea laboratory in the world used by NEEMO

**arithmetic-logic unit**—the part of the central processing unit that performs arithmetic and logical operations

**ARPAnet**—a project of the Advanced Research Projects Agency of the U.S. Department of Defense (1969); an attempt to create both a national network of scientists and a communications system that could withstand nuclear attack; later became the Internet

**arrhythmia monitor**—a device that monitors heart rate

**ARTEMIS**—a robotic system that works with the simulation software KISMET; allows a surgeon to perform minimally invasive surgery while viewing three screens that show the view presented by the endoscope and simulations

**artificial intelligence**—the branch of computer science that seeks to make computers simulate human intelligence

**assignment**—the amount the insurance company pays

**assistive technology**—see *adaptive technology*

**augmentative communication device**—a device that helps those who cannot speak or whose speech is incomprehensible to communicate

**augmented reality surgery**—(enhanced reality surgery) makes use of computer-generated imagery to provide the surgeon with information that would otherwise be unavailable; these images may be either fused with the image on the monitor or projected directly onto the patient's body during the operation, allowing the doctor to virtually see inside the patient

**authorization**—permission by the insurance carrier for the provider to perform a medical procedure

**automated endoscopic system for optimal positioning (AESOP)**—introduced in 1994 by Computer Motion Inc., it is the first FDA-cleared surgical robot; originally developed for the space program, AESOP is now used as an assistant in endoscopic procedures

**automatic recalculation**—refers to the fact that when one value in a spreadsheet is changed, any cell that refers to it is automatically changed

**avatar**—virtual body

**Baby CareLink**—originated in Massachusetts. Its purpose was to compare high-risk, premature infants receiving traditional care with an experimental group, which in addition to traditional care received a telemedicine link to the hospital while the babies were hospitalized and for 6 months after. The addition of telemedicine to the care of premature babies has been so successful that Baby CareLink is now used throughout the United States

**BabySim**—a human patient simulator; teaches the skills needed to work with infants

**balance billing**—bucket billing (or balance billing) is specific to health care office environments, where each insurer must be billed and payment received before the patient is billed

**bandwidth**—a measure of the capacity of transmission media to carry data; the broader the bandwidth, the faster the medium

**bar-code scanner**—direct-entry scanning input device; reads the universal product code (UPC)

**binary digit (bit)**—a one or a zero; binary digits are used to represent data and information in the computer

**bioinformatics**—the application of information technology to biology

**biometric keyboard**—a keyboard that can identify a typist by fingerprints

**biometric methods**—ways of identifying a user by some physical characteristic; include fingerprints, hand prints, retina or iris scans, lip prints, facial thermography, and body odor sensors

**biometrics**—the science that measures body characteristics; enables security devices to identify a user by these characteristics

**biomicroscopes**—used for diagnosis of cataracts

**Biomove 3000**—for stroke patients; helps to stimulate the muscles to avoid atrophy and increase both the range of motion and blood circulation

**biotechnology**—discipline that sees the human body as a collection of molecules and seeks to understand and treat disease in terms of these molecules

**bit (binary digit)**—binary digit (1 or 0)

**Bluetooth**—a wireless technology that can connect digital devices from computers to medical devices to cell phones

**Body Browser**—from an Internet window, the user can look into the human body, rotate it, and zoom in or out; peel back layers; and look at bones, muscles, or blood vessels

**body odor sensor**—a biometric device enabling the identification of user by odor

**bonding**—involves the application of a material to the tooth that can be shaped and polished

**boot**—load the operating system into memory

**botnet**—comprised of a collection of automatic software robots; can remove software or send spam

**BrainGate Neural Interface System**—for ALS (Lou Gehrig's disease); the system involves implanting a chip in the brain that will convert brain cell impulses to computer signals

**bucket billing**—see *balance billing*

**Cable Communications Policy Act (1984)**—protects the personal information of customers of cable service providers

**capitated plan**—a physician is paid a fixed fee (the capitation), and the physician is paid regardless of the amount of treatment he or she provides

**case**—the condition for which the patient visits the doctor

**CD (compact disk)**—optical disks, CDs (compact disks), or DVDs (digital video disks) store data as pits and lands burnt into a plastic disk

**CD-ROM (compact disk-read-only memory)**—optical disk created at a factory that can be read, but not written to; lasers are used to create pits and lands to store data

**cell phone**—wireless device that allows text messaging, music, videos, and, of course, telephone calls

**Centers for Disease Control and Prevention**—www.cdc.gov maintains several departments concerned with occupational safety and health

**Centers for Medicare and Medicaid Services (CMS)**—government insurance plans are administered by the federal Centers for Medicare and Medicaid Services (CMS), formerly the Health Care Financing Administration (HCFA)

**CenterWatch**—maintains a Web site that lists current clinical trials in the United States; includes a database of trials that are looking for volunteers, as well as information on completed trials and educational resources

**central processing unit (CPU)**—contains the arithmetic-logic unit and control unit

**CHAMPUS**—covers medical necessities for those eligible: retired military, dependents of those on active duty, retired, or dead military

**CHAMPVA**—covers the immediate families of veterans who are totally disabled; surviving spouse and children of a veteran who died from a service-related disability; widow and children of a veteran who was permanently disabled; and the surviving spouse and children of a member of the military who died in the line of duty

**channel**—medium used to connect the nodes on a network

**charge**—the amount a patient is billed for the provider's service

**Children's Online Privacy Protection Act 2000**—requires Web sites targeting children aged 13 or under to get parental consent to gather information on the children

**CINAHL (Cumulative Index to Nursing and Allied Health Literature)**—a database specifically geared to the needs of nurses and other professionals in 17 allied health fields, including dental hygiene,

occupational therapy, and radiology; includes an index of 1,000 journals from 1982 to the present; bibliographic citations of books, pamphlets, software, and standards of practice; abstracts or full text of articles where they are available; journals; and descriptions of Web sites of interest

**claim**—a request to an insurance company for payment for services

**clearinghouse**—practices that submit electronic claims use a clearinghouse—a business that collects insurance claims from providers and sends them to the correct insurance carrier

**C-Leg**—computerized lower leg prosthesis

**climate change**—see Global Warming

**clinical**—relating to or based on work done with real patients; of or relating to the medical treatment that is given to patients in hospitals, clinics, etc.

**clinical application**—the use of information technology for direct patient care; includes patient monitoring, interventional radiology, surgery, and electronic prosthetics

**clinical decision support (CDS)**—(also referred to as clinical decision-support systems [CDSS]) computer programs (also called expert systems) that help health care professionals in making diagnoses by analyzing patient data

**clinical decision-support systems (CDSS)**—(also referred to as clinical decision support [CDS]) computer programs (also called expert systems) that help health care professionals in making diagnoses by analyzing patient data

**clinical information system (CIS)**—uses computers to manage clinical information

**Clinical Pharmacology**—a database of the latest drug information

**ClinicalTrials.gov**—launched in February 2000; lists 105,168 clinical trials in 174 countries; is searchable by disease and location—for example, cancer AND Los Angeles

**cloud computing**—allows many users to have secure access to all of their applications (for example, documents, chat, e-mail, blogs, presentations, video, calender, pictures, addressbook, and training spreadsheets) from their multiple network devices (smartphones, laptops, desktops, tablets, etc)

**CMS-1500**—the most widely accepted claim form (formerly called HCFA-1500)

**code of conduct**—internal company policy that attempts to safeguard information and guarantee privacy

**Combat Methamphetamine Epidemic Act (2005)**—a new part of the USA Patriot Act that requires anyone who buys cough medicine containing pseudoephedrine to present photo ID

**communications software**—application software that allows the connection of one computer to other computers

**Composite International Diagnostic Interview (CIDI)**—a tool for diagnosing mental disorders

**Composite International Diagnostic Interview-Auto (CIDI-Auto)**—a computerized version of CIDI; can be self-administered

**computed tomography (CT)**—an imaging technique that involves taking a series of X-rays at different angles from which the computer constructs a cross-sectional image

**computed tomography colonography (CTC)**—a virtual colonoscopy

**computer**—an electronic device that can accept data (raw facts) as input, process or alter them in some way, and produce useful information as output

**Computer Abuse Amendments Act 1994**—makes it a crime to "gain unauthorized access to a computer system [used in interstate commerce] with the intent to obtain anything of value, to defraud the system, or to cause more than $1000 worth of damage." This applies to any computer linked to the Internet. It specifically prohibits the transmission of viruses. (Note: Section 1030 was amended on October 26, 2001, by the USA Patriot Act antiterrorism legislation)

**computer-aided detection**—automatically reads radiographic scans immediately, before the radiologist reads them

**computer-assisted surgery**—makes use of computers, robotic devices, and/or computer-generated images in the planning and carrying out of surgical procedures

**computer-assisted trial design (CATD)**—software that allows the simulation of clinical drug trials before the actual trials begin

**Computer-based Training in Cognitive Behavioral Therapy (CBT4CBT)**—a computer program designed to treat addiction

**Computer Fraud and Abuse Act 1984 (amended in 1994)**—prohibits unauthorized access to federal computers

**computer information systems**—used in some hospitals and other health care facilities to help manage and organize relevant patient, financial, pharmacy, laboratory, and radiological information

**computer literacy**—familiarity with and knowledge about computers, the Internet, and the World Wide Web; the ability to use computers to perform tasks in one's own field

**Computer Matching and Privacy Protection Act 1988 (amended in 1990)**—limits the use of computer matching

**computerized functional electrical stimulation (CFES or FES)**—a technique involving the use of low-level electrical stimulation; has been used for many years in pacemakers and other implanted devices; now used to strengthen paralyzed muscles with simulated exercise; low-level electrical stimulation is applied directly to muscles that cannot receive these signals from the brain because of spinal cord injury

**computerized medical instruments**—contain microprocessors and provide direct patient services such as monitoring, administering medication, or treatment

**computerized physician order entry system (CPOE)**—a doctor enters a prescription electronically and it is checked against a hospital database of patients' allergies and drug interactions.

**cone beam CT (CBCT)**—more precisely focuses a beam of radiation on a tumor; can be attached to the machine delivering radiation, creating three-dimensional images so that doctors can compare the latest images with the earlier images they used to plan the treatment

**connectivity**—the fact that computers can be connected to each other

**control unit**—the part of the central processing unit that controls processing following the instructions of a program; it directs the movement of electronic signals between parts of the computer

**cookies**—small programs put on a user's hard drive every time a Web site is visited

**co-payment**—the part of the charge for which the patient is responsible

**CoreValve**—currently in clinical trials; used in minimally invasive heart surgery; made of a special alloy and heart material from a pig; threaded through the blood vessels to the aortic valve using X-ray guidance; once implanted, it expands and becomes an entirely new valve

**corneal topography**—uses a computer to create an accurate three-dimensional map of the cornea, so the health care professional can see the shape and power of the cornea

**cosmetic dentistry**—attempts to create a more attractive smile

**CPT (current procedural terminology)**—codes laboratory tests, treatments, and other procedures

**CRKP (carbapenem-resistant *Klebsiella pneumoniae*)**—a deadly bacterium; carbapenems have been the "antibiotic of last resort," working when no other antibiotic could; as CRKP spread, it became more and more resistant to antibiotics, even carbapenem; CRKP can cause pneumonia, bloodstream infections, and infections in wounds and surgical sites

**cyber knife**—a device that compensates for patient movement and can be used to treat brain and spinal tumors with radiosurgery

**cybertherapist**—a simulated human, programmed to act like a therapist

**cybertherapy**—use of virtual worlds in therapy

**data accuracy**—correctness and currency of information

**Databank for Cardiovascular Disease**—at Duke University, a highly specialized expert system that combines computer monitoring with extensive collections of information on cardiac patients

**database**—a large organized collection of information that is easy to maintain, search, and sort

**database management software (DBMS)**—application software that allows the user to enter organized lists of data and easily edit, sort, and search them

**da Vinci**—robot (Intuitive Surgical, Inc.) was first cleared for assisting in surgery in 1997, for performing some surgeries in 2000, and for performing cardiac surgery, such as mitral valve repair in November 2002; it performs minimally invasive surgeries

**deductible**—a certain amount the patient is required to pay each year before the health insurance begins paying

**Deepwater Horizon oil spill**—on April 20, 2010, the Deepwater Horizon oil rig exploded in the Gulf of Mexico immediately killing 11 human beings; among the first effects was the spill of tens of thousands of barrels of oil a day into the Gulf, effectively polluting the water, damaging the shoreline, and killing wildlife; the spill was not stopped for 85 days

**demineralize**— deterioration of the enamel of the teeth caused by acids

**denial-of-service attack**—also called an e-mail bomb; sends so much e-mail to one address that the server stops working

**dental implants**—used to replace missing teeth; computers help plan the exact placement of the implant

**dental informatics**—combines computer technology with dentistry to create a basis for research, education, and the solution of real-world problems in oral health care using computer applications

**DentSim**—a program that uses virtual reality; its purpose is to teach technical dexterity to dental students; a small pilot study has been completed

**deoxyribonucleic acid (DNA)**—a nucleic acid molecule containing genetic instructions for living things

**diffusion tensor imaging (DTI)**—a new MRI-related imaging technique; it shows the white matter of the brain, the connections between parts of the brain, so that these are not damaged during surgery

**digital imaging and communications in medicine (DICOM)**—the standard communication protocols of imaging devices are called DICOM

**digital imaging fiber optic transillumination (DIFOTI)**—involves using a digital camera to obtain images of teeth illuminated with laser light; the images are analyzed using computer algorithms

**digital video disk (DVD)**—optical medium with enormous storage capacity (several gigabytes)

**digitize**—to translate into zeroes and ones that the computer can understand

**digitizing tablet**—a direct-entry input device, pointing device; the user works on a tablet on the desk (instead of directly on the screen) with a stylus

**direct access storage device**—a secondary storage device that allows reading from or writing to any part of the storage medium (disk)

**direct-entry devices**—input devices including scanning and pointing devices and sensors

**disk drive**—storage device in which a medium (disk) is inserted; the drive includes a motor to spin the disk and a read/write head that reads data from or writes it to the disk

**distance (or telepresence) surgery**— surgery performed by robotic devices controlled by surgeons at another site

**DRG (diagnosis-related group)**—code used for diagnosis; hospital reimbursement by insurers is based on a formula using DRGs

**Driver Privacy Protection Act 1997**— limits disclosure of personal information in Motor Vehicles records

**dual X-ray absorptiometry (DEXA) scan**—a special kind of low-radiation X-ray that shows changes in the rays' intensity after passing through bone; doctors can see small changes in bone density from the amount of change in the X-ray

**electrical conductance**—currently used to diagnose cavities. An electric current is passed through a tooth, and the tooth's resistance is measured. A decayed tooth has a different resistance reading than a healthy tooth

**electronic aids to daily living (EADL)**— (formerly called environmental control systems [ECS]) help physically challenged people control their environments

**Electronic Communications Privacy Act of 1986**—prohibits government agencies from intercepting electronic communications without a search warrant. It also prohibits individuals from intercepting e-mail. However, there are numerous exceptions, and the courts have interpreted this to allow employers to access employees' e-mail. This law does not apply to communications within an organization

**electronic dental chart**—dental chart in an electronic form; standardized, easy to search, and easy to read. It will integrate practice management tasks (administrative applications) with clinical information

**electronic health record (EHR)**— electronic record of patient health information generated by one or more encounters in any care delivery setting

**electronic media claim (EMC)**—is an electronically processed and transmitted claim

**electronic medical record (EMR)**—in a computerized office, the information that was gathered and entered onto a patient information form will then be entered into a computer into electronic medical records. This will form the patient's medical record

**electronic remittance advice (ERA)**— accompanies the response to an electronic claim to an insurance company

**electronic spreadsheet**—application software that allows the user to store and manipulate numbers

**eLegs exoskeleton**—a bionic device that helps paraplegics walk; it is wearable and artificially intelligent

**e-mail bomb**—also called a denial-of-service attack; sends so much e-mail to one address that the server stops working

**embedded computer**—a single-purpose computer on a chip of silicon, which is embedded in anything from appliances to humans. An embedded computer may help run your car, microwave, pacemaker, or watch

**encounter form (superbill)**—list of diagnoses and procedures common to a practice

**encryption**—used to protect information from unauthorized users; involves encoding of messages

**endodontics**—dental specialty that diagnoses and treats diseases of the pulp

**endoluminal surgery**—one form of minimally invasive robotic surgery is called endoluminal surgery. Endoluminal surgery does not require incisions. It is also called natural orifice surgery

**endoscope**—a thin tube with a light source that either allows a direct view into the body or is connected to a minuscule camera that projects an image of the surgical site onto a monitor

**environmental control system (ECS)**— now called electronic aids to daily living (EADL)

**epidemic**—an excess in the number of cases of a given health problem

**epidemiology**—the study of diseases in populations by collecting and analyzing statistical data

**e-prescribing (electronic prescribing)**— the use of computers and software to enter prescriptions and send them to pharmacies electronically

**expansion boards**—circuit boards that are plugged into the expansion slots on the main circuit board; they include the electronic circuitry needed by add-on hardware

**expansion slots**—slots in the main circuit board that allow expansion boards to be inserted

**expert system**—a program that attempts to make computers mimic human expertise in limited fields; uses a database of numerous facts and rules about how decisions are made; also called decision support system

**explanation of benefits (EOB)**—the response of an insurance company to a paper claim includes an explanation of benefits (EOB), which explains why certain services were covered and others not

**Explorable Virtual Human**—will include authoring tools that engineers can use to build anatomical models that will allow students to experience how real anatomical structures feel, appear, and sound

**extranet**—a corporate intranet connected to other intranets outside the corporation

**EYESI surgical simulator**—allows doctors to learn new surgical skills and techniques for eye surgery

**facial structure scan**—a biometric method that identifies users by facial structure

**facial thermography**—a biometric method that identifies users by the heat generated by their faces

**Fair and Accurate Credit Transaction Act of 2003 (FACTA)**—added new sections to the federal Fair Credit Reporting Act intended to help consumers fight identity theft; accuracy, privacy, limits on information sharing, and new consumer rights to disclosure are included

**Fair Credit Reporting Act of 1970**—a federal law that regulates credit agencies; it allows you to see your credit reports to check the accuracy of information and to challenge inaccuracies

**fax machine**—a direct-entry input device, scanning device; scans the text or image and converts it to electronic signals that are sent over telephone lines; the receiving fax machine converts it back into text and images

**fee-for-service plans**—health insurance plans that are not restricted to a network of providers; they do not need referrals to specialists

**fetal monitor**—measures fetal heart rate

**fiber optic camera**—analogous to the endoscope used in surgery. It is used to view an area of the mouth that is normally difficult to see

**fiber optic transillumination**—finds early lesions (affecting enamel) but is limited in diagnosing advanced caries

**field**—each record in a table is made up of related fields. One field holds one piece of information, such as a patient's last name, Social Security number, or chart number

**file**—a practice can store all of its data and information in a database file stored

on a computer. Within the file, there can be several tables

**financial information system (FIS)**—is concerned with the financial details of running a hospital

**Financial Modernization Act 1999**—governs collection and disclosure of customers' personal financial information by financial institutions

**fingerprint**—biometric method of identification

**firewall**—software used to protect LANs from unauthorized access through the Internet

**firmware**—a computer program that is embedded in a hardware device

**focused ultrasound surgery**—in the early experimental stages; uses sound waves to raise the temperature of cancerous tissue until it dies; also being examined as a way to stop massive bleeding

**Food and Drug Administration (FDA)**—federal agency in the Department of Health and Human Services in charge of reviewing, approving, and regulating the purity of food and the safety and effectiveness of drugs

**fraud**—includes such crimes as using a computer program to illegally transfer money from one bank account to another or printing payroll checks to oneself

**fraudulent dialer**—can connect the user with numbers without the user's knowledge; the dialer may connect the user's computer to an expensive 900 number. The user will be totally unaware until he or she receives the telephone bill

**functional electrical stimulation (FES or CFES)**—see *computerized functional electrical stimulation*

**functional MRI (fMRI)**—measures small metabolic changes in an active part of the brain. fMRI identifies brain activity by changes in blood oxygen

**gamma knife**—bloodless surgical device; works by delivering 201 focused beams of radiation directly at a brain tumor, killing the tumor and sparing the surrounding tissue

**gamma knife surgery**—bloodless surgery using a gamma knife

**GDx Access**—uses an infrared laser to measure the thickness of the retinal nerve fiber. It is used for the early detection of glaucoma

**Genetic Information Nondiscrimination Act (2008) (GINA)**—basic purpose is to protect people from discrimination

by health insurers and employers based on genetic information

**global warming**—our planet is warming, and we are helping to make it happen by adding more heat-trapping gases, primarily carbon dioxide ($CO_2$), to the atmosphere. Global warming is already having a devastating effect on the earth and on human health: More intense heat waves lead to more heat-related deaths. Asthma and eczema in children and adults have been linked to global warming

**graphical user interface (GUI)**—an operating environment or interface used by Windows and Macintosh OS that allows users to interact with the computer by clicking on icons with a mouse

**guarantor**—the person responsible for payment of a medical bill; it may be the patient or a third party

**hacker**—a proficient computer user without authorized access to systems

**hand print**—biometric method of identification used to restrict access to computers

**hard copy**—printed output

**hardware**—the physical components of a computer

**HCFA-1500 (now CMS-1500)**—the most commonly accepted claim form

**head mouse**—input device that moves the cursor according to the user's head motions

**Health Care Financing Administration (HCFA) (now CMS)**—administers government health plans

**Healthfinder**—a listing of "sites 'hand-picked' . . . by health professionals"

**Health Information Technology for Economic and Clinical Health Act (HITECH) of 2009**—part of the ARRA, funds ONCHIT, and is "designed to . . . provide the necessary assistance and technical support to providers, enable coordination and alignment within and among states, establish connectivity to the public health community in case of emergencies, and assure the workforce is properly trained and equipped to be meaningful users of electronic health records"

**health insurance exchanges (HIEs)**—marketplaces "that allow individuals and small-business owners to pool their purchasing power to negotiate lower rates"

**Health Insurance Portability and Accountability Act (HIPAA)**—in 1996, Congress passed the Health Insurance

Portability and Accountability Act (HIPAA). Guidelines to protect electronic medical records were developed by the Department of Health and Human Services. By encouraging the use of the electronic medical record and facilitating the sharing of medical records among health care providers, it can assure continuity of care and thus save lives

**health maintenance organization (HMO)**—a patient who uses a health maintenance organization (HMO) pays a fixed yearly fee and must choose among an approved network of health care providers and hospitals

**Heidelberg retinal tomograph (HRT)**—uses lasers to scan the retina resulting in a three-dimensional description. This technique can detect glaucoma before any loss of vision

**HELEN (HELp Neuropsychology)**—a computerized program that contains diagnostic analyses that keep track of specific tests and tasks performed by the stroke patient

**HERMES**—an FDA-cleared computer operating system that controls all the electronic equipment in the operating room, coordinating the endoscope and robotic devices

**HIV**—see Human Immunodeficiency Syndrome

**Homeland Security Act**—expands and centralizes the data gathering allowed under the Patriot Act

**hospital information system (HIS)**—attempts to integrate the administrative and clinical functions in a hospital. Ideally, the HIS includes clinical information systems, financial information systems, laboratory information systems, nursing and pharmacy information systems, picture archiving and communication systems, and radiology information systems

**human-biology input device**—uses sensors to interpret body movements and characteristics, allowing the user's body to be used as an input device

**Human Genome Project (HGP)**—international project (begun in 1990) seeking to understand the human genetic makeup; to find the location of the 100,000 or so human genes; and to read the entire genetic script, all three billion bits of information, by the year 2005

**human immunodeficiency virus (HIV)**—the virus that causes AIDS

**human patient simulators (HPS)**—programmable mannequins on which

students can practice medical and dental procedures

**ICD (International Classification of Disease; ICD-9-CM or 10)**—codes 1,000 diseases

**identity theft**—involves someone using your private information to assume your identity

**iHealth Record**—a personal medical record that the patient can create and maintain at no cost. It is available at some doctors' offices

**ILIAD**—a program that provides hypothetical cases for the student to evaluate. The student's diagnostic abilities are then compared to the computer's

**image scanner**—a direct-entry input device, scanning device; can scan whole pages of graphics and text and digitize them so that the computer can process them

**image-guided (or directed) surgery**—surgery guided by computer-generated images of the surgical field, not a direct view

**iMedConsent**—an electronic informed consent program used by the VA and 190 U.S. hospitals

**indemnity plan**—fee-for-service health insurance plan

**information technology (IT)**—includes computers, communications networks, and computer literacy

**Innova**—can image fine vessels and cardiovascular anatomy, producing three-dimensional images of the vascular system, bone, and soft tissue

**input device**—a device that translates data into a form the computer can process (bits)

**input/output device**—a device that contains a monitor for output and a keyboard for input

**intensity-modulated radiation therapy (IRIS)**—a linear accelerator that "shapes and varies the intensity of radiation beams"

**interactive videoconferencing**—(teleconferencing) allows doctors and patients to consult in real time, at a distance

**interapy**—Internet-based therapy

**Internet (interconnected network)**—a global network of networks, connecting innumerable smaller networks, computers, and users

**INTERNIST**—medical expert system used as decision-support system to help in diagnosis

**interoperability**—the connection of people and diverse computer systems

**interventional radiology**—the use of the tools of radiology to treat conditions that once required surgery

**intranet**—a private corporate network that uses the same structure as the Internet and the same TCP/IP protocols

**intraoral fiber optic camera**—allows both patient and dentist to get a close-up tour of the patient's mouth. A fiber optic device is aimed at an area of the patient's mouth, and the image appears on the screen

**iPad**—a tablet computer with many health-related applications

**iPhone**—a smartphone with many health-related applications

**iris scan**—a biometric method of identification used to restrict access to computers

**iStan**—a human patient simulator; completely wireless; designed around a human-like skeleton; its arms, neck, spine, and hips move; its skin looks and feels human; it can sweat, breathe, drool, cry, and bleed; its eyes are "fully reactive"

**key field**—uniquely identifies each record in a table

**keyboard**—an input device

**keylogging**—can be used by anyone to track anyone else's keystrokes

**KISMET**—simulation software used in surgery

**Kurzweil scanner**—a direct-entry input device, scanning device, and also an output device; scans printed text and reads it aloud to the user

**laboratory information systems (LIS)**—use computers to manage both laboratory tests and their results

**laparoscope**—endoscope used for abdominal surgery

**laser (light amplification by stimulated emission of radiation)**—delivers light energy. There are several uses of lasers in dentistry. Low-level lasers can find pits in tooth enamel that may become cavities. The FDA has approved laser machines for drilling and filling cavities; lasers also reduce the bacteria in the cavity; lasers are also used in surgery

**LASIK**—eye surgery that uses lasers to correct vision by changing the shape of the cornea

**light illumination**—several methods use light to help diagnose tooth disease.

To find decay, a bright light is used to illuminate the tooth, revealing color differences

**light pen**—direct-entry input device, pointing device; allows the use of a pen-like device to identify exact points to draw on the screen

**line-of-sight system**—allows you to use your body as an input device; the user's eyes can point to a part of the screen; a camera and computer can identify the area you are looking at

**lip print**—biometric method of identification used to restrict access to computers

**local area network (LAN)**—a small private network that spans a room or building

**LOINC (Logical Observation Identifiers, Names, and Codes)**—standardizes laboratory and clinical codes

**LUMA Cervical Imaging System**—helps detect cervical cancer

**magnetic diskette**—storage medium that stores data as magnetic spots

**magnetic ink character recognition (MICR)**—technology used only by banks to read the magnetic ink characters at the bottoms of checks

**magnetic resonance imaging (MRI)**—an imaging technique that uses computer technology to produce images of soft tissue within the body that could not be pictured by traditional X-rays; can produce images of the insides of bones; uses computers and a very strong magnetic field and radio waves to generate mathematical data from which an image is constructed

**magnetic tape**—sequential access storage medium; magnetic tape was widely used as secondary storage in the 1950s and 1960s; now used mainly for backup and archives

**main circuit board**—motherboard

**mainframe**—large, fast computer designed for multiple users; used for input/output intensive tasks

**malware**—includes different forms of malicious hardware, software, and firmware

**managed care**—a type of health insurance that requires the patient to choose among a network of providers

**meaningful use (of electronic health records [EHRs])**—under the ARRA, meaningful use refers to meeting a required 15 criteria, and meeting 5 out of 10 other criteria. EHRs must include patient demographics, vital signs, up-to-date problem lists, active medication lists, and allergy lists, among other things

**MEDCIN**—provides 250,000 codes for such things as symptoms, patient history, physical examinations, tests, diagnoses, and treatments. MEDCIN codes can be integrated with other coding systems

**Medicaid**—jointly funded, federal-state health insurance for certain low-income and needy people

**medical informatics**—the use of computers and computer technology in health care and its delivery

**Medical Information Bureau**—now known as the MIB Group, Inc.

**Medicare**—a government plan that serves people age 65 years and over and disabled people with chronic renal disorders

**medication reconciliation**—concerns identifying the most accurate list of a patient's medications

**Medi-Span**—a database of information on drug/drug interactions and drug/food interactions

**MEDLARS (Medical Literature Analysis and Retrieval System)**—a collection of 40 computerized databases containing 18 million references, available free via the Internet; can be searched for bibliographical lists or for information

**MEDLINE**—a comprehensive online database of current medical research including publications from 1966 to the present; it contains 8.5 million articles from 3,700 journals; 31,000 citations are added each month

**Medscape**—provides a collection of medical journals online

**memory**—temporary storage area used during processing; internal storage made up of RAM and ROM

**METI LiVE**—lets the user create hospitals or disasters using several patient simulators

**MIB Group, Inc.**—(formerly the Medical Information Bureau) comprised of 470 insurance companies; its database contains health information on about 15 million Americans and Canadians

**microcomputer**—personal computer (PC), designed for use by one person at a time

**microdialysis**—a technique that attempts to look at the body's response to an implant at the cellular level

**microprocessor**—a tiny computer on a chip; contains millions of miniaturized transistors

**MIDAS**—see Models of Infectious Disease Agent Study

**MINERVA**—a robot developed to perform stereotactic neurosurgical procedures

**minicomputer**—a smaller, less expensive version of the mainframe; designed for multiple users

**minimally invasive dentistry**—emphasizes prevention and the least possible intervention

**minimally invasive surgery (MIS)**—surgery performed through small incisions

**Models of Infectious Disease Agent Study (MIDAS)**—a collaboration of research and informatics groups to develop computational models of the interactions between infectious agents and their hosts, disease spread, prediction systems, and response strategies, according to the NIH

**Modular Prosthetic Limb (MPL)**—a mind-controlled prosthetic limb currently being developed by DARPA and several universities

**monitor**—screen

**motherboard**—main circuit board of the computer

**MotionMonitor**—a real-time computer-based system that objectively measures joint motion in a patient for a therapist

**mouse**—a direct-entry input device, pointing device; used to select items from a menu and position the insertion point

**MRSA (methicillin-resistant *Staphylococcus aureus*)**—a staphylococcal infection resistant to many antibiotics

**MYCIN**—an expert system used as a decision-support system to help in the diagnosis and treatment of bacterial infections

**myoelectric limbs**—artificial limbs containing motors and responding to the electrical signals transmitted by the residual limb to electrodes mounted in the socket

**nanotechnology**—a nanometer is one-billionth of a meter. Nanotechnology works with miniscule materials the size of atoms and molecules. It holds promise for regenerative medicine

**national drug codes (NDCs)**—developed by the FDA, they identify drugs

**National Electronic Disease Surveillance System (NEDSS)**—(part of the Public Health Information Network) will promote "integrated surveillance systems that can transfer . . . public health, laboratory and clinical data . . . over the Internet." This would be a national electronic surveillance system that would allow epidemics to be identified quickly

**National Information Infrastructure Protection Act 1996**—establishes penalties for interstate theft of information and for threats against networks and computer system trespassing

**Nationwide Health Information Network (NHIN)**—the infrastructure that would allow communication between RHIOs

**NDM-1 (New Delhi metallo-beta-lactamase-1)**—an enzyme that makes bacteria resistant to antibiotics

**NEEMO (NASA Extreme Environment Mission Operation)**—a series of NASA missions in which groups of scientists live in Aquarius

**neonatal monitor**—monitors infant heart and breathing rates

**network**—computers and other hardware devices linked together via communications media

**NeuroArm Robot**—developed at the University of Calgary in Canada; two-armed robot controlled by a surgeon sitting at a console; unlike other surgical robots, it can operate in an MRI, with near real-time image guidance; its arms can be moved 50 microns at a time—a microscopic scale

**neuromodulation**—a field that helps treat disorders of the central nervous system including chronic pain

**Neuromove**—for stroke patients; helps to stimulate the muscles to avoid atrophy and increases both the range of motion and blood circulation

**neuroprosthesis**—in 2006, a new implantable device using FES—a neuroprosthesis—was developed. It uses "low levels of electricity in order to activate nerves and muscles in order to restore movement"

**New Medicines in Development**—a database that provides information on newly approved drugs and drugs awaiting approval

**nursing information systems (NIS)**—are supposed to improve nursing care by using computers to manage charting, staff scheduling, and the integration of clinical information

**Online Privacy Protection Act (2005)**—requires the Federal Trade Commission to prescribe regulations to protect the privacy of personal information collected from and about individuals who are not covered by the Children's Online Privacy Protection Act of 1998 on the Internet, to provide greater individual control over the collection and use of that information, and for other purposes

**open architecture**—computer design that allows hardware devices to be added by plugging expansion boards into expansion slots on the main circuit board

**operating system**—the system software that controls the basic operation of the computer hardware, managing the resources of the computer including input and output, the execution of programs, and processor time; provides the user interface

**optical biometry**—in cataract surgery, the eye's lens is replaced by an intraocular lens (IOL). The measurements used to determine which IOL to use are determined by calculations referred to as optical biometry

**optical card**—holds about 2,000 pages of data

**optical character recognition (OCR)**—direct-entry input device, scanning device; reads printed characters

**optical disk**—secondary storage device on which data are represented by pits and lands burnt in by a laser

**optical mark recognition (OMR)**—direct-entry input device, scanning device; reads marks on paper

**Optomap Panoramic200**—can examine the retina without dilation using low-powered red and green lasers

**osseointegration**—a technology that allows the integration of living bone with titanium implants

**output devices**—hardware that presents information in a form a human user can comprehend

**page scanner**—a direct-entry input device that digitizes printed text

**pandemic**—a global disease outbreak to which everyone is susceptible

**Parkinson's disease**—involves damage to brain cells that hamper brain communication having to do with balance, movement, walking, and speech

**PARO**—a therapeutic robot developed in Japan; looks and feels like a little furry seal

**password**—a secret code assigned to (or chosen by) an authorized user

**patient aging report**—used to show a patient's outstanding payments

**patient day sheet**—lists the day's patients, chart numbers, and transactions

**Patient Protection and Affordable Care Act (2010)**—expands health insurance coverage to 32 million more people by requiring them to buy health insurance. It also expands Medicaid coverage and reforms current insurance practices. U.S. citizens and legal residents would be required to buy "minimal essential coverage"

**payment day sheet**—a grouped report organized by providers

**payments**—made by a patient or an insurance carrier to the practice

**PDUFA (Prescription Drug User Fee Act)**—requires drug companies to pay fees to support the drug review process

**PediaSim**—a programmable human patient simulator of a child used for teaching purposes

**pen-based system**—direct-entry input device, pointing device; allows handwritten input

**periodontics**—concerned with diagnosing and treating diseases of the gums and other structures supporting the teeth. Periodontal disease is caused by bacteria

**personal computer (PC)**—microcomputer

**personal digital assistant (PDA)**—handheld computer

**personal health record (PHR)**—is a person's health information in electronic form. It belongs to the individual and is available to him or her on any Web-enabled device

**personal identification number (PIN)**—a secret code assigned to (or chosen by) an authorized user

**pharmacy information systems (PIS)**—monitor drug allergies and interactions and fill and track prescriptions. They also track inventory and create patient drug profiles

**phishing**—sending fraudulent messages via e-mail or instant message that purport to be from a legitimate source such as a social network or IT administrator; the user is directed to a fake Web site and asked to enter information

**physiological monitoring systems**—monitor physiological processes; analyze blood and other fluids

**Physiome Project**—project attempting to develop accurate and complete human physiological models, which may in the future be used as simulated patients in drug trials

**picture archiving and communication systems (PACS)**—manage digital images. Digital images are immediately available on the monitor and can be shared over a network

**PLATO (Programmed Logic for Automatic Teaching Operations)**—an early (1960s) simulation program for nurses

**plotter**—output device that produces hard copy; used for graphics, such as maps and architectural drawings

**pointing devices**—input devices including the mouse, trackball, light pen, and touch screen

**polio**—a contagious virus that can cause paralysis and even death. It became very rare in the United States in the second half of the 20th century

**port**—socket, usually on the back of the computer

**positron emission tomography (PET)**—an imaging technique that uses radioisotope technology to create a picture of the body "in action"; uses computers to construct images from the emission of positive electrons (positrons) by radioactive substances administered to the patient

**Postoperative Expert Medical System (POEMS)**—an expert system that focuses on patients who become sick while recovering from surgery

**practice**—a group of health care practitioners in business together

**practice analysis report**—generated on a monthly basis; a summary total of all procedures, charges, and transactions

**practice management software**—software that enables an office to do administrative tasks such as scheduling and accounting electronically

**Pre-Existing Conditions Insurance Plan**—provides insurance for people with pre-existing conditions at the same rates as healthy people would pay

**preferred provider organization (PPO)**—a patient with PPO insurance can seek care within an approved network of health care providers who have agreed with the insurance company to lower their charges and accept assignment

**printer**—output device that produces hard copy

**privacy**—the ability to control personal information and the right to keep it from misuse

**Privacy Act (1974)**—prohibits disclosure of government records to anyone except the individual concerned, except for law enforcement purposes; it also prohibits the use of information except for the purpose for which it was gathered; it deals with the use and disclosure of Social Security numbers

**procedure day sheet**—a grouped report organized by procedure

**processing unit**—manipulates data

**processor (system unit)**—contains the CPU and memory; does the actual manipulation of data

**program**—step-by-step instructions; also called software

**prosthetic devices**—replacement limbs and organs

**protocols**—technical standards governing communication between computers

**public health**—is where the largest numbers of lives are saved, usually by understanding the epidemiology of a disease—its patterns, where and how it emerges and spreads—and attacking it at its weak points. This can lead to prevention by means of public health measures like better sanitation or providing cleaner water. It can also lead to the development and widespread distribution of vaccinations

**public health informatics**—supports public health practice and research with information technology

**PubMed**—search engine for Medline

**puff straw**—an input device that allows people to control the mouse with their mouths

**pulmonary monitor**—measures blood flow through the heart and respiratory rate

**radio frequency identification (RFID) tag**—radio frequency identification tags are becoming more and more common. RFID tags can be incorporated into products; they receive and send a wireless signal

**radiology information systems (RIS)**—manage patients in the radiology department including scheduling appointments, tracking film, and reporting results

**random-access memory (RAM)**—the part of temporary, volatile internal storage that holds the work you are currently doing while you are doing it, including the program and data you are using; the operating system must be in RAM for other programs to run

**rational drug design**—a technique that uses computers to model molecules and develop chemical compounds that will bind to the target molecule and inhibit or stimulate it; used in the development of drugs that are used for Alzheimer's disease, hypertension, and AIDS

**Raven**—a 50-pound, mobile surgical robot used on NEEMO

**read-only memory (ROM)**—part of internal memory; firmware; permanent instructions that the user normally cannot change

**Real ID Act of 2005**—"directly imposes prescriptive federal driver's license standards" by the federal government on the states. This law requires every American to have an electronic identification card; however, by 2011, according to some sources, the Real ID Act had "been put in limbo after 25 states adopted legislation opposing it"

**record**—a table is made up of related records; each record holds all the information on one item in the table

**regional extension centers (RECs)**—more than 60 RECs will give technical help and information to further the adoption of EHRs

**regional health information organizations (RHIOs)**—regional cooperation is being fostered through the establishment of regional health information organizations (RHIOs) in which data could be shared within a region

**relational database**—organized collection of related data

**remineralize**—repair damage to the tooth's enamel using phosphate and fluoride

**remote monitoring device**—transmits signals over communications lines, making it possible for patients to be monitored at home or in ambulances

**retina scan**—a biometric method of identifying users

**ribonucleic acid (RNA)**—made in the nucleus of a cell, but not restricted to the nucleus. It is a long coiled-up molecule whose purpose is to take the blueprint from DNA and build our actual proteins

**Right to Financial Privacy Act (RFPA) (1978)**—establishes procedures for the federal government to follow when looking at bank records. RFPA amended due to the USA Patriot Act of 2001: to permit the disclosure of financial information to any intelligence or counterintelligence agency in any investigation related to international terrorism (October, 2001)

**RNA interference (RNAi)**—a new technology aimed at drug development

**ROBODOC**—a computer-controlled, image-directed robot used in hip-replacement surgery

**robot**—a programmable machine that can manipulate its environment

**SARS**—see Severe Acute Respiratory Syndrome

**SATELLIFE**—founded in 1989, its purpose was to deliver journals and other information to health care workers in developing areas

**scanning devices**—direct-entry input devices; include fax machines, optical character recognition, optical mark recognition, magnetic ink character recognition, and image scanners

**schedule of benefits**—a list of those services that the insurance carrier will cover

**scientific visualization**—the process of graphically representing the results of numerical calculations

**screen reader software**—used with page scanners and synthesizers; tells the speech synthesizer what to say, for example, to read the text description of an icon

**SDILINE (Selective Dissemination of Information Online)**—contains only the latest month's additions to MEDLINE

**search engine**—software that allows you to search the Web

**secondary storage devices**—include disk drives and tape drives that, with their media, allow the more permanent storage of data, programs, and information than primary storage

**secondary storage media**—include disks and tape, which provide more permanent storage than random-access memory

**security**—measures attempting to protect computer systems (including hardware, software, and information) from harm and abuse; the threats may stem from many sources including natural disaster, human error, or crime

**sensor**—a direct-entry input device that collects data directly from the environment and sends it to a computer; used to collect patient information for clinical monitoring systems

**severe acute respiratory syndrome (SARS)**—a form of pneumonia caused by a virus that was identified in 2003; leads to difficulty in breathing and can cause death

**Simantha**—a life-size patient simulator for cardiologists; includes monitors that mimic displays in angiographic suites and multimedia characters

**SimCoach**—developed by the U.S. Army; a cybertherapist; will conduct interviews with veterans and their families to see what problems they are experiencing

**simulation software**—software that attempts to recreate a real situation

**simulations**—computers can create what-if scenarios or simulations of what would happen to an infectious disease if something else happened

**single-photon emission computed tomography (SPECT)**—an imaging technique that, like the PET scan, shows movement; less precise and less expensive than PET

**smart card**—includes a microprocessor and memory and holds about 30 pages of data; used as a debit card

**smart glasses**—glasses developed at the University of Arizona that will soon be able to automatically change focus

**smartphone**—a cell phone with built-in applications and Internet access

**SNOMED (Systematized Nomenclature of Medicine)**— "provides a common language that enables a consistent way of capturing, sharing, and aggregating health data"

**Social Security Protection Act of 2004**—amended the Social Security Act and the Internal Revenue Code of 1986 to provide additional safeguards for Social Security and Supplemental Security Income

**Socrates**—system that allows long-distance mentoring of surgeons in real time

**soft (digital) copy**—output on a monitor or voice output

**SoftScanR**—now in clinical trials; it is meant to be a diagnostic tool that will complement mammography

**software**— programs; the step-by-step instructions that tell the computer what to do

**software piracy**—unauthorized copying of copyrighted software

**solid-state memory devices**—include flash memory cards used in notebooks, memory sticks, and very compact key chain devices; they have no moving parts, are very small, and have a high capacity. USB flash drives have a huge capacity for information

**special-purpose application**—the use of information technology for applications not included in clinical or administrative applications, such as drug design and education

**speech recognition**—is useful for people who do not have the use of their hands and for the vision impaired. It promises that you can give computer commands or dictate text

**speech synthesizer**—a device with a processor, memory, and output capability, which turns digital data into speech-like sounds, allowing the computer to talk

**SpineAssist**—a robot that can be clamped on a patient's back; doctors take a picture of where the spine surgery will take place and a computer plans the robot's path; the robot creates a three-dimensional map of a patient's spine, making it possible for the surgeons to plan "exactly where to place pins or make incisions"; following the path, SpineAssist drills into the patient's vertebrae

**Spybot Search and Destroy software**—can remove malware, adware, spyware, fraudulent dialers, and keyloggers from your computer

**spyware**—software that can be installed without the user's knowledge to track their actions on a computer

**Starbright World**—a network linking seriously ill children in 100 hospitals in the United States (1998); children in the networked hospitals can play games, chat, send and receive e-mail, and receive medical information

**stem cells**—cells that can develop into different types of body cells; theoretically, they can repair the body. As a stem cell divides, the new cells can stay stem cells or become another kind of cell

**stereotactic radiosurgery**—gamma knife surgery; used to treat brain tumors

**store-and-forward technology**—technique in which the data to be sent are digitized, stored, and transmitted over a telecommunications network

**superbill**—encounter form

**superbugs**—antibiotic-resistant bacteria

**supercomputer**—the fastest, largest, most expensive computer at any time; used for complex processor-intensive, scientific tasks such as weather forecasting and weapons research

**syndromic surveillance**—uses health-related data that precede diagnosis and signal a sufficient probability of a case or an outbreak

**system software**—programs that control hardware operations and interact between the applications and the computer; includes the operating system, utility programs, and language translators

**system unit**—processor, contains the CPU and memory

**table**—in a relational database, each table holds related information

**tablet computer**—a computer contained in a touch screen

**telecommunications network**—network using telephone lines as media

**teleconferencing**—may involve anything from a conference call to a meeting between people who are not in the same place, but who can see and hear each other via video and audio equipment. It may also involve sharing documents on monitors and being able to work on them cooperatively

**teledentistry**—programs to help dentists access specialists in order to improve patient care

**teledermatology**—the practice of dermatology using telecommunications networks

**telehealth**—includes telemedicine and other health-related activities using telecommunications lines and computers, including education, research, public health, and administration of health services

**telehome care**—involves the monitoring of vital signs from a distance via telecommunications equipment and the replacement of home nursing visits with videoconferences

**telemedicine**—the delivery of health care over telecommunications lines

**teleneurology**—neurology was slower to use telemedicine than other specialties. Now, however, e-mail and video-conferencing are replacing the letter and telephone call. One of the first subspecialties to use telemedicine in neurology is stroke diagnosis

**telenursing**—involves teletriage and the telecommunication of health-related data, the remote house call, and the monitoring of chronic disease

**teleoncology**—use of telemedicine to treat cancer

**telepathology**—the transmission of microscopic images over telecommunications lines

**telepharmacy**—the linking of the prescribing doctor's office with the dispensing pharmacy via telecommunications lines

**telepresence surgery**—see *distance surgery*

**telepsychiatry**—the delivery of therapy using telecommunications lines

**teleradiology**—the sending of radiological images in digital form over telecommunications lines

**telespirometry**—monitoring system used by asthmatic patients; it is designed to transmit over the telephone to a remote location

**telestroke**—a program that connects small local hospitals with stroke experts. When a stroke victim appears at the local hospital, the doctors do CT scans and forward them to stroke specialists

**teletriage**—telemedicine application in which calls are screened and directed to the proper services

**telewound care**—treating chronic wounds using telemedicine; telewound care can benefit from the use of both store-and-forward and videoconferencing technology

**text telephones**—Computers can be used as text telephones and can send and receive e-mail.

**theft of information**—unauthorized access to and use of information

**theft of services**—unauthorized use of services such as cable TV

**tonometers**—measure eye pressure

**touch screen**—a direct-entry input device, pointing device; a screen that can receive input through touch; used at ATMs, in airports, in stores, in restaurants, and in kiosks in malls

**Tracey visual function analyzer**—measures how well you can see by measuring how your eye focuses light. These data help in surgical or laser vision correction. Computers are also used to custom design contact lenses

**transactions**—charges, payments, and adjustments

**transmission-control protocol/Internet protocol (TCP/IP)**—the protocols that govern the Internet

**TRICARE**—the U.S. health program for armed service members and their families

**Trojan horse**—appears to be a normal program such as computer game but "conceals malicious functions"

**tsunami**—"a series of traveling ocean waves of extremely long length generated by disturbances associated primarily with earthquakes occurring below or near the ocean floor" (weather.gov)

**UB-4**—it is a claim form

**ultrafast CT**—a variation of the traditional CT scan; may be used in place of a coronary angiogram to examine coronary artery blockages. Compared to a coronary angiogram, the ultrafast CT is painless, less dangerous, noninvasive, and less expensive

**ultrasound**—an imaging technique that uses no radiation; uses very high-frequency sound waves and the echoes they produce when they hit an object to generate information that is used by a computer to create a two-dimensional moving image on a screen; used to examine a moving fetus, to study blood flow, and to diagnose gallstones and prostate disease

**uniform resource locator (URL)**—address of a Web page

**universal product code (UPC)**—bar code that appears on products for sale

**USA Patriot Act (2001)**—gives law-enforcement agencies greater power to monitor electronic and other communications, with fewer checks

**user interface**—(operating environment) defines how the user communicates with the computer

**vaccination**—protects people against infection

**vector-borne diseases**—is a disease transmitted to a human or animal host by a tic, mosquito, or other arthropod that carries the bacteria or virus. According to the CDC, vector-borne diseases are emerging and reemerging

**Vesalius Project**—a project that is creating models of anatomical regions and structures to be used in teaching anatomy

**Video Privacy Protection Act (1988)**—prohibits video rental stores from revealing what tapes you rent

**Video Voyeurism Act** (2004)—would prohibit video voyeurism in the maritime and territorial jurisdiction of the United States

**virtual environment**—technology used to provide surgeons with realistic accurate models on which to teach surgery and plan and practice operations

**Virtual Hospital**—a comprehensive and authoritative Web site maintained by the University of Iowa

**Virtual Human Embryo**—a project that is digitizing some of the 7,000 human embryos lost in miscarriages that have been kept by the National Museum of Health and Medicine of the Armed Forces Institute of Pathology since the 1880s

**virtual reality (VR)**—technology that allows the computer to create an environment that seems real but is not; used in planning and teaching surgical and other procedures

**virus**—a program, attached to another file, that replicates itself and may do damage to your computer system

**Visible Human Project**—a computerized library of human anatomy at the National Library of Medicine, seeking to create accurate, three-dimensional representations of the male and female body.

The project began in the late 1980s. It now contains images of 1,800 cross-sections of a male cadaver (39 years old) and 5,000 of a female cadaver (59 years old) stored in a computer and accessible over the Internet

**vision input**—input via a digital camera

**vision replacement therapy (VRT)**—retrains the brain. Using dots on a computer screen, the aim is to stimulate peripheral vision. This therapy can be effective years after the stroke occurred

**voice recognition**—is the ability of a software program to receive and interpret dictation and carry out spoken commands

**WAND**—Students can use a wand to create three-dimensional structures from two-dimensional structures or from segmented slices. Students will be able to build and palpate organs

**Web-based Depression and Anxiety Test (WB-DAT)**—computer-guided therapy, found effective in diagnosing anxiety disorders and depression

**Web browser**—software needed to browse the Web

**Web page**—Web site

**Web site**—files in which information on the Web is stored

**West Nile Virus**—first appeared in the 1930s; it is a form of encephalitis or brain inflammation; it cycles between mosquitoes and birds; infected birds will infect mosquitoes, which can spread the disease to humans; can be diagnosed by MRIs

**what-if scenarios**—computers can create what-if scenarios or simulations of what would happen to an infectious disease if something else happened

**WHONET**—an information system developed to support the World Health Organization's (WHO) goal of global surveillance of bacterial resistance to antimicrobial agents

**wide area network (WAN)**—a network that may span a state, country, or even the world

**Wi-Fi**—a wireless technology that allows you to connect a PDA (and other devices) to a network (including the Internet), if you are close enough to a Wi-Fi access point

**word-processing software**—application software that allows the user to create, edit, format, save, retrieve, and print text documents

**worker's compensation**—a government program that covers job-related illness or injury

**World Health Organization (WHO)**—the directing and coordinating authority for health within the United Nations system

**World Wide Web (WWW) or Web**—the part of the Internet that is most accessible and easiest to navigate, organized as sites with hyperlinks to one another

**X-ray**—a traditional imaging technique that uses high-energy electromagnetic waves to produce a two-dimensional picture on film; does not produce good images of all organs and cannot see behind bones

**ZEUS**—a robotic surgical system that will make possible minimally invasive microsurgery; has three interactive robotic arms, one of which holds the endoscope, whereas the other two manipulate the surgical instruments; the surgeon, sitting at a console, controls them; includes a feedback system so that the surgeon "feels" the tissue

# Index